Manual of Breast Diseases

Manual of Breast Diseases

Edited by

Ismail Jatoi, M.D., PH.D., F.A.C.S.
Chief, General Surgery Service
U.S. Army Hospital
Heidelberg, Germany;
Associate Professor of Surgery
Uniformed Services University of the Health Sciences
Bethesda, Maryland

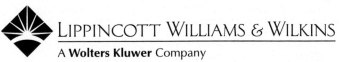

LIPPINCOTT WILLIAMS & WILKINS
A **Wolters Kluwer** Company
Philadelphia • Baltimore • New York • London
Buenos Aires • Hong Kong • Sydney • Tokyo

Acquisitions Editor: Jonathan Pine
Developmental Editor: Lisa Consoli
Production Editor: Emily Lerman
Manufacturing Manager: Tim Reynolds
Cover Designer: Christine Jenny
Compositor: Maryland Composition
Printer: Edwards Brothers

© **2002 by LIPPINCOTT WILLIAMS & WILKINS**
530 Walnut Street
Philadelphia, PA 19106 USA
LWW.com

Printed in the USA

Library of Congress Cataloging-in-Publication Data

Manual of breast diseases / edited by Ismail Jatoi.
   p. ; cm.
   Includes bibliographical references and index.
   ISBN 0-7817-2950-5
   1. Breast—Diseases—Handbooks, manuals, etc. 2. Breast—Cancer—Handbooks, manuals, etc. I. Jatoi, Ismail, 1955–
   [DNLM: 1. Breast Diseases. WP 870 M294 2001]
   RG491 .M363 2001
   618.1′9—dc21

                                                              2001038466

---

10 9 8 7 6 5 4 3 2 1

Contents

Contributing Authors

Deborah N. Ader, PH.D., *Director, Behavioral and Prevention Research Program, Rheumatic Diseases Branch, National Institute of Arthritis and Musculoskeletal and Skin Research, National Institutes of Health, Bethesda, Maryland*

Odysseus Argy, M.D., *Instructor, Department of Surgery, Boston University School of Medicine, Boston, Massachusetts; President, Odyssey Health Communications, Inc., South Dartmouth, Massachusetts*

Lawrence W. Bassett, M.D., *Iris Cantor Professor of Breast Imaging, Department of Radiological Sciences, University of California at Los Angeles School of Medicine, Los Angeles, California*

Vence L. Bonham, Jr., J.D., *Associate Professor, Department of Medicine, Michigan State University, East Lansing, Michigan*

R. Phillip Burns, M.D., *Chairman and Professor, Department of Surgery, University of Tennessee College of Medicine—Chattanooga Unit, Chattanooga, Tennessee*

Saundra S. Buys, M.D., *Professor, Department of Medicine, University of Utah Health Sciences Center, Huntsman Cancer Institute, Salt Lake City, Utah*

Blake Cady, M.D., F.A.C.S., *Professor, Department of Surgery, Brown University School of Medicine; Director, Breast Health Center, Women & Infants Hospital of Rhode Island, Providence, Rhode Island*

Maureen A. Chung, M.D., PH.D., *Assistant Professor, Department of Surgery, Brown University School of Medicine; Surgical Oncologist, Breast Health Center, Women & Infants Hospital of Rhode Island, Providence, Rhode Island*

Joseph P. Crowe, M.D., *Director, Breast Center, Department of General Surgery, Cleveland Clinic Health Systems, Cleveland, Ohio*

Jill R. Dietz, M.D., *Associate Staff, Department of General Surgery, The Cleveland Clinic Foundation, Cleveland, Ohio*

Stephen S. Falkenberry, M.D., *Women & Infants Hospital of Rhode Island; Assistant Professor, Department of Obstetrics and Gynecology, Brown University School of Medicine, Providence Rhode Island*

Patricia A. Ganz, M.D., *Professor, University of California at Los Angeles Schools of Medicine and Public Health; Director, Division of Cancer Prevention and Control Research, Jonsson Comprehensive Cancer Center, Los Angeles, California*

Paul E. Goss, M.D., PH.D., *Professor, Department of Medicine, University of Toronto; Director, Breast Cancer Prevention Program, Princess Margaret Hospital, University Health Network, Toronto, Ontario, Canada*

Dawn M. Grabrick, PH.D., *Research Associate, Health Sciences Research, Mayo Clinic, Rochester, Minnesota*

William J. Gradishar, M.D., *Associate Professor, Department of Medicine, Robert H. Lurie Comprehensive Cancer Center, Northwestern University Medical School, Chicago, Illinois*

Ruth Heimann, M.D., PH.D., *Associate Professor and Director of Breast Program, Department of Radiation and Cellular Oncology, The Pritzker School of Medicine, The University of Chicago; Head, Breast Service in Radiotherapy, Department of Radiation and Cellular Oncology, The University of Chicago Hospitals, Duchossois Center for Advanced Medicine, Chicago, Illinois*

Anne Christine Hoyt, M.D., *Assistant Professor, Department of Radiological Sciences, University of California at Los Angeles School of Medicine, Los Angeles, California; Chief of Breast Imaging, Department of Radiology, Olive—View UCLA Medical Center, Sylmar, California*

Kevin S. Hughes, M.D., F.A.C.S., *Surgical Director, Breast Screening Program, Massachusetts General Hospital, Boston, Massachusetts*

Ismail Jatoi, M.D., PH.D., F.A.C.S., *Chief, General Surgery Service, U.S. Army Hospital, Heidelberg, Germany; Associate Professor of Surgery, Uniformed Services of the University of the Health Sciences, Bethesda, Maryland*

Roy A. Jensen, M.D., *Associate Professor, Department of Pathology, Cell Biology, and Cancer Biology, Vanderbilt University Medical Center; Attending Surgical Pathologist, Department of Pathology, Vanderbilt University Hospital, Nashville, Tennessee*

Craig Lawson, M.D. *Assistant Professor, Department of Anatomy, St. Louis University School of Medicine, St. Louis, Missouri*

Verity H. Livingstone, M.D., *Associate Professor, Department of Family Practice, Faculty of Medicine, University of British Columbia, Vancouver, British Columbia, Canada*

R.T. Osteen, M.D., *Associate Professor, Department of Surgery, Harvard Medical School; Surgeon, Department of Surgery, Brigham and Women's Hospital, Boston, Massachusetts*

Janet Rose Osuch, M.S., M.D., *Professor, Department of Surgery, Michigan State University, East Lansing, Michigan*

David L. Page, M.D., *Professor, Departments of Pathology and Preventive Medicine, Vanderbilt University Medical Center, Nashville, Tennessee*

Edith A. Perez, M.D., *Professor of Medicine, Department of Hematology/Oncology, Mayo Medical School; Director, Clinical Research and Breast Cancer Program, Department of Hematology/Oncology, Mayo Clinic, Jacksonville, Florida*

Joseph Ragaz, M.D., F.R.C.P.(C). *Department of Medical Oncology, British Columbia Cancer Agency, Vancouver, British Columbia, Canada*

Constance A. Roche, M.S.N., R.N., C.S., *Nurse Practitioner, Breast Screening Program, Massachusetts General Hospital, Boston, Massachusetts*

Christy A. Russell, M.D., *Associate Professor, Department of Medicine, University of Southern California School of Medicine; Chief of Medicine, USC-Norris Comprehensive Cancer Center, Los Angeles, California*

Carol E.H. Scott-Connor, M.D., PH.D., M.B.A., *Professor and Head, Department of Surgery, University of Iowa College of Medicine; Staff Physician, Department of Surgery, University of Iowa Hospitals and Clinics, Iowa City, Iowa*

Thomas A. Sellers, PH.D., *Professor, Health Sciences Research, Mayo Clinic, Rochester, Minnesota*

Michele A. Shermak, M.D., *Assistant Professor, Department of Plastic Surgery, Johns Hopkins Medical Institutions; Faculty, Department of Plastic Surgery, Johns Hopkins Bayview Medical Center, Baltimore, Maryland*

Jean F. Simpson, M.D., *Professor, Department of Pathology, Vanderbilt University School of Medicine; Director, Anatomic Pathology, Department of Pathology, Vanderbilt University Medical Center, Nashville, Tennessee*

Kathrin Strasser, M.D., *Fellow, Department of Medicine, University of Toronto, Toronto, Ontario, Canada*

Vickie L. Venne, M.S., *Genetic Counselor, University of Utah, Huntsman Cancer Institute, Salt Lake City, Utah*

John T. Vetto, M.D., F.A.C.S., *Associate Professor, Department of Surgery, Section of Surgical Oncology, Oregon Health Sciences University, Portland, Oregon*

Laura E. Witherspoon, M.D., *Assistant Professor, Department of Surgery, University of Tennessee College of Medicine—Chattanooga Unit; Active Staff, Department of Surgery, Erlanger Medical Center, Chattanooga, Tennessee*

Preface

In recent years, physicians from various disciplines have developed an interest in breast diseases. General surgeons, internists, family practitioners, gynecologists, radiologists, and oncologists frequently encounter patients with breast diseases, and the management of these diseases often requires a multidisciplinary approach. This manual is intended to serve as a practical guide for physicians of various specialties. The aim was to provide a general overview of breast diseases, both benign and malignant, and to highlight controversial issues that are of particular relevance to many physicians.

The management of breast diseases should be predicated on *evidence-based medicine*. Large, randomized prospective trials have provided useful information concerning the effectiveness of breast cancer screening and chemoprevention. Additionally, numerous trials have addressed the impact of systemic therapy, radiotherapy, and variations in local therapy on breast cancer mortality. These trials have clearly had a beneficial effect. Several industrialized countries are now reporting reductions in breast cancer mortality, and this trend is expected to continue in the years ahead. In this manual, many of these landmark clinical trials are discussed in considerable detail. Whenever applicable, the results of these trials should serve as a basis for clinical management.

Ismail Jatoi, M.D., PH.D., F.A.C.S.

Acknowledgments

I am deeply indebted to my mentors who, over the years, have been a source of inspiration: the late Dr. Rene Wegria, the late Dr. George E. Block, Dr. Victor Richards, and Professor Michael Baum.

I am grateful to the contributors to this manual, who spent a great deal of time and effort in writing concise reviews. Each chapter in this book is not only informative, but provides the contributors' personal perspective on controversial issues. I also thank the editorial staff of Lippincott Williams & Wilkins for their valuable assistance. This manual has required the collaborative effort of many individuals, and I hope that it makes an important contribution to the care of patients with breast diseases.

1

Anatomy and Physiology of the Breast

Craig Lawson

The mammary glands are modified sweat glands in structure and function and whose site of origin determines certain morphologic features. Their modified structure differs from that of either merocrine- or apocrine-type sweat glands. Their modified function is to provide the newborn infant with specialized nutrients. Their superficial origin accounts for the absence of a true fibrous capsule or sheath surrounding the glands. The glands do not benefit from a specialized vascular supply or innervation, as all these needs are derived from existing structures serving the thoracic wall.

GROSS ANATOMY

The mammary glands are found within the breasts, situated on the anterior thoracic wall. In an adult nulliparous woman, the mammary gland typically extends from the second or third rib to the sixth or seventh costal cartilage and from the lateral sternal border to slightly beyond the anterior axillary fold. The gland has a convex, lens-like shape. The portion of the gland extending along the lateral part of the pectoralis major is known as the *axillary tail* (of Spence). The mammary sinus is the midline, external to the sternum, between the two breasts. The surface of the gland is smooth and slightly curved. Its flattened cranial border does not demonstrate a sharp demarcation from the anterior thoracic wall, but laterally and inferiorly, its borders are well defined. The greatest prominence of the gland occurs at the nipple. The pigmented region surrounding the nipple is the *areola*. The gland protrudes 3.5 to 7 cm from the chest wall but is entirely contained in subcutaneous fascia. The gland averages 10 to 12 cm in craniocaudal dimension, slightly less in transverse diameter. The mammary glands of a nonlactating women each weigh approximately 200 g; lactating mammary glands may weigh as much as 500 g each.

The human breast is unique in its conical or hemispherical shape: In many mammals, even other primates, the breast is relatively flat. The flattened form is maintained during pregnancy and lactation. It is interesting that the intermixture of epithelial and stromal elements occurs in such a manner that no surgical plane of dissection is known to exist within the gland (1).

The smooth conical breasts of a nulliparous woman often become hemispheric with an increase in connective tissue content. In older age or in a state of malnutrition or emaciation, the breasts may become reduced to a flattened disk.

In girls, the mammary glands remain relatively undeveloped until the age of puberty, when the breasts show a rapid increase in size. This rapid growth period is followed by a much longer period of gradual enlargement. With each menstrual cycle, the gland undergoes proliferative changes with subsequent regression. Through the years, a progressive enlargement takes place in most women, also in part because of increased deposition of adipose cells.

After lactation, the breasts tend to become more pendulous in character. After repeated pregnancies, they may become elongated. In addition to changes brought about by breast-feeding, other factors may play a role in the shape of the breast, including cultural differences, mechanical support, diet, and body habitus. The appearance from middle age onward also must take into account diminution of hormonal support.

The mammary gland contains a blend of epithelial glandular tissue, the parenchyma, and supporting connective tissue, the stroma. The essential part of each breast is a disc-shaped mass of glandular tissue that is white or reddish white in color. The gland is thickest opposite the nipple and thins toward the periphery. Each mammary gland is composed of 15 to 20 lobes, each lobe an irregular flattened pyramid of glandular tissue whose apex is directed toward the nipple and whose base radiates toward the periphery (Fig. 1.1) (2). Each lobe has a collecting duct that opens by a tapered opening at the tip of the nipple. The lactiferous ducts (segmental ducts) run parallel to each other in the nipple but ramify in a radial fashion at the nipple base. Beneath the areola, a short segment of the lactiferous duct is dilated from a typical 1- to 2-mm diameter to a diameter of 4 to 5 mm. This short dilated segment constitutes the lactiferous sinus and, thus formed, becomes a reservoir for contents delivered through the duct system. Distally, the diameter of each lactiferous duct is reduced by branching (into subsegmental ducts). Each terminal branch ends in a tubulosaccular structure (Fig. 1.1, inset). Numerous acini open into a common duct and constitute a lobule, and all the lobules that drain through the same excretory duct comprise a lobe. Anastomoses between lobes have not been demonstrated.

The mammary stroma constitutes the connective tissue of the gland. Each part of the parenchyma, lobes, lobules, and acini is surrounded by loose connective tissue. The entire gland also is invested by connective tissue; however, it is not sufficiently organized to form a true capsule. This investment is derived from the fibrous tissue of the subcutaneous layer. The adipose content of the subcutis underlies the skin and, being interspersed between connective tissue strands, imparts a smoothness to the skin over the mammary gland. As occurs elsewhere in the body, bundles of collagen from the hypodermis attach to and blend with the skin. Such collagenous bundles are often particularly well developed over the upper part of the breast and have been called the *suspensory ligaments* (of Cooper).

Nipple and Areola

The nipple is cylindrical or rounded with a fissured tip that accommodates approximately 20 openings from the lactiferous ducts (Fig.1.2). The skin of the nipple is characteristically pigmented, wrinkled, and roughened by small papillae. The nipple typically extends outward 10 to 12 mm from the areola and has no adipose tissue

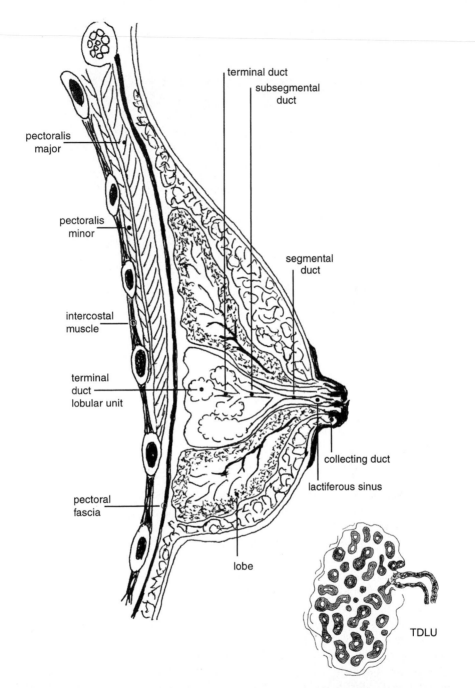

FIG. 1.1. Sagittal section through the breast of a woman of reproductive age. Three lobes are depicted in this diagram, but only one shows the basic structures, including a collecting duct, lactiferous sinus, segmental (lactiferous) duct, subsegmental duct, and terminal duct. Inset: Enhancement of the terminal duct–lobular unit (TDLU) from the larger diagram. Schematic shows typical arrangement of terminal duct and acinar profiles in nonlactating gland.

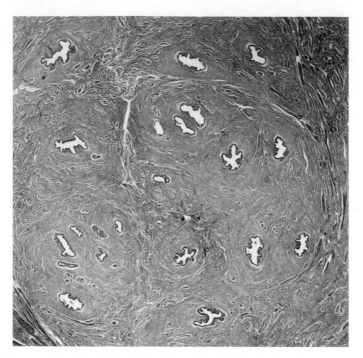

FIG. 1.2. Cross-section through the nipple. Approximately 20 collecting ducts are present in this section. The stroma is densely packed with smooth muscle bundles. Hematoxylin and eosin, ×15. (Reproduced from Tavassoli FA. *Pathology of the breast,* 2nd ed. Stamford, CT: Appleton & Lange, 1999, with permission.)

within it. The nipple has neither hairs nor sweat glands. Sebaceous glands are numerous, and their secretions protect the skin of the nipple. In the deeper parts of the nipple, smooth muscle forms a loose layer that is continuous with the smooth muscle of the areola. The muscle fiber arrangement is principally circular, but some fibers are also arranged vertically, interlacing among the lactiferous and collecting ducts. The circular muscle fibers appear to cause nipple erection, making it narrower and firmer. Through prolonged contraction, the muscle acts as a sphincter on the excretory ducts; by cyclic contraction, the muscle tends to empty the lactiferous sinus. The areola is covered by pigmented skin, the color of which varies with the individual complexion, but it always darkens in pregnancy. The size of the areola shows considerable variation, its diameter ranging from 15 to 60 mm. Following lactation, the pigmentation diminishes, but it usually never returns completely to the virginal or pregestational color. Sebaceous and areolar glands produce elevations of the skin and areola. The areolar glands (of Montgomery) are rudimentary milk glands that enlarge and are pronounced during pregnancy. The dermis under the areola lacks adipose cells but does contain a layer of smooth muscle. The muscle fibers are mainly circular, and the layer is continuous with that of the nipple. Hair follicles are sometimes present at the edge of the areola.

Innervation

Innervation of the skin of the breast is accomplished through cutaneous nerves of the thorax. The lateral cutaneous branches of intercostal nerves two through six (T2–6) provide lateral mammary branches on the axillary side of the gland. Anterior cutaneous branches of intercostal nerves T2 through T5 supply medial mammary branches to the sternal side of the gland. The skin over the uppermost parts of the gland is supplied by branches from supraclavicular nerves (cervical nerves C3–4). Nerves to mammary parenchyma include both sensory and sympathetic fibers. The sympathetic fibers pass to glandular tissue, smooth muscle of the areola, nipple, and blood vessels.

Vascular Supply

The arterial supply of the mammary gland, although robust, is not derived from a single source. The principal vascular supply of the breast enters the gland from its superolateral and superomedial borders. Only scant vascularity is derived from the inferior aspect of the gland. Anterior perforating branches from the internal thoracic artery emerge through the intercostal spaces (and muscles) at the lateral sternal border. The second, third, fourth, and occasionally fifth perforating arteries supply the medial and deep parts of the gland through medial mammary branches. Lateral mammary branches are derived from the lateral thoracic artery and must sweep around the lateral border of the pectoralis major to reach the gland. Intercostal arteries also provide some anterior and lateral branches that supply the mammary gland. The branches derived from the intercostal system accompany corresponding branches from intercostal nerves to the gland. The blood supply to the deep aspect of the gland is provided by the pectoral branches from the thoracoacromial trunk.

The venous drainage within the gland is by way of both superficial and deep plexuses that, for the most part, have an arrangement similar to the arterial distribution. The venous outflow from the gland is mainly to the internal thoracic, lateral thoracic, and upper intercostal veins. Some vessels drain to veins at the base of the cervical region.

Lymphatic Drainage

The lymphatic drainage of the mammary gland is of great importance in view of the development of neoplasias within the gland and the subsequent dissemination of malignant cells through the lymphatic system (Fig. 1.3) (3,4). The thoracic wall has a superficial lymphatic network associated with the cervical region above and the abdominal region below it. The lymphatics of the skin of the breast are a part of this system, but they have a special distribution with respect to the nipple and areola. A thick network of cutaneous lymph capillaries is connected to the surrounding cutaneous plexus and also is united by small channels to a subdermal subareolar plexus. At the edge of the areola, the subareolar plexus becomes thinned and changes character to become the circumareolar plexus. The circumareolar plexus becomes continuous with the general lymphatic network of the skin over the breast.

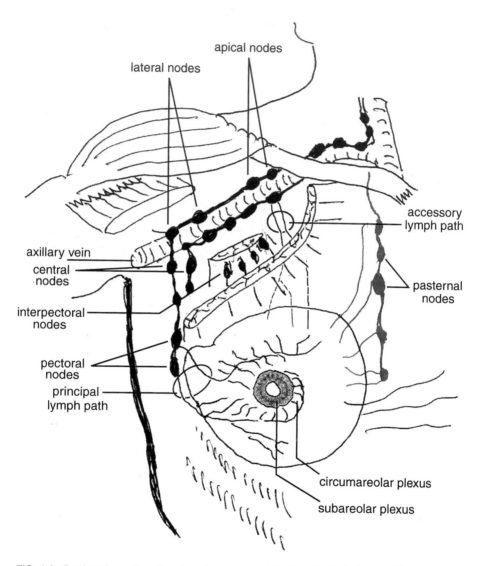

FIG. 1.3. Depicts the axillary lymph node groups and the lymphatic drainage of the mammary gland. The internal thoracic (parasternal) group of nodes is shown in silhouette.

The subareolar lymphatic plexus receives converging lymphatic channels from the mammary gland. Lymphatic vessels from the perilobular and interlobular areas, in addition to those of the lactiferous ducts, pass to the subareolar lymphatic plexus.

The principal axillary path from the mammary gland follows two routes (5,6). From the subareolar plexus, a lateral lymphatic trunk runs transversely outward toward the axillary lymph nodes. The medial and inferior lymphatic trunk curves below the areola, receives a tributary from the lower part of the gland, and proceeds laterally to the base of the axilla. After winding around the anterior axillary fold, both channels terminate in the pectoral group of axillary nodes. Other collecting vessels of this principal lymph path terminate directly in the central or the lateral group of axillary nodes.

Some lymphatic channels emerge from the gland periphery, perforate the pectoralis major muscle and then follow branches of the thoracoacromial vessels to apical axillary nodes. Other collecting vessels turn around the lower border of the pectoralis major and ascend between the pectoral muscles to reach apical axillary nodes. Interpectoral nodes (of Rotter) are found along these accessory paths (7). From the circumareolar plexus, a group of lymphatic vessels pass toward the midline in company with anterior perforating branches of the internal thoracic vessels. These channels perforate muscle at the sternal border and penetrate the thoracic wall to terminate in the internal thoracic (parasternal) lymphatic chain. These nodes are found deep to the sternum along the course of internal thoracic vessels, opposite intercostal spaces.

Axillary Nodes

The axillary lymph nodes consist of from 20 to 30 nodes, arranged in a pure anatomical perspective as five subgroups (Fig. 1.3). They are the lateral, pectoral, subscapular, central, and apical groups (8). The importance of the axillary nodes cannot be overstated because they serve as the major pathway for dissemination of mammary carcinomas (4). They receive about 75% of the lymph flow from each mammary gland compared with approximately 25% for the internal thoracic nodes.

The lateral group of nodes lies medial and posterior to the distal part of the axillary artery and vein. Efferent channels from this group carry lymph to the central and apical axillary nodes and sometimes to the inferior deep cervical lymph nodes.

The pectoral group of nodes is found along the course of the lateral thoracic vessels, adjacent to the axillary border of the pectoralis minor. The nodes in this group receive drainage from the anterolateral thoracic wall, skin, and muscles of the abdomen above the umbilicus and most of the mammary gland. Efferent vessels from this group drain to the central and apical nodes.

The subscapular group is arranged along the subscapular vessels. These nodes receive drainage from the skin and posterior thoracic wall, including the scapular region and lower posterior cervical area. Their efferent channels converge on the central axillary node group.

The central group of nodes resides within the axillary fat. These nodes are found at a level traversed by the intercostobrachial nerve (lateral cutaneous branch of T2). The nodes of this group often are noted to be among the largest of those found within the axilla, but their number is typically inversely proportional to their size. Afferent channels to this group come from lymphatics of the brachium and mammary gland, but the majority of lymph is derived from the preceding lymph node groups.

The apical nodes are found at the axillary apex, along the axillary artery and vein, adjacent to the cranial border of the pectoralis minor. Afferents to the apical group come from all other axillary node groups, from lymph channels that accompany the cephalic vein and from lymph channels at the edge of the mammary gland. The efferent channels from the apical group usually are gathered into a single trunk (subclavian lymphatic trunk) that terminates on the right side at the junction of the internal jugular and subclavian veins. On the left side, the subclavian lymph trunk joins the thoracic duct or separately enters the junction of internal jugular and subclavian veins.

For indicating the level of metastatic progression to a surgeon, pathologists commonly report axillary lymph node involvement in a different manner. In this technique, the presence or absence of metastasis is noted in any of three levels, where nodes may be found along the path from the breast to the apical group. In this scheme, level I nodes are found along the axillary border of the pectoralis minor. Level II nodes lie dorsal to the pectoralis minor and between its medial and lateral borders. Level III nodes are found medial to the sternal border and superior to cranial border of the pectoralis minor.

Asymmetry

It is the rule rather than the exception that there is some variation in the size and symmetry of a patient's breasts. The left breast is usually larger than the right. If slight, the differences may not have been noted by the patient. How much a difference in size or degree of asymmetry must be present for the patient to feel abnormal is difficult to state and will vary from patient to patient. A more delicate distinction involves how much variance between breasts may be normal but may be interpreted as unattractive by a patient (9). Occasionally, patients with gross asymmetry will not consider intervention and thus be well adjusted to appearance, whereas rare patients with slight degrees of asymmetry will be devastated and report an unacceptable body image (10).

In general, it appears that the threshold for either acceptability or seeking reparative action will differ for each patient. Although input from parents, spouse, surgeon, and psychiatrist should be considered, ultimately, the patient probably ought to be the one who determines what she finds acceptable.

Questions occasionally arise as to what structure in form, number, or position constitutes an anomaly versus a variation. It is generally agreed that differences in size (of normal breast) or length of extension into the axilla are so common as to be regarded as variation. True anomalies of the breast include those instances in which breast tissue is absent or hypoplastic or where there are accessory breasts or nipples.

Classification of Asymmetry

A number of different conditions may produce an asymmetrical appearance to the breasts. These conditions include developmental abnormalities, tumors, surgery, radiation, trauma, and others. Abnormalities of development account for the greatest percentage of asymmetrical breasts. Simon et al. (11) modified the four anatomic categories established by Maliniac (12) to produce a complete classification scheme as follows:

1. One breast hypoplastic, the other normal sized
2. Both breasts hypoplastic but unequal in size
3. One breast hypertrophic, the other normal
4. Both breasts hypertrophic and unequal in size
5. One breast hypoplastic, the other hypertrophic
6. Unilateral hypoplasia of thorax, pectoral muscles, and breast

Amastia

Amastia is defined as the absence of the breast. The complete absence of one or both breasts is a rare anomaly, but it can occur in siblings (13–15). Various series have examined this condition in both women and men, although the condition is more common in women (16). The condition is usually unilateral.

In a considerable proportion of cases of amastia, there is an associated absence or underdevelopment of ipsilateral structures of the shoulder, thorax, or brachium (17). Many patients with an underlying defect in the pectoral musculature, however, have a normal ipsilateral breast (18). Several cases of mother and daughter affectation are recorded, and in rare instances, the defect has been traced through successive generations (19).

Polymastia and Polythelia

The presence of additional mammary tissue is called *polymastia*, and the presence of additional nipples is termed *polythelia*. Most accessory glandular tissue is found in the axilla, caudal mammary border, or vulva (Fig. 1.4).

Incomplete regression or persistence of tissues associated with the milk line results in accessory mammary tissue in approximately 2% to 3% of adult women. Accessory breasts or nipples occurs in from 1% to 2% of white subjects but is reported with an increased frequency in Asians, 1.7% in Japanese males, and 5.1% in Japanese females (20). The presence of accessory breast tissue is an anomaly that shows a hereditary pattern; there are reports of familial transmission (21,51).

Accessory breast tissue may occur as any combination of the standard components of the breast: acinar or ductal elements, the areola, or the nipple. It also may occur as any single component. The most frequent combination is a reduced nipple and small areola. Bilateral accessory breast tissue also is found.

Whereas it may be true that accessory breast tissue is not important physiologically, it is important to remember that accessory breast tissue may be subject to the same kinds of benign and malignant processes that occur in breast tissue that is normally situated (22–26). It also may be misdiagnosed, resulting in needless excision with attendant surgical risks.

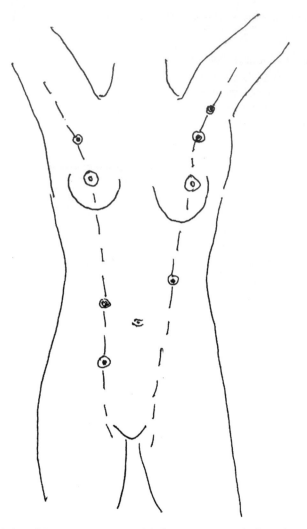

FIG. 1.4. A depiction of the "milk line" in an adult. Supernumerary nipples or breasts may persist anywhere along these lines, which extend from the axilla to the inguinal region.

MICROSCOPIC ANATOMY

The mammary gland is histologically classified as a compound tubuloalveolar gland. The mammary gland in an adult woman is sometimes called a *resting* gland to distinguish it from one that is in the process of active growth (as in pregnancy) or one that is functioning in lactation.

The nipple, areola, and principal ostia of the collecting ducts are covered by a stratified squamous type epithelium. Within a few millimeters of the surface, lactiferous and segmental ducts become lined by a pseudostratified columnar epithelium. Deeper still, the distal portions of the segmental ducts, subsegmental ducts and acini

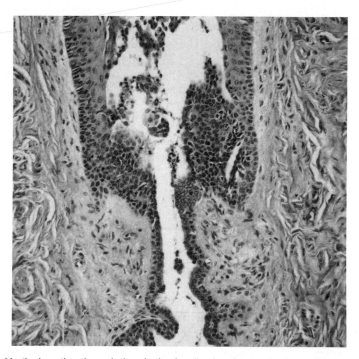

FIG. 1.5. Vertical section through the nipple. A collecting duct is shown close to its opening on the nipple surface. Squamous epithelium is seen (top) undergoing transition to two epithelial layers (bottom). Hematoxylin and eosin, × 160. (Reproduced from Tavassoli FA. *Pathology of the breast,* 2nd ed. Stamford, CT: Appleton & Lange, 1999, with permission.)

are lined by a low columnar to cuboidal epithelium (Fig. 1.5). The lining epithelium is supported on its basal surface by a second layer of epithelial cells, which have a flattened, almost squamoid appearance. These are a distinct cell type: the *myoepithelial cells.* Myoepithelial cells contain myofilaments and have nuclei that are found oriented perpendicular to the long axis of the duct. The myoepithelial cells lie against the basal lamina. External to the basal lamina, each terminal duct and acinus is surrounded by delicate collagen fibers, a few scattered fibroblasts, and lymphocytes.

Considering a lobe from the deepest parts of the gland outward, the portion of the duct that leaves an acinus is called the *terminal duct* (Fig. 1.1, inset). Many terminal ducts join one another to form the subsegmental duct. Subsegmental ducts join one another other to form a segmental duct. Segmental ducts are also known as *lactiferous ducts,* whose proximal portion demonstrates a dilated segment, the *lactiferous sinus.* The portion of the duct system external to the lactiferous sinus is called the *collecting duct,* and each lobe of the breast is represented by such a collecting duct opening on the nipple. Three-dimensional stereo microscopy has supported our traditional understanding of the branching pattern of the mammary gland (27).

The principal pathophysiologic unit of the mammary gland is the terminal duct–lobular unit (TDLU) (Fig. 1.6A). The TDLU is separately recognized (and emphasized)

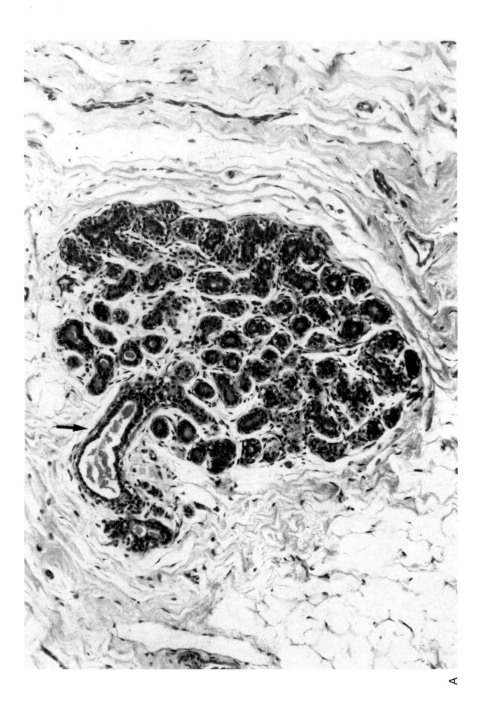

A

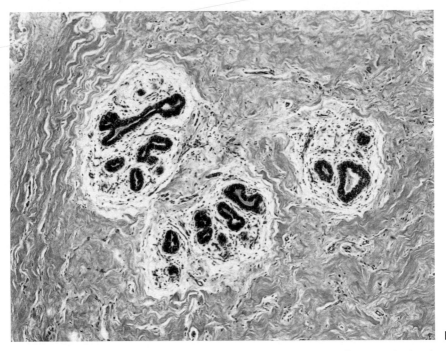

FIG. 1.6. *Continued.* **B:** Photomicrograph from a 13-year-old girl showing an underdeveloped lobule. Note the abundant intra- and interlobular stroma. Hematoxylin and eosin, × 40. (A: Reproduced from Tavassoli FA. *Pathology of the breast,* 2nd ed. Stamford, CT: Appleton & Lange, 1999, with permission.)

because it has a well-defined lobular histologic appearance, it is surrounded a cuff of myxoid-like connective tissue, and there is an absence of elastic fibers (28). The larger ducts have a sparsity of specialized connective tissue but do demonstrate abundant elastic fibers. Recognizing the concept of the TDLU, and its implications, will enhance the understanding of many pathological lesions that occur in the breast.

IMMUNOHISTOCHEMISTRY

In general, the two epithelial cell types of the mammary gland have distinctive immunohistochemical profiles with few similarities but several important differences. Both epithelial cell types (i.e., epithelial and myoepithelial) demonstrate immunoreactivity for various keratins, epithelial membrane antigen, milk-fat globule

FIG. 1.6. A: Photomicrograph shows a terminal duct (*arrow*) leading to a TDLU from a 26-year-old woman. The intralobular stroma is sparse. Hematoxylin and eosin, × 100.

membrane antigen, α-lactalbumin, and S-100 (29). Epithelial cells demonstrate immunoreactivity for many cytokeratins, especially cytokeratin 7. Whereas cytokeratins other than cytokeratin 7 show more or less immunoreactivity for breast epithelial cells, cytokeratin 20 does not stain these cells. There is inconsistent immunoreactivity for S-100 in lining epithelium (compared with the myoepithelial cell layer); so this agent is not a reliable immunohistochemical marker.

Myoepithelial cells demonstrate moderate to weak reactivity for the cytokeratins, especially cytokeratin 14, but not for the acidic cytokeratins 18 and 19. Myoepithelial cells are weakly positive for S-100 immunostain, but they display strong reactivity for actin (29,30). Thus, an epithelial versus myoepithelial cell lineage can be clearly distinguished through application of the actin immunostain (and controls). S-100 is not as reliable an antibody for separating these two cell types. In addition, although the glandular cells display strong immunoreactivity for estrogen and progesterone receptor, myoepithelial cells do not react with either immunostain. The fetal breast epithelial cell antibody *bcl-2* also stains adult epithelial cells, but myoepithelial cells show no immunoreactivity to this agent (31,32).

Application of the proliferation antibody Ki-67 to structurally normal mammary epithelium demonstrates higher proliferation rates during the luteal phase of the cycle than does epithelium sampled during the proliferative phase (1,33,34). The application of chromogranin immunostain has demonstrated a scattered population of endocrine cells in the normal mammary gland (35,36). Their role in breast physiology is not clear. The myoepithelial cells rest on a basal lamina, which is easily demonstrable with routine histochemical stains but also with immunohistochemical reagents for laminin and type IV collagen (37,38).

EMBRYOLOGY AND DEVELOPMENT OF THE BREAST

The mammary gland is derived primarily from epidermal thickenings that develop along the ventral surface of the body, the so-called milk line. These bilateral tissue ridges form during the sixth week of embryonic life between the upper and lower limb buds. The line can be visualized in the adult as extending from the axilla to the anterior aspect of the inguinal region (Fig. 1.4).

A number of globular primordia arise during fetal development along this line, but by the ninth week of gestation, typically one pair of papilla in the pectoral region produce the nipple buds. Other primitive nipple structures that may have formed usually regress and eventually undergo complete involution (39).

During the second trimester of fetal life, cords of squamous cells from the epithelial surface invade the nipple bud, and primary mammary ducts develop from these downgrowths (39). The cords and buds eventually become hollow and develop continuous lumina. At the time of birth, usually only the primitive nipple and rudimentary lactiferous ducts are present at the level of the fifth intercostal space in the midclavicular line. The lactiferous ducts begin to radiate outward from a small area in the region of the nipple and areola. Collecting ducts eventually open onto the nipple from a small sinusoidal dilatation, the lactiferous sinus. This area becomes elevated and forms the nipple. Pigmentation develops in the nipple and the areola.

At birth, breast development is far from complete. Numerous biochemical mediators must act synergistically to stimulate the development and maturation of the mammary ductal and acinar target cells. Growth and branching of mammary ducts occur at a slow rate during prepubertal life. In the male, mammary development typically stops at this stage. In the female, development of the mammary glands dramatically increases at puberty with branching of ducts, scattered formation of acinar buds, and a concomitant proliferation of interductal stroma.

During adolescence, stromal growth is responsible for most of the increase in breast size. In the glandular portion of the breast, ductal structures are present, but acini are usually not found (Fig. 1.6B).

It is only with the onset of pregnancy that the breast achieves complete structural maturation and full functional activity. From each acinar bud, numerous true secretory units develop and form grape-like clusters. As a result, there is a reversal of the previous stromal–glandular proportions in the breast. Thus, by the end of pregnancy, the mammary gland is composed almost entirely of acinar units separated by small amounts of connective tissue.

Following a lactational cycle, the acinar tissue undergoes regression and atrophy, ductal structures shrink, and the whole breast diminishes remarkably in size. Complete regression to a pregestational size, however, typically does not occur for most women.

At the time of menopause, acini and ducts undergo regressive changes with further loss of both intralobular and interlobular connective tissue. Eventually, acinar structures may be almost completely absent from the female breast. The appearance that remains, of variously sized ductal structures, may resemble the morphologic pattern of the male breast, but most women, even in postmenopause, will have enough estrogenic stimulation to maintain occasional remnants of acinar structures (11). A more detailed account of the histomorphologic changes that accompany development, gestation, puberty, lactation, and menopause has been given (40).

PHYSIOLOGY

The functional activity of the mammary glands represents a dynamic process that begins during fetal life, progresses through the reproductive years, and terminates with regressive–atrophic changes after menopause. The process involves many repetitive physiologic cycles and peaks (in a morphologic sense) with lactation after pregnancy.

The mammary glands serve as a target organ for a variety of hormones and chemical modulators that have active or permissive roles in breast physiology. The various endocrine secretions are important for mammogenesis (breast development), lactogenesis (the process that establishes the secretory state), and galactopoiesis (the production of milk).

Optimal development and mammary function involve an exquisite balance between the endocrine, nervous, and reproductive systems. Estrogen, progesterone, and prolactin play active roles in breast physiology. Estrogen and progesterone synergistically drive the process of development, with estrogen stimulating the ductal structures and progesterone stimulating the lobular units. Estrogen and progesterone exert maximal effects when prolactin is present (41). Estrogen stimulates mammary epithelial stem cell division, but for the process to continue, prolactin, insulin, and growth hormone must be present (Fig. 1.7)(42). Sensitization of acinar epithelial cells by cortisol, insulin, and thyroxine permits final differentiation into milk producing cells (43). Other hormones, including human placental lactogen, stimulate ductal epithelial cells (44).

During fetal mammary development, the milk ridge appears in the sixth week. The persistence of the nipple in the pectoral region is succeeded by the development of primitive duct structures. At first, development appears independent of hormonal influences, but by the end of the first trimester, gender differences in the breast become apparent. For such differentiation to occur, estrogen and testosterone are required. The absence of the testosterone receptor, as in testicular feminization syndrome, or exposure of the fetus to androgenic interference, will result in a female histomorphology in the gland.

At birth and in the immediate postnatal period, breast tissue is responsive to multiple hormonal stimuli. Transfer of maternal hormones across the placenta may cause a transient mammary hyperplasia in the newborn (45). Occasionally, the hyperplastic tissue persists for weeks or months (46). Because the hyperplastic breast primordium is not pathologic, it should not be excised because its removal will produce an ipsilateral amastia. The phenomenon of transient hyperplasia is eliminated when pituitary prolactin declines and is followed by involution of the newborn mammary epithelium.

During the childhood years, there is only minimal branching of segmental ducts. Acini are not formed under normal circumstances. At puberty, the hypothalamus produces gonadotropin-releasing hormone, which stimulates the production of follicle-stimulating hormone and luteinizing hormone. When the ovarian cellular apparatus is stimulated, follicular maturation begins and estradiol is produced. This stimulates mammary growth, and thelarche takes place. Premature thelarche occurs as an aberrant response of mammary tissue to endogenous hormones. It results in a subareolar discoid thickening histologically characterized by ductular proliferation in a background of thickened connective tissue.

For a short time, the breast is stimulated primarily by estrogen, which causes ductal growth and arborization, an increase in the periductal connective tissue, and concomitant increase in vascularity. Once ovulation takes place, progesterone from the corpus luteum stimulates terminal duct–acinar development. A longitudinal study by Marshall and Tanner described mammary development in adolescent girls as proceeding through five stages (47).

During the reproductive years, mammary tissue demonstrates repeated cyclic

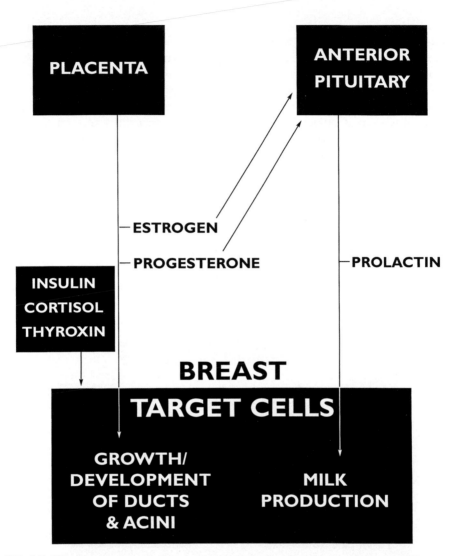

FIG. 1.7. This figure outlines the hormonal control of mammary gland development during pregnancy and lactation. Milk production is prevented during pregnancy by inhibition of prolactin. When estrogen and progesterone are withdrawn after delivery of the placenta, the barrier to milk production is removed.

changes, indicative of the hormonal fluctuations during the menstrual cycle (48). Vogel et al. categorized the histologic alterations of the mammary gland into five phases and correlated them with five stages of the menstrual cycle (49). Generally, in the proliferative phase of the cycle, estrogen stimulates epithelial mitoses, increased density of connective tissue, and the presence of nonvacuolated myoepithelial cells.

In the luteal phase, progesterone secretion results in the formation of an edematous stroma, absence of epithelial mitotic activity, and vacuolated myoepithelial cells. Prolactin levels also increase, and in conjunction with steroid and metabolic hormones, acinar cells demonstrate secretory activity.

During an ovulatory cycle, many women normally experience breast fullness and tenderness. In this situation, breast volume is enhanced by increased blood flow, increased volume of extracellular fluid, and ductal–acinar differentiation. Toward the end of a menstrual cycle, regressive changes occur in the breast. During menses, the lobules become smaller and acinar lumina narrow.

The state of gestation is characterized by significant alterations to the hormonal balance. A large increment in steroids occurs from the fetoplacental unit. Prolactin

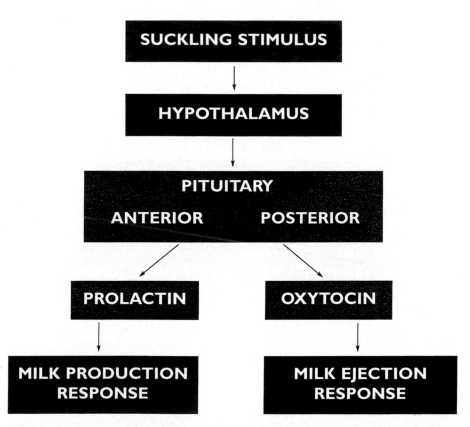

FIG. 1.8. Schematic to show how lactation occurs in a two-stage process. Milk production is stimulated by prolactin, whereas milk ejection is stimulated by oxytocin. The act of suckling is the event that triggers this neuroendocrine reflex.

and growth hormone are the most important pituitary hormones stimulating mammary growth. Human placental lactogen and human chorionic somatomammotropin appear and stimulate a dramatic increase of acini per lobule and induction of secretory activity. Pregnancy also is characterized by increased free cortisol and hyperinsulinemia. Although lactogenesis takes place, lactation typically does not occur during pregnancy. It is hypothesized that estrogen, progesterone, and other inhibiting mediators act as a barrier to prevent the full effect of prolactin on mammary epithelium (Fig. 1.7). Once parturition has occurred and the placenta is delivered, the withdrawal of estrogen and progesterone removes any metabolic barrier that can block the effect of prolactin and lactation will occur.

The act of nursing helps to maintain high levels of prolactin release via a neuroendocrine reflex (Fig. 1.8). Sensory nerve endings in the breast, activated by suckling, relay impulses to the hypothalamus, turning off the secretion of prolactin-inhibiting hormone. The suckling stimulus also may increase the secretion of prolactin-releasing hormone. Suckling thus results in the release of prolactin from the anterior pituitary, which promotes the secretion of milk from the gland.

Suckling also stimulates the reflex secretion of oxytocin from the posterior pituitary (Fig. 1.8). This hormone is produced in the hypothalamus and stored in the posterior pituitary. When released, it results in the milk (ejection) letdown reflex. Oxytocin stimulates contraction of smooth muscle around the lactiferous sinus and thus aids the expression of milk. Oxytocin also stimulates the contraction of uterine smooth muscle as well, helping women who breast-feed regain uterine muscle tone faster than women who bottle-feed. When cessation of suckling takes place, lactation usually stops.

With termination of ovarian function at menopause, mammary regression and involution take place (16). At first, there is mild to moderate loss of mammary epithelium as well as loss of terminal duct–acinar units (Fig. 1.9A). In the lobules, both epithelial and myoepithelial layers become attenuated, lumina are obliterated, the basal lamina thickens, and hyalinization of the surrounding stroma occurs. Subsequently, there is significant atrophy of glandular tissue and a corresponding increase in adipose deposition and eventual predominance of hyalinized connective tissue nodules (Fig. 1.9B). The loss of lobular units is most significant and typically decreases to approximately one-third to one-fourth of the number seen during the reproductive years (19). In the final stage of breast involution, one may find only scattered duct profiles and rare islands of small acini (Fig. 1.9C) (50).

In summary, physiologic mediators act synergistically to stimulate structural and functional development of breast cells. The process begins during fetal life, continues imperceptibly through childhood, is dramatically enhanced at puberty, and undergoes repeated proliferative and secretory cycles during the reproductive years. If pregnancy takes place, a lactation cycle intervenes with significant secretory changes, followed by structural and functional involution. More complete regressive changes leading to atrophy in the acinar–ductal system are seen after menopause.

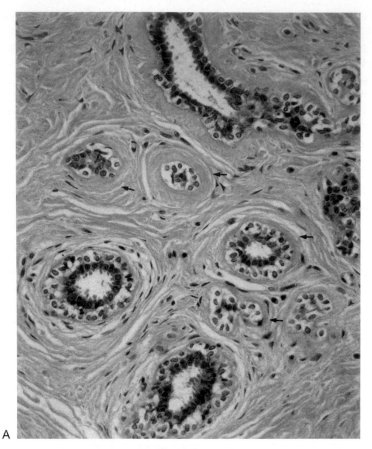

A

FIG. 1.9. A: Photomicrograph showing an early stage in postmenopausal involution. The process begins with periductal thickening of the basal lamina (*arrows*). Hematoxylin and eosin, ×250.

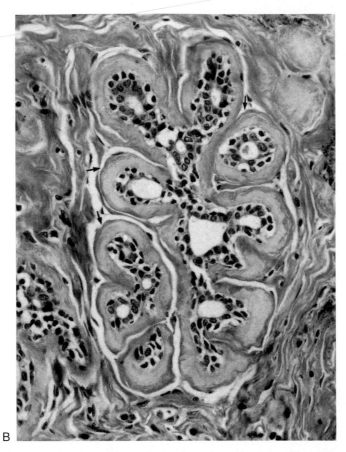

B

FIG. 1.9. *Continued.* **B:** Photomicrograph showing more advanced periductal fibrosis (*arrows*) with reduction of luminal diameters. Hyalinization of basal lamina is evident. Hematoxylin and eosin, ×250.

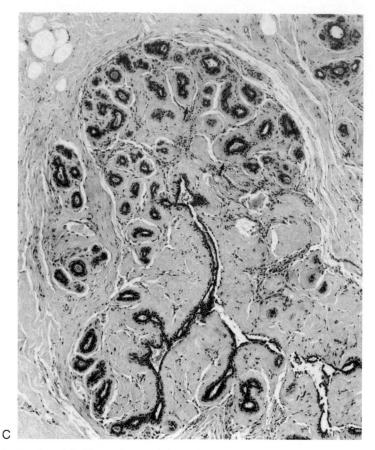

C

FIG. 1.9. *Continued.* **C:** Photomicrograph from a later stage in postmenopausal involution. The acini in this lobule show various stages in the involutional process. In some areas, there is complete fibrosis from the basal lamina to the edge of the lobule. Hematoxylin and eosin, × 160. (Reproduced from Tavassoli FA. *Pathology of the breast,* 2nd ed. Stamford, CT: Appleton & Lange, 1999, with permission.)

ACKNOWLEDGMENT

It was my good fortune to have worked with Mrs. Sandy Turck for three years. She continues to amaze me with her adaptability, perseverance, and professionalism. I gratefully acknowledge her advice and assistance with respect to the graphics and artwork contained in this manuscript.

REFERENCES

1. Going JJ, Anderson TJ, Battersby B, et al. Proliferative and secretory activity in human breast during natural and artificial menstrual cycles. *Am J Pathol* 1988;130:193–204.
2. Cowie AT. Overview of the mammary gland. *J Invest Dermatol* 1974;63:2–9.
3. Hultborn AL, Hulten B, Roos M, et al. Effectiveness of axillary lymph node dissection in modified radical mastectomy with preservation of pectoral muscles. *Ann Surg* 1974;179:269–272.
4. Pickren JW. Lymph node metastasis in carcinoma of the female mammary gland. *Bulletin of Roswell Park Memorial Institute* 1956;1:79–90.
5. Goss CM, ed. *Anatomy of the human body,* 39th ed. Philadelphia: Lea & Febiger, 1973.
6. Hultborn KA, Larsson LG, Ragnhult I. The lymphatic drainage from the breast to the axillary and parasternal lymph nodes: studies with the aid of colloid Au-198. *Acta Radiol* 1955;43:52–64.
7. Egan RL, McSweeney MB. Intramammary lymph nodes. *Cancer* 1983;51:1838–1842.
8. Woodburne RT. *Essentials of human anatomy,* 7th ed. New York: Oxford University Press, 1983.
9. Hueston JT. Unilateral agenesis and hypoplasia: difficulties and suggestions. In: Goldwyn RM, ed. *Plastic and reconstructive surgery of the breast.* Boston: Little, Brown and Company, 1976.
10. Schonfeld WA. Body-image disturbances in adolescents with inappropriate sexual development. *Am J Orthopyschiatry* 1964;34:493–499.
11. Simon BE, Hoffman S, Kahn S. Treatment of asymmetry of the breasts. *Clin Plast Surg* 1975;2: 375–390.
12. Maliniac JW. *Breast deformities and their repair.* New York: Grune & Stratton, 1950.
13. Deaver JB, McFarland J. *The breast.* Philadelphia: P. Blakiston's Son & Co, 1917.
14. Kowlessar M, Orti E. Complete breast absence in siblings. *Am J Dis Child* 1968;15:91–92.
15. Rees TD. Mammary asymmetry. *Clin Plast Surg* 1975;2:371–374.
16. Hutson SW, Cowen PN, Bird CC. Morphologic studies of age related changes in normal human breast and their significance in the evolution of mammary cancer. *J Clin Pathol* 1985;38:281–287.
17. Trier WC. Complete breast absence: case report and review of the literature. *Plast Reconstr Surg* 1965;36:430–439.
18. Pers M. Alasias of the anterior thoracic wall, the pectoral muscle and the breast. *Scand J Plast Reconstr Surg* 1968;2:125–135.
19. Haagensen CD. *Diseases of the breast,* 3rd ed. Philadelphia: WB Saunders, 1986.
20. Iwai T. A statistical study on the polymastia of the Japanese. *Lancet* 1907;2:753–759.
21. Klinkerfuss GH. Four generations of polymastia. *JAMA* 1924;82:1247–1251.
22. Cogswell AD, Czerny EW. Carcinoma of accessory breast of the axilla. *Am Surg* 1961;27:388–390.
23. Dyess DL, Tucker JA, Ferrar JJ. Carcinoma in a supernumerary nipple/breast complex: case report and review of the literature. *Breast Dis* 1995;8:77–84.
24. Levin M, Pakarakas HA, Chang M, et al. Primary breast carcinoma of the vulva: a case report and review of the literature. *Gynecol Oncol* 1995;56:448–451.
25. Noronha AJ. Cystic disease in supernumerary breasts. *Br J Surg* 1936;24:143–147.
26. Shrotria S, Gilchik MW. Axillary accessory breasts: a clinicopathological study of 35 patients with axillary masses. *Breast Disease* 1994;7:43–52.
27. Moffat DF, Going JJ. Three dimensional anatomy of complete duct systems in human breast: pathological and developmental implications. *J Clin Pathol* 1996;49:48–52.
28. Tavassoli FA. *Pathology of the breast,* 2nd ed. Stamford, CT: Appleton & Lange, 1999.
29. Jarish ED, Nagel RB, Kaufmann M, et al. Differential diagnosis of benign epithelial proliferations and carcinomas of the breast using antibodies to cytokeratins. *Hum Pathol* 1988;19:276–289.
30. Egan MJ, Newman J, Crocker J, et al. Immunohistochemical localization of S-100 protein in benign and malignant conditions of the breast. *Arch Pathol Lab Med* 1987;111:28–31.
31. Leek RD, Kaklamanis L, Pezzella F, et al. bcl-2 in normal human breast and carcinoma, association

with estrogen receptor-positive, epidermal growth factor receptor-negative tumors and *in situ* cancer. *Br J Cancer* 1994;69:135–139.

32. Nathan B, Anbazhagan R, Clarkson P, et al. Expression of *bcl-2* in the developing human fetal and infant breast. *Histopathology* 1994;24:73–76.

33. Ferguson DJP, Anderson TJ. Morphological evaluation of cell turnover in relation to the menstrual cycle in the resting human breast. *Br J Cancer* 1981;44:177–181.

34. Potten CS, Watson RJ, Williams CT, et al. The effect of age and the menstrual cycle upon proliferative activity of the normal human breast. *Br J Cancer* 1988;58:163–170.

35. Bussolati G, Gugliotta P, Sapino A, et al. Chromogranin reactive endocrine cells in argyrophilic carcinomas (''carcinoids'') and normal tissue of the breast. *Am J Pathol* 1985;120:186–192.

36. Satake T, Matsuyama M. Endocrine cells in a normal breast and non-cancerous breast lesion. *Acta Pathol Jpn* 1991;41:874–878.

37. Charpin C, Lissitzky JC, Jacquemier J, et al. Immunohistochemical detection of laminin in 98 human breast carcinomas: a light and electron microscopic study. *Hum Pathol* 1986;17:355–365.

38. Monteagudo C, Merino MJ, San-Juan J, et al. Immunohistochemical distribution of type IV collagenase in normal, benign, and malignant breast tissue. *Am J Pathol* 1990;136:585–592.

39. Moore KL. *The developing human, clinically oriented embryology.* Philadelphia: WB Saunders, 1988.

40. Salazar H, Tobon H, Josimovich JB. Developmental, gestational and postgestational modifications of the human breast. *Clin Obstet Gynecol* 1975;18:113–137.

41. Reyniak JV. Endocrine physiology of the breast. *J Reprod Med* 1979;22:303–309.

42. Speroff L, Glass RH, Kase NG. *Clinical gynecology endocrinology and infertility.* Baltimore: Williams & Wilkins, 1973.

43. Ceriani RL. Proceedings: hormones and other factors controlling growth in the mammary gland: a review. *J Invest Dermatol* 1974;63:93–108.

44. McManus MJ, Welch CW. The effect of estrogen, progesterone, thyroxine and human placental lactogen on DNA synthesis of human breast ductal epithelium maintained in athymic nude mice. *Cancer* 1984;54:1920–1927.

45. Newton M. Human lactation. In: Kon SK, Cowie AT, eds. *Milk: the mammary gland and its secretion.* New York: Academic Press, 1961.

46. Van Winter JT, Noller KL, Zimmerman D, et al. Natural history of premature thelarche in Olmsted County, Minnesota, 1940–1984. *J Pediatr* 1990;116:278–280.

47. Marshall WA, Tanner JM. Variations in pattern of pubertal changes in girls. *Arch Dis Child* 1969; 44:291–303.

48. Longacre TA, Bartow SA. A correlative morphologic study of human breast and endometrium in the menstrual cycle. *Am J Surg Pathol* 1986;10:382–393.

49. Vogel PM, Georgiade NG, Fetter BF, et al. The correlation of histological changes in the human breast with the menstrual cycle. *Am J Pathol* 1981;104:23–34.

50. Cowan DF, Herbert TA. Involution of the breast in women aged 50 to 104 years. A histological study of 102 cases. *Surg Pathol* 1989;2:323–334.

51. Cellini A, Offidavi A. Familial supernumerary nipples and breasts. *Dermatology* 1992;185:56–58.

2

Congenital and Developmental Abnormalities of the Breast

Michele A. Shermak

DEVELOPMENT OF THE BREAST

Development of the mammary glands begins in the embryo, and further development occurs into adulthood. During the fifth week of fetal development, primitive milk streaks, also known as *galactic bands*, form. These are single, thickened ridges of ectoderm that extend bilaterally from the axillary to the inguinal region. Each band consolidates to form a mammary ridge on the thorax, and the remaining band regresses. At 6 to 8 weeks, a primary bud forms, with thickening of the mammary anlage, which penetrates into the chest wall mesenchyme. The primary mammary bud gives rise to secondary buds that extend into the surrounding connective tissue and become the lactiferous ducts and their branches. Between 12 and 16 weeks of development, mesenchymal cells differentiate into the smooth muscle of the nipple–areolar complex (NAC), and branches link to future secretory alveoli. The secondary mammary anlage then develops with differentiation of hair follicles and sweat glands. Between 20 and 30 weeks, placental sex hormones induce canalization of the branched epithelial tissues. By 32 to 40 weeks, the parenchyma differentiates into alveolar and lobular structures. The epidermis at the origin of the mammary gland becomes depressed, forming a shallow mammary pit onto which the lactiferous ducts open. The breast bud becomes palpable at 34 weeks, measuring approximately 3 mm at 36 weeks of age and 4 mm to 10 mm by 40 weeks (Fig. 2.1). Soon after birth, the nipple rises because of proliferation of the mesenchyme underneath, and the areola becomes pigmented. Under the influence of maternal hormones that pass into the placenta, male and female neonates may secrete colostral milk, also known as *witch's milk*, up to 4 to 7 days postpartum. Neonates also may demonstrate hyperplasia of the breast, which generally regresses spontaneously within a few weeks or months (1–3).

Intrauterine development progresses autonomously and is governed by epithelial–mesenchymal signaling, unlike development in puberty and pregnancy, which depends on hormonal stimulation (4). Various growth factors mediate the signals. Transforming growth factor-α (TGF-α) stimulates ductal and lobuloalveolar development. TGF-β affects canalization of ductal structures and suppression of lactation (3,5). Laminin-5 aids in hemidesmosome attachment and signaling (6). Hepatocyte growth factor/scatter factor enhances ductal end bud size, numbers, and branching

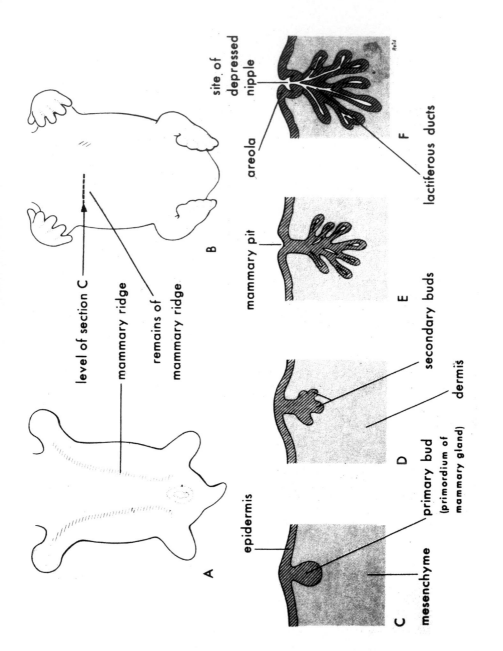

A

level of section C

mammary ridge

remains of
mammary ridge

B

epidermis

primary bud
(primordium of
mammary gland)

mesenchyme

C

secondary buds

dermis

D

mammary pit

E

site of
depressed
nipple

areola

lactiferous ducts

F

(7). It is mitogenic for luminal cells and morphogenic to myoepithelial cells (8). The presence of matrix metalloproteinase and the absence of tissue inhibitor of metalloproteinases allow necessary disruption of basement membrane and the involution process after weaning (9). BCL-2 and parathyroid hormone-related protein are other factors that signal the growth and development of the mammary gland (10, 11).

Before puberty, it is not unusual to have nodular growth of one or both breasts in either sex. Nodules are typically soft, mobile, and uniform, and they tend to disappear spontaneously after a few weeks or months; so observation is recommended. Biopsy of the prepubertal breast may irreversibly hinder later development (12).

Breast development (*thelarche*) in girls is usually the first sign of sexual maturation. The female mammary glands remain underdeveloped until puberty. At puberty, the breasts rapidly grow and mature under the influence of elevated estrogen, progesterone, and prolactin levels and growth hormones, including luteinizing and follicular-stimulating hormone (LH and FSH), which stimulate estrogen secretion as well as hypothalamic gonadotropin-releasing hormone (3). Thyroxine also plays a regulatory role (12). Elevated estrogen levels stimulate ductal growth and branching, whereas progesterone influences lobular and alveolar development. The volume and elasticity of the connective tissues increase, as do the vascularity and fat deposition. Progressive enlargement of the breasts occurs. The average age of thelarche is 11.2 years, ranging from 9 to 14 years of age. Other signs of puberty typically follow the onset of thelarche. The mammary glands in males normally undergo no postnatal development.

The female breasts again enlarge during pregnancy, with proliferation and creation of new glandular tissue under the influence of luteal and placental sex steroids, placental lactogen, prolactin, and chorionic gonadotropin (3). Prolactin levels in particular elevate to three to five times higher than normal during the second and third trimesters (3). Breast enlargement becomes apparent with increased weight and dilatation of superficial veins. The areola enlarges and becomes deep brown to black, with diminution of color postpartum. Areolar sebaceous glands enlarge and secrete an oily substance that provides a protective lubricant for the areola and nipple. Increasing breast size in the latter half of pregnancy is associated with increasing dilatation of the alveoli with colostrum, as well as hypertrophy of myoepithelial cells, connective tissue, and fat. Increased glandular tissue may be associated with increased nodularity. This nodularity must be followed closely because breast cancer has developed in the pregnant breast. By the end of pregnancy, the breasts produce and secrete colostrum under the influence of prolactin.

FIG. 2.1. Embryonic development of the mammary glands. **A:** Ventral view of a 28-day embryo, with regression of the mammary ridge by 6 weeks, as represented in **B**. **C–F:** Cross-sections of the developing breast bud from 6 weeks to birth. (From Moore KL. *The developing human.* Philadelphia: WB Saunders, 1988:426, with permission.)

The breasts become more edematous and nodular over the menstrual cycle because of hormonal changes. Nodularity is a manifestation of the proliferation of lobules of the breast under hormonal stimulation (12).

Faulty developmental processes result in deformities of the breast. The absent or incomplete development of the breasts is often the result of complete or imperfect suppression of the breast anlage in the embryo. Accessory breasts or nipples represent failure of regression of the galactic bands. Abnormal signaling and hormonal stimulation also can result in developmental deviations, particularly when considering premature thelarche, gigantomastia at puberty or pregnancy, or gynecomastia. Sequelae that result from these developmental mishaps are elucidated more specifically in this chapter.

ANATOMY OF THE BREAST

The breasts are situated superficial to the pectoralis major muscle and are hemispheric in shape with an elliptic base in the average young woman. Although breasts vary markedly in size, they normally extend between the second and sixth ribs vertically and horizontally between the lateral edge of the sternum and the midaxillary line. The average diameter is 10 to 12 cm. Breast tissue projects toward the axilla as the axillary tail of Spence.

The three major components of the breast include skin, subcutaneous tissue, and breast tissue, including parenchyma and supporting stroma. The breast gland is firmly adherent to the skin by suspensory ligaments of Cooper. These fibrous bands, which traverse and support the breast, connect the skin and the deep fascia overlying the pectoralis major muscle.

Lactiferous ducts open on the nipple, and each drains a lobe. The lobes are arranged radially around the breast. Each lobe consists of 20 to 40 lobules, separated by connective tissue and fat. Each lobule contains 10 to 100 alveoli. Under the areola, each lactiferous duct has a dilated portion called the *lactiferous sinus* in which milk accumulates during lactation.

The arterial supply of the breast includes the internal mammary and lateral thoracic arteries as well as lateral and anterior cutaneous branches of the intercostal arteries from interspaces 3, 4, and 5 and subdermal vessels. Venous drainage flows primarily into the axilla, with further drainage into the internal thoracic, lateral thoracic, and intercostal veins. Most of the lymph drains into superficial and axillary nodes. The second to sixth intercostal nerves, chiefly the fourth lateral intercostal nerve, innervate the breast gland and overlying skin.

PREMATURE THELARCHE

Premature thelarche describes isolated unilateral or bilateral breast development before any other pubertal changes occur. Development is considered to be early in white girls younger than 7 years of age and in African-American girls less than 6 years of age (13). Premature thelarche usually becomes manifest within the first 2 years of life and spontaneously regresses over a period of 6 months to 6 years (14–16). The earlier the presentation, the greater the likelihood of spontaneous regression (17,18). It is important to distinguish premature thelarche from precocious puberty, a more serious disorder that originally presents with premature thelarche but ultimately causes progressive secondary sexual development, accelerated growth, skeletal maturation, early epiphyseal fusion, and short adult stature.

Premature thelarche is a benign, self-limited condition that occurs sporadically and rarely progresses to central precocious puberty. No more than 18% of these girls ultimately develop precocious puberty (17). Tenore et al. performed a study to predict which patients progressed to precocious puberty. With a 6-month follow-up, those who had elevated LH, bone age, and growth velocity proceeded to develop precocious puberty (16). No relationship has been shown between premature thelarche and maternal obstetric problems, exposure to medications, diet, or prenatal infections (19). Girls with premature thelarche are otherwise medically and sexually normal.

It is important to take a detailed history in these patients. The possibility of endocrine disorders resulting from hypothalamic lesions, ovarian granulosa cell tumors, follicular cysts, adrenocortical tumors, syndromic and medicinal etiologies must be excluded (20). Kabuki makeup syndrome with hypothalamopituitary dysfunction includes premature thelarche as part of its constellation of findings, which also includes short stature and partial growth hormone deficiency (21,22). Rubinstein-Taybi syndrome with neuroblastoma also has associated premature thelarche (23).

The cause of premature thelarche is unknown. Reports conflict about whether growth hormone regulation is altered if the breast tissue has highly sensitive receptors, if ovarian cysts intermittently release estrogen, or if there are increased circulating hormone levels. Studies have cited normal regulation of the hypothalamopituitary–gonadal axis, with normal basal prolactin, LH, FSH, sex hormone-binding globulin protein, and thyroxine-binding globulin levels (16,24,25). Normal growth hormone levels and hormonal regulation support the idea that premature thelarche results from hypersensitive receptors in the breast not present in other target tissues.

Other studies report differences in the hormonal milieu of patients, suggesting that premature thelarche is an incomplete form of precocious sexual development. An ultrasensitive recombinant cell bioassay revealed that girls younger than 3 years with premature thelarche had significantly higher estradiol levels than age-matched controls (26). Mean basal FSH and the response of FSH to LH-releasing hormone (LHRH) stimulation were significantly higher than prepubertal controls, whereas LH remained stable (14,17,27–29). Pulsatile secretion of LH and FSH during sleep and after LHRH stimulation was also higher than in controls (30).

Various diagnostic tests are available to differentiate premature thelarche from precocious puberty patients. Pelvic ultrasonography demonstrates larger average uterine and ovarian volumes in precocious puberty compared with girls with premature thelarche and controls (31,32). One report indicated a higher likelihood of ovarian follicular cysts in girls with premature thelarche (33), whereas another report emphasized the more cystic character of the ovaries of precocious puberty patients (32). Breast contact thermography differentiates premature thelarche from precocious puberty because patients with precocious puberty exhibit thermographic signs of vascularization not found in patients with premature thelarche (34).

In most cases of premature thelarche, there are no other problems of sexual development or function. It is strongly recommended that all girls with this condition be monitored clinically for accelerated pubertal progression. There are no predictive clinical or laboratory tests that can identify at-risk patients. Sympathetic reassurance may be offered because in most instances the condition spontaneously regresses.

GYNECOMASTIA

Gynecomastia describes the proliferation of glandular breast tissue in a male; this term derives from the Greek *gyne*, meaning associated with women, and *mastia*, or breast. True gynecomastia is pathologically defined by the presence of hypertrophied breast glandular tissue. A firm, rubbery, disc-like mound of tissue is palpable beneath the NAC. *Pseudogynecomastia* refers to enlargement of the male breast caused primarily by fatty infiltration. Mixed gynecomastia is a combination of true and pseudogynecomastia. Breast enlargement in gynecomastia is most frequently bilateral (9:1) and nontender, although tenderness may be associated (Fig. 2.2).

Asymptomatic gynecomastia commonly occurs in healthy males and presents in three different age groups (35). The first peak occurs in the neonatal period with passage of maternal estrogens, affecting between 60% and 90% of all newborns. The second peak occurs during puberty, affecting 60% to 70% of 10- to 13-year-old boys. Breast enlargement and tenderness typically regress within 1 to 3 years in this age group. The final peak is in adult men aged between 50 and 80 years. There is no racial difference in prevalence.

Causative factors range from physiologic to endocrine to exogenous; most cases are of idiopathic origin (25%). Cirrhosis and malnutrition (8%), primary hypogonadism (8%), testicular tumor (3%), secondary hypogonadism (2%), hyperthyroidism (1.5%), and renal disease (1%) are conditions that often result in gynecomastia. Exogenous medications account for 10% to 20% of all cases (35–37).

Gynecomastia results from a relative imbalance of serum estrogen and androgen (testosterone) levels, more specifically, elevated estrogen levels, decreased androgen levels, androgen receptor abnormalities, and hormonally hypersensitive breast tissue. Neoplasms, medications, and systemic disease can elevate estrogen levels. Decreased androgen levels are a component of normal aging and hence increase the frequency of gynecomastia in older men. The gynecomastia workup includes a complete history and physical examination. Diagnostic testing may follow depending on suspicious findings. Physical examination must include a detailed examination of the breasts, axillae for adenopathy, and testes for enlargement, atrophy, or neoplasm. Whereas asymmetric gynecomastia is common, the examiner must rule out breast cancer. A breast examination revealing a unilateral, eccentric, hard, fixed mass should raise the suspicion of breast cancer. Other physical findings indicating cancer include

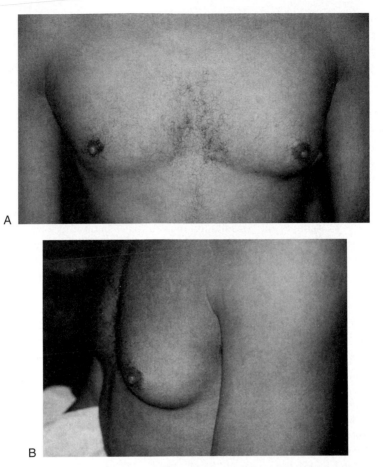

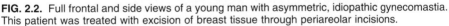

FIG. 2.2. Full frontal and side views of a young man with asymmetric, idiopathic gynecomastia. This patient was treated with excision of breast tissue through periareolar incisions.

dimpled skin, nipple retraction, nipple discharge, and axillary adenopathy (38,39). Mammography and diagnostic biopsy, either fine needle or excisional, are necessary if cancer is suspected. Although breast cancer in men constitutes fewer than 1% of all cancers in men and fewer than 1% of all cases of breast cancer in the United States, sizable series exist (39).

Laboratory studies are often not indicated, particularly in the pubertal patient, because gynecomastia typically resolves spontaneously. Screening is performed to rule out systemic disease and neoplastic processes. Elevated serum human chorionic gonadotropin may indicate a germ cell tumor. Urinary 17-ketosteroids and serum dihydroepiandrosterone sulfate are associated with adrenal cancer. Serum estradiol is elevated in Leydig cell tumors. Serum testosterone and gonadotropins are low in cases of hypogonadism. Serum prolactin may be associated with pituitary tumor.

Karyotypic analysis is useful to rule out Klinefelter syndrome. The *BRCA-2* gene has been associated with both female and male breast cancer and may serve as a future screening test (35,36,39).

Most patients with gynecomastia pursue treatment because of embarrassment about their feminine appearance. Both medical and surgical treatments are available. Medical treatment is less invasive but often ineffective. The first steps include removal of any potentially causative medications (i.e., spironolactone, cimetidine) and treatment of any underlying systemic conditions (i.e., hyperthyroidism, obesity). The basis of other medical treatments is hormonal manipulation, which has associated side effects and is transient. Testosterone and danazol increase androgen levels; clomiphene citrate and tamoxifen are antiestrogens; and testolactone is an aromatase inhibitor (35,36).

Patients are referred to the plastic surgeon after endocrine workup or failure of medical therapy or simply for consultation regarding aesthetic improvement. Prior to 1980, the only surgical option available was sharp excision of the breast and fatty tissue. The more recent introduction of liposuction has allowed improved treatment of gynecomastia. Used either in conjunction with surgical excision or alone, lipoplasty allows improved contour with decreased operative risk and morbidity (40–43).

Gynecomastia is a prevalent problem in the male population. Although functionally benign, breast enlargement causes sufficient embarrassment for many men to pursue treatment.

TUBULAR OR TUBEROUS BREASTS

Rees and Aston first reported the tubular breast deformity in 1976. They described the condition in which the female breast resembles the shape of a tuberous plant root and provided recommendations for treatment (44). The condition may be unilateral or bilateral, and the exact incidence is unknown (45,46). The breast has normal function but abnormal morphology. Features of the fully developed syndrome include skin envelope deficiency, hypoplastic breast tissue, decreased vertical and horizontal breast diameter, ptosis, a hypertrophic areola, and a raised inframammary fold. With the narrowed transverse breast diameter and base constriction, the breast appears to herniate into an oversized and protuberant areola (47) (Fig. 2.3). As a result of the breast's appearance, another name for the tubular breast is the *Snoopy-nose deformity,* and in the more remote past, the deformity was described as the *nipple-type breast* (48,49).

Patients consult a plastic surgeon to correct their deformity. The tubular breast deformity presents a challenging reconstructive problem that requires attention to the skin and the breast tissue. Treatment objectives include expanding the base circumference and the skin of the lower hemisphere, releasing constricting skin tightness at the areolar junction, lowering the inframammary fold, increasing breast volume and height, and decreasing areolar size (47,49,50).

Surgical correction varies according to the level of deformity. Treatment by simple

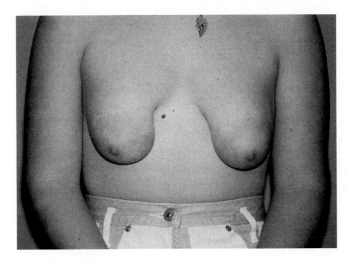

FIG. 2.3. Classic case of tubular breast deformity with narrowed base diameter and pseudo-herniated breast tissue through an enlarged nipple–areolar complex.

augmentation mammaplasty accentuates the deformity, increasing the protuberance of the nipple and areola ("Snoopy nose") (44). Rees and Aston described telescoping the herniated nipple back, with areolar skin reduction and placement of a retromammary implant. The posterior capsule of the breast might require radial incisions for expansion and redraping. Strategic periareolar incisions camouflage the correction (44). The plastic surgery literature describes various internal maneuvers to reshape the constricted breast tissue (51). Tissue expansion such as that used for breast reconstruction after mastectomy improves skin deficiency and broadens the breast mound. In a second-stage procedure, the expander would be replaced with a permanent implant (46,52).

IDIOPATHIC ASYMMETRY

The initiation of thelarche may occur on one side and proceed at a faster rate for unknown reasons. In most cases, both breasts become relatively equal in volume by the end of puberty (12). A small degree of breast asymmetry is not uncommon or abnormal; however, a marked inequality of the breast volume can be noticeable. Hueston noted that patients experience difficulty in concealing asymmetry greater than 33% with everyday attire (53). Pitanguy found noticeable asymmetry in 4% of his series of 1,400 patients he evaluated for all types of mammaplasty procedures (54).

Idiopathic breast asymmetry is classifiable into six categories: unilateral hypoplasia, asymmetrical hypoplasia, unilateral hyperplasia, asymmetric hyperplasia, hyperplasia/hypoplasia, and hypoplasia associated with chest-wall deformities. Unilateral hypoplasia is the most common and may vary from the minimal idiopathic form to

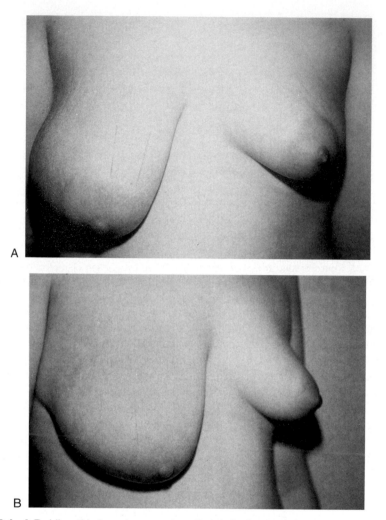

FIG. 2.4. A,B: Idiopathic breast asymmetry with tubular breast deformity in combination with contralateral breast hypertrophy.

severe Poland syndrome (55,56). Associated with breast hypoplasia is a small and cephalad-located NAC; in rare instances, the NAC is absent (55) (Fig. 2.4). Several etiologies of breast asymmetry have been described, including abnormal development with differential end-organ response to hormonal stimulation, tumors, medications, and iatrogenic causes, including operations, radiation and trauma. Asymmetry may be a manifestation of a syndrome such as Stein–Leventhal syndrome (57,58).

Breast asymmetry may cause physical discomfort in addition to the psychological distress stemming from the obvious deformity. Early surgical correction may be

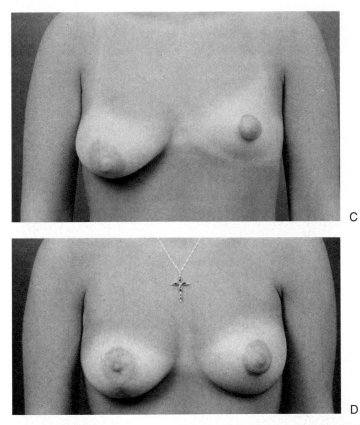

FIG. 2.4. *Continued.* **C:** Idiopathic breast asymmetry with unilateral hypoplasia. **D:** This patient opted for single stage augmentation on the affected side with a circumareolar mastopexy performed on the contralateral side for symmetry. (Photos C and D courtesy of Dr. Bernard Chang, with permission.)

warranted. Postponing corrective surgery for adolescents with significant asymmetry may be psychologically detrimental and unnecessary (59,60).

Plastic surgeons use reconstructive techniques to create improved symmetry. Hypoplastic breasts are augmented and may require tissue expansion as a first stage (Fig. 2.5). Initial attempts at reconstruction with just an implant often lead to suboptimal results because of the high incidence of scar contracture, poor contour, a superiorly displaced NAC, and untreated infraclavicular concavity. Tissue expansion preceding placement of a permanent implant allows descent and expansion of the hypoplastic breast and NAC, as well as expansion of the deficient soft-tissue envelope (55). In particularly young patients, the expansion process may take place over years until the opposite, unaffected breast reaches maturity. Placement of a permanent implant follows when growth of the unaffected breast has ceased over 2 years (55). In more severe cases of hypoplasia, the latissimus may be transposed over top

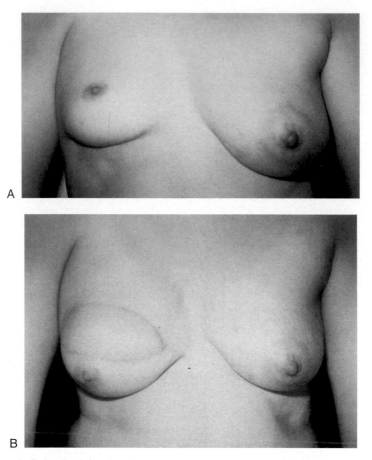

FIG. 2.5. A: Poland's deformity with hypoplastic breast and absent anterior axillary fold as a result of absent pectoralis major muscle. **B:** A latissimus musculocutaneous flap was performed to reconstruct the involved breast. No implant was necessary.

of the implant to improve contour and decrease the risk of contracture. Correction or camouflage of underlying chest-wall deformities may be necessary. The unaffected breast, although normal, may have ptosis requiring a mastopexy to achieve more perfect symmetry.

Hyperplastic breasts present a somewhat easier reconstructive problem. Breast reduction corrects the deformity. Again, contralateral maneuvers on the unaffected breast may be necessary to achieve symmetry.

Breast cancer has been reported in a unilateral hypomastic breast; so cancer must be considered when a suspicious mass is present (61).

POLAND SYNDROME

Poland syndrome is a variant of breast asymmetry with unilateral hypomastia or amastia and associated with ipsilateral upper limb deformities. The syndrome was named by Clarkson in 1962 after he operated on a patient in a case similar to one described by Alfred Poland in 1841 (62). Poland's initial description of the syndrome in the *Guy's Hospital Report* was limited to deficiencies of the chest-wall muscles and ipsilateral syndactyly, findings he discovered as a medical student from anatomic cadaver dissections (3,63,64).

Since Poland's initial report, the constellation of findings associated with the syndrome has greatly expanded. Clinical manifestations are highly variable and rarely are all features found in an individual patient. There is no correlation between the severity of findings in the chest wall and upper limbs. Characteristic findings include brachysyndactyly; hypoplasia or absence of the breast, nipple, or both; deficient subcutaneous tissue with dense adhesions from the chest to the skin; absent pectoralis major muscle or deficient sternal head; absent pectoralis minor muscle; absent costal cartilages 2 through 4 or 3 through 5; abnormal subclavian vein; absent or maldeveloped latissimus, deltoid, supraspinatus and infraspinatus muscles; and maldeveloped rectus abdominis muscle or intercostal muscles (62). A patient with two or more findings qualifies as having Poland syndrome (64). The full-blown syndrome includes shortening of the entire hemithorax with a low-riding clavicular head, cartilage agenesis and malformation, an abnormally high insertion of the rectus abdominis muscle, and paradoxical motion of the thinned chest wall over areas of rib agenesis with lung herniation through the chest-wall defect. The chest-wall defect is of physiologic importance in children who play contact sports (65,66).

The estimated incidence of Poland syndrome is 1 in 20,000 to 1 in 32,000 births (64). The right breast is affected more than the left (75%), and males are affected more than females (3:1), although female patients may be more likely to seek treatment (62). No cases of bilateral Poland syndrome have been reported. Renal hypoplasia, leukemia, and Möbius syndrome are reportedly associated with Poland syndrome (66,67).

Poland syndrome is sporadic and appears to develop secondary to an intrauterine insult. One theory is that it develops from ischemia related to hypoplasia of the subclavian artery (64,68). Another theory is related to abnormal migration of embryonic tissues. In a 9-mm embryo, the limb bud that forms the pectoralis muscle develops; by the time it becomes a 15-mm embryo, the bud splits into clavicular, pectoral, and sternal components. Faulty attachment or failure of attachment of this primitive limb bud to the upper rib cage and sternum would explain the Poland deformity (64,67).

The diagnosis of Poland syndrome is made through physical examination, but underlying defects may be defined more specifically by two-dimensional and three-dimensional computed tomography (CT) and magnetic resonance imaging (64,68, 69). These modalities are particularly useful when planning reconstruction to determine the presence of muscles of interest. CT is also useful in assessing chest-wall deformities. Angiography may also assist in assessing ipsilateral vascular anatomy (68).

Male patients will pursue treatment secondary to their perception of asymmetry and lack of soft-tissue fill of the upper chest wall, whereas female patients are additionally concerned about hypoplasia or absence of the ipsilateral breast (66).

The goal of treatment is to reconstruct a natural-appearing breast and chest wall. Treatment includes camouflage or correction of the underlying deformity.

To correct the Poland deformity, the innervated latissimus muscle with or without overlying skin may be transposed anteriorly to fill out a deficient chest wall, simulate an absent pectoralis muscle, and recreate the anterior axillary fold (70–72) (Fig. 2.5). Studies have demonstrated that rotating the latissimus prior to puberty does not impair development (i.e., scoliosis or rib deformities) (65,68,73). A contralateral microvascular latissimus may be considered in patients with ipsilateral latissimus deficiency, but preoperative angiography would be recommended because the thoracodorsal (recipient) vessels may be deficient as well (68).

Autologous rib grafting may be performed to reconstruct severe chest-wall concavity and absent ribs. Normal rib below the chest wall defect or from the contralateral side is harvested and attached to the sternum. The latissimus then is mobilized to fill out the thinned soft tissue (64–66). The goal is to correct abnormal position and rotation of the sternum as well as replace aplastic ribs. Reports remark on improved aesthetic and functional outcome after autogenous chest wall reconstruction (65,74).

In the absence of a functional deficit from chest-wall defects, camouflage techniques are preferred (66). Standard or custom breast implants may camouflage underlying deformities of the breast and chest wall (75,76). Sculpting plaster and plastic to form a symmetric shape with the unaffected side creates a moulage of the desired chest-wall contour. The model then is transformed into a prototype composed of silicone rubber to replace the missing ribs and chest wall cartilage, whereas a silicone gel prosthesis simulates the contour and texture of the absent breast. Autogenous tissue may be combined with implant reconstruction to provide the best result in more severe deformities and to hide prominent custom implants. Using an implant also may aid in preventing noticeable progressive latissimus atrophy, which has been reported to occur (62). Even in cases without complete correction, there is marked postoperative improvement in self-image (62,63).

A case was reported in which breast cancer was diagnosed in the affected side of a patient with Poland syndrome; therefore, suspicious breast masses in these patients require the usual monitoring and workup (77).

POLYMASTIA AND POLYTHELIA

Polymastia refers to accessory breast tissue, and *polythelia* refers to supernumerary nipples (Fig. 2.6). Polymastia and polythelia develop as a result of incomplete regression of the primitive milk lines. Accessory tissue is located anywhere along the course of the primitive milk line, from the axilla to the groin. Other sites are rare but have been reported and may relate to displaced breast tissue (78).

Supernumerary nipples are present in other mammalian species; so Darwin described the condition in humans or other primates as *atavistic*, an evolutionary throwback. He used this condition to support his theory that humans evolved from lower animals (79–81). The *Hox* genes have been associated with development of struc-

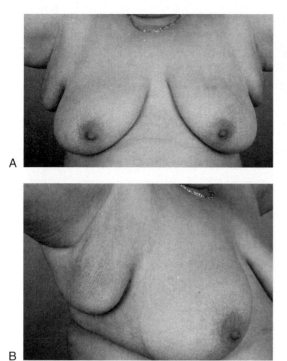

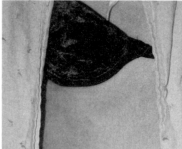

FIG. 2.6. A: Patient with polymastia with accessory axillary breast tissue. **B:** Side view of same patient. (Photos courtesy of Dr. Joseph P. Delozier, with permission) **C:** Patient presenting with polythelia.

tures out of place and time, and so mutations in these genes have been targeted as the underlying etiologic factor (81).

Polythelia is the most commonly found breast deformity, whereas polymastia is far less common. Accessory mammary tissue has been reported to occur in up to 6% of the population, more frequently in women and in the axilla (79,80,82–84). Inheritance may be autosomal dominant with incomplete penetrance, but sporadic cases represent the more common situation (81,82,85).

Patients with polythelia may have other associated anomalies. Polythelia has been strongly linked with nephrologic–urologic anomalies, including obstructive uropathies, renal agenesis, renal cell carcinoma, and supernumerary kidneys. Such anomalies are found in approximately 8% to 15% of patients with polythelia (82,86). An association with cardiac anomalies also has been described, including congenital defects and conduction disturbances (83,87–89). The renal and cardiac systems develop when the mammary ridges regress and thicken to form the mammary anlage. Polythelia in association with underlying rib defects also has been described (84). Rarely, polythelia has been associated with faulty limb and facial development (90–92). The presence of polythelia in children should prompt consideration of polythelia-associated conditions. Such investigation ought to include thorough physical examination, urinalysis, and renal ultrasound. Because of a higher likelihood of developing renal malignancy, urinalysis should be done at routine medical visits over time in these patients (82).

Polythelia is commonly an incidental finding in an otherwise healthy person. Often patients consult a physician because they are concerned about a pigmented lesion and are otherwise asymptomatic. A supernumerary nipple may resemble a pigmented nevus, skin tag, or fibroma (Fig. 2.6C). Whereas accessory breast or nipple structures vary in appearance, they are identifiable by the following: They are congenital, located on the embryonic milk line, have a nipple-like appearance with pigment like the primary nipples, and are at least 5 mm large. Multiple nipples have been reported to occur within one areola (93,94). Histopathologic analysis confirms the diagnosis, along with the presence of pilosebaceous units, smooth muscle, and mammary glands (95).

The nipple may connect to glandular tissue or the ductal system, and so pain and swelling may be experienced during menstruation or pregnancy (particularly with axillary polymastia), and lactation may occur. Although these changes are rarely of any consequence, accessory mammary tissue may undergo neoplastic changes and carcinomatous degeneration. When a mass is noted along the milk line, accessory breast tissue must be considered and may require workup to rule out cancer (79).

Surgical intervention is generally requested for aesthetic reasons. Accessory tissue may be excised for discomfort from tenderness, lactation, or psychological embarrassment. In the rare instance when cancer does occur in accessory tissue, surgical excision is obviously mandatory.

AMASTIA AND ATHELIA

Amastia, absence of the breast, is an unusual condition resulting from failure of development of the mammary ridges. The first recorded reference to amastia was in ''The Song of Solomon'' in the *Bible*: ''We have a little sister, and she hath no breast: What shall we do for our sister in the day when she shall be spoken for?'' (1) The fictional Amazonian nation was composed of independent women who removed one of their breasts to gain a competitive advantage in archery. In 1939, Froriep first reported a case of amastia (96).

Amastia has been reported as an isolated finding and a syndromic component. Trier reviewed the literature extensively in 1965 and noted three presentations after reviewing 43 patients: bilateral amastia with congenital ectodermal defects, unilateral amastia, and bilateral amastia with variable associated anomalies. Associated abnormalities include cleft palate, hypertelorism, anomalous pectoralis muscles, upper-limb deformities, and abnormalities of the genitourinary tract (96). Syndromes with amastia include ectodermal dysplasia, an autosomal dominant hereditary disease, and Mayer–Rokitansky–Kuster–Hauser syndrome with vaginal–uterine agenesis (97–99). Familial cases have been reported, and inheritance is believed to be autosomal dominant in those cases (1,96,100).

Athelia is also an extremely rare condition. Absence of the nipples, like amastia, has been reported as a dominant trait in some families and as a finding in various syndromes, including the family of ectodermal dysplasias (101,102). Athelia is a component of Al Awadi/Raas–Rothschild syndrome, a lethal autosomal recessive facio-skeletal–genital syndrome (103). Athelia also has been described as part of the scalp-ear-nipple (SEN) syndrome, an autosomal dominant condition with aplasia cutis congenita, posterior scalp nodules, and malformed ears. A case was reported in which the patient had choanal atresia and athelia that was likely induced by methimazole treatment for hyperthyroidism in the pregnant mother (104).

Plastic surgical reconstruction of the breast and nipple is performed to treat amastia and athelia. A report describing placement of an implant in an amastia patient noted anomalous vascular supply to the chest-wall skin with fibrosis. After subcutaneous dissection and placement of a breast prosthesis, the patient's skin fared poorly, with recovery after implant removal decreasing overlying skin tension. The researcher who reported this case deduced that faulty breast development resulted in anomalous vascular inflow to the skin overlying the pectoralis muscle and that caution is necessary in reconstruction in these patients, who may have unpredictably complicated outcomes (99).

SYMMASTIA

Symmastia describes medial confluence of the breasts, producing a web across the midline (Fig. 2.7). This entity has been described minimally in the literature. As one plastic surgeon wrote, this is "an uncommon breast condition that is not of monumental importance to plastic surgery" (104). It is more commonly an iatrogenic problem in patients who have undergone bilateral augmentation mammaplasty.

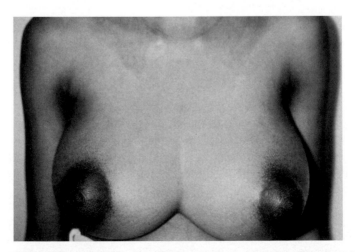

FIG. 2.7. Patient with symmastia with medial confluence of breasts. (Photo courtesy of Dr. Robert J. Spence, with permission.)

Surgical treatment varies with presentation (104). In thin patients with normally sized breasts, an inferior dart may be created to separate the confluence and better define cleavage. In patients with larger breasts, reduction mammaplasty is performed in conjunction with design of skin flaps to tack down the confluence. Liposuction is another option for treatment.

INVERTED NIPPLES

Sir Ashley Cooper first described this entity in 1840. Inverted nipples occur when the tight, shortened deep tissues retract the nipple. Developmentally, this entity originates from a lack of proper elevation of the nipple from proliferation of the mesenchyme underlying the future nipple areola complex (105).

Inverted nipples are found in about 2% of the female population and are most frequently bilateral (105,106). Although most cases are congenital, acquired causes occur as the result of scarring from mastitis, partial mastectomy, and prior drainage procedures (105,107,108). Syndromes such as Robinow syndrome and carbohydrate-deficient glycoprotein syndrome include inverted nipples in their constellation of findings (109,110).

Concerns related to inverted nipples range from aesthetic to functional to psychological. Women with this condition may have difficulty breast-feeding. Numerous plastic surgical techniques have been introduced for correction of the inverted nipple (111–115). Nipple sensory change, scarring, vascular compromise, obliteration of the ductal system with faulty lactation, and incomplete correction, as well as a high rate of recurrence may complicate correction (105).

IATROGENIC BREAST DEFORMITIES

Iatrogenic and acquired origins of breast deformities warrant discussion because they must be considered when obtaining the history from patients. Failure of complete breast development may be the result of injury to the breast in the prepubertal period.

Trauma, incisions, infection or radiation to the young female breast may lead to subsequent scarring restricting breast growth. Two cases of dog-bite injuries to the breast were reported in girls, one who suffered from scarring and limited development of the involved breast (116). Seatbelt injuries cause compression to skin and underlying fat and may result in breast atrophy and asymmetry (117) (Fig. 2.8). Radiation therapy to the chest wall to treat childhood malignancies ultimately may lead to impaired breast development as well (118).

Breast and pectoral muscle maldevelopment has been reported in children who have undergone anterolateral and posterolateral surgical incisions through the third and fourth intercostal space, an approach used for congenital heart surgery. Anterolateral thoracotomies resulted in 60% of the patients subsequently having a greater than 20% discrepancy in volume of the breast and pectoral muscles on the ipsilateral

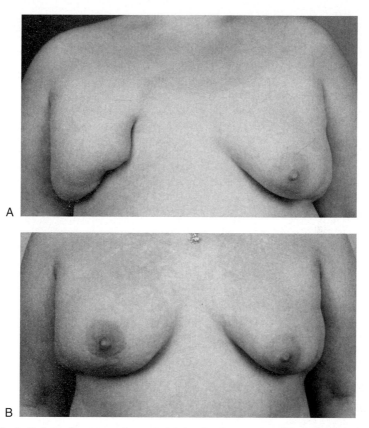

FIG. 2.8. A: Patient after traumatic seatbelt injury leading to ischemia of right medial breast. **B:** Same patient after complex reconstruction with implant augmentation. (Photos courtesy of Dr. Joseph P. Delozier, with permission.)

and unaffected sides as reported in a retrospective study from the Children's Hospital of Pittsburgh. This is a noticeable difference in size. In addition, three patients were unable to nurse their infants when they reached adulthood. Cadaver dissections revealed the presence of breast bud tissue more than 1.5 cm from the NAC, placing it at risk for devascularization and amputation with thoracic procedures (119).

Great caution must be exercised when creating incisions around the prepubertal breast. Because breast malignancies are so rare in prepubertal patients, biopsy of a suspicious mass is warranted only after a reasonable observation period.

Burns, as well as surgical incisions of the chest wall, can result in growth disruption in the prepubertal patient (Fig. 2.9). For burn cases, careful tangential excision to viable tissue with skin grafting ultimately can result in normal growth (120). Burns to the chest wall may require skin grafting or local skin flaps to allow the release necessary for continued breast development (121). Scald injuries of the ante-

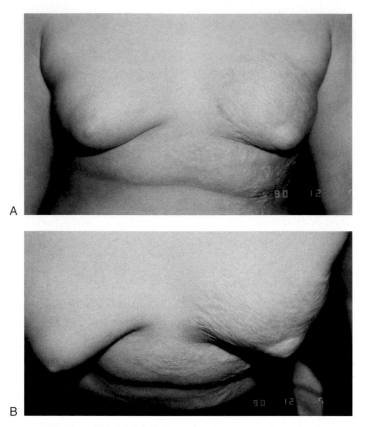

FIG. 2.9. A: Frontal view of patient with left breast burn and constricting scar leading to asymmetry. **B:** Bird's-eye view. (Photos courtesy of Dr. Robert J. Spence, with permission.)

rior chest to deep second- and third-degree levels do not burn actual mammary tissue, but scarring of the skin will restrict breast growth and development; so scar excision and skin grafting are recommended (122).

Nodular deformities in the breast have been described after core needle biopsy and diagnosed as reactive spindle cell nodules. These are benign masses resulting from an exuberant reparative response and myofibroblast influx after needle trauma (123).

Constrictive scarring of the chest over young breast tissue requires release to allow breast growth. If the breast bud has been traumatized, definitive breast reconstruction may be considered once the unaffected breast reaches its mature size. If only the NAC is injured, it may be reconstructed with local flaps and tattooed to match the contralateral side.

GIGANTOMASTIA

Virginal

Virginal gigantomastia occurs infrequently in adolescent girls and is manifested by bilateral, excessively large breasts that have a tendency for further growth (Fig. 2.10) Growth is dramatic in both rate and volume. The breasts may be asymmetric or grow at different rates (124). Unlike adult women with macromastia who complain primarily of back pain, bra grooving, and hygienic problems, adolescent girls have additionally profound psychosocial symptoms. These include loss of self-esteem, eating disorders, and difficulties with athletics. These girls wear clothes that camouflage their appearance, and they shy away from peer interactions. Psychological embarrassment should not be underestimated (125,126).

Gigantomastia is induced by an exaggerated response to normal hormonal levels, such that the breast is hypersensitive to levels of circulating estrogen, which are elevated during puberty. Others propose that the liver does not adequately deactivate

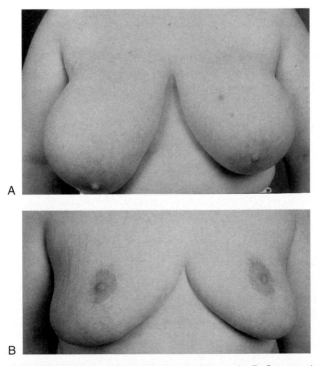

FIG. 2.10. A: Adolescent patient with asymmetric gigantomastia. **B:** Same patient after bilateral reduction mammaplasty. (Photos courtesy of Dr. Joseph P. Delozier, with permission.)

hormones. Disorders leading to exogenous hormone production, such as adrenal, ovarian, or pituitary tumors, must be ruled out. Familial cases have been described, but generally virginal hypertrophy is sporadic (127).

Virginal hypertrophy occurs in healthy, normal girls. Pathology is limited to the breast with otherwise normal systemic growth and development (127). Examination reveals diffuse firmness, venous engorgement, nodularity, and occasional discrete, rubbery masses. Axillary adenopathy does not occur. (124) Patients also present with typical findings of macromastia, including bra grooving, altered posture, and intertrigo.

Unilateral breast enlargement in this patient population is more commonly due to fibroepithelial tumors, including fibroadenomas, which prove to be larger in adolescents, or cystosarcoma phylloides (124). Patients with discrete breast masses present strong concern and require malignancy workup.

There is no need to perform hormonal assays because levels of estrogen, gonadotropins, urinary 17-ketosteroid, and hydroxysteroid are normal. The number of estrogen and progesterone receptors in the breast tissue is normal as well (124).

Histologically, stromal hypertrophy with epithelial proliferation, fibrosis, glandular hyperplasia, cystic degeneration of the lactiferous ducts, interstitial edema, and the presence of fat lobules may be evident. (124,127,128)

Although it is preferable to delay surgery until the breast is fully matured, earlier treatment may be mandated by overwhelming physical and psychological symptoms. Surgical consultation is recommended at an early age to answer concerns and provide information and assurance. Surgical options include breast reduction or subcutaneous mastectomy. Breast reduction surgery is favored as the primary treatment, and volumes of 1,800 to 8,000 g have been resected from each breast (125,129). Unfortunately, there is a tendency to recurrence postoperatively (125,130). As long as the patient is aware of the risk of relapse and need for further surgery, breast reduction is the first surgical alternative. If recurrence after reduction is a problem, the more definitive treatment of gigantomastia is mastectomy, followed by breast reconstruction with tissue expansion and ultimate placement of a permanent implant. When to operate must be balanced by the adverse effects of macromastia on a developing psyche and personality of a teenaged girl.

Postoperative hormonal treatments prevent recurrent breast growth after surgical resection has been tried. The use of the antiestrogen dydrogesterone (Gynorest, BIAM, France) at a dosage of 10 mg daily has helped to prevent recurrence without hindering ovulation (126). Synthetic progesterone, Provera (Pharmacia & Upjohn, Kalamazoo, MI), with its competitive action against estrogens, inhibits LH, which decreases estrogen secretion (128). Danazol blocks estrogen receptors (131). Tamoxifen also has been prescribed (132). These medications may be given up to 6 months after surgery. Many surgeons, however, prefer to avoid hormonal manipulation in pubertal patients because of the unknown long-term effects on growth and development (124,127).

Gravid

This entity, though more rare, is similar to virginal hypertrophy, except that rapidly progressive gigantomastia occurs during pregnancy. Macromastia may be evident prior to pregnancy, but it is exacerbated by pregnancy. Normal thelarche takes place at puberty. Gravid gigantomastia may occur after normal, unaffected pregnancies, but subsequent pregnancies will more likely result in similar gigantomastia. Like virginal hypertrophy, gravid gigantomastia is related to end-organ hypersensitivity to elevated circulating hormone levels, including estrogen and prolactin (133,134). A serum factor, like an autoimmune antibody that interferes with the normal hormone-receptor complex, has been proposed (135).

Because of extreme growth, patients experience severe pain, skin ulceration, and imminent infection from the wounds. Breasts are tense, firm, and may demonstrate large superficial veins and peau d'orange skin changes. Erosion of veins under excoriated skin threatens hemorrhage (136).

Either breast reduction or mastectomy is recommended for these patients. Patients may qualify for breast surgery at the time of pregnancy, although there is a risk for miscarriage and teratogenicity with anesthesia. Some opt for therapeutic abortion, a radical but curative choice.

Bromocriptine has been prescribed after delivery to induce involution and, in some patients, during gestation to delay surgical therapy. It lowers the secretion of prolactin from the pituitary, or it may act directly on the breast (135). Bromocriptine may have teratogenic effects, including intrauterine growth retardation (137).

Drug-Induced

Some cases of gigantomastia are induced by medications. Hormonal therapy, corticosteroids, marijuana, D-penicillamine, cimetidine, and the antiepileptic sulpiride may lead to unilateral or bilateral gigantomastia (1,127,128) (Fig. 2.11). A kidney

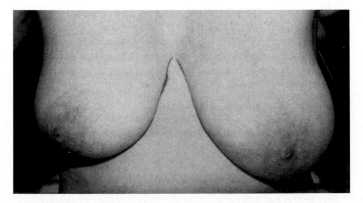

FIG. 2.11. Penicillamine-induced unilateral gigantomastia.

transplant patient with benign breast lumps and gigantomastia was reportedly taking cyclosporine, prednisolone, and calcium antagonists (138). Medications either stimulate hormones or act locally.

CONCLUSION

Because our culture places great importance on breasts and fuels a pervasive fear of breast cancer, persons with breast and chest-wall deformities harbor strong concerns. Many of these deformities are congenital and based on faulty developmental processes. The breast deformity may be a marker for other underlying systemic disorders, principally involving the genitourinary and cardiac systems. The relationship is based on parallel developmental processes in the embryo. Some breast deformities are iatrogenic, and the potential for damage to the developing breast bud must be considered when performing surgery on the chest of a prepubertal patient.

Although rarely of functional importance, obvious breast deformities may generate devastating psychological effects, causing isolation and withdrawal from social situations. These patients benefit from early consultation with physicians to address their concerns and direct them to treatment to reconstruct their deformity. The reconstructive breast surgeon aims to preserve nipple sensation and erectility, ductile function, and blood supply to the skin and gland while creating necessary symmetry and a more normal appearance. The patient's self-esteem is often much improved after surgery, even if exact symmetry is not attained.

REFERENCES

1. Bland KI, Romrell LJ. Congenital and acquired disturbances of breast development and growth. In: Bland KI, Copeland EM, eds. *The breast: comprehensive management of benign and malignant diseases.* Philadelphia: WB Saunders, 1998;214–232.
2. Moore KL. *The developing human.* Philadelphia: WB Saunders, 1988:426–428.
3. Osborne MP. Breast development and anatomy. In: Harris JR, Lippman ME, Morrow M, et al., eds. *Diseases of the breast.* Philadelphia: Lippincott–Raven Publishers, 1996:1–14.
4. Robinson GW, Karpf AB, Kratochwil K. Regulation of mammary gland development by tissue interaction. *J Mammary Gland Biol Neoplasia* 1999;4:9–19.
5. Osin PP, Anbazhagan R, Bartkova J, et al. Breast development gives insights into breast disease. *Histopathology* 1998;33:275–283.
6. Stahl S, Weitzman S, Jones JC. The role of laminin-5 and its receptors in mammary epithelial cell branching morphogenesis. *J Cell Sci* 1997;110:55–63.
7. Yant J, Buluwela L, Niranjan B, et al. *In vivo* effects of hepatocyte growth factor/scatter factor on mouse mammary gland development. *Exp Cell Res* 1998;241:476–481.
8. Niranjan B, Buluwela L, Yant J, et al. HGF/SF: a potent cytokine for mammary growth, morphogenesis and development. *Development* 1997;121:2897–2908.
9. Werb Z, Ashkenas J, MacAuley A, et al. Extracellular matrix remodeling as a regulator of stromal-epithelial interactions during mammary gland development, involution and carcinogenesis. *Brazil J Med Biol Res* 1996;29:1087–1097.
10. Nathan B, Anbazhagan R, Clarkson P, et al. Expression of BCL-2 in the developing human fetal and infant breast. *Histopathology* 1994;24:73–76.
11. Dunbar ME, Wysolmerski JJ. Parathyroid hormone-related protein: a developmental regulatory molecule necessary for mammary gland development. *J Mammary Gland Biol Neoplasia* 1999;4:21–34.

12. Neinstein LS. Breast disease in adolescents and young women. *Pediatr Clin North Am* 1999;46: 607–629.
13. Kaplowitz PB, Oberfield SE. Reexamination of the age limit for defining when puberty is precocious in girls in the United States: implications for evaluation and treatment. *Pediatrics* 1999;104: 936–941.
14. Ilicki A, Prager LR, Kauli R, et al. Premature thelarche – natural history and sex hormone secretion in 68 girls. *Acta Paediatr Scand* 1984;73:756–762.
15. Pasquino AM, Pucarelli I, Passeri F, et al. Progression of premature thelarche to central precocious puberty. *J Pediatr* 1995;126:11–14.
16. Tenore A, Franzese A, Quattrin T, et al. Prognostic signs in the evolution of premature thelarche by discriminant analysis. *J Endocrinol Invest* 1991;14:375–381.
17. Verrotti A, Ferrari M, Morgese G, et al. Premature thelarche: a long-term follow-up. *Gynecol Endocrinol* 1996;10:241–247.
18. Volta C, Bernasconi S, Cisternino M, et al. Isolated premature thelarche variant: clinical and auxological follow-up of 119 girls. *J Endocrinol Invest* 1998;21:180–183.
19. Mills JL, Stolley PD, Davies J, et al. Premature thelarche: natural history and etiologic investigation. *Am J Dis Child* 1981;135:743–745.
20. Arisaka O, Arisaka M, Kitamure Y, et al. Precocious breast development: a case of unilateral hyperplasia of the adrenal cortex. *Eur J Pediatr* 1985;143:308–310.
21. Devriedt K, Lemli L, Craen M, et al. Growth hormone deficiency and premature thelarche in a female infant with Kabuki makeup syndrome. *Horm Res* 1995;43:303–306.
22. Tutar HE, Ocal G, Ince E, et al. Premature thelarche in Kabuki make-up syndrome. *Acta Paediatr Jpn* 1994;36:104–106.
23. Ihara K, Kuromaru R, Takemoto M, et al. Rubinstein-Taybi syndrome: a girl with a history of neuroblastoma and premature thelarche. *Am J Med Genet* 1999;83:365–366.
24. Abe K, Matsuura N, Nohara Y. Prolactin response to thyrotropin-releasing hormone in children with gynecomastia, premature thelarche and idiopathic precocious puberty. *Tohoku J Exp Med* 1984;142:283–288.
25. Wenick GB, Chasalow FI, Blethen SL. Sex hormone-binding globulin and thyroxine-binding globulin levels in premature thelarche. *Steroids* 1988;2:543–550.
26. Klein KO, Mericq V, Brown-Dawson J, et al. Estrogen levels in girls with premature thelarche compared with normal prepubertal girls as determined by an ultrasensitive recombinant cell bioassay. *J Pediatr* 1999;134:190–192.
27. Garibaldi LR, Aceto T Jr, Weber C. The pattern of gonadotropin and estradiol secretion in exaggerated thelarche. *Acta Endocrinol* 1993;128:345–350.
28. Pescovitz OH, Hench KD, Barnes KM, et al. Premature thelarche and central precocious puberty: the relationship between clinical presentation and the gonadotropin response to luteinizing hormone-releasing hormone. *J Clin Endocrinol Metab* 1988;67:474–479.
29. Wang C, Zhong CQ, Leung A, et al. Serum bioactive follicle-stimulating hormone levels in girls with precocious sexual development. *J Clin Endocrinol Metab* 1990;70:615–619.
30. Beck W, Stubbe P. Pulsatile secretion of luteinizing hormone and sleep-related gonadotropin rhythms in girls with premature thelarche. *Eur J Pediatr* 1984;141:168–170.
31. Haber HP, Wollmann HA, Ranke MB. Pelvic ultrasonography: early differentiation between isolated premature thelarche and central precocious puberty. *Eur J Pediatr* 1995;154:182–186.
32. Stanhope R, Abdulwahid NA, Adams J, et al. Studies of gonadotrophin pulsatility and pelvic ultrasound examinations distinguish between isolated premature thelarche and central precocious puberty. *Eur J Pediatr* 1986;145:190–194.
33. Nakamure M, Okabe I, Shimoizumi H, et al. Ultrasonography of ovary, uterus and breast in premature thelarche. *Acta Paediatr Jpn* 1991;33:645–648.
34. Frejaville E, Pagni G, Cacciari E. Breast contact thermography for differentiation between premature thelarche and true precocious puberty. *Eur J Pediatr* 1988;147:389–391.
35. Carlson HE. Current concepts: gynecomastia. *N Engl J Med* 1980;303:795–799.
36. Braunstein GD. Current concepts: gynecomastia. *N Engl J Med* 1993;328:490–495.
37. Aiache AE. Male chest correction: pectoral implants and gynecomastia. *Clin Plast Surg* 1991;18: 823–828.
38. Rigg BM. Morselization suction: a modified technique for gynecomastia. *Plast Reconstr Surg* 1991; 88:159–160.

39. Aiache AE. Surgical treatment of gynecomastia in the body builder. *Plast Reconstr Surg* 1989;83: 61–66.
40. Davidson BA. Concentric circle operation for massive gynecomastia to excise the redundant skin. *Plast Reconstr Surg* 1979;63:350–354.
41. Botta SA. Alternatives for the surgical correction of severe gynecomastia. *Aesthetic Plast Surg* 1998;22:65–70.
42. Khan JI, Ho-Asjoe M, Frame JD. Pectoralis major ruptures postsuction lipectomy for surgical management of gynecomastia. *Aesthetic Plast Surg* 1998;22:16–19.
43. Teimourian B, Pearlman R. Surgery for gynecomastia. *Aesthetic Plast Surg* 1983;7:155–157.
44. Rees TD, Aston SJ. The tuberous breast. *Clin Plast Surg* 1976;3:339–347.
45. Toranto IR. Two-stage correction of tuberous breasts. *Plast Reconstr Surg* 1981;67:642–647.
46. Versaci AD, Rozzelle AA. Treatment of tuberous breasts utilizing tissue expansion. *Aesthetic Plast Surg* 1991;15:307–312.
47. Dinner MI, Dowden RV. The tubular/tuberous breast syndrome. *Ann Plast Surg* 1987;19:414–420.
48. Teimourian B, Adham MN. Surgical correction of the tuberous breast. *Ann Plast Surg* 1983;10: 190–193.
49. Longacre JJ. Correction of the hypoplastic breast with special reference to reconstruction of the nipple type breast with local dermo-fat pedicle flaps. *Plast Reconstr Surg* 1954;14:431–441.
50. Elliott MP. A musculocutaneous transposition flap mammaplasty for correction of the tuberous breast. *Ann Plast Surg* 1988;20:153–157.
51. Williams G, Hoffman S. Mammoplasty for tubular breasts. *Aesthetic Plast Surg* 1981;5:51–56.
52. Scheepers JH, Quaba AA. Tissue expansion in the treatment of tubular breast deformity. *Br J Plast Surg* 1992;45:529–532.
53. Hueston JT. Unilateral agenesis and hypoplasia: difficulties and suggestions. In: Goldwyn RM, ed. *Plastic and reconstructive surgery of the breast*. Boston: Little, Brown and Company, 1976: 361–373.
54. Pitanguy I. Surgical treatment of breast hypertrophy. *Br J Plast Surg* 1967;20:78–85.
55. Argenta LC, VanderKolk C, Friedman RJ, et al. Refinements in reconstruction of congenital breast deformities. *Plast Reconstr Surg* 1985;76:73–80.
56. Smith KJ, Palin WE, Katch V, et al. Surgical treatment of congenital breast asymmetry. *Ann Plast Surg* 1986;17:92–101.
57. Sandsmark M, Amland PF, Samdal F, et al. Clinical results in 87 patients treated for asymmetrical breasts. *Scand J Plast Reconstr Hand Surg* 1992;26:321–326.
58. Wapner I, Rabinowitz B, Snyderman R. Asymmetrical breasts in an adolescent. *Plast Reconstr Surg* 1988;81:813.
59. Harris DL. Self-consciousness of disproportionate breast size: a primary psychological reaction to abnormal appearance. *Br J Plast Surg* 1983:36:191–195.
60. Corso PF. Plastic surgery for the unilateral hypoplastic breast. *Plast Reconstr Surg* 1972;50: 134–141.
61. Funicello A. De Sandre R, Salloum L, et al. Infiltrating ductal carcinoma of the hypomastic breast: a case report. *Am Surg* 1998;64:1037–1039.
62. Marks MW, Argenta LC, Izenberg PH, et al. Management of the chest-wall deformity in male patients with Poland's syndrome. *Plast Reconstr Surg* 1991;87:674–681.
63. Ravitch MM. Poland's syndrome–a study of an eponym. *Plast Reconstr Surg* 1977;59:508–512.
64. Shamberger RC, Welch KJ. Surgical treatment of thoracic deformity in Poland's syndrome. *J Pediatr Surg* 1989;24:760–766.
65. Haller JA, Colombani PM, Miller D, et al. Early reconstruction of Poland's syndrome using autologous rib grafts combined with a latissimus muscle flap. *J Pediatr Surg* 1984;19:423–429.
66. Seyfer AE, Icochea R, Graeber GM. Poland's anomaly. *Ann Surg* 1988;208:776–782.
67. Urschel HC, Byrd S, Sethi SM, et al. Poland's syndrome: improved surgical management. *Ann Thorac Surg* 1984;37:204–211.
68. Beer GM, Kompatscher P, Hergan K. Poland's syndrome and vascular malformations. *Br J Plast Surg* 1996;49:482–484.
69. Hurwitz DJ, Stofman G, Curtin H. Three-dimensional imaging of Poland's syndrome. *Plast Reconstr Surg* 1994;94:719–723.
70. Hester TR, Bostwick J. Poland's syndrome: correction with latissimus muscle transposition. *Plast Reconstr Surg* 1982;69:226–233.

71. Fodor PB, Khoury F. Latissimus dorsi muscle flap in reconstruction of congenitally absent breast and pectoralis muscle. *Ann Plast Surg* 1980;4:422–425.
72. Ohmori K, Takada H. Correction of Poland's pectoralis major muscle anomaly with latissimus dorsi musculocutaneous flaps. *Plast Reconstr Surg* 1980;65:400–404.
73. Anderl H, Kerschbaumer S. Early correction of the thoracic deformity of Poland's syndrome in children with the latissimus dorsi muscle flap: long term follow-up of two cases. *Br J Plast Surg* 1986;39:167–172.
74. Kuan HZ. Restoration of the defect in the anterior rib cage in Poland's syndrome. *Plast Reconstr Surg* 1988;82:196–198.
75. Hochberg J, Ardenghy M, Graeber GM, et al. Complex reconstruction of the chest wall and breast utilizing a customized silicone implant. *Ann Plast Surg* 1994;32:524–528
76. Lavey E, Apfelberg DB, Lash H, et al. Customized silicone implants of the breast and chest. *Plast Reconstr Surg* 1982;69:646–651.
77. Havlik RJ, Sian KU, Wagner JD, et al. Breast cancer in Poland syndrome. *Plast Reconstr Surg* 1999;104:180–182.
78. Leung W, Heaton JP, Morales A. An uncommon urologic presentation of a supernumerary breast. *Urology* 1997;50:122–124.
79. Grossl NA. Supernumerary breast tissue: historical perspectives and clinical features. *South Med J* 2000;93:29–32.
80. Johnson CC, Felson B, Jolles H. Polythelia (supernumerary nipple): an update. *South Med J* 1986; 79:1106–1108.
81. Schmidt H. Supernumerary nipples: prevalence, size, sex and side predilection – a prospective clinical study. *Eur J Pediatr* 1998;157:821–823.
82. Casey HD, Chasan PE, Chick LR. Familial polythelia without associated anomalies. *Ann Plast Surg* 1996;36:101–104.
83. Goedert jj, McKeen EA, Javadpour N, et al. Polythelia and testicular cancer. *Ann Intern Med* 1984; 101:646–647.
84. Deshpande SN, Jagtap SR, Thatte RL. An unusual case of congenital chest wall deformity with polymastia and absence of part of the lung. *Br J Plast Surg* 1989;42:484–486.
85. Toumbis-Ioannou E, Cohen PR. Familial polythelia. *J Am Acad Dermatol* 1994;30:667–668.
86. Urbani CE, Betti R. Accessory mammary tissue associated with congenital and hereditary nephrourinary malformations. *Int J Dermatol* 1996;35:349–352.
87. Cohen PR, Kurzrock R. Miscellaneous genodermatoses: Beckwith-Wiedemann syndrome, Birt-Hogg-Dube syndrome, familial atypical multiple mole melanoma syndrome, hereditary tylosis, incontinentia pigmenti, supernumerary nipples. *Dermatol Clin* 1995;13:211–230.
88. Kahn SA, Wagner RF. Polythelia and unilateral renal agenesis. *Cutis* 1982;30:225–226.
89. Mate K, Horvath J, Schmidt J, et al. Polythelia associated with disturbances of cardiac conduction. *Cor Vasa* 1979;21:112–116.
90. Sabry MA, Al-Saleh Q, Al-Saw'an R, et al. Right upper limb bud triplication and polythelia, left sided hemihypertrophy and congenital hip dislocation, facial dysmorphism, congenital heart disease, and scoliosis: disorganization-like spectrum or patterning gene defect? *J Med Genet* 1995;32: 555–556.
91. Wittebol-Post D, Hennekam RC. Blepharophimosis, ptosis, polythelia and brachydactyly (BPPB): a new autosomal dominant syndrome? *Clin Dysmorphol* 1993;2:346–350.
92. Zohar Y, Laurian N. Bifid condyle of the mandible with associated polythelia and manual anomalies. *J Laryngol Otol* 1987;101:1315–1319.
93. Abramson DJ. Bilateral intra-areolar polythelia. *Arch Surg* 1975;110:1255.
94. Hawtof DB. Intra-areolar polythelia. *Plast Reconstr Surg* 1969;43:96–98.
95. Pellegrini JR, Wagner RF. Polythelia and associated conditions. *Am Fam Physician* 1983;28: 129–132.
96. Trier WC. Complete breast absence. *Plast Reconstr Surg* 1965;36:431–439.
97. Amesse L, Yen FF, Weisskopf B, et al. Vaginal uterine agenesis associated with amastia in a phenotypic female with a de novo 46,XX,t(8;13)(q22.1;q32.1) translocation. *Clin Genet* 1999;55: 493–495.
98. Breslau-Siderius EJ, Toonstra J, Baart JA, et al. Ectodermal dysplasia, lipoatrophy, diabetes mellitus, and amastia: a second case of the AREDYLD syndrome. *Am J Med Genet* 1992;44:374–377.
99. Taylor GA. Reconstruction of congenital amastia with complication. *Ann Plast Surg* 1979;2: 531–534.

100. Rich MA, Heimler A, Waber L, et al. Autosomal dominant transmission of ureteral triplication and bilateral amastia. *J Urol* 1987;137:102–105.
101. Burck U, Held KR. Athelia in a female infant–heterozygous for anhidrotic ectodermal dysplasia. *Clin Genet* 1981;19:117–121.
102. Tsakalakos N, Jordaan F, Taljaard JJF, et al. A previously undescribed ectodermal dysplasia of the tricho-odonto-onychial subgroup in a family. *Arch Dermatol* 1986;122:1047–1053.
103. Mollica F, Mazzone D, Cimino G, et al. Severe case of Al Awadi/Raas-Rothschild syndrome or new, possibly autosomal recessive facio-skeleto-genital syndrome. *Am J Med Genet* 1995;56: 168–172.
104. Spence RJ, Feldman JJ, Ryan JJ. Symmastia: the problem of medial confluence of the breasts. *Plast Reconstr Surg* 1984;73:261–269.
105. Lee H-B, Roh T-S, Chung Y-K, et al. Correction of inverted nipple using strut reinforcement with deepithelialized triangular flaps. *Plast Reconstr Surg* 1998;102:1253–1258.
106. Park HS, Yoon CH, Kim HJ. The prevalence of congenital inverted nipple. *Aesthetic Plast Surg* 1999; 23:144–146.
107. Kurihara K, Maezawa N, Yanagawa H, et al. Surgical correction of the inverted nipple with a tendon graft: hammock procedure. *Plast Reconstr Surg* 1990;86:999–1003.
108. Teimourian B, Adham MN. Simple technique for correction of inverted nipple. *Plast Reconstr Surg* 1980;65:504–506.
109. Lorenzetti MH, Fryns JP. Inverted nipples in Robinow syndrome. *Genet Couns* 1996;7:67–69.
110. Young G, Driscoll MC. Coagulation abnormalities in the carbohydrate-deficient glycoprotein syndrome: case report and review of the literature. *Am J Hematol* 1999;60:66–69.
111. Aiache A. Surgical repair of the inverted nipple. *Ann Plast Surg* 1990;25:457–460.
112. el Sharkawy AG. A method for correction of congenitally inverted nipple with preservation of the ducts. *Plast Reconstr Surg* 1995;95:1111–1114.
113. Hamilton JM. Inverted nipples. *Plast Reconstr Surg* 1980;65:507–509.
114. Pribaz JJ, Pousti T. Correction of recurrent nipple inversion with cartilage graft. *Ann Plast Surg* 1998;40:14–17.
115. Wolfort FG, Marshall KA, Cochran TC. Correction of the inverted nipple. *Ann Plast Surg* 1978; 1:294–297.
116. Miyata N, Abe S. Dog-bite injuries to the breast in children: deformities to secondary sex characteristics and their repair in an extended follow-up. *Ann Plast Surg* 1999;43:542–545.
117. Matthews RN, Khan FT. A seat belt injury to the female breast. *Br J Plast Surg* 1998;51:653.
118. Rosenfield NS, Haller JO, Berdon WE. Failure of development of the growing breast after radiation therapy. *Pediatr Radiol* 1989;19:124–127.
119. Cherup LL, Siewers RD, Futrell JW. Breast and pectoral muscle maldevelopment after anterolateral and posterolateral thoracotomies in children. *Ann Thorac Surg* 1986;41:492–497.
120. Al-Qattan MM, Zuker RM. Management of acute burns of the female pediatric breast: delayed tangential excision versus spontaneous eschar separation. *Ann Plast Surg* 1994;33:66–67.
121. McCauley RL, Beraja V, Rutan RL, et al. Longitudinal assessment of breast development in adolescent female patietns with burns involving the nipple-areolar complex. *Plast Reconstr Surg* 1989; 83:676–680.
122. Kunert P, Schneider W, Flory J. Principles and procedures in female breast reconstruction in the young child's burn injury. *Aesthetic Plast Surg* 1988;12:101–106.
123. Gobbi H, Tse G, Page DL, et al. Reactive spindle cell nodules of the breast after core biopsy or fine-needle aspiration. *Am J Clin Pathol* 2000;113:288–294.
124. Netscher DT, Mosharrafa AM, Laucirica R. Massive asymmetric virginal breast hypertrophy. *South Med J* 1996;89:434–437.
125. Cardoso de Castro C. Subcutaneous mastectomy for gigantomastia in an adolescent girl. *Plast Reconstr Surg* 1977;59:575–578.
126. Denk MJ. Topics in pediatric plastic surgery. *Pediatr Clin North Am* 1998;45:1479–1506.
127. Kupfer D, Dingman D, Broadbent R. Juvenile breast hypertrophy: report of a familial pattern and review of the literature. *Plast Reconstr Surg* 1992;90:303–309.
128. Gliosci A, Presutti F. Virginal gigantomastia: validity of combined surgical and hormonal treatments. *Aesth Plast Surg* 1993;17:61–65.
129. Samuelov R, Siplovich L. Juvenile gigantomastia. *J Pediatr Surg* 1988;23:1014–1015.
130. McMahan JD, Wolfe JA, Cromer BA, et al. Lasting success in teenage reduction mammaplasty. *Ann Plast Surg* 1995;35:227–231.

131. Taylor RJ, Cumming DC, Corenblum B. Successful treatment of D-penicillamine-induced breast gigantism with danazol. *BMJ* 1981;282:362–363.
132. Morimoto T, Komaki K, Mori T. Juvenile gigantomastia: report of a case. *Surg Today* 1993;23: 260–264.
133. Kullander S. Effect of 2 br-alpha-ergocryptin (CB 154) on serum prolactin and the clinical picture in a case of progressive gigantomastia in pregnancy. *Ann Chir Gynaecol* 1976;65:227–233.
134. Wolner-Hanssen P, Palmer B, Sjoberg NO, et al. Gigantomastia. *Acta Obstet Gynecol Scand* 1981; 60:525–527.
135. Gargan TJ, Goldwyn RM. Gigantomastia complicating pregnancy. *Plast Reconstr Surg* 1987;80: 121–124.
136. Moss WM. Gigantomastia with pregnancy: a case report with review of the literature. *Arch Surg* 1968;96:27–32.
137. Hedberg K, Karlsson K, Linstedt G. Gigantomastia during pregnancy: effect of a dopamine agonist. *Am J Obstet Gynecol* 1979;133:928–931.
138. Cervelli V, Orlando G, Giudiceandrea F, et al. Gigantomastia and breast lumps in a kidney transplant recipient. *Transplant Proc* 1999;31:3224–3225.

3

Nipple Discharge

Jill R. Dietz and Joseph P. Crowe

Nipple discharge is an uncommon complaint of women seeking medical care for breast problems. The reported incidence in this population of patients is between 3% and 7.4% (1–4). As screening, breast cancer awareness, and breast self-examination become more widespread, it is likely that more women will present with this symptom. Whereas most of these patients will have a benign process, nipple discharge can be the sole sign of cancer in 1% of patients (3). The patient with nipple discharge is often more challenging to the breast clinician than is the patient with breast cancer. The evaluation and treatment of nipple discharge vary greatly in practice and in the literature, causing confusion for both patients and physicians. Differentiating between physiologic and pathologic nipple discharge is critical to identify patients in need of a diagnostic workup and treatment plan.

ANATOMY AND PHYSIOLOGY

A review of the anatomy and physiology of the human mammary ductal system is helpful in understanding the etiology of nipple discharge. The female breast has approximately 15 to 20 lobes that radiate from the nipple. Each lobe is composed of glands (lobules) and branching milk ducts. The breast milk is produced in the terminal ductal lobular units (TDLU), which empty into a branching ductal network that leads to the proximal duct. The proximal ducts converge toward the areola and empty into the nipple. The mammary ducts are lined by actively dividing epithelial cells that slough on a regular basis. The nipple orifices of nonlactating women usually are blocked by a keratin plug that prevents the leakage of normal ductal secretions. During pregnancy, the ductal system proliferates and secretions are produced in response to large increases in estrogen, progesterone, and prolactin (which is released by the anterior pituitary gland). After parturition, lactation is promoted by persistently elevated levels of prolactin and rapidly declining levels of estrogen and progesterone. The nursing infant causes further release of prolactin via the suckling reflex, thus stimulating milk production. These same hormones that promote and sustain breast-feeding also contribute to nipple discharge in nonlactating women.

DEFINITION

Nipple discharge is fluid that flows or is expressed from the mammary ducts and is present in a very small percentage of women. Nipple secretions are found within the ductal system and are by-products of the epithelial cells that are undergoing cellular turnover. These physiologic secretions are generally not evident to most women because they are blocked by the keratin plug and eventually reabsorbed. Using a suction aspirating device, Goodson and King found secretions, or nipple aspirate fluid (NAF), in up to 81.2% of asymptomatic women (4). Another study showed that between 24.7% and 88.4% of women could have nipple secretions extracted using a nipple-aspirating device (5). These and other studies confirmed that the ability to aspirate nipple secretions is influenced by age, race, parity, and hormonal status but is successful in most patients (5–8). Although nipple secretions are considered normal, the mammary ducts are the origin of most breast cancers, making the fluid secreted by the ducts a point of interest for researchers.

Many studies have been done on aspirated nipple secretions to examine cellular changes and biochemical composition (7–12). NAF contains cholesterol and other steroids, immunoglobulin, lactose, fatty acids, and α-lactalbumin. Exogenous compounds such as caffeine, nicotine, pesticides, and other drugs also are found in nipple secretions (11). The color of NAF, which can vary from white to dark green, is related to the cholesterol, lipid peroxide, and estrogen content (12). The normal cellular makeup of NAF consists of foam cells, a few epithelial cells, and other cells of hematogenous origin (13,14).

When secretions become abundant or persistent enough that they discharge spontaneously from the duct orifice, they are known as *nipple discharge*. Nipple discharge generally is separated into physiologic and pathologic discharge. Physiologic discharge can be caused by exogenous or endogenous hormones, medications, direct stimulation, stress, or endocrine abnormalities. Although the cause of the hormonal influence may be pathologic, as is the case with prolactinoma, the ductal system itself has no abnormality; so the resultant discharge is classified as physiologic. Most physiologic discharge is bilateral and nonspontaneous and involves multiple ducts (Fig. 3.1). These characteristics result from the central effect of an outside

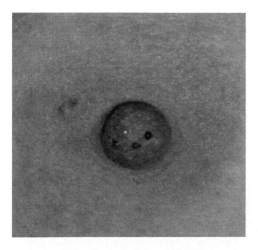

FIG. 3.1. Classic presentation of physiologic nipple discharge.

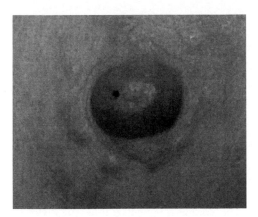

FIG. 3.2. Classic presentation of pathologic nipple discharge.

influence on the breast. The color of the discharge can vary from milky to yellow, gray, brown, or dark green, depending on the composition and cause of the physiologic discharge. As with NAF, darker discharges are associated with higher levels of estrogens and cholesterol (12). There is rarely a pathologic abnormality involved with this type of discharge, and localization procedures are not necessary.

Pathologic nipple discharge is caused by an abnormality of the duct epithelium. It is typically unilateral and from a single duct. The discharge is spontaneous or at least easily expressible. The patient often notices the discharge after a warm shower, which likely removes the keratin plug. The fluid collects in the dilated duct (Fig. 3.2) and in the ampulla and subsequently is released when the plug is removed or the duct is expressed. The color of the discharge is usually clear, serous, or bloody, although pathologic nipple discharge can present as other colors. This type of discharge tends not to be affected by the menstrual cycle or hormonal status. Although some women seek care when they first notice the discharge, many will delay until the discharge becomes socially embarrassing or bloody. Although most of these women will have a benign etiology for their nipple discharge, all patients with pathologic nipple discharge need a thorough evaluation to rule out cancer.

INCIDENCE

Over the last 5 years, we have evaluated 17,560 patients in our breast center; 691 (4%) complained of nipple discharge. This finding corresponds with other series in which the reported incidence of nipple discharge in women seeking breast care ranges from 3% to 7.4% (1,15,16). The incidence is likely underreported because many women do not seek medical care for this symptom. In a recent series of more than 50,000 patients seeking breast care, nipple discharge was more common in younger women, but the incidence of bloody nipple discharge increased with age. Patients with nipple discharge had a higher relative risk for cancer than the asymptomatic population, and patients with nipple discharge associated with a mass or skin change had an even higher relative risk of cancer. In this series, bloody nipple discharge was associated with a high cancer risk, although cancer also was found in milky and serous fluid. Rarely were bilateral, multicentric discharges found to be caused by cancer (16). Breast cancer was found to be the etiology of the nipple discharge in 4% to 14.3% of cases in several series (2,3,15,17–21). The number of breast cancers presenting with it has dropped over the last few decades. In the series by Copeland and Higgins in the 1950s, 25 of 67 patients with nipple discharge had breast cancer (22). The decrease in the incidence of cancer presenting in this way is likely due to the earlier detection of breast cancer and smaller tumors at the time of diagnosis secondary to better awareness and improved screening.

The series of 20,000 patients by Chaudary et al. showed that the age distribution for patients with cancer as a cause of their nipple discharge was similar to the age distribution for breast cancer in general. The youngest patient in this series was 32 years old, and the mean age of patients with discharge was 53.2 years (3). As with breast cancer in general, increasing age presents as a risk factor for having cancer as the cause of nipple discharge.

The incidence of breast cancer increases when the nipple discharge is associated with an abnormal mammogram (23). Although most patients with pathologic nipple discharge have normal mammograms, suspicious radiologic findings should be evaluated with stereotactic or core biopsy prior to duct excision. If minimally invasive biopsy is not available, the mammographic abnormality will need to be evaluated at the time of duct excision.

The incidence of cancer for patients with nipple discharge associated with a mass is also higher than that for patients with nipple discharge alone (15). One study showed that the incidence of carcinoma for patients with discharge and a mass was 61.5% compared with 6.1% for patients with discharge alone (24). The palpable abnormality should be addressed prior to undertaking a procedure for the discharge by either fine needle aspiration (FNA) or core biopsy, if possible.

Even though the most significant cause of nipple discharge is cancer, most cases have a benign etiology. Many studies do not differentiate the exact histology of benign lesions, although it is clear that papillomatosis or papillomas are responsible for a large percentage of pathologic nipple discharge. Other causes are duct ectasia, epithelial hyperplasia, and fibrocystic changes (3,15,18,23).

CHARACTERISTICS AND ETIOLOGY

Discharge from the nipple can present as a spectrum of signs, from a tiny opaque drop during breast examination to alarming bloody discharge that stains the patients clothing. The presentation and history are important in categorizing the discharge as either *physiologic* or *pathologic*. This grouping system is helpful in determining both the evaluation and treatment necessary for that patient. Table 3.1 shows the classic presentation of each type of nipple discharge.

Physiologic nipple discharge has various presentations and etiologies. Table 3.2 reviews the most common causes of physiologic nipple discharge. More than 75%

TABLE 3.1. *Characteristics of pathologic and physiologic nipple discharge*

Characteristic	Physiologic	Pathologic
Laterality	Bilateral	Unilateral
No. of ducts	Multiple	One
Spontaneity	Expressed	Spontaneous
Color	Multicolored, milky, gray green, brown, yellow	Bloody, serous, clear

of nipple discharges are physiologic in nature and do not require surgical intervention (2). The evaluation and treatment of physiologic nipple discharge should be focused on identifying the external factor that is stimulating the breasts.

Galactorrhea is physiologic discharge from the nipple that resembles breast milk but occurs in a patient who is not lactating. The discharge is a thin, watery milk-like substance that usually arises from both breasts. The most common scenario is a postpartum woman who continues to have discharge from one or both breasts long after she stopped breast-feeding. She may have some concern regarding the discharge and may attempt to repeatedly express the fluid. The continued stimulation of the nipple causes further discharge, perpetuating the cycle. Other sources of nipple stimulation, such as the friction of clothing, or nipple involvement during intimacy, also can aggravate the symptom. Again, explaining to the patient the likely etiology of the discharge and offering reassurance are usually sufficient.

Thin, milky discharge can occur around menarche and menopause, when the breasts are exposed to extreme hormonal variation. The discharge is self-limited and simply requires reassuring the patient. Nipple discharge also can be seen in newborns as a result of maternal hormones that cross the placental barrier prior to parturition. After delivery, the precipitous drop in estrogen and progesterone levels associated with the high neonatal prolactin levels cause stimulation of the infant's breast tissue. This discharge, commonly referred to as *witch's milk*, lasts only a few weeks (25).

Galactorrhea can result from an increase in prolactin levels. Most often, the levels are elevated because of medication, although the most significant cause is a pituitary

TABLE 3.2. *Causes of physiologic nipple discharge*

Hormonal variation
Pregnancy/postlactational
Mechanical stimulation
Galactorrhea
Duct ectasia
Bloody discharge of pregnancy
Infection (Zuska's disease)
Montgomery gland discharge
Fibrocystic change

TABLE 3.3. *Causes of galactorrhea (hyperprolactinemia)*

Postlactational
Mechanical stimulation
Stress
Chest trauma or surgery
Pituitary and hypothalamic tumors
Ectopic prolactin (bronchogenic carcinoma)
Chronic renal failure
Hypothyroidism
Acromegaly
Cushing disease
Lactogenic drugs
   Estrogens
   Progestins
   Long-term opiate use (e.g., morphine, cocaine)
   Phenothiazines (e.g., Compazine, Thorazine)
   Antidepressants (e.g., Elavil, Prozac, Paxil)
   Antipsychotics (e.g., Clozaril)
   Antihypertensives (e.g., Aldomet, Calan)
   Butyrophenones (e.g., Haldol)
   Thioxanthenes (e.g., Navane)
   Benzodiazepines (e.g., Valium)
   Other commonly prescribed drugs (e.g., Tagamet, Isoniazid,
     Danocrine, Reglan)

adenoma that secretes prolactin. Prolactinoma should be expected if the patient has the classic triad of symptoms: amenorrhea, galactorrhea, and infertility. The tumor arises from the anterior pituitary gland and can become quite large causing symptoms of diplopia from compression of the optic chiasm. Prolactinomas can erode into the floor of the pituitary fossa, and this may be evident on a plain lateral radiograph of the skull. If a prolactinoma is suspected, a prolactin level should be drawn, which will be abnormal (> 30 ng/mL). Screening nipple discharge patients with prolactin levels is not cost-effective considering that fewer than one in 1,000 cases are due to a pituitary adenoma (26). If a tumor is found, it can be treated successfully with a dopamine agonist, which will also eliminate the discharge. Occasionally, surgical excision of the tumor may be necessary.

Other rare causes of galactorrhea are listed in Table 3.3, along with the categories of medications that have been known to cause nipple discharge. Thoracic surgery or chest trauma has been reported to cause nipple discharge. The injury stimulates the afferent thoracic nerves and the hypothalamic–pituitary axis, resulting in increased prolactin release, which, in turn, stimulates nipple discharge (1).

Opalescent physiologic discharges, which are multicolored and nonserous, emanate from one or both breasts and usually from multiple ducts. The discharge may be evident only with vigorous expression by the patient, or it may be easily expressed and copious. Creamy white, tan, or yellow discharge may present next to a duct producing a brown, dark green or blackish discharge. Although this type of discharge is often alarming to the patient, it is quite unlikely for it to be associated with an intraductal lesion. When duct excision is done for this type of discharge, histology often shows normal breast tissue, duct ectasia, or fibrocystic changes. Most patients with physiologic discharge are willing to have follow-up after being reassured of the benign nature of the discharge. On rare occasion, the patient may request surgery to eliminate copious discharge. If the discharge is associated with pain and fibrocystic changes, the patient should be informed that it is not likely that the surgery will decrease her pain. It also may result in decreased nipple sensation and the inability to breast-feed, particularly if bilateral excisions are required. If an underlying cause for the nipple discharge can be identified, it can be addressed, for example, by a medication change or cessation of hormones.

Communication of cysts with ductal structures appears to be responsible for nipple discharge in some instances. In these situations, the cyst, often presenting as a mass, may disappear with the onset of discharge. Whenever a patient presents with nipple discharge and an associated mass, the mass must be evaluated. In this case, aspirated cyst fluid characteristics will likely correlate to the nipple discharge, and no further evaluation is necessary. A ductogram may show communication with the cyst. Although this is an interesting finding, a ductogram is not necessary if there is clinical evidence that the cyst is related to the discharge. If the problem persists, the cyst should be treated and evaluation for the discharge initiated.

Some breast infections present with purulent and malodorous nipple discharge. This condition is treated like other breast infections. Large abscess cavities may be apparent and should be drained. Cellulitis in association with nipple discharge may be indicative of a deep abscess cavity. If it is unclear whether an abscess has formed, an ultrasound may be useful. Otherwise, conservative treatment with an antibiotic that has adequate gram-positive coverage is appropriate initial therapy. The discharge itself may be a useful source to test for microbiology and sensitivities. Squamous metaplasia of lactiferous sinuses (Zuska's disease) is a chronic condition of periareolar abscess with sinus formation, and it can result in intermittent nipple discharge and infection. Excision of the entire ductal system on the affected side, including the sinus tract, is often beneficial and is associated with the fewest recurrences (27).

Duct ectasia is a condition that results in poor emptying of ductal secretions, stagnation, and inflammation of the ducts (Fig. 3.3). The associated nipple discharge can present spontaneously or require vigorous expression to elicit a thick, white discharge. Bilateral, multiduct involvment varying in color is the most common presentation. The drainage is thought to be secondary to increased glandular secretions resulting from chronic inflammation (28). Whereas the condition itself does not require surgery, ductal ectasia can present as pathologic nipple discharge, and the inability to rule out carcinoma may be an indication for a ductal excision. The cause of the inflammation is unknown, and the blocked ducts can become secondarily infected. Surgery is necessary to treat recurrent infections or, in the case of pathologic discharge, to distinguish it from malignant conditons (25,29).

Occasionally, women who are in their third trimester of pregnancy or who are postpartum will experience bloody nipple discharge. Although it is common to have a milky discharge at this time, bloody discharge is rare, often unilateral, and may

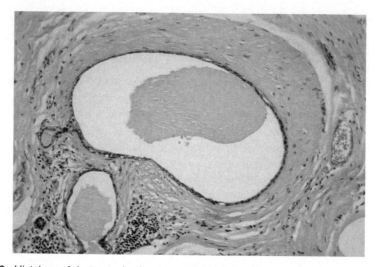

FIG. 3.3. Histology of duct ectasia showing a dilated duct with surrounding inflammation.

be expressible from multiple ducts. The bloody discharge often is noted after an abrupt increase in breast size associated with the pregnancy. In women who have asymmetric breast growth during pregnancy, bloody nipple discharge more often is associated with the larger breast (30). The discharge can accompany normal lactation and is often alarming to the patient, who may be concerned about breast cancer or the blood harming her nursing infant. The bleeding is usually minimal and self-limited and is unlikely to cause a problem for the nursing infant. Most case reports describe resolution of the bleeding by the third month after delivery. Cytologic evaluation of nipple discharge in pregnant or postpartum patients often reveals abnormal-appearing cells that are the result of normal epithelial changes during lactation. These cells may be falsely interpreted as arising from cancer, and therefore, cytologic examination of this discharge must be interpreted with caution. This bloody discharge of pregnancy and lactation is an unusual circumstance in which it may be reasonable to postpone or at least delay further evaluation (31). It must be appreciated that if the discharge is associated with a mass or persists as a unilateral, single duct discharge, then further evaluation is needed.

Montgomery gland discharge presents from the large areolar sebaceous glands known as Montgomery's tubercles and is not truly nipple discharge. This type of discharge usually occurs at times of extreme changes in hormonal status, such as menarche or menopause. The discharge has characteristics of physiologic discharge because it is commonly found coming from many glands and is either serous or opaque. This type of discharge requires reassurance unless infection occurs; in the latter case, antibiotic therapy and occasionally, excision of the infected gland are indicated (32).

Nipple discharge in the male patient is treated similarly to that in females. Puberty

TABLE 3.4. *Causes of pathologic
nipple discharge*

Papilloma
Papillomatosis
Papillary cancer
Ductal carcinoma *in situ*
Invasive ductal carcinoma
Duct ectasia
Ductal epithelial hyperplasia
Cysts/fibrocystic disease

in adolescents and the same drugs and medical conditions that stimulate gynecomastia in men can cause nipple discharge. The evaluation should include mammography in addition to careful history and physical examination. A biopsy should be done if any suspicious mass or mammographic abnormality is found. A recent series reported clinical gynecomastia in 35.5% of male patients with breast cancer. This rate is well above the general incidence of gynecomastia, suggesting it as a risk factor for cancer development (33). In the series of 6,200 patients reported by Leis, 5 of 24 (20.8%) men diagnosed with cancer had nipple discharge as the presenting symptom. Evaluation is mandatory for male patients with pathologic nipple discharge, especially when associated with a mass, because of the increased risk of cancer and decreased survival rate of male patients with invasive breast cancer (15).

Pathologic nipple discharge is caused by an intraductal abnormality and is therefore typically a unilateral finding. Although it is possible for the pathology to involve more than one ductal system, the typical presentation is consistent discharge from a single duct orifice. The discharge can be watery and clear, serosanguinous, dark brown old blood, or bright blood. Occasionally, reports of carcinoma with other types of discharge, such as milky, have been reported, but this is distinctly unusual (16,34). Table 3.4 reviews the common etiologies of pathologic nipple discharge.

Papilloma

A large percentage of pathologic nipple discharge is attributed to papillomas or papillomatosis (Fig. 3.4). Papillomas are often found centrally in the subareolar region. Solitary papillomas arise from the larger ducts compared with the smaller, often multiple papillomas, which are more peripherally located and arise from the TDLU. Peripheral papillomas can occur bilaterally and have a higher recurrence rate after excision than the solitary central variety. Multiple, peripheral papillomas present with pathologic nipple discharge less frequently than do central papillomas (1,35).

In the past, there has been much controversy over whether papillomas are premalignant. It is generally accepted that central, solitary papillomas have little malignant potential, although they should be completely excised to avoid recurrence (36). In contrast, papillomas arising in small, more peripheral ducts can be associated with

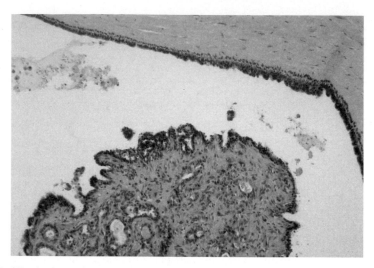

FIG. 3.4. Histologic section through an intraductal papilloma showing the vascular stroma with epithelial lining.

cancer. Ohuchi et al. reconstructed ductal excision specimens from patients with pathologic nipple discharge and found that cancer was associated with 37.5% of peripheral papillomas but not with central papillomas (37). Anatomic studies of the human breast have shown that abnormal, premalignant proliferation of the epithelium occurs more frequently in the TDLU (38). Patients with nipple discharge who are found to have peripheral lesions on ductography should be considered for a preoperative localizing procedure to guide the surgeon during surgical biopsy. These patients should also have careful follow-up because the risk of recurrence or development of cancer is higher than that for central lesions (36).

Carcinoma

One percent of all breast cancers have nipple discharge as the only symptom (Fig. 3.5) (3). Approximately one in ten cases of pathologic nipple discharge will have cancer as the etiology and the incidence increases if the discharge is bloody. The rationale for investigation in patients with pathologic nipple discharge is to rule out cancer as the source. Although numerous diagnostic tests are available that correlate with the malignant potential of a lesion, no single test can rule out carcinoma.

Fibrocystic Disease

Several series reported that fibrocystic disease is a common histologic finding in many duct-excision specimens from patients with pathologic nipple discharge. In cases where fibrocystic change or normal breast tissue is reported, it is important

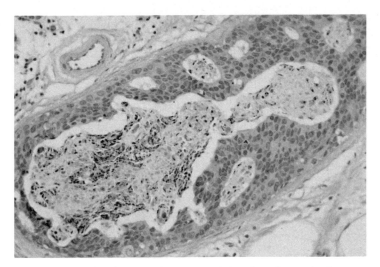

FIG. 3.5. Histologic representation of ductal carcinoma *in situ*.

to ensure that all the excised tissue is analyzed or that the correct tissue was excised. Some papillomas are only 1 to 2 mm in size and could be missed easily with the sampling error of serial sectioning. A high suspicion for a missed papilloma should remain when the histologic diagnosis of fibrocystic change is reported for duct-excision specimens.

DIAGNOSTIC EVALUATION

History and Physical Examination

Many diagnostic tests are available to evaluate patients with nipple discharge. Before embarking on any of these, a full history must first be taken including the patient's age, gynecologic and sexual history, and use of medication and hormones. Pertinent medical history, such as previous endocrine problems or chest trauma, should also be ascertained. The characteristics of the discharge must be noted, including laterality, spontaneity, number of ducts involved, color, and consistency. Physical examination should include a breast examination to assess for palpable masses, lymphadenopathy, skin changes, and nipple inversion or lesions. The information obtained from a careful history and a confirming physical examination will frequently lead to a diagnosis and limit the tests needed prior to duct excision.

Mammography

If it is determined that the patient has physiologic nipple discharge, no additional procedures are needed. Mammography is reserved for patients in the appropriate age group if physiologic discharge is the presenting symptom. All patients with pathologic nipple discharge should undergo mammographic evaluation regardless of age. Still, mammography is often normal in cases of discharge associated with cancer. Fung et al. found that only 2 of 15 patients with cancer causing nipple discharge had mammograms suggestive of malignancy (39). Mammography may identify a separate or associated lesion that may alter the course of management. Mammographic abnormalities associated with nipple discharge increase the likelihood of a malignancy (23). If a mammographic abnormality is visualized, this finding takes precedence and a stereotactic or ultrasound-guided core biopsy should be performed. If a minimally invasive biopsy is not done, then a needle localization excisional biopsy should be performed.

Magnetic Resonance Imaging

Magnetic resonance imaging is being used more often as an additional diagnostic tool for breast diseases. It is particularly useful in young women with dense breast tissue where more conventional tests such as mammography and ultrasound have a lower sensitivity. Magnetic resonance galactography has been developed as an additional tool for patients with pathologic nipple discharge and can be useful for identifying the extent of the disease. It may provide information in suspected cancer cases where breast conservation will be attempted (40).

Ultrasound

Ultrasound has been used for patients with pathologic nipple discharge to view dilated ducts. This technique also has been used with saline lavage of the discharging duct to dilate and obtain cytology from the duct under echographic guidance (41, 42). Chung et al. compared ultrasound to ductography and found that ultrasound is superior for defining small 0.5-cm lesions and to evaluate multiple ductal systems. Ductography remains superior to ultrasound for visualizing the extent of abnormality within a ductal system and for detection of microcalcifications (43). High-resolution ultrasound is performed at 13 to 15 MHz and has a higher sensitivity for the diagnosis of intraductal pathology than conventional ultrasound (75% vs. 30%). Although it has a lower specificity than conventional ultrasound performed at 7.5 MHz, high-resolution ultrasound appears to be better for evaluating proximal ducts (44). If an identified peripheral lesion can be visualized by ultrasound, needle localization or ultrasound-guided FNA can be performed. The sensitivity of cytologic examination of ultrasound-guided FNA is only 50%, however, and duct excision is warranted to remove the lesion (45). Localizing tests for peripheral lesions will assist the surgeon in excising the lesion but may be dependent on the availability of instrumentation and radiologic personnel at an individual institution.

Occult Blood

Testing nipple discharge for occult blood has been evaluated in many studies. Bloody or heme-positive discharge has been associated with an increased incidence of cancer (46). In one large series, discharge was tested for occult blood using a Bili-labstix reagent strip. All patients with the eventual diagnosis of cancer tested positive even though fewer than half were grossly bloody (3). If the discharge is pathologic by characteristics, it should be evaluated even if it is heme-occult negative.

Cytology

Many physicians will send nipple discharge for cytologic evaluation. In a large screening study in which cytology was performed on more than 20,000 patients with nipple discharge, only 0.2 % were either positive or suspicious for malignancy. In this same series, 61 of 404 detected cancers had nipple discharge. In these 61 cases, cytology findings were 24 negative, 18 positive, 7 suspicious, and 12 atypical for a sensitivity of 60.7 % (47). The ability to detect malignancy by cytologic examination of nipple discharge ranges from 45% to 82% (15,16,48–50). Nipple discharge cytology has a 0.9% to 2.6% false-positive rate (15,50). Cytology alone should not be used to determine whether surgical excision is necessary because of the high false-negative and false-positive rates. In cases of positive nipple cytology and mammographic changes suggestive of malignancy, a definitive surgical procedure may be justified (51). It is likely, however, that the mammographic abnormality will be biopsied during the workup and thus establish the diagnosis. For patients with pathologic nipple discharge and no mass or mammographic abnormality, a surgical biopsy to obtain a tissue diagnosis should be performed prior to the definitive procedure. Duct excision provides tissue for histologic diagnosis and usually is performed in most cases of pathologic nipple discharge regardless of the cytology findings.

Cytology examination is not recommended for pregnant patients because of the difficulty in differentiating normal from abnormal proliferative changes (31). Lesions of the nipple with or without associated discharge can be evaluated by cytology. The crust of the lesion is removed, and the base of the lesion is scraped and applied to a slide (48). An alternate method for assessing nipple lesions is a punch biopsy, which also can be done in the office. Positive cytology in cases of pathologic nipple discharge or nipple lesions can be helpful, but in cases in which the clinical evaluation is suspicious without positive cytology or if cytology is positive without a corresponding high level of clinical suspicion, tissue biopsy is required (Fig. 3.6).

Biochemical Markers

Several researchers have addressed the role of biochemical markers in nipple discharge in an attempt to diagnose breast cancer. Certain lactic dehydrogenase isoenzyme levels have been elevated in the nipple discharge of patients with breast cancer. The test is relatively simple and inexpensive but is associated with a false-negative rate in cases where a cancer is in another area of the breast and not associated with the discharge (52). Immunoassays for carcinoembryonic antigen (CEA) have

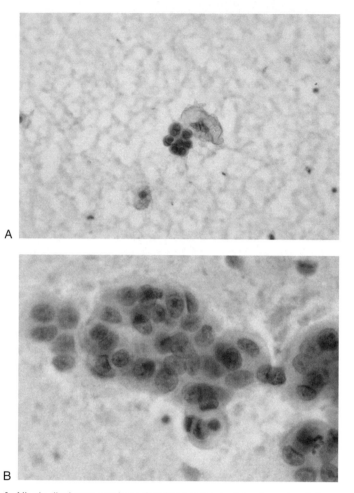

FIG. 3.6. A: Nipple discharge cytology showing benign ductal cells and proteinaceous material. **B:** Nipple discharge cytology showing malignant cells.

been done using small nitrocellulose-backed disks placed on the nipples of cancer patients. Nipple secretions from 94% of the patients with cancer had significantly higher levels of CEA than from those without cancer. This difference was not apparent in healthy controls (53). Several studies of NAF and abnormal discharge using immunoassays for CEA show similar trends, whereas others show no difference (54–56). Using a modified breast pump to obtain NAF, Sauter et al. found that decreased levels of prostatic-specific antigen were associated with an increased breast cancer risk (8). In a recent study, Liu et al. found that nipple fluid basic fibroblast growth factor was significantly increased in breast cancer patients over controls (57). These tests using nipple discharge or secretions could aid in the diagno-

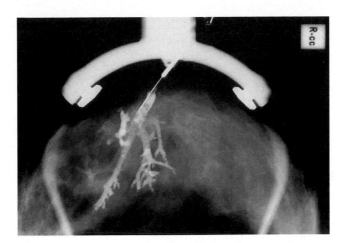

FIG. 3.7. Ductogram showing the typical lobulated appearance of a benign intraductal papilloma.

sis of breast cancer but are currently not accurate enough to rule out carcinoma or negate the need for biopsy.

Ductal Imaging

Ductography, or galactography, has proven useful for preoperative localization of intraductal lesions (58,59) (Fig. 3.7). Because of the significant false-negative rate, however, most physicians believe the decision to operate should not be based solely on the results of ductography (18,20). The ability of ductography to distinguish between benign and malignant disease remains limited (43,60). A recent study reported an increase in the duct excision yield of neoplastic growths from 67% to 100% by using preoperative ductography (61). This procedure can be performed easily by inserting a 30-gauge blunt-tip needle into the discharging duct orifice and instilling 0.1 to 1.5 mL of water-soluble contrast. Mammograms are taken in two views and will show a filling defect or duct cutoff in most circumstances (17). In cases where the ductal lesion is far from the nipple, ductography can be combined with preoperative needle localization to assist the surgeon with the excision (61, 62). Other techniques combine preoperative ductography with methylene-blue dye injection to assist the surgeon in removing the lesion (61,63).

Standard ductography via the nipple is not possible in many patients who have had previous duct surgery with retained or new duct lesions or for patients who have dilated ducts that cannot be accessed through the nipple. In these cases, percutaneous ductography has been described using ultrasound guidance. This procedure allows for identification and localization of the lesion to assist with surgical excision (64).

Despite the advances in diagnostic and radiologic techniques, patients with pathologic nipple discharge frequently come to surgical excision. Because there are no tests that can adequately differentiate benign from malignant intraductal lesions, removal of the lesion is necessary (24).

SURGICAL EVALUATION AND TREATMENT

Surgery for pathologic nipple discharge can be a less than satisfying procedure. Duct excision typically is performed blindly because the intraluminal pathology cannot be visualized directly during surgery. Duct excision can cause decreased sensation to the nipple and prevent the ability to breast-feed, depending on the extent of dissection. The surgeon must judge the amount of tissue to be excised to ensure adequate removal of the lesion without unnecessary destruction of normal breast tissue. Benign or normal pathology findings could result from not excising the lesion, from the pathologist not identifying the lesion within the specimen, or possibly from a truly negative pathology.

Various techniques for surgical removal of the mammary ducts have been described. A major duct excision removes all or most of the subareolar ductal tissue through either a circumareolar or radial incision (15,65). Traditionally, this approach was used for pathologic nipple discharge prior to the availability of localizing procedures. It is still useful in cases of copious physiologic discharge for which the patient requests surgery or for cases where localizing attempts are unsuccessful or show multiple duct involvement. After the incision is made, the ducts are encircled and tied off as they enter the nipple. The subareolar tissue is coned out for several centimeters to remove all apparent ductal tissue. The recurrence rate of nipple discharge after this procedure is low (15). The relatively large circumareolar incision necessary to perform a major duct excision disrupts the nerve supply to the nipple and can leave the patient with numbness and the inability to nurse on that side. Care must be taken to avoid cautery burn to the undersurface of the nipple to limit the possibility of nipple necrosis (66).

A more limited or segmental duct resection can be performed by cannulating the discharging duct with a probe. The tissue is removed from around the probe deep within the breast. The goal is to remove an entire ductal system from the nipple to the TDLU. This is useful in cases where localizing attempts have failed and the location of the lesion is unknown or for deep lesions. A circumareolar incision is commonly made in the quadrant of the discharging duct (67). A flap is created undermining to the nipple, and the dilated or blue duct is encircled. It is important to dissect into the nipple to remove the proximal duct tissue to prevent recurrent discharge (66). A useful adjunct to this procedure is preoperative ductography combined, if necessary, with needle localization for a deep abnormality. The proximal duct is removed with the assistance of a probe or blue dye while the deep lesion is identified by excising the tissue around the localizing wire (62). Duct excision using a lacrimal probe guide has the advantage of identifying the proximal portion of the discharging duct. The probe, however, can enter the wrong duct at a bifurcation or may be unable to be advanced to the level of the pathology. Blue dye will stain the entire ductal system if it is placed in the abnormal duct, but it does not direct the surgeon to the lesion itself.

The treatment of breast cancer presenting as nipple discharge has traditionally been mastectomy. Many series suggest that intraductal cancer presenting as nipple discharge is more extensive and has a higher recurrence rate than does ductal *carcinoma in situ* in other areas of the breast (68–71). Ito et al. found that in 26 patients with nonpalpable breast cancer associated with nipple discharge who were treated with duct–lobular segmentectomy, only one patient had microscopic residual disease found in the follow-up mastectomy specimen. These findings suggest that segmental duct resection is an adequate surgery for nonpalpable cancers presenting with nipple discharge (72). Most series suggest that negative margins may not guarantee complete excision of the cancer. At the very least, radiation therapy and close follow-up are essential for cancer patients presenting with discharge who are undergoing segmental duct excision (68).

Microdochectomy is a procedure that removes the abnormal duct while preserving surrounding normal breast tissue (73). The technique involves identifying and cannulating the discharging duct preoperatively by ductography. Blue dye is injected into the abnormal ductal system through the cannula placed during the preoperative ductography. The duct is dissected from the nipple toward the distal ducts removing only the blue-stained duct tissue. This technique has been described as using a transareolar incision, which is a radial incision through the nipple, but a small curvilinear incision within the areola also can be used. This technique has the benefit of removing the discharging duct while preserving the normal ducts in an effort to limit sensation loss and retain the ability to breast-feed.

Mammary Ductoscopy

Mammary ductoscopy allows direct visualization of the intraductal lesion by passing a small endoscope through the nipple into the ductal system after the duct orifice is dilated. The ability to enter the ductal system and directly visualize ductal abnormalities has distinct advantages. The intraductal pathology can be visualized during the excision, and the scope itself directs the surgeon to the lesion. This enables adequate removal of the lesion while preserving surrounding normal tissue. Ductoscopy enables the surgeon to identify the abnormality within the specimen and assists the pathologist in locating the lesion (Fig. 3.8).

Mammary ductoscopy has been under investigation for longer than a decade. Initial attempts were not encouraging. The scopes were too large to be inserted into the nipple with ease or to maneuver through the smaller ducts, and smaller fiberoptic scopes had poor optics and no working channel (74–78). Several years ago, we collaborated with a company that produced a more useful mammary ductoscope that was 1.2 mm in diameter with a 350 μ working channel to allow for air insufflation and saline irrigation during visualization (Acueity, Larkspur, CA) (Fig. 3.9). The working channel provides ductal dilatation, enables sampling of intraductal lesions, and allows irrigation of discharge and debris, thus providing a clear image. Our

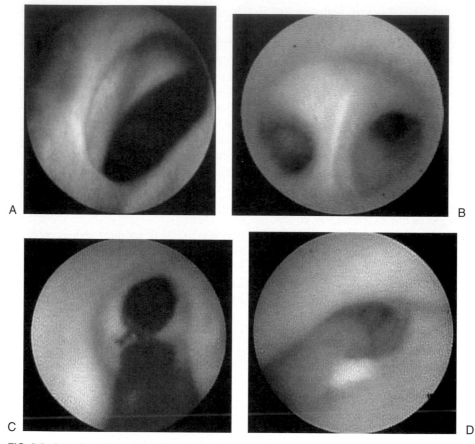

FIG. 3.8. Intraductal images through the mammary ductoscope. **A:** Normal duct. **B:** Duct bifurcation. **C:** Bloody discharge. **D:** Intraductal papilloma.

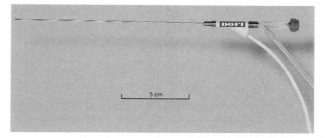

FIG. 3.9. The mammary ductoscope produced by DOFI (now Acueity, Larkspur, CA).

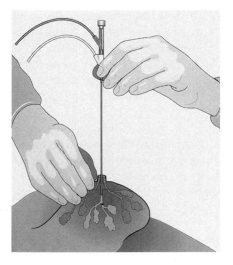

FIG. 3.10. Representation of the mammary ductoscopy technique.

earliest feasibility studies utilized mastectomy specimens and the 1.2-mm prototype ductoscope by Acueity (Larkspur, CA) (79). Visualization into the proximal ducts was possible in 81% of specimens, whereas successful ductoscopy into the distal ducts and bifurcations occurred in 52%. The same study demonstrated a 100% success rate for mammary ductoscopy in specimens with nipple discharge. Since this study, a phase 1 clinical trial of more than 30 patients with pathologic nipple discharge was conducted using either a 0.9-mm or 1.2-mm ductoscope with a working channel. In the operating room, at the time of duct excision, mammary ductoscopy was able to visualize an intraductal abnormality in 90% of the patients (Fig. 3.10). Ductoscopy successfully revealed the intraductal abnormality in six patients in whom preoperative ductography was unsuccessful or failed to identify the lesion. Synchronous, unsuspected deep lesions also were identified during ductoscopy; these likely would have been missed using standard duct excision. Mammary ductoscopy may limit the extent of surgery necessary to excise intraductal pathology, as well as more accurately identifying the lesions to be removed. Although no adverse affects were seen with ductoscopy-assisted duct excision, more studies and longer follow-up are needed to show a decrease in complication rates and preserved breast-feeding ability over standard surgical technique. As technical advances are made, the possibility of removal and treatment of intraductal pathology is on the horizon.

FOLLOW-UP

Carcinoma of the ipsilateral breast following duct excision has been reported in a number of series (3,23,68,80). Many of these patients were found to have benign disease or no pathologic diagnosis at the original surgery. In these cases, it is likely that the lesion causing the discharge was not removed during the first procedure.

These cancers typically present as masses rather than recurrent nipple discharge because of the interruption of the ductal system at the time of the original duct excision. For patients with nipple discharge in whom pathology was not found at duct excision and for patients with peripheral papillomas, close follow-up is essential. Patients undergoing breast conservation who have *in situ* carcinomas as the cause of their nipple discharge also should have postoperative radiation therapy and close mammographic and clinical follow-up (68).

Nipple discharge, in most patients with this symptom, is a physiologic discharge that usually does not require further evaluation. Spontaneous, clear or bloody, single-duct discharge needs a workup, and most of these patients need surgery to rule out carcinoma. Advances in technology and the ability to access the ductal system allow for more options in the diagnosis and treatment of nipple discharge and other intra-ductal pathology.

REFERENCES

1. Haagensen DD. *Diseases of the breast,* 2nd ed. Philadelphia: WB Saunders, 1971;102–104.
2. Devitt JE. Management of nipple discharge by clinical findings. *Am J Surg* 1985;149:789–792.
3. Chaudary M, Millis R, Davies G, Hayward JL. Nipple discharge: the diagnostic value of testing for occult blood. *Ann Surg* 1982;196:651–655.
4. GoodsonWH, King EB. Discharges and secretions of the nipple. In: Bland KI, Copeland EM, eds. *The breast: comprehensive management of benign and malignant diseases,* 2nd ed. Philadelphia: WB Saunders, 1998:51–74.
5. Petrakis NL, Mason L, Lee R. Association of race, age, menopausal status, and cerumen type with breast fluid secretion in nonlactating women as determined by nipple aspiration. *J Natl Cancer Inst* 1975;54:829–834.
6. Wynder EL, Lahti H, Laakso K et al. Nipple aspirates of breast fluid and the epidemiology of breast disease. *Cancer* 1958;56:1473–1478.
7. Sartorius OW, Smith HS, Morris P, et al. Cytological evaluation of breast fluid in the detection of breast diseases. *J Natl Cancer Inst* 1977;59:1073–1080.
8. Sauter ER, Daly M, Linahan K, et al. Prostate-specific antigen levels in nipple aspirate fluid correlate with breast cancer risk. *Cancer Epidemiol Biomarkers Prev* 1996;5:967–970.
9. King EB, Chew KC, Petrakis NL, et al. Nipple aspirate cytology for the study of breast cancer precursors. *J Natl Cancer Inst* 1983;71:1115–1121.
10. Wrensch MR, Petrakis NL, Gruenke LD, et al. Factors associate with obtaining nipple aspirate fluid: analysis of 1428 women and literature review *Breast Cancer Res Treat* 1990;15:39–51
11. Petrakis NL. Physiologic, biochemical, and cytologic aspects of nipple aspirate fluid. *Breast Cancer Res Treat* 1986;8:7–19.
12. Petrakis NL, Lee RE, Miike R, et al. Coloration of breast fluid related to concentration of cholesterol, cholesterol epoxides, estrogens and lipid peroxides. *Am J Clin Pathol* 1988;89:117–120.
13. Papanicolaou GN, Bader GM, Holmquist DG. Exfoliative cytology of the human mammary gland and its value in the diagnosis of cancer and other diseases of the breast. *Cancer* 1958;11:337–409.
14. King EB, Barrett D, King MC, Petrakis NL. Cellular composition of the nipple aspirate specimen of breast fluid: the benign cells. *Am J Clin Pathol* 1975;64:728–738.
15. Leis HP Jr. Management of nipple discharge. *World J Surg* 1989;13:736–742.
16. Ciatto S, Bravetti, P, Cariaggi P. Significance of nipple discharge clinical patterns in selection of cases for cytologic examination. *Acta Cytol* 1986;30:17–20.
17. Tabar L, Dean PB, Pentek Z. Galactography: the diagnostic procedure of choice for nipple discharge. *Radiology* 1983;149:31–38.
18. DiPietro S, Coopmans D, Bergonzi S, et al. Nipple discharge as a sign of preneoplastic lesion and occult carcinoma of the breast: clinical and galactographic study in 103 consecutive patients. *Tumori* 1979;65:317–324.

19. Kindermann G, Paterok E, Weishaar J, et al. Early detection of ductal breast cancer: the diagnostic procedure for pathologic discharge from the nipple. *Tumori* 1979;65:555–562.
20. Dawes LG, Bowen C, Luz VA, et al. Ductography for nipple discharge: no replacement for ductal excision. *Surgery* 1998;124:685–691.
21. Paterok EM, Rosenthal H, Sabel M. Nipple discharge and abnormal galactogram: results of a long-term study (1964–1990). *Eur J Obstet Gynecol Reprod Biol* 1993;50:227–234.
22. Copeland M, Higgins T. Significance of discharge from the nipple in nonpuerperal mammary conditions. *Ann Surg* 1960;151: 638–648.
23. Carty NJ, Mudan SS, Ravichandran D, et al. Prospective study of outcome in women presenting with nipple discharge. *Ann R Coll Surg Engl* 1994;76:387–389.
24. Gulay H, Bora S, Kilicturgay S, et al. Management of nipple discharge. *J Am Coll Surg* 1994;178: 471–474.
25. Arnold G, Neiheisel M. A comprehensive approach to evaluating nipple discharge. *The Nurse Practitioner* 1997;22:96–111.
26. Newman HF, Klein M, Northrup JD, et al. Nipple discharge: frequency and pathogenesis in an ambulatory population. *NY State J Med* 1983;83:928–935.
27. Zuska JJ, Crile G Jr, Ayres WW. Fistulas of lactiferous ducts. *Am J Surg* 1951;81:312–317.
28. Fiorica JV. Nipple discharge. *Obstet Gynecol Clin North Am* 1994;21:453–460.
29. Dixon JM, Anderson TJ, Lumsden AB, et al. Mammary duct ectasia. *Br J Surg* 1983;70:601–603.
30. Lafreniere R. Bloody nipple discharge during pregnancy and /or lactation: a rational for conservative treatment. *J Surg Oncol* 1990;43:228–230.
31. Kline TS, Lash SR. The bleeding nipple of pregnancy and postpartum period: a cytologic and histologic study. *Acta Cytol* 1964;8:336–340.
32. Heyman RB, Rauh JL. Areolar gland discharge in adolescent females. *J Adolesc Health* 1983;4: 285–286.
33. Cutuli B, Dilhuydy JM, DeLaFontan B, et al. Ductal carcinoma in-situ in the male breast: analysis of 31 cases. *Eur J Cancer* 1997;33:35–38.
34. Bauer RL, Eckhert KH Jr, Nemoto T. Ductal carcinoma in situ-associated nipple discharge: a clinical marker for locally extensive disease. *Ann Surg Oncol* 1998;5:452–455.
35. Cardenosa G, Eklund GW. Benign papillary neoplasms of the breast: mammographic findings. *Radiology* 1991;181:751–755.
36. Carter D. Intraductal papillary tumors of the breast. *Cancer* 1977;39:1689–1692.
37. Ohuchi N, Abe R, Kasai M. Possible cancerous change of intraductal pappilloma of the breast. *Cancer* 1984;54:605–611.
38. Wellings SR, Jensen HM, Marcum RG. An atlas of subgross pathology of human breast with special reference to possible precancerous lesions. *J Natl Cancer Inst* 1975;55:231–273.
39. Fung A, Rayter Z, Fisher C, et al. Preoperative cytology and mammography in patients with single-duct nipple discharge treated by surgery. *Br J Surg* 1990;77:1211–1212.
40. Yoshimoto M, Kasumi F, Iwase T, et al. Magnetic resonance galactography for a patient with nipple discharge. *Breast Cancer Res Treat* 1997;42:87–90.
41. Teboul M. A new concept in breast investigation: echo-histological acino-ductal analysis or analytic echography. *Biomed Pharmacother* 1988;42:289–296.
42. Feige C. Dynamic morpho-cyto-echography and the echographic galactoscopy endoductal sample: intrinsic and extrinsic markers in the detection of breast cancers. *Ultrasound Med Biol* 1988;14: 97–108.
43. Chung SY, Lee KW, Park KS, Bae SH. Breast tumors associated with nipple discharge: correlation of findings on galactography and sonography. *Clin Imaging* 1995;19:165–171.
44. Cilotti A, Campassi C, Bagnlesi P, et al. Pathologic nipple discharge: high resolution versus conventional ultrasound in the evaluation of ductal disease. *Breast Disease* 1996;9:1–13.
45. Sardanelli F, Imperiale A, Zandrino F, et al. Breast intraductal masses: ultrasound guided fine needle aspiration after galactography. *Radiology* 1997;204:143–148.
46. Seltzer MH, Perloff LJ, Kelley RI, Fitts WT Jr. The significance of age in patients with nipple discharge. *Surg Gynecol Obstet* 1970;131:519–522.
47. Takeda T, Matsui A, SatoY, et al. Nipple discharge cytology in mass screening for breast cancer. *Acta Cytol* 1990;34:161–164.
48. Dunn JM, Lucarotti E, Wood SJ, et al. Exfoliative cytology in the diagnosis of breast disease. *Br J Surg* 1995;82:789–791.

49. Florio M, Manganaro T, Pollicino A, et al. Surgical approach to nipple discharge a ten-year experience. *J Surg Oncol* 1999;71:235–238.
50. Knight DC, Lowell D, Heimann A, et al. Aspiration of the breast and nipple discharge cytology. *Surg Gynecol Obstet* 1986;163:415–420.
51. Ranieri E, Virno F, D'Andrea M, et al. The role of cytology in differentiation of breast lesions *Anticancer Res* 1955;15:607–612.
52. Kawamoto M. Breast cancer diagnosis by lactate dehydrogenase isoenzymes in nipple discharge. *Cancer* 1994;73:1836–1841.
53. Imayama IS, Mori M, Ueo H, et al. Presence of elevated carcinoembryonic antigen on absorbent disks applied to nipple area of breast cancer patients. *Cancer* 1996;78:12229–12234.
54. Inaji H, Yayoi E, Maeura Y, et al. Carcinoembryonic antigen estimation in nipple discharge an adjunctive tool in the diagnosis of early breast cancer. *Cancer* 1987;60:3008–3013.
55. Nishiguchi T, Hishimoto T, Funahashi S, et al. Clinical usefulness of carcinoembryonic antigen measurement in nipple discharge as an adjunctive tool for diagnosis of breast cancer. *Jpn J Clin Pathol* 1992;40:67–72.
56. Fortova L, Garber JE, Sadowsky NL, et al. Carcinoembryonic antigen in breast nipple aspirate fluid. *Cancer Epidemiol Biomarkers Prev* 1998;7:195–198.
57. Liu Y, Wang JL, Chang H, et al. Breast-cancer diagnosis with nipple fluid bFGF [Letter]. *Lancet* 2000;356:567.
58. Baker KS, Davey DD, Stelling CB. Ductal abnormalities detected with galactography: frequency of adequate excisional biopsy. *Am J Roentgenol* 1994;162:821–824.
59. Ciatto S, Bravetti P, Berni D, et al. The role of galactography in the detection of breast cancer. *Tumori* 1988;74:177–181.
60. Rongione AJ, Evans BD, Kling KM, et al. Ductography is a useful technique in evaluation of abnormal nipple discharge. *Am Surg* 1996;62:785–788.
61. Van Zee KJ, Perez GO, Minnard E, et al. Preoperative ductography increases the diagnostic yield of major duct excision for nipple discharge. *Cancer* 1998;82:1874–1880.
62. Cardenosa G, Doudna C, Eklund GW. Ductography of the breast: techniques and findings. *Am J Roentgenol* 1994;162:1081–1087.
63. Saarela AO, Kiviniemi HO, Rissanen TJ. Preoperative methylene blue staining of galactographically suspicious breast lesions. *Int Surg* 1997;82:403–405.
64. Hussain S, Lui DM. Ultrasound guided percutaneous galactography. *Eur J Radiol* 1997;24:163–165.
65. Urban JA. Excision of the major duct system of the breast. *Cancer* 1963;16:516–520.
66. Srivastava A, Griwan MS, Samaiyar SS, et al. A safe technique of major mammary duct excision. *J R Coll Surg Edinb* 1995;40:35–37.
67. Jardines L. Management of nipple discharge. *Am Surg* 1996;62:119–122.
68. Bauer RL, Eckhert KH Jr, Nemoto T. Ductal carcinoma in situ-associated nipple discharge: a clinical marker for locally extensive disease. *Ann Surg Oncol* 1998;5:452–455.
69. Solin LJ, Recht A, Fourquet A, et al. Ten-year results of breast-conserving surgery and definitive irradiation for intraductal carcinoma of the breast. *Cancer*1991;68:2337–2344.
70. Fowable BL, Solin LJ, Goodman RL. Results of conservative surgery and radiation for intraductal noninvasive breast cancer *Am J Clin Oncol* 1987:10:110–111.
71. Recht A, Danoff B, Solin LJ, et al. Intraductal carcinoma of the breast: results of treatment with excisional biopsy and radiation. *J Clin Oncol* 1985;3:1339–1343.
72. Ito Y, Tamaki Y, Nakano Y, et al. Nonpalpable breast cancer with nipple discharge: how should it be treated? *Anticancer Res* 1997;17:791–794.
73. Tan W, Lim T C. Transareolar dye-injection microdochectomy. *Am Surg* 1992;58:404–408.
75. Okazaki A, Hirata K, Okazaki M, et al. Nipple discharge disorders: current diagnostic management and the role of fiber-ductoscopy. *Eur Radiol* 1999;9:583–590.
75. Love S, Barsky S. Breast duct endoscopy to study stages of cancerous breast disease. *Lancet* 1996; 348:997–999.
76. Berna J, Garcia-Medina V, Kuni C. Ductoscopy: a new technique for ductal exploration. *Eur J Radiol* 1991;12:127–129.
77. Makita M, Sakamoto G, Akiyama F, et al. Duct endoscopy and endoscopic biopsy in the evaluation of nipple discharge. *Breast Cancer Res Treat* 1991;18:179–188.
78. Okazaki A, Okazaki M, Asishi K, et al. Fiberoptic ductoscopy of the breast: a new diagnostic procedure for nipple discharge. *Jpn J Clin Oncol* 1991;21:188–193.
79. Dietz JR, Kim JA, Malycky JL, et al. Feasibility and technical considerations of mammary ductoscopy in human mastectomy specimens. *The Breast Journal* 2000; 6: (3)161–165.
80. Urban JA, Egeli RA. Nonlactational nipple discharge. *CA Cancer J Clin* 1978;28:131–140.

4

Mastalgia

Deborah N. Ader

Epidemiologic and clinical research consistently show that 60% to 70% of women experience some degree of breast pain (1–5). Articles and book chapters on mastalgia (or *mastodynia*, as it is sometimes called) are virtually unanimous in stating that pain is the most common breast-related presenting complaint in primary care or specialty clinics. Appropriate assessment of these complaints will reveal that most are unrelated to serious pathology and insufficiently severe to require treatment. Paradoxically, however, it is also true that most women with moderately severe to severe mastalgia do not present with this complaint and may reveal it only when directly asked (2–6). Mastalgia can be a significant source of anxiety, discomfort, and disruption of normal activities, and relationships (2,7–11). In addition, elevated use of mammography has been reported among young women with mastalgia (2,3, 6,12).

This chapter presents an overview of mastalgia, including a brief summary of the state of knowledge about its prevalence and etiology. Based on the literature, recommendations for assessment and discussion of treatment options are presented. In addition, despite the relative dearth of research into psychological, behavioral, or social factors in mastalgia, relevant biopsychosocial issues are raised. Cyclical mastalgia is emphasized because it is by far the most prevalent form of mastalgia and has received more research and clinical attention in the literature than the varieties of noncyclic mastalgia.

CATEGORIES OF MASTALGIA

Cyclic Mastalgia

Cyclic mastalgia (CM) is characterized by its relationship to the menstrual cycle, usually beginning 2 to 14 days before onset of menses and remitting at or within 2 to 3 days of onset of menses. Minor discomfort lasting a few days premenstrually is both common and mild enough to be considered normal; however, some women experience significant pain and tenderness lasting 5 to 14 days or longer each month. This pain can be (but is not necessarily) accompanied by swelling; in some women, bra cup increases by one to two sizes during each episode (13). The pain is most commonly reported in the upper and outer quadrants of the breasts and can be unilateral or bilateral. By definition, cyclical mastalgia occurs only in premenopausal women and ends at menopause. Onset can occur at any age. A recent study of 120

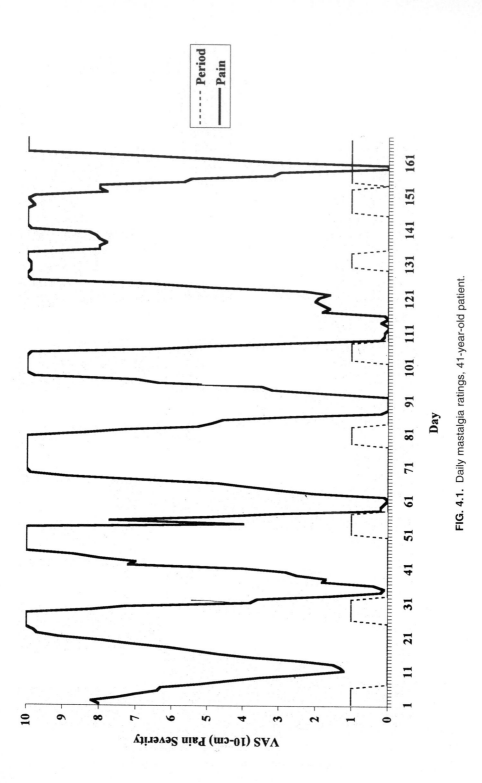

FIG. 4.1. Daily mastalgia ratings, 41-year-old patient.

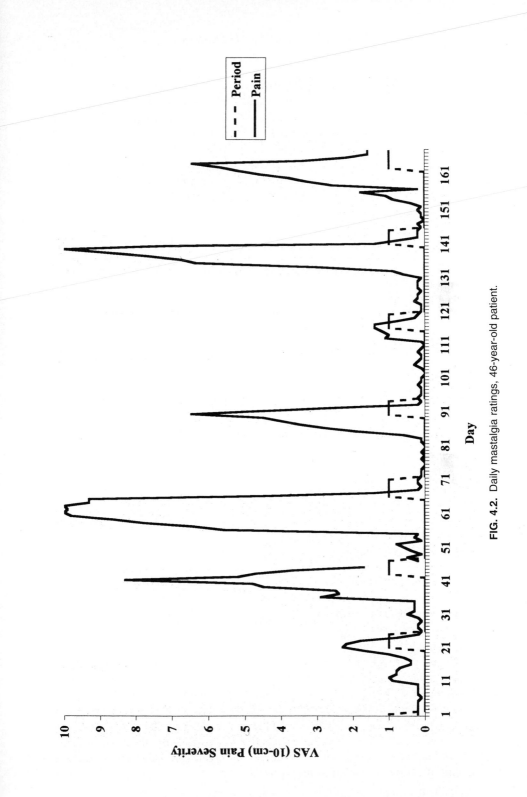

FIG. 4.2. Daily mastalgia ratings, 46-year-old patient.

patients with severe cyclical mastalgia found a median onset age of 34 years (range, 12–51 years) (10). Younger age at onset is associated with a prolonged course (10, 14). Most women experience pain for at least 5 years; in a combined group of women with CM and non-CM, median duration was 12 years (range, 1 month to 38 years) (10). Severity of mastalgia appears to increase with age (5,14).

Studies in which women chart their breast pain daily for several months have demonstrated variability in the severity of the condition from month to month (15); to date, no research has investigated why mastalgia is severe and prolonged in some cycles and not in others. Figures 4.1 and 4.2 show the pattern of breast pain for two participants in a 6-month daily prospective study of mastalgia (15).

Noncyclic Mastalgia

About a third of mastalgia overall, and 6% to 10% of severe mastalgia, is unrelated to the menstrual cycle (14,16,17). The pain can be constant or intermittent, unilateral or bilateral and located anywhere in the breast. Women with non-CM tend to be older, on average, than women with CM, with pain onset common in the thirties and forties (e.g., one study reported a median onset of 41 years; range, 19–63 years, in a sample of 55 women with non-CM) (10). One of the most common forms of non-CM is not true breast pain at all but chest-wall pain.

ETIOLOGICAL FACTORS AND ASSOCIATED DISORDERS

Hormones

Sex hormones are almost certain to play some role in producing cyclical mastalgia. Hyperestrogenism has been proposed, but research has failed to demonstrate consistently any abnormality in circulating estrogen levels or in relative estrogen levels as a result of impaired progesterone secretion (18–21); however, elevated levels of the estrogen-induced protein pS2 have been found in the breast secretions of women with severe CM (22).

Basal prolactin levels are generally normal in women with mastalgia (18,19,23); however, some researchers have demonstrated prolactin hyperresponsiveness to stimulation with thyrotropin-releasing hormone (TRH), at least in a subset of women with cyclical mastalgia (7,19,23,24).

Some researchers have suggested that normal levels of sex hormones may have elevated activity in women with CM (22,23,25). Suggested mechanisms have included abnormalities of fatty acid metabolism (25), abnormal levels of sex hormone binding globulin, or increased tissue sensitivity to prolactin (23). Mastalgia is common among women with diets high in fat, especially saturated fat (13, 26,27). Women with CM have been found to have elevated levels of saturated fatty acids and low levels of polyunsaturated essential fatty acids (EFAs), particularly the n-6 fatty acids (25). These fatty acids bind to estrogen receptor sites; decreased levels may increase the amount of estrogen binding in breast tissue.

Non-CM is most often of unknown etiology; however, in a number of cases, the pain is actually musculoskeletal in origin. Other identifiable causes of non-CM include injury or trauma, sclerosing adenosis, duct ectasia, and cysts. In addition, mastalgia is a frequent effect of hormone replacement therapy (HRT). Otherwise, there is no known hormonal etiology in this form of breast pain.

Cancer

Clinically, it is widely believed that little or no relationship exists between mastalgia and cancer. Otherwise undetected cancer or precancerous changes, however, have been reported in 7% to 11% of cases in which breast pain was the only complaint (4,28). It is not clear whether subclinical or early cancer causes the pain, but this possibility cannot be ruled out. Equally important, from a public health point of view, is the possibility that a long-term history of mastalgia is associated with elevated risk for developing breast cancer. A small but growing body of research suggests this relationship may exist.

Women with CM may be more likely to develop fibrocystic changes than those without CM (29,30), and it has been established that some fibrocystic changes (i.e., atypical ductal hyperplasia) are associated with significantly increased risk for developing breast cancer (31–34). Increased risk of cancer or fibroadenoma has been reported in women with a history of premenstrual breast pain or swelling (35–37). A study in which women with axillary node-negative breast cancer and healthy age-matched controls prospectively recorded breast symptoms (in the noncancerous breast for cases and in the matched breast for controls) found a significantly higher prevalence of mastalgia among the cases (38). Deschamps et al. (39) found a significantly elevated risk of mammary dysplasia involving 50% or more of the breast parenchyma in women with mastalgia, with a particularly strong association between dysplasia and cyclical mastalgia in premenopausal women. Additional studies examining patterns of hormonal reactivity (40) and mammography (41) yielded results suggesting elevated breast cancer risk in women with CM.

Psychological Factors

Historically, psychological etiologies (e.g., fear of cancer, sexual or sex role conflict, neurosis) have been suggested in mastalgia (42–45). No data to support a psychogenic etiology exist, however, and systematic research into the possible contribution of psychological factors has not been conducted. Two studies found elevated anxiety and depression among women with mastalgia (9,46), but it is not possible to determine whether anxiety and depression were associated with development of mastalgia, were results of having this pain disorder, or had no causal relationship. Past references to psychogenic etiology have tended to be anecdotal and simplistic; nevertheless, psychological, social, or behavioral factors are likely to play some role in mastalgia. Such factors may affect the physiologic functions that produce the disorder, may influence whether cyclic breast changes are perceived as painful or distressing, and certainly determine whether treatment is sought.

ASSESSMENT

History and Prospective Symptom Rating

Table 4.1 lists suggested information to be obtained when taking an initial history of a patient with mastalgia. Asking patients specifically about mastalgia frequency, duration, and severity can be helpful in identifying women whose pain should be assessed further; however, retrospective reporting of pain has only low to moderate validity (47). Prospective daily rating of pain for at least 2 months, using scales such as the Cardiff Breast Pain Chart or a visual analog scale (VAS), yields more valid and reliable data than retrospective reporting (Figs. 4.3 and 4.4) (15,47). The information obtained enables the clinician to confirm whether the mastalgia is cyclic or noncyclic and can facilitate patient–physician decisions regarding the risk-to-benefit ratio of available treatment options. Daily ratings require minimal time and effort, and patients, feeling that their concerns are taken seriously, often will faithfully provide these ratings. In addition, patients who perform daily ratings over several cycles may find a spontaneous remission or improvement in symptoms or realize that their symptoms are neither prolonged nor severe enough routinely to warrant the cost, risks, and discomforts of treatment. These women usually will require no further medical attention for mastalgia (Table 4.1)

A subset of women will produce daily ratings showing moderate or severe levels of pain for several days or even weeks each month. Women who indicate that their mastalgia interferes with normal functioning require treatment. For patients who do not report interference with daily activities, recommendations regarding when treatment is warranted vary slightly in terms of the severity and monthly duration used as cutoff points. These recommendations are based on opinion more than on the systematic collection of data (e.g., who responds best to treatment, whose mastalgia is most likely to spontaneously remit). A synthesis of current practice recommendations is presented in Table 4.2.

TABLE 4.1. *Information to obtain when evaluating breast pain*

Is pain constant or intermittent? If intermittent, is it perimenstrual?
How many months/years has the pain pattern been present?
Was there any identifiable trigger or major event preceding onset of the pain (e.g., injury, surgery, pregnancy, childbirth, new medication, etc.)?
If the pain is cyclical or intermittent, how long does each episode last?
How severe is the pain?
Is the patient concerned that the pain may be related to cancer or other disease?
Is the pain sufficiently severe and prolonged to be distressing in itself, and/or to interfere with normal activities?
What medications, nutritional supplements, dietary changes, behavioral changes, or alternative therapies has the patient attempted on her own and did any seem effective?

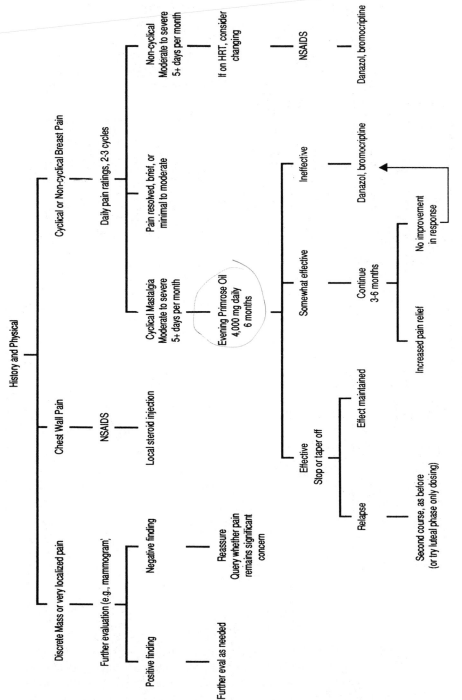

FIG. 4.3. Recommendations for managing mastalgia.

Daily   Breast   Pain   Chart

Name: _____

Record the amount of breast pain you experience each day by drawing a line at the point on the scale that best represents your pain level for the day. Please write the date for each day, the time at which you are recording your pain, and check the space under P for each day that you have your period.

DATE   TIME   P

____   ____   ___   _____

                      No Pain   Extremely Severe Pain

____   ____   ___   _____

                      No Pain   Extremely Severe Pain

____   ____   ___   _____

                      No Pain   Extremely Severe Pain

____   ____   ___   _____

                      No Pain   Extremely Severe Pain

____   ____   ___   _____

                      No Pain   Extremely Severe Pain

____   ____   ___   _____

                      No Pain   Extremely Severe Pain

____   ____   ___   _____

                      No Pain   Extremely Severe Pain

FIG. 4.4. Daily breast pain chart.

Physical Examination

A complete breast examination should be done to rule out the presence of other breast disorders. Women with non-CM should be examined carefully to determine whether the pain is true breast pain or musculoskeletal in origin. With the patient lying on her side, the breast can be moved away from the chest wall, and tenderness beneath the breast at midchest can be assessed to determine whether costochondritis

TABLE 4.2. *Criteria for considering treatment of mastalgia*

Significant disruption of normal functioning results and/or
Pain is moderate to severe *and*
Has been present for **at least** 6 months *and*
Lasts at least 5–7 days each month *and*
Other disorders requiring further evaluation or treatment have been
ruled out

is the true source of pain (48). Lateral chest-wall pain should be assessed using palpation, especially just below the axilla (49).

Mammography should be considered for appropriate candidates. Many patients are concerned more about the possibility that the pain may be associated with breast cancer than they are bothered by the pain itself and may be seeking reassurance that they do not have cancer. Research indicates, however, that mammography is over-used in women with mastalgia. In an obstetric/gynecologic clinic sample, 18% of young women (i.e., younger than 36 years) with recent symptoms and 32% of young women with recent severe levels of CM reported having had a mammogram (compared with 7% of asymptomatic women) (2). Similar overuse of mammography, especially in young women with mastalgia, was demonstrated in breast clinic patients and in an epidemiologic sample as well (3,6,12). Duijm et al. found mastalgia alone to be the reason for mammography in 15% of their sample of 6,864 women undergoing mammography and found few radiologic abnormalities associated with the mastalgia (50). These researchers suggest that there is little diagnostic value in ordering mammograms for women whose only breast symptom or sign is pain. Whereas many patients may be seeking reassurance that their mastalgia does not indicate cancer, the use of mammography to provide such reassurance in young women (assuming mastalgia and care-seeking are the only reasons for ordering the mammogram) is not recommended. Indeed, Britain's Royal College of Radiologists specifically states that mammography is not indicated for mastalgia (51).

Breast examination may reveal cysts and nodules or fibrocystic changes. Although physicians commonly tell women with complaints of breast pain that their pain is a result of fibrocystic changes or "fibrocystic disease," (2) the evidence does not support that causal relationship, especially with CM (29). Most women develop fibrocystic breast changes, but only a subset will develop severe mastalgia. In some cases, one or more discrete, painful cysts can be identified, and aspiration of these cysts may provide relief (52). About 50% of CM cases exist without associated fibrocystic changes, and, conversely, women with cysts can be asymptomatic (8,30, 53–58). Studies are inconsistent in their results regarding the relationship between the mammographic, endocrinologic, or histologic findings associated with fibrocysts and a pattern of mastalgia (7,42,59,60). On the other hand, as mentioned, there is some evidence that CM is associated with elevated risk for fibrocystic changes (29, 30). Researchers have alternately suggested that cyclical breast changes associated with pain may lead to development of fibrocysts or that fibrocysts and pain are different, albeit often coexisting, factors in benign breast disorders (7,43).

Premenstrual Syndrome

Mastalgia is a common symptom of premenstrual syndrome (PMS), and women with clinically significant breast pain are more likely than those without CM to have other somatic and affective symptoms that vary with the menstrual cycle (6,15). Most women with CM, however, do not meet diagnostic criteria for PMS (15). CM may differ from PMS not only in its presentation but also in aspects of its etiology and in effective treatment approaches. Thus, simply labeling the mastalgia as PMS is not helpful to the patient. Nevertheless, assessing for PMS or referring the patient to a practitioner with expertise in PMS evaluation and treatment may be indicated when a history reveals multiple complaints and possible mood disturbance.

TREATMENT

About 10% to 18% of women with breast pain have symptoms of a severity and duration that warrant treatment (1,2,61). These women are significantly more likely to ask a physician about their pain and to raise this issue at multiple visits than are women with lower levels of CM (2).

Numerous interventions have been tried for CM, with varying results. The most common is simply reassurance that the patient does not have any malignancy; in many cases, patients request no further treatment (1,61–64). In addition, wearing a fitted support bra can provide substantial relief (65). The disorder shows a relatively high rate of responding to placebo, ranging from 19% to 30% (1,66), at least in the initial month or two of treatment. Thus, treatment claims derived from uncontrolled studies must be interpreted with caution.

Patients are often counseled to reduce or eliminate consumption of methylxanthines (e.g., coffee, chocolate), with mixed results (54,59,67,68). Reducing dietary fat appears to help some patients (13,67). Some studies report useful effects of vitamin A (69,70), vitamin B_6 (63), vitamin E (16), and beta carotene (71); unfortunately, these trials were not adequately controlled. Placebo-controlled trials failed to find significant treatment effects for vitamin B_6 (72) or vitamin E (73). Although diuretics are often recommended, or tried independently by CM sufferers (2), little evidence substantiates the effectiveness of this approach. Preece and colleagues showed that mastalgia is unrelated to total body water (74). Over-the-counter analgesics and nonsteroidal antiinflammatory medications are not generally useful in women with true breast pain, but they may be helpful in some cases of chest-wall pain. Severe cases of chest-wall pain may require the injection of steroids. Some success was reported with the use of topical nonsteroidal antiinflammatory gel for diffuse chest-wall pain (75).

Suggesting caffeine reduction or elimination and dietary changes to patients who have not independently attempted these changes is a worthwhile first line of intervention that involves little cost or risk. These recommendations should be presented in a realistic manner, however. For example, the patient could be told "some women find that reducing caffeine or reducing fat intake is helpful; would you be willing to give it a try for several months and see how you feel?'' This approach is preferable to strong directives, given the weakness of the empirical support for these measures.

Figure 4.5 is a chart showing the most common results of an initial history and physical and listing suggested treatment approaches for chest-wall pain, CM, and non-CM. Obtaining daily pain ratings is not essential but is highly recommended for the reasons discussed already. Use of a support bra and dietary changes can (and probably should) be attempted before medication is prescribed. No systematic studies on modifying or eliminating hormone replacement therapy (HRT) with regard to mastalgia have been reported, and so any decisions about altering HRT because of significant non-CM should be considered with careful attention to the risks and benefits in each case. Details regarding the medications suggested for mastalgia are discussed below and summarized in Table 4.3.

Mastalgia often persists or recurs for many years, necessitating multiple courses of treatment or switching from one treatment to another. Another suggested approach has been to maintain chronically relapsing patients on a continuous low-dose regimen (10); however, no studies of this approach have been reported.

Hormonal Therapies

Danazol, bromocriptine, and tamoxifen have been shown in double-blind, controlled studies to be effective in treating cyclical mastalgia; danazol is currently the only medication that is approved by the U.S. Food and Drug Administration for this indication. The sample size, study design, dosages used, and treatment duration in controlled trials are shown in Table 4.3. In all trials, the tested therapy was significantly better than placebo in reducing mastalgia. Danazol produced a useful response (usually defined as at least a 50% reduction in pain) in 60% to 80% of patients, bromocriptine in about 50% to 65%, and tamoxifen in 70% to 90%. Unfortunately, nontrivial adverse effects and risks are associated with all three medications, and relapse occurs in many or most patients within several months of terminating treatment (21,55,60,76–86). The most common adverse effects are listed in Table 4.4. Rea and colleagues found that women with CM whose prolactin response to TRH was elevated (i.e., at least triple the upper normal limit) were significantly more likely to show improvement or remission of mastalgia when treated with bromocriptine than women whose prolactin response was normal. These researchers suggested testing prolactin response to TRH injection to determine whether bromocriptine is the best treatment (23) (Tables 4.3 and 4.4).

Although non-CM is not known to have a hormonal component, many women with this disorder do respond well to treatment with danazol, bromocriptine, or tamoxifen, albeit at a significantly lower rate than women with CM (49,84,87,88)

Treatment of mastalgia has been attempted with other hormonal agents as well as those already listed, including norethisterone; progesterone (oral, vaginal, or topical) (89–91), lynestrenol (92), gestrinone (93,94), buserelin (95), goserelin (96), thyroid hormone (97), testosterone (98), and oral contraceptives, with some success. Much

DAILY BREAST PAIN CHART

Date Chart Issued [ ][ ][ ]   D/M/Y

Patient Number [ ][ ][ ][ ]

Patient Initials [ ][ ]

Please record the amount of breast pain you experience each day by shading in each box as illustrated

■ Severe pain

◧ Mild/moderate pain

⊡ No pain

For example:- If you get severe breast pain on the fifth of the month, then shade in completely the square under 5.

Please note the date your period starts each month with the letter 'P'.

Day of Month

Month	1	2	3	4	5	6	7	8	9	10	11	12	13	14	15	16	17	18	19	20	21	22	23	24	25	26	27	28	29	30	31

PLEASE BRING THIS CARD WITH YOU ON EACH VISIT

FIG. 4.5. Daily breast pain chart.

TABLE 4.3. *Double-blind, placebo-controlled studies of pharmacotherapy for cyclical mastalgia*

Author(s), year (reference no.)	n	Design	Months	(mg)/day
Danazol				
Dhont et al., 1979 (106)	25	2	2	400
Mansel et al., 1982 (78)	28	1	3	200
Doberl et al., 1984 (55)	30	2	6	100–200
Gorins et al., 1984 (107)	38	1	3	400
Hinton et al., 1986 (104)	21	2	3	300
Ramsey, 1988 (77)	80	2	3	400
Kontostolis et al., 1997 (86)	61	2	6	200
Bromocriptine				
Mansel et al., 1978 (101)	29	1	6	5
Blichert-Toft et al., 1979 (102)	10	1	2	2.5–5.0
Durning and Sellwood, 1982 (103)	38	1	2	1.25–5.0
Parlati et al., 1988 (19)	26	2	3	2.5–7.5
Hinton et al., 1986 (104)	19	2	3	5.0
Dogliotti and Mansel, 1989 (60)	272	2	3–6	5.0
Nazli et al., 1989 (105)	50	1	3–6	2.5–7.5
Tamoxifen				
Fentiman et al., 1986 (84)	60	1	3	20
Messinis and Lolis, 1988 (85)	36	2	6	10
Kontostolis et al., 1997 (86)	61	2	6	10
Grio et al., 1998 (108)	88	2	—	10
Evening primrose oil				
Preece et al., 1982 (109)	41	1	3–6	3,000
Pye et al., 1985 (110)	46	2	4	4,000
Gateley et al., 1992 (99)	36	2	2–4	4,000

1, crossover design; 2, parallel design.

TABLE 4.4. *Common adverse effects of therapeutic agents for mastalgia*

Danazol, 30%–100%
    Menstrual irregularities   Acne
    Bloating   Nausea
    Weight gain   Hot flashes
    Depression   Malaise
    Decreased voice pitch   Muscle cramps
Bromocriptine, 35%–70%
    Dizziness   Vomiting
    Nausea   General malaise
Tamoxifen, 26%–42%
    Hot flashes   Vaginal discharge
    Menorrhagia   Nausea
    General malaise   Urticaria
    Alopecia   Weight gain
    Depression/irritability

of this literature suffers from methodologic problems, however, most notably the absence of placebo-control groups. Most findings in controlled research with these agents do not indicate a significant benefit over placebo (gestrinone and vaginal progesterone, however, were each effective in one well-controlled study and were tolerated well by patients) (90,93). One study compared the prevalence of mastalgia between 346 women using parenteral progesterones for contraception with 1,150 age-matched controls. The women using Depo-Provera had significantly less cyclical mastalgia than the controls, and it decreased significantly over time with continued use of the contraceptive. Although not a treatment trial per se, this study suggests parenteral progesterones should be investigated further as a potentially effective treatment for cyclical mastalgia (5).

Evening Primrose Oil

Evening primrose oil (EPO), extracted from the seeds of *Oenothera biennis*, is a source of the EFA gamma-linolenic acid, a precursor of prostaglandin E_1. Although the mechanism of action of EPO has not been established, research with this agent and from studies using antiestrogens strongly implicate fatty acids in this disorder (25,67,99). It has been suggested that low levels of n-6 EFAs may result in an exaggerated effect of normal levels of hormone and that supplementation with EFAs may return reactivity to normal levels (25).

Goodwin et al. (67), in a review of therapies for CM, categorized EPO as a "definitely effective" treatment. Information from three double-blind, placebo-controlled trials of EPO is shown in Table 4.3. Studies suggest that EPO produces a useful clinical response in 44% to 59% of patients. In Britain, EPO is one of the most widely prescribed therapeutic agents for mastalgia (100). EPO has not been systematically evaluated in the United States, where it is available over-the-counter as a nutritional supplement. EPO has a slower, less dramatic effect than the antiestrogens, but a virtual absence of adverse effects and serious risks make it an attractive alternative to hormonal therapies. As with other therapies, relapse eventually occurs in most patients after treatment is terminated.

CONCLUSION

Mastalgia has been under-recognized, under-researched, and under-treated in the United States, and it presents a challenge to both clinicians and scientists. Adequate evaluation, in addition to a basic history and physical examination, should include asking the patient to make prospective daily ratings of the pain for at least two or three cycles to establish its timing, duration, and severity. This type of evaluation is likely to allay anxiety in many cases and will identify patients with severe mastalgia warranting therapy. If behavioral measures such as wearing a well-fitting support bra and decreasing methylxanthine and fat consumption fail to alleviate symptoms, the patient can be offered EPO or danazol as a treatment option or antiinflammatory steroid injection for costochondritis. The availability of well-designed, placebo-controlled trials supporting the use of EPO is limited, and the cost of this nutritional supplement, which health insurance will not defray, is substantial. Danazol is well established as an effective treatment and may be less expensive for women with health insurance, but it has significant adverse effects. There remains a need for further systematic study of the mastalgias and for development of more effective, lower-risk treatment options.

REFERENCES

1. Gateley CA, Mansel RE. Management of cyclical breast pain. *British Journal of Hospital Medicine* 1990;43:330–332.
2. Ader DN, Browne MW. Prevalence and impact of cyclical mastalgia in a U.S. clinic-based sample. *Am J Obstet Gynecol* 1997;177:126–132.
3. Ader DN, Shriver CD. Cyclical mastalgia: prevalence and impact in an outpatient breast clinic sample. *J Am Coll Surg* 1997;185:466–470.
4. Bejanga BI, Marcus E, Djukom CD, et al. How confounding are breast pain confounders? *J R Coll Surg Edinb* 1997;42:386–388.
5. Euhus DM, Uyehara C. Influence of parenteral progesterones on the prevalence and severity of mastalgia in premenopausal women: a multi-institutional cross-sectional study. *J Am Coll Surg* 1997;184:596–604.
6. Goodwin PJ, Miller A, Del Giudice ME, et al. Breast health and associated premenstrual symptoms in women with severe cyclic mastopathy. *Am J Obstet Gynecol* 1997;176:998–1005.
7. Ayers JW, Gidwani GP. The "luteal breast": hormonal and sonographic investigation of benign breast disease in patients with cyclic mastalgia. *Fertil Steril* 1983;40:779–784.
8. Rasmussen T, Tobiassen T. Patient characteristics and age-dependent sub-populations in severe fibrocystic breast disease: the Hjorring project. *Acta Obstet Gynecol Scand Suppl* 1984;123:151–155.
9. Ramirez AJ, Jarrett SR, Hamed H, et al. Psychosocial adjustment of women with mastalgia. *The Breast* 1995;4:48–51.
10. Davies EL, Gateley CA, Miers M, et al. The long-term course of mastalgia. *J R Soc Med* 1998;91:462–464.
11. Cheung KL. Management of cyclical mastalgia in oriental women: pioneer experience of using gamolenic acid (Efamast) in Asia. *Aust N Z J Surg* 1999;69:492–494.
12. Ader DN, South-Paul J, Adera PT, et al. Cyclical mastalgia: prevalence and associated health and behavioral factors. *J Psychosom Obstet Gynecol* 2001;22:71–81.
13. Boyd NF, McGuire V, Shannon P, et al. Effect of a low-fat high-carbohydrate diet on symptoms of cyclical mastopathy. *Lancet* 1988;2:128–132.
14. Wisbey JR, Kumar S, Mansel RE, et al. Natural history of breast pain. *Lancet* 1983;2:672–674.
15. Ader D, Shriver C, Browne M. Cyclical mastalgia: premenstrual syndrome or recurrent pain disorder? *J Psychosom Obstet Gynecol* 1999;20:198–202.
16. Khanna AK, Tapodar J, Misra MK. Spectrum of benign breast disorders in a university hospital. *J Indian Med Assoc* 1997;95:5–8.
17. BeLieu R. Mastodynia. *Obstet Gynecol Clin North Am* 1994;21:461–477.
18. Watt-Boolsen S, Eskildsen PC, Blaehr H. Release of prolactin, thyrotropin, and growth hormone in women with cyclical mastalgia and fibrocystic disease of the breast. *Cancer* 1985;56:500–502.
19. Parlati E, Travaglini A, Liberale I, et al. Hormonal profile in benign breast disease. Endocrine status of cyclical mastalgia patients. *J Endocrinol Invest* 1988;11:679–683.
20. Walsh PV, McDicken IW, Bulbrook RD, et al. Serum oestradiol-17 beta and prolactin concentrations during the luteal phase in women with benign breast disease. *Eur J Cancer Clin Oncol* 1984;20:1345–1351.
21. Gorins A, Cordray JP. Hormonal profile of benign breast disease and premenstrual mastodynia. *Eur J Gynaecol Oncol* 1984;5:1–10.
22. Harding C, Tetlow A, Howell A, et al. Target organ sensitivity. In: Mansel RE, ed. *Recent developments in the study of benign breast disease*. London: The Parthenon Publishing Group, 1997:49–58.

23. Rea N, Bove F, Gentile A, et al. Prolactin response to thyrotropin-releasing hormone as a guideline for cyclical mastalgia treatment. *Minerva Med* 1997;88:479–487.
24. Kumar S, Mansel RE, Hughes LE, et al. Prolactin response to thyrotropin-releasing hormone stimulation and dopaminergic inhibition in benign breast disease. *Cancer* 1984;53:1311–1315.
25. Horrobin DF, Manku MS. Premenstrual syndrome and premenstrual breast pain (cyclical mastalgia): disorders of essential fatty acid (EFA) metabolism. *Prostaglandins Leukot Essent Fatty Acids* 1989; 37:255–261.
26. Horrobin DF. Nutritional and medical importance of gamma-linolenic acid. *Prog Lipid Res* 1992; 31:163–194.
27. Goodwin PJ, Miller A, Del Giudice ME, et al. Elevated high-density lipoprotein cholesterol and dietary fat intake in women with cyclic mastopathy. *Am J Obstet Gynecol* 1998;179:430–437.
28. Preece PE, Baum M, Mansel RE, et al. Importance of mastalgia in operable breast cancer. *BMJ* 1982;284:1299–1300.
29. Jorgensen J, Watt BS. Cyclical mastalgia and breast pathology. *Acta Chir Scand* 1985;151:319–321.
30. Simard A, Vobecky J, Vobecky JS, et al. Case-control study of fibrocystic breast disease. *Rev Epidemiol Sante Publique* 1993;41:84–89.
31. Dupont WD, Page DL. Risk factors for breast cancer in women with proliferative breast disease. *N Engl J Med* 1985;312:146–151.
32. Hendler FJ. Breast diseases and the internist. *Am J Med Sci* 1987;293:332–347.
33. Dixon JM. Cystic disease and fibroadenoma of the breast: natural history and relation to breast cancer risk. *Br Med Bull* 1991;47:258–271.
34. Fiorica JV. Fibrocystic changes. *Obstet Gynecol Clin North Am* 1994;21:445–452.
35. Plu-Bureau G, Thalabard JC, Sitruk-Ware R, et al. Cyclical mastalgia as a marker of breast cancer susceptibility: results of a case-control study among French women. *Br J Cancer* 1992;65:945–949.
36. Sitruk WR, Thalabard JC, Benotmane A, et al. Risk factors for breast fibroadenoma in young women. *Contraception* 1989;40:251–268.
37. Wynder EL, MacCornack RA, Stellman SD. The epidemiology of breast cancer in 785 United States Caucasian women. *Cancer* 1978;41:2341–2354.
38. Goodwin PJ, De Boer G, Clark RM, et al. Cyclical mastopathy and premenopausal breast cancer risk: results of a case-control study. *Breast Cancer Res Treat* 1995;33:63–73.
39. Deschamps M, Band PR, Coldman AJ, et al. Clinical determinants of mammographic dysplasia patterns. *Cancer Detect Prev* 1996;20:610–619.
40. Rose DP, Boyar AP, Cohen C, et al. Effect of low-fat diet on hormone levels in women with cystic breast disease. I. Serum steroids and gonadotropins. *J Natl Cancer Inst* 1987;78:623–626.
41. Leinster SJ, Whitehouse GH, Walsh PV. Cyclical mastalgia: clinical and mammographic observations in a screened population. *Br J Surg* 1987;74:220–222.
42. Atkins HJB. Chronic mastitis. *Lancet* 1938;1:707–712.
43. Patey DH. Two common non-malignant conditions of the breast: the clinical features of cystic disease and the pain syndrome. *BMJ* 1949;1:96–99.
44. Preece PE, Mansel RE, Hughes LE. Mastalgia: psychoneurosis or organic disease? *BMJ* 1978;1: 29–30.
45. Ashley B. Mastalgia. *Lippincott's Primary Care Practitioner* 1998;2:189–93.
46. Downey HM, Deadman JM, Davis C, et al. Psychologic characteristics of women with cyclical mastalgia. *Breast Disease* 1993;6:99–105.
47. Tavaf-Motamen H, Ader DN, Brown MW, Shriver CD. Clinical evaluation of mastalgia. *Arch Surg* 1998;133:211–213.
48. Dixon JM. Managing breast pain. *Practitioner* 1999;243:484–486,488–489, 491.
49. Maddox PR, Harrison BJ, Mansel RE, et al. Non-cyclical mastalgia: an improved classification and treatment. *Br J Surg* 1989;76:901–904.
50. Duijm LE, Guit GL, Hendriks JH, et al. Value of breast imaging in women with painful breasts: observational follow up study. *BMJ* 1998;317:1492–1495.
51. Royal College of Physicians. *Making the best use of a Department of Clinical Radiology: guidelines for doctors*, 4th ed. London: Royal College of Radiologists, 1998.
52. DeVane GW. Breast dysfunction: galactorrhea and mastalgia. In: Blackwell RE, Grotting JC, eds. *Diagnosis and management of breast disease*. Cambridge, MA: Blackwell Science, 1996:19–76.
53. Deschamps M, Hislop TG, Band PR, et al. Study of benign breast disease in a population screened for breast cancer. *Cancer Detect Prev* 1986;9:151–156.

54. Drukker BH, deMendonca WC. Fibrocystic change and fibrocystic disease of the breast. *Obstet Gynecol Clin North Am* 1987;14:685–702.
55. Doberl A, Tobiassen T, Rasmussen T. Treatment of recurrent cyclical mastodynia in patients with fibrocystic breast disease: a double-blind placebo-controlled study—the Hjorring project. *Acta Obstet Gynecol Scand Suppl* 1984;123:177–184.
56. Estes NC. Mastodynia due to fibrocystic disease of the breast controlled with thyroid hormone. *Am J Surg* 1981;142:764–766.
57. Humphrey LJ, Estes NC. Aspects of fibrocystic disease of the breast: treatment with danazol. *Postgrad Med J* 1979;5:48–51.
58. Scott EB. Fibrocystic breast disease. *Am Fam Physician* 1987;36:119–126.
59. Russell LC. Caffeine restriction as initial treatment for breast pain. *Nurse Pract* 1989;14:36–37.
60. Dogliotti L, Mansel RE. Bromocriptine treatment of cyclical mastalgia/fibrocystic breast disease: update on the European trial. *Br J Clin Pract Symp Suppl*1989;68:26–32.
61. Maddox PR, Mansel RE. Management of breast pain and nodularity. *World J Surg* 1989;13: 699–705.
62. Fentiman IS. Mastalgia mostly merits masterly inactivity [Editorial]. *Br J Clin Pract* 1992;46:158.
63. McFayden IJ, Forrest AP, Chetty U, et al. Cyclical breast pain—some observations and the difficulties in treatment. *Br J Clin Pract* 1992;46:161–164.
64. Murtagh J. Mastalgia. *Aust Fam Physician* 1991;20:818–819.
65. Wilson MC, Sellwood RA. Therapeutic value of a supporting brassiere in mastodynia. *BMJ* 1976; 2:90.
66. Mansel RE. The clinical assessment of mastalgia. *Br J Clin Pract Symp Suppl* 1989;68:17–20.
67. Goodwin PJ, Neelam M, Boyd NF. Cyclical mastopathy: a critical review of therapy. *Br J Surg* 1988;75:837–844.
68. Minton JP, Abou-Issa H. Neuroendocrine theories of the etiology of benign breast disease. *World J Surg* 1989;13:680–684.
69. Brocq P, Stora C, Bernheim L. De l'emploi de la vitamine A dans le traitement des mastoses. *Ann Endocrinol* 1956;17:193–200.
70. Band PR, Deschamps M, Falardeau M, et al. Treatment of benign breast disease with vitamin A. *Prev Med* 1984;13:549–554.
71. Santamaria L, DellOrti M, Bianchi SA. Beta-carotene supplementation associated with intermittent retinol administration in the treatment of premenopausal mastodynia. *Boll Chim Farm* 1989;128: 284–287.
72. Smallwood J, Ah KD, Taylor I. Vitamin B6 in the treatment of pre-menstrual mastalgia. *Br J Clin Pract* 1986;40:532–533.
73. Ernster VL, Goodson WHD, Hunt TK, et al. Vitamin E and benign breast "disease": a double-blind, randomized clinical trial. *Surgery* 1985;97:490–494.
74. Preece PE, Richards AR, Owen GM, et al. Mastalgia and total body water. *BMJ* 1975;4:498–500.
75. Kollias J, Sibbering DM, Blamey RW. Topical non-steroidal anti-inflammatory gel for diffuse chest wall pain in mastalgia patients. In: Mansel RE, ed. *Recent developments in the study of benign breast disease*. London: The Parthenon Publishing Group, 1997:119–124.
76. Watts JF, Butt WR, Logan ER. A clinical trial using danazol for the treatment of premenstrual tension. *Br J Obstet Gynaecol* 1987;94:30–34.
77. Ramsey SG. The treatment of symptomatic benign breast disease with danazol. *Aust N Z J Obstet Gynaecol* 1988;28:299–304.
78. Mansel RE, Wisbey JR, Hughes LE. Controlled trial of the antigonadotropin danazol in painful nodular benign breast disease. *Lancet* 1982;1:928–930.
79. Deeny M, Hawthorn R, McKay HD. Low dose danazol in the treatment of the premenstrual syndrome. *Postgrad Med J* 1991;67:450–454.
80. Meden VH, Vujic D. Bromocriptine (Bromergon, Lek) in the management of premenstrual syndrome. *Clin Exp Obstet Gynecol* 1992;19:242–248.
81. Andersch B. Bromocriptine and premenstrual symptoms: a survey of double blind trials. *Obstet Gynecol Surv* 1983;38:643–646.
82. Mansel RE, Dogliotti L. European multicentre trial of bromocriptine in cyclical mastalgia. *Lancet* 1990;335:190–193.
83. Shaaban MM, Morad F, Hassan AER. Treatment of fibrocystic mastopathy by an antiestrogen, tamoxifen. *Int J Gynaecol Obstet* 1980;18:348–350.

84. Fentiman IS, Caleffi M, Brame K, et al. Double-blind controlled trial of tamoxifen therapy for mastalgia. *Lancet* 1986;1:287–288.
85. Messinis IE, Lolis D. Treatment of premenstrual mastalgia with tamoxifen. *Acta Obstet Gynecol Scand* 1988;67:307–309.
86. Kontostolis E, Stefanidis K, Navrozoglou I, et al. Comparison of tamoxifen with danazol for treatment of cyclical mastalgia. *Gynecol Endocrinol* 1997;11:393–397.
87. Gateley CA, Maddox PR, Mansel RE, et al. Mastalgia refractory to drug treatment. *Br J Surg* 1990; 77:1110–1112.
88. Gateley CA, Miers M, Mansel RE, et al. Drug treatments for mastalgia: 17 years experience in the Cardiff Mastalgia Clinic. *J R Soc Med* 1992;85:12–15.
89. Maddox PR, Harrison BJ, Horobin JM, et al. A randomised controlled trial of medroxyprogesterone acetate in mastalgia [see comments]. *Ann R Coll Surg Engl* 1990;72:71–76.
90. Nappi C, Affinito P, Di CC, et al. Double-blind controlled trial of progesterone vaginal cream treatment for cyclical mastodynia in women with benign breast disease. *J Endocrinol Invest* 1992; 15:801–806.
91. Plu-Bureau G, Le MG, Thalabard JC, et al. Percutaneous progesterone use and risk of breast cancer: results from a French cohort study of premenopausal women with benign breast disease. *Cancer Detect Prev* 1999;23:290–296.
92. Kubista E, Muller G, Spona J. [Treatment of mastopathies with cyclic mastodynia. Clinical results and hormonal profiles]. *Rev Fr Gynecol Obstet* 1987;82:221–227.
93. Peters F. Multicentre study of gestrinone in cyclical breast pain. *Lancet* 1992;339:205–208.
94. Coutinho EM, Azadian BG. Treatment of fibrocystic disease of the breast with gestrinone, a new trienic synthetic steroid with anti-estrogen, anti-progesterone properties. *Int J Gynaecol Obstet* 1984; 22:363–366.
95. Klijn JG, van Geel B, de Jong FH, et al. The relation between pharmacokinetics and endocrine effects of buserelin implants in patients with mastalgia. *Clin Endocrinol (Oxf)* 1991;34:253–258.
96. Hamed H, Caleffi M, Chaudary MA, et al. LHRH analogue for treatment of recurrent and refractory mastalgia. *Ann R Coll Surg Engl* 1990;72:221–224.
97. Peters F, Pickardt CR, Breckwoldt M. Thyroid hormones in benign breast disease: normalization of exaggerated prolactin responsiveness to thyrotropin-releasing hormone. *Cancer* 1985;56: 1082–1085.
98. Holland P, Gately CA. Drug therapy of mastalgia. What are the options? *Drugs* 1994;48:709–716.
99. Gateley CA, Maddox PR, Pritchard GA, et al. Plasma fatty acid profiles in benign breast disorders. *Br J Surg* 1992;79:407–409.
100. Pain JA, Cahill CJ. Management of cyclical mastalgia. *Br J Clin Pract* 1990;44:454–456.
101. Mansel RE, Preece PE, Hughes LE. A double blind trial of the prolactin inhibitor bromocriptine in painful benign breast disease. *Br J Surg* 1978;65:724–727.
102. Blichert-Toft M, Anderson AN, Henriksen OB, et al. Treatment of mastalgia with bromocriptine: a double-blind cross-over study. *BMJ* 1979;1:237.
103. Durning P, Sellwood RA. Bromocriptine in severe cyclical breast pain. *Br J Surg* 1982;69:248–249.
104. Hinton CP, Bishop HM, Holliday HW, et al. A double-blind controlled trial of danazol and bromocriptine in the management of breast pain. *Br J Clin Pract* 1986;40:326–330.
105. Nazli K, Syed S, Mahmood MR, Ansari F. Controlled trial of the prolactin inhibitor bromocriptine (Parlodel) in the treatment of severe cyclical mastalgia. *Br J Clin Pract* 1989;43:322–327.
106. Dhont M, van Eyck J, Delbeke L, et al. Danazol treatment of chronic cystic mastopathy: a clinical and hormonal evaluation. *Posgrad. Med. J* 1979;55:66–70.
107. Gorins A, Perret F, Tournant B, et al. A French double-blind crossover study (danazol versus placebo) in the treatment of severe fibrocystic breast disease. *Eur J Gynaecol Oncol* 1984;5:85–89.
108. Grio R, Cellura A, Geranio R, et al. Clinical efficacy of tamoxifen in the treatment of premenstrual mastodynia. *Minerva Ginecol* 1998;50:101–103.
109. Preece PE, Hanslip JI, Gilbert L, et al. Evening primrose oil (Efamol) for mastalgia. In: Horrobin DF, ed. *Clinical uses of essential fatty acids.* Montreal: Eden Press, 1982:147–154.
110. Pye JK, Mansel RE, Hughes LE. Clinical experience of drug treatments for mastalgia. *Lancet* 1985; 2:373–377.

5

Management of Common Lactation and Breast-feeding Problems

Verity H. Livingstone

Lactation is a physiologic process under neuroendocrine control; breast-feeding is a technical process by which milk is transferred from the maternal breast to the infant. Success depends on maternal health, adequate mammogenesis, unimpeded lactogenesis, successful galactopoiesis, effective milk transfer, and appropriate quality and quantity of daily milk intake. Each phase of lactation and breast-feeding is influenced by multiple predisposing, facilitating, or impeding biopsychosocial factors: puberty, pregnancy, childbirth, breast stimulation and drainage, maternal milk ejection reflex, maternal and infant breast-feeding technique, frequency and duration of suckling, and the pattern of breast use. All these factors are influenced by other factors such as maternal knowledge, attitude, motivation, mood, and health; infant health and behavior; and support from family, friends, and health care professionals.

The concept of breast-feeding kinetics as developed by Livingstone conveys the idea that there is a dynamic interaction between a breast-feeding mother and her infant over time (1). Most disorders of lactation are iatrogenic because of impeded establishment of lactation or inadequate ongoing stimulation and drainage of the breast. Most breast-feeding difficulties are due to a lack of knowledge, poor technical skills, or a lack of support. Almost all problems are reversible. Prevention, early detection, and management should become a routine part of the maternal and child health care.

PRENATAL PERIOD

Prenatal breast-feeding goals are to assist families make an informed choice about infant feeding, to prepare women cognitively and emotionally for breast-feeding, to identify and modify risk factors to lactation and breast-feeding, and to offer anticipatory guidance. These goals can be achieved by providing prenatal breast-feeding education and by performing a prenatal lactation assessment (2,3).

Informed Choice

Health professionals must assist families in making an informed decision by discussing the recommended infant-feeding guidelines, including benefits of breast-feeding and the risks of breast milk substitutes (4,5). Exclusive breast-feeding for the first 6 months is recommended, with the timely introduction of table foods around 6 months. Child-lead weaning should occur after the first year.

Benefits of Breast-feeding

To the Infant

- Human milk is species specific; it is the ideal nutrition because the protein and fat content are uniquely suited to the needs of the infant. It also provides protection against iron and vitamin deficiencies (6,7).
- Breast milk contains more than 100 biologically active ingredients. It offers immunologic protection to an otherwise immunodeficient neonate. The enteromammary immune cycle provides specific maternal antibodies to infant antigens. It protects against otitis media, gastroenteritis, respiratory tract infections, other bacterial and viral diseases, inflammatory bowel disease, allergies, necrotizing enterocolitis, and childhood leukemias and lymphomas (8–10).
- Breast-feeding provides a close interaction between mother and infant and helps the two develop a strong, positive emotional bond, which has long-term psychological advantages (11).
- The action of breast-feeding facilitates correct jaw and dental development (12).
- The incidence of sudden infant death is lower in breast-fed infants (13).

To the Mother

- Breast-feeding provides psychological satisfaction and close maternal bonding between mother and infant. It offers a regular opportunity to sit and relax during the often exhausting early parenting period (14,15).
- Using breast-feeding as the sole nourishment activity causes lactation amenorrhea, which is an effective and reliable method of birth control and child spacing (16, 17).
- Prolonged breast-feeding decreases the risks of premenopausal breast cancer by 50% and also decreases the risks of ovarian cancer and osteoporosis (18–21).
- It reduces postpartum anemia.

To Society

- Breast milk is a natural resource that is replenished and does not leave waste.
- The future of a society depends on the health of its children.
- Breast-feeding is the most health-promoting, disease-preventing, and cost-effective activity mothers can do.

The Hazards of Infant Formula

Inadequate nutrition: Infant formulas may contain inadequate or excessive micronutrients. They lack essential fatty acids known to be vital for myelination and proper brain and retinal development. Some formulas contain excess vitamin D (22).

Contaminants: A variety of contaminants—including life-threatening bacterial contaminants, excessive aluminium, lead, and iodine—have been identified, and many brands of formula have been withdrawn because of these discoveries (23).

Impaired cognitive development: Several well-controlled studies have reported significantly lower intelligence quotient scores and poorer development in children who lack breast milk in their diet (24–26).

Allergies: More formula-fed infants develop wheezing, diarrhea, prolonged colds, and allergies to milk and soya than infants who were not exposed to formula early in life (27–29).

Morbidity and mortality: The added risk of bottle-feeding can account for 7% of infants hospitalized for respiratory infections and, in the United States, formula-fed infants have a tenfold risk of being hospitalized for any bacterial infection. They have more than double the risk of contracting lower respiratory tract infections, and otitis media is up to three to four times more prevalent (30–32). Formula-fed infants have a higher incidence of childhood cancers and inflammatory bowel diseases in adulthood. Formula feeding accounts for 2% to 26% of insulin-dependent diabetes mellitus in children (33,34).

Costs: It costs approximately $150 per month to formula-feed an infant fully; therefore, many infants in low-income families are at risk for receiving low-cost and inappropriate alternative fluids and the early introduction of table foods. It is also time consuming to purchase and prepare formula.

Prenatal Education

Breast-feeding is a learned skill that should be taught prenatally; physicians can use models in their offices to help reinforce the learning process. Industry-developed literature on infant feeding should not be distributed because it gives mixed messages to breast-feeding families (35,36).

Prenatal Lactation Assessment

Lactation is essential for the survival of most mammalian species and can be considered the final stage of the reproductive cycle. Mammogenesis begins in the embryo and continues throughout life, with active growth phases during puberty and pregnancy. It is controlled by a complex hormonal milieu. Clinical signs of successful mammogenesis are breast growth, increased breast sensitivity, and the excretion of a colostrum-like fluid by the end of pregnancy. Failure of mammogenesis presents clinically as a lack of or an abnormality in breast growth and development during puberty or pregnancy.

Screening for Risk Factors

During the prenatal period, physicians have an opportunity to screen women for certain biological, psychological, and social risk factors that might interfere with mammogenesis, successful lactation, or breast-feeding. A formal *prenatal lactation assessment* should be performed in the third trimester as a routine component of antenatal care for all women.

Maternal Biological Risk Factors for Successful Lactation

- Anatomically abnormal breasts, including hypoplastic or conical breasts, may never lactate adequately because of insufficient glandular development associated with failure of mammogenesis (37).
- Breast surgery, including reduction mammoplasty, may interfere with glandular or lactiferous duct function (38).
- Certain endocrinopathies, including thyroid, pituitary, and ovarian dysfunction and relative infertility, may interfere with lactation (39,40).
- Chronic maternal illnesses, such as diabetes mellitus, systemic lupus erythematosus, and hypertension, may cause maternal fatigue but usually do not affect lactation.
- Women with physical disabilities usually can breast-feed, but they may have to be given guidance and assistance with regard to safe, alternative nursing positions.
- Complications of pregnancy such as gestational diabetes, pregnancy-induced hypertension, and preterm labor may result in early maternal infant separation, which can interfere with the initiation of lactation.
- Maternal infections such as hepatitis, human immunodeficiency virus (HIV), or cytomegalovirus may be transmitted to the infant *in utero*, but the added viral load through breast milk is probably clinically insignificant. In industrial countries, it would seem prudent to advise HIV-positive women not to breast-feed (41,42).
- Women who abuse substances such as street drugs or alcohol should be informed about the risks and counseled about abstinence. If the abuse continues, the women should be advised not to breast-feed. Smoking is not advisable, but when considering breast-feeding, the risks of contaminated breast milk and the risks of artificial feeding must be weighed against the benefits of human milk (43,44). Breast-feeding should therefore be recommended in spite of smoking.
- A previous unsuccessful breast-feeding experience may herald future problems.
- Previous or chronic psychiatric disorders, including depression, may recur in the postpartum period and interfere with maternal parenting abilities. These mothers need extra help during the early postpartum period.

Infant Biological Risk Factors for Successful Lactation

Several infant factors interfere with the establishment of lactation and breast-feeding. These include neonatal illness, which necessitates early maternal/infant separation, and sucking, swallowing, or breathing disorders. Some factors can be identified or predicted prenatally.

Psychological Risk Factors

There is interplay between the many forces that influence a woman's choice of feeding methods (45,46).

Beliefs: Many women have preconceived ideas about feeding their infants. They may have anxieties and concerns over their ability to breast-feed, they may believe their breasts are too small or their nipples too large, or they may fear the consequences of altered breast appearance. They may have had previous unsuccessful breast-feeding experiences or family members who offer negative advice. It is important to clarify beliefs surrounding breast-feeding.

Attitudes: The physician should explore the woman's attitudes toward breast-feeding, returning to work, and breast-feeding in public. Prenatal exploration of these areas helps families start addressing their own attitudes.

Knowledge and skills: The physician should explore the woman's knowledge by asking what she knows about infant feeding and how she is planning to feed her infant.

Social Risk Factors

Women are more likely to succeed in breast-feeding if they have support from their family and friends. In the prenatal phase, the goal is to help to foster a positive emotional environment among family, friends, and community.

Family support: Throughout history, women have been supported in their decision to breast-feed by grandmothers, sisters, close friends, or doulas. Nowadays, with the disintegration of the traditional family, lack of support often culminates in abandonment of breast-feeding (47).

Peer support: Single teenaged mothers experience considerable peer pressure to continue the carefree life of youth, and they may opt for the perceived freedom of bottle-feeding rather than the commitment to breast-feeding. Peer support programs have been shown to be an effective way of helping to increase the duration of breast-feeding.

Community support: Many women are embarrassed about breast-feeding in public. A prenatal discussion around the issue of breast-feeding in public may help. Employment outside the home need not be a reason for stopping breast-feeding; planning, flexibility, and good child care can go a long way toward enabling a mother to maintain lactation during prolonged hours of separation.

Prenatal Breast Examination

After reviewing the woman's history, a careful breast examination should be performed.

Size and Symmetry

It is not until pregnancy that the full maturation of the mammary glands occurs. Lactogenic hormones, including estrogen, progesterone, prolactin, insulin, thyroid, and growth hormones, trigger the development of the mammary epithelial cells, acinar glands, and lactiferous ducts. By 16 weeks' gestation, lactation can occur. The breasts should have enlarged by at least one or two bra cup sizes. Variations in breast appearance or asymmetry may indicate lactation insufficiency and therefore should be noted; future milk synthesis should be closely monitored. Scars give clues to potential glandular, ductal, or nerve disruption.

Nipple Graspability

For infants to latch and suckle effectively, they should be able to grasp the nipple and areola tissue and form a teat. The areola can be gently pinched to assess its elasticity and graspability. Nipples may protrude, pseudoprotrude, remain flat, pseudoinvert, or truly invert. They may be large or small. There is no evidence to support nipple preparation such as nipple stretching exercises or the use of nipple shells because the anatomy of the nipple and areola is not altered by prenatal exercises (48). The action of sucking by the infant helps to draw out the nipple and form a teat during the process of breast-feeding. It is only true inverted nipples that may impede correct latching and suckling. The Nipplette (Avent, Suffolk, England) was designed to help correct inverted nipples prenatally. Cutting off the needle end of a 20-mL syringe and reversing the plunger can make a simplified version. The flange end of the syringe can be placed over the nipple and gentle suction applied to draw out the nipple slowly. There are no data to confirm that the syringe works, but clinical experience suggests that it may be useful in helping to make the nipple area more graspable (49). There is no need to apply lotions or oils to the breasts to soften the skin, and normal daily bathing with soap is recommended.

Anticipatory Guidance

After completing a careful history and physical examination, the following anticipatory guidance should be offered.

- Avoid medicated or interventional labor. Soon after natural childbirth, infants exhibit an instinctive rooting behavior to locate and latch onto the breast. Medications and complications of childbirth may interfere with this neurodevelopmental behavior (50,51).
- Initiate breast-feeding or breast pumping as soon as possible following complete delivery of the placenta because it is this early breast stimulation that initiates lactation (4,15,52,53).
- Breast-feed or pump on demand, every 2 to 3 hours because regular breast drainage and stimulation facilitates lactogenesis (54,55).

- Practice rooming and bedding in for 24 hours per day. Maternal–infant separation impedes regular breast drainage and stimulation (56–58).
- Combined mother and infant nursing care enables the institution of patient-centered teaching (59).
- Relieve engorgement early to prevent involutional atrophy of acinar cells (60).
- Avoid routine supplementation because it causes ''breast confusion'' by removing an infant's hunger drive, thereby decreasing breast stimulation and drainage (61, 62).
- Avoid rubber nipples and pacifiers. If infants are demonstrating hunger cues by sucking, they are hungry. Offering a pacifier is not an appropriate maternal response to these infants' cues. The infant should suckle on the breast frequently to establish successful lactation (63).
- Exclusive breast-feeding ensures that the infant receives adequate colostrum, including secretary immunoglobulin A (IgA) and other unique hormonal factors that contribute to the infant's health, growth, and development (64).
- Avoid formula because it predisposes the neonate to potential allergies and other risk factors associated with artificial foods. The immature gut is not designed to digest cow milk or soya milk (65).
- Review the availability of community resources postpartum; close follow-up in the postpartum period is crucial for successful breast-feeding (66).

INTRAPARTUM PERIOD

Establishing Lactation

Breast-feeding should be considered the fourth stage of labor; childbirth is not complete until the infant is latched on to the breast and suckling, thus triggering lactogenesis. Soon after delivery, neonates exhibit a natural locating reflex and can find the nipple themselves, if permitted. Once the nipple is located, they root, latch onto it, and suckle instinctively. Studies have shown that this process may take 60 to 120 minutes and that the locating and suckling instinct can be impaired if foreign objects are inserted into neonate's mouths soon after birth or if the infant is sedated secondarily to maternal medication (67).

Early suckling is crucial for four reasons. First, it allows an imprinting to occur as the neonate learns to grasp and shape a teat and suckle effectively while the nipple and areola are still soft and easily grasped. Second, the neonate ingests a small amount of colostrum, which has a high content of maternal secretary IgA, which acts as the first immunization to the immuno-immature neonate. Third, following parturition and the delivery of an intact placenta, the inhibitory effects of the hormones of pregnancy are removed, and the prolactin receptors in the mammary gland become responsive. Fourth, early suckling stimulates the release of lactotrophs including prolactins, which trigger the onset of milk synthesis. Frequent episodes of breast stimulation cause surges of prolactin, which maintain lactogenesis. Clinical signs of successful lactogenesis are fullness of the breasts postpartum with the production of colostrum initially and then a gradual change to transitional milk and mature milk within about 36 to 48 hours (68,69).

Galactopoiesis is the process of ongoing milk synthesis. It follows successful mammogenesis and unimpeded lactogenesis. The rate of milk synthesis varies throughout the day and between mothers. It is controlled by regular and complete drainage and is primarily an autocrine action. Recent studies suggest that ongoing milk synthesis is inhibited by the buildup of local suppressor peptides; regular suckling removes this inhibition (69,70). Prolactin surges stimulate the breast alveoli to actively secrete milk, and oxytocin causes the myoepithelial cells surrounding the glands and the ductules to contract and eject milk down the ducts to the nipples. These contractions effectively squeeze the fat globules across the cell membrane into the ducts. As a feed progresses, the quality and quantity of milk produced change. The fore milk, at the beginning of the feed, is composed mainly of milk that has collected between feeds, and it has lower fat and higher whey content than hind milk. The fat content increases throughout a feed, but the volume of milk ingested decreases (71). Serum prolactin levels should increase several-fold following suckling; lack of a prolactin response may be significant. Prolactin levels fall over the first 4 to 6 weeks, and the suckling induced prolactin surges are markedly reduced by 3 months, virtually disappearing by 6 months, and yet lactation can continue (40, 72).

Factors that Help to Establish Lactation

Following childbirth, mothers and neonate should remain together, skin to skin, to allow the process of breast-feeding to begin. Neonates instinctively know how to locate the breast and suckle, but mothers must be taught.

The World Health Organization and the United Nations Children's Fund recognized the importance of successful establishment of breast-feeding in the hospital, and they launched the global Baby Friendly Hospital Initiative in 1992. This is an educational quality assurance program for hospitals based on the joint statement "Protecting, Supporting and Promoting Breastfeeding—The Special Role of Maternity Services," which outlines ten simple steps designed to protect these delicate physiologic processes (73) (Fig. 5.1).

Factors that Interfere with Lactation

Insufficient maternal milk is the most common reason given for stopping breast-feeding in the early weeks. The cause is often iatrogenic resulting from mismanagement during the critical early phase. Many maternal and infant factors contribute to lactation failure, including premammary gland, mammary gland, and postmammary gland causes.

Failure of Mammogenesis

In the normal course of events, mammogenesis begins in the embryo and continues throughout life with active growth phases during puberty and pregnancy. Mammo-

Every facility providing maternity services and care for newborn infants should:

1.   Have a written breastfeeding policy that is routinely communicated to all health care staff.

2.   Train all health care staff in skills necessary to implement this policy.

3.   Inform all pregnant women about the benefits and management of breastfeeding.

4.   Help mothers initiate breastfeeding within a half hour of birth.

5.   Show mothers how to breastfeed and how to maintain lactation even if they should be separated from their infants.

6.   Give newborn infants no food or drink other than breast milk, unless medically indicated.

7.   Practice rooming in - allow mothers and infants to remain together 24 hours a day.

8.   Encourage breastfeeding on demand.

9.   Give no artificial teats or pacifiers (also called dummies or soothers) to breastfeeding infants.

10.   Foster the establishment of breastfeeding support groups and refer mothers to them on discharge from the hospital or clinic.

FIG. 5.1. Ten steps to successful breast-feeding. (From Protecting, promoting, and supporting breastfeeding: the special role of maternity services. A joint WHO/UNICEF statement. Geneva: WHO, 1989, with permission.)

genesis is controlled by a complex hormonal milieu that cannot be covered in depth in this article. The hormones involved include the pituitary hormones: prolactin, adrenocorticotropic hormone, growth hormone, thyrotropin, follicle-stimulating hormone, and luteinizing hormone. In addition, steroid hormones from the ovary, adrenal glands, and placenta, plus thyroid hormones and insulin, contribute to mammary growth and function either directly or indirectly (74).

Failure of mammogenesis presents clinically as a lack of, or an abnormality in, breast growth and development during puberty, adulthood, or pregnancy and may be due to any or a combination of the following factors:

Preglandular Failure

The most common cause of premammary glandular failure is a deficiency of mammary growth stimulating hormones, but other possibilities include the presence of biologically inactive hormones or antibodies to the hormones preventing their normal action (75). Pathological conditions associated with disrupted production can be hypothalamic or pituitary in origin. Destruction of the hypothalamus can occur as a result of encephalitis, infiltration of tumor following lymphocytic hypophysitis, or idiopathic causes (76). Pituitary causes include space-occupying lesions, hyperplasia, empty sella syndrome, acromegaly, pituitary stalk section, and Sheehan syndrome (77). A pregnancy-specific mammary nuclear factor (PMF) has been identified which is stimulated by progesterone. PMF may suppress genes involved in mammary gland development (39).

Glandular Failure

Glandular failure is defined as lack of mammary gland response to normal lactogens during pregnancy. A PMF imbalance or end-organ receptor failure, such as estrogen or prolactin mammary gland receptor deficits, may occur. The regulatory factors involved in development of the myoepithelial cells prior to lactation are not well understood.

Failure of Lactogenesis

Lactogenesis, or the initiation of lactation, occurs close to parturition. It is under endocrine control of the pituitary gland via prolactin and other lactogenic hormones. The decline of placental hormones following delivery of an intact placenta, associated with early and frequent suckling, are the major triggers to establishing milk synthesis. Clinical signs of lactogenesis are increase in breast size and the production of colostrum. Failure of lactogenesis presents clinically as lack of breast engorgement and lack of colostrum production.

Preglandular

Preglandular causes of failure of lactogenesis include an intrinsic lack of lactogenic hormones, biologically inactive lactogens, or lactogenic antibodies (78). In addition to the pituitary and hypothalamic pathologies, factors predisposing to a reduction in pituitary hormone production in the postpartum period, in particular prolactin, include drugs such as bromocriptine and retained placental fragments (79). The latter demonstrates the inhibitory effect of estrogen and progesterone on the initiation of lactogenesis.

Glandular

Glandular causes include a lack of mammary gland responsiveness to lactogenic hormones, including plasma membrane receptor deficits or faulty gene transcription (80).

Postglandular

Postglandular causes relate to a delay in the initiation of breast-feeding. The length of delay that becomes significant has not been clarified, but it undoubtedly plays a role. Subsequent infrequent breast stimulation acts as an extrinsic inhibitor of lacto-genic hormone release in the early postpartum period (81). The use of supplementary feeding with formula, which is routine in some hospitals, may have a detrimental effect on milk synthesis in a mother who planned exclusively to breast-feed after hospital discharge (82). Unrelieved engorgement is also recognized as having a negative feedback effect on milk synthesis. This condition may be due to the buildup of inhibitor factors in the milk or to pressure effects by the milk volume.

Failure of Galactopoiesis

The action of many hormones is involved in the maintenance of lactation. Prolactin plays the major role. Prolactin levels fall over the first 4 to 6 weeks, and the suckling induced prolactin surges are markedly reduced by 3 months, virtually disappearing by 6 months, and yet lactation can continue. Failure of galactopoiesis presents clini-cally as lack of copious milk production. Causes of failure of galactopoiesis include the following.

Preglandular

An intrinsic lack of lactogenic hormones is one cause. Contributing factors to reduced milk synthesis include certain drugs, smoking, or superimposed pregnancy.

Glandular

Glandular causes include unresponsiveness to lactogenic hormones or secondary to failure of mammogenesis or lactogenesis.

Postglandular

Postglandular causes of failure include inadequate breast stimulation leading to an extrinsic lack of lactogenic hormones and inadequate breast drainage due to inefficient or infrequent breast-feeding. The result may be a lack of removal and a buildup of local inhibitor factors, which block milk synthesis (70).

The most common cause of lactation failure is a delay in early and frequent breast simulation and inadequate drainage, which commonly occurs when mothers and infants are separated because of existing or anticipated health problems. Newborns usually suckle effectively when they are positioned appropriately at the breast; how-ever, the maternal physiological ability to lactate rapidly declines if both breasts are not stimulated quickly following parturition and drained every 2 or 3 hours. There is a window for the initiation of lactation, and studies have shown that the duration of lactation correlates inversely with the time of the first breast stimulation. The extrinsic lack of prolactin surges fail to trigger and maintain lactation (83).

Inadequate drainage as a result of infrequent suckling or ineffective breast-feeding techniques leads to the lack of removal of the milk and a buildup of local inhibitor factors in the retained milk which shuts down ongoing milk synthesis. Involution of the glands commences, leading to premature weaning. After delivery, there is considerable vascular and lymphatic congestion in the breast tissue, leading to a rise in interductal pressure. If unrelieved, the engorgement impedes the intraductal flow of milk and reduces circulation, rapidly causing pressure atrophy at the alveoli and inhibiting the establishment of a good milk supply. Impairment to milk drainage as a result of lactiferous duct outlet obstruction also may occur following mammoplasty or surgical reconstruction of the breast, although newer surgical techniques attempt to maintain the integrity of the lactiferous ducts (84–86). Neifert et al. found a threefold increase in the risk of lactation insufficiency in women who had undergone breast surgery compared to women without surgery (38). Where there was a periareolar incision, the risk was five times greater than when there was no history of breast surgery.

Breast fullness or engorgement may prevent infants from latching effectively. This leads to sore nipples, caused by tongue trauma, inadequate breast stimulation, drainage, and insufficient milk intake by the infant. If the breast milk intake is low, the infant remains hungry and may receive formula supplement and become satiated. The net result is milk retention, impeded lactogenesis, and maternal unhappiness. Hot compresses and manual expression of milk before latching helps to improve the attachment, and cold compresses reduce swelling after feeds (87,88).

The fluid requirements of healthy newborn infants are minimal for the first few days. Neonates drink 7 to 20 mL of colostrum per feed initially, and they do not require extra fluids. Prelacteal and complementary feeds may upset the process of lactogenesis by removing the neonate's hunger drive and decreasing the frequency of breast stimulation and drainage (62,89). Night sedation may offer a temporary respite, but the lack of breast-feeding at night can impede lactogenesis because of irregular breast stimulation and drainage (90).

If frequent efficient breast-feeding is not possible, for example, if a mother is separated from her sick infant, she should be shown how to express her milk regularly, either by hand or by using a breast pump, to ensure complete breast drainage and prevent milk stasis. Contrary to popular belief, this does not lead to an excessive milk synthesis but prevents early and irreversible involution. A minimum of 100 minutes pumping per 24 hours is needed to maintain adequate prolactin levels. Short, frequent pumpings are most effective (91).

Milk Transfer

Milk is transferred from the breast by the infant during breast-feeding, in combination with the maternal milk ejection reflex. The rate of transfer of milk from the breast to the infant depends on various factors, including milk synthesis and the volume of pooled milk, the strength and frequency of the milk ejection reflex, and the technical process of breast-feeding (92). The milk ejection reflex, or *letdown*, is stimulated by oxytocin released from the posterior pituitary following direct nipple stimulation and via hypothalamic triggering. It causes smooth-muscle contractions and propels milk through the ducts and out of the nipple pores. The character of the reflex varies between women and over time; some mothers have a well-developed letdown, whereas others have a slow, irregular reflex. Either way, confidence facilitates the ejection reflex and anxiety may impede it (92,93).

Factors that Help Milk Transfer

Basic Breast-feeding Skills

Breast-feeding is a technical process of transferring milk from the breast. It depends on careful positioning and attachment of the infant to the breast and on an intact suckling ability of the infant. Parenting starts at birth; therefore, hospital staff should encourage mothers to assume this role as soon as possible. Mothers should be shown how to breast-feed (59,94) (Fig. 5.2).

Positioning. The mother should be sitting comfortably with her arms and back supported and her feet raised on a small stool. The infant should be placed on her lap, facing the uncovered breast; a pillow may help raise up the baby. Breast-feeding is easier if two hands are used to start with. The breast should be cupped with one hand underneath using the thumb and fingers to shape the breast to form an oval that matches the shape of the mouth, lifting the breast up slightly while directing the nipples toward the infant's mouth. The other hand is used to support the infant's shoulders and back of the head. The infant's arms should be free to embrace the breast and the body held very close to the mother, stomach to stomach.

Attachment. The latching technique involves brushing the nipple against the infant's upper lip and waiting until the infant roots, lifting his or her head and opening the mouth wide. This often requires ''teasing the baby'' and encouraging the mouth to open wider than before. When the mother can see the gaping mouth, she should quickly draw the baby forward over the nipple and onto areola tissue. The amount of areola available to the mouth depends on the size of the areola and on the neonate's gape. It is incorrect to assume that all the areola tissue should be covered. The lips should be everted or flanged and placed well behind the nipple base. The chin is extended into the breast and the nose is adjacent to it. Young infants do not have the ability to maintain their position at the breast alone, and so the mother must continue to sandwich her breast and support the infant's head and shoulders, throughout the duration of the feed. Older infants are able to latch and maintain themselves more easily and suckle comfortably in an elbow crook.

Suckling. An infant who is correctly latched and has a mouthful of soft breast tissue will draw the nipple and the areola tissue to the junction of the hard and soft palate to form a teat and then will initiate suckling. The more elastic and extensible the breast tissue, the easier it is for the young infant. A fixed, retracted, or engorged nipple and areola tissue make it harder for this to occur. Ultrasound studies show how the gums and jaws are positioned over pressure receptors in the lactiferous ducts and trigger milk ejection. The jaw is raised and the gums compress the lactifer-

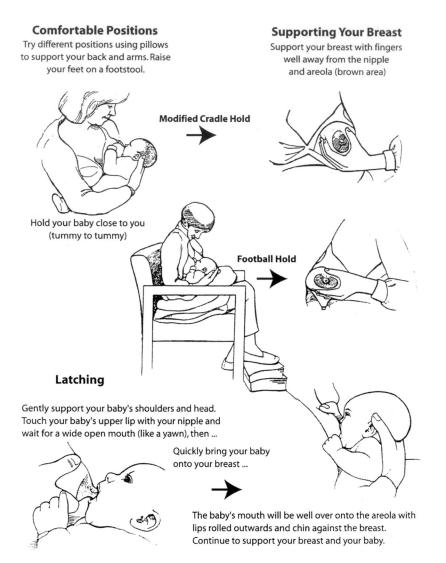

Comfortable Positions
Try different positions using pillows to support your back and arms. Raise your feet on a footstool.

Supporting Your Breast
Support your breast with fingers well away from the nipple and areola (brown area)

Modified Cradle Hold

Hold your baby close to you (tummy to tummy)

Football Hold

Latching

Gently support your baby's shoulders and head. Touch your baby's upper lip with your nipple and wait for a wide open mouth (like a yawn), then ...

Quickly bring your baby onto your breast ...

The baby's mouth will be well over onto the areola with lips rolled outwards and chin against the breast. Continue to support your breast and your baby.

FIG. 5.2. Comfortable positions for breast-feeding.

ous sinuses under the areola; the tongue protrudes over the lower gums, grooves and undulates in a coordinated manner to strip out milk from the teat, and draws milk into the mouth. The cheeks and tongue help to form a bolus of milk. The jaw lowers, and the soft palate elevates to close the nasopharynx; a slight negative pressure is created, and the milk is effectively transferred and swallowed in a coordinated manner (95–98).

Factors Impeding Milk Transfer

The milk ejection reflex is a primitive one and is not easily blocked. The effects of adrenaline can reduce it temporarily if the mother is subjected to sudden unpleasant or extremely painful physical or psychological stimuli. This could include embarrassment or fear, inducing a stress reaction with the release of adrenaline, which can cause vasoconstriction and impede the action of oxytocin. Over time, however, this inhibition seems to be overcome. The strength and frequency of the ejection reflex depend on hypophysial stimulation of the posterior pituitary and suckling pressure on the lactiferous ducts, causing oxytocin release. The more milk that has pooled between feeds, the more is ejected with the initial let down. The character of this reflex varies between women and over time; some mothers have a well-developed ejection reflex, whereas others have a slow, irregular reflex. Confidence facilitates the ejection reflex, and anxiety may impede it (72,93).

Inefficient milk transfer may be the result of poor maternal breast-feeding technique in positioning the infant at the breast or in facilitating his or her attachment because of a lack of knowledge or maternal or infant physical disabilities. In addition, improper positioning and attachment lead to decreased breast stimulation and inadequate drainage, which result in decreased milk production and decreased milk intake. Simple correction of the position and latch is often the only remedy needed to improve the quality of the feed.

Inefficient milk transfer also may result from poor neonate suckling technique either because of an inability to grasp the nipple correctly or because of a suck, swallow, or breath disorder. Large, well-defined nipples may entice the neonate to suckle directly on the nipple, resulting in sore nipples and ineffective milk transfer. Retrognathia, cleft lip or palate, an uncoordinated, weak, flutter, or a bunched-up tongue may interfere with effective sucking dynamics, often because the jaw fails to compress the lactiferous ducts or the tongue and cheeks are unable to create the necessary negative pressure to draw in the milk (99). These infants may benefit from suck training, but clinical experience suggests that as the mandible elongates and facial muscles strengthen, the dynamics of sucking improve naturally (100,101). *Ankyloglossia* (tongue-tie) is an important cause of suckling difficulties. The tethered tongue is unable to protrude over the gum and cannot move upward; the teat is not stripped correctly, and less milk is transferred. The nipple often becomes traumatized and sore. The infant may not thrive, and milk production decreases because of inadequate drainage. A simple surgical release of the frenulum is required and should be done as soon as possible when clinically indicated; after a few weeks, it is often difficult to alter the way these infants suckle (102,103).

Milk Intake

Over the first few days, the infant drinks small volumes of colostrum of 7 to 20 mL per feed. This rapidly increases to approximately 760 to 840 mL per day, with approximately seven or eight feeding episodes. The milk intake per feed is about 80 to 120 mL. Breasts have a great capacity to yield milk and can produce double this amount. If necessary, a woman can feed from one breast exclusively (104).

Frequency

Infants are able to recognize hunger and should be fed according to their cues. Most newborns breast-feed every 2 to 3 hours, causing frequent surges of prolactin, which help to ensure full lactation. Mothers who have a low milk supply should be encouraged to breast-feed frequently to ensure good drainage and stimulation.

Duration

Studies show that the duration of a breast-feed varies between mother–infant pairs. The rate of milk transfer is not uniform. Some breast-feeding pairs have a rapid milk transfer and, hence, a very short feed. This is because of the large amount of milk that has collected in the breasts since the previous feed and the well-established milk ejection reflex. Others have long feeds because milk ejection is poor, the breast-feeding technique is relatively ineffective, or milk production is slow and the pooled milk volume is low, which consequently leads to a slowed milk transfer. Previously held beliefs that most of the feed is taken in the first few minutes or that both breasts should be used at each feed fail to recognize the uniqueness of each nursing pair. The total volume of milk intake also varies and seems to depend on total fat and caloric content. Infants recognize satiation and spontaneously stop suckling when they are full. A high-fat, low-volume feed may have a different duration than the lower-fat, high-volume feed. The exact mechanism of control has not been fully elucidated (105).

Pattern of Breast Use

The quality and quantity of milk intake depend on the pattern of breast use. Between feeds, milk is synthesized and collects in the lactiferous ducts. This low-fat milk is readily available at the start of each feed. As the feed progresses, the volume of milk the infant drinks will decrease, but the quality increases as more fat is passed into the milk. The infant should remain at the first breast until the rate of flow of milk is no longer sufficient to satisfy the infant. The second breast should then be offered.

Factors that Help Milk Intake

To establish lactation, both breasts should be offered at each feed. The removal of colostrum facilitates ongoing lactogenesis. When lactation is well established, the first breast should be comfortably drained before switching to the second. This will prevent milk stasis and results in a balanced milk production and optimum infant growth. Mothers with a high milk yield may feed unilaterally, whereas mothers with a slow rate of milk synthesis should feed bilaterally. When the rate of milk transfer is rapid, the infant may gag, choke, and pull away from the breast; frequent burping is recommended in this situation, as is manual expression of some milk before attaching the infant.

Factors that Impair Milk Intake

A "happy to starve" infant that sleeps for long periods may fail to thrive because of inadequate daily milk intake. A pause in feeding after a few minutes of sucking may be interpreted incorrectly as the infant having had enough, leading to early termination of the feed. A crying, discontented infant may be given a pacifier to prolong the time between feeds. A mother also may be under the impression that only one breast should be used at each feed and choose not to feed off the second side even though the neonate is still hungry. Newborns frequently pause while feeding, and these episodes may last several minutes. Problems arise when a mother terminates a feed or switches to the other side prematurely because to do so alters the quality and quantity of the milk consumed.

Maternal Psychosocial Health

The psychological and social health of the mother is crucial throughout all stages of breast-feeding. A mother who is ambivalent about breast-feeding and who lacks support may allow her infant fewer chances to suckle, thereby inhibiting lactogenesis and galactopoiesis. A mother who lacks confidence or knowledge may interpret any breast-feeding infant problem as being due to insufficient milk; a consequent move to bottle-feeding compounds the problem. Lack of support from family and friends can negatively influence her endeavors (106,107).

In-hospital Risk Assessment

Some mothers and infants are at high risk for lactation and breast-feeding difficulties. As discussed previously, several biopsychosocial risk factors can be identified prenatally, and this information should be readily available in hospital. A routine in-hospital breast-feeding risk assessment should be performed (108) (Fig. 5.3).

Newborns often lose weight within the first few days as the result of normal physiologic fluid losses (109). If breast-feeding is successfully established, this weight loss should be no greater than about 7%. Excessive weight loss may imply inadequate food intake and deserves a detailed clinical breast-feeding assessment. The underlying cause is usually easy to elucidate and management can be directed toward either increasing the rate of maternal milk synthesis, improving milk transfer, or increasing the daily quantity or quality of milk intake (1, 110).

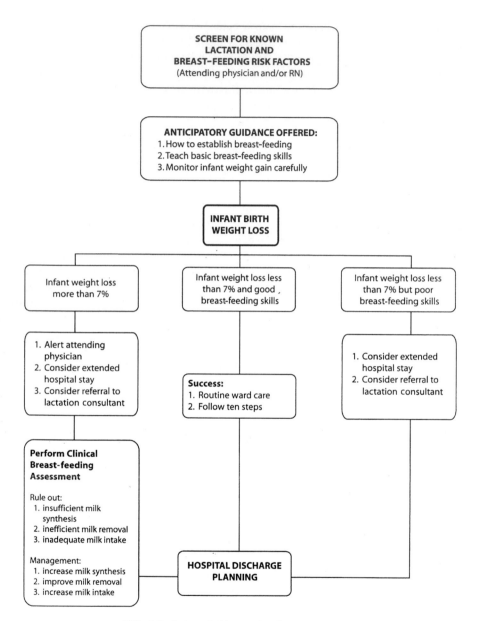

FIG. 5.3. In-hospital breast-feeding assessment.

If the neonate's weight continues to fall, additional calories must be provided either as the mother's own breast milk, pasteurized donor breast milk, or formula. Some neonates have preexisting difficulties grasping and suckling at the breast. In these situations, wide-based rubber nipples and thin silicone nipple shields are useful suck training devices that encourage normal biomechanical jaw excursions.

Hospital Discharge Planning

Hospital stays are short. Discharge planning enables a physician to review the stages of lactation and breast-feeding and allows early identification of potential or actual problems. All mothers should be taught the signs that their baby is breast-feeding well and instructed to call for advice if they have concerns (Fig. 5.4). If an infant has lost more than 7% of his or her birth weight at the scheduled hospital

By three or four days of age, your baby:

- has wet diapers: at least 4-5 noticeable times (looks or feels wet) in twenty-four hours (pale and odorless urine)
- has at least 2-3 bowel movements in twenty-four hours (color progressing from brownish to seedy mustard yellow and at least the size of a loonie).
- breastfeeds at least 8 times in twenty-four hours.
- is content after most feedings.

Other signs that suggest your baby is breast-feeding well are:

- You can hear your baby swallowing during feeding.
- Your breasts are full before feedings and soft after feedings.
- Your baby is only drinking breast milk.

If any one of these signs is **not** present after your baby is 3 or 4 days old or if you are having problems, please **call for help**.

Physician/Midwife: _____   Community Health Nurse: _____

If your baby is breast-feeding well, **make an appointment within the first week** for you and your baby to see either your Family Physician, Midwife, or Community Health Nurse.

Birth Weight: _____   Discharge Weight: _____
            Weight at One Week: _____

FIG. 5.4. Signs that your infant is breast-feeding well (first 3 weeks).

discharge, or if the mother–infant pair has known risk factors for breast-feeding difficulties, a delayed discharge or early community follow-up for breast-feeding assistance would be appropriate. All other mothers and infants should be reassessed within 1 week of birth (111).

POSTPARTUM PERIOD

Clinical Breast-feeding Assessment

Lactation and breast-feeding difficulties manifest in many ways, including infant problems such as failure to thrive, colic, fussiness, early introduction of supplements, or maternal concerns such as breast discomfort, sore cracked nipples, engorgement mastitis, or postpartum depression. Different clinical complexes of symptoms and signs or syndromes reflect the normal variations in maternal lactation ability and infant breast-feeding ability. These symptoms and signs are not diagnostic. Diagnosis and problem solving starts with a detailed history and physical examination of both mother and infant, including breast-feeding history and observation. Once the etiology and pathophysiology have been elucidated, successful management depends on sound knowledge of the anatomy of the breast, the physiology of lactation, and the mechanics of infant suckle combined with a clear understanding of breast-feeding kinetics (112,113).

The rate of breast milk synthesis varies throughout the day and between mothers. It depends on a variety of central and local factors, including direct breast stimulation and breast drainage (68,114,115). A 20-minute period of breast stimulation causes peak prolactin surges that take approximately 2 hours to decline to baseline levels (72). Milk synthesis occurs during this period and is followed by a quiescent period. Irregular breast drainage results in a lack of removal and local buildup of inhibition that decreases milk synthesis. In clinical practice, approximately 15% of mothers have a high rate of milk synthesis of 60 mL per hour or more (hyperlactation), and about 15% of mothers have a low rate of synthesis of 10 mL per hour or less (hypolactation) (Fig. 5.5).

Insufficient Milk Syndrome

The most common reason given for abandoning breast-feeding in the early postpartum period is insufficient milk. The etiology is multifactorial, but most causes are reversible if the mother receives accurate breast-feeding management advice early in the postpartum period. A small percentage are irreversible (Fig. 5.6).

If the mother is having difficulties breast-feeding or if the infant's weight is continuing to fall or is more than 7% below birth weight, a careful evaluation is required. This involves a detailed clinical breast-feeding assessment incorporating maternal and infant history, and breast-feeding history and includes a careful maternal and infant examination. Observation of breast-feeding is required to assess positioning, latching, suckling and swallowing. An accurate test feed followed by esti-

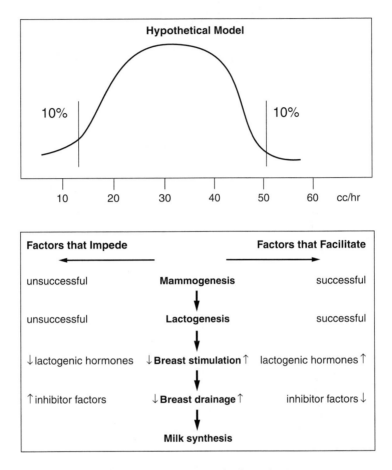

FIG. 5.5. Rate of maternal milk synthesis.

mating residual milk in the breasts by pumping are helpful measurements when assessing maternal milk yield and infant milk intake. Caution must be taken when using standard office scales due to their unreliability in measuring small volume changes (116–118). Other causes of infant failure to thrive should always be considered (Fig. 5.7).

In broad terms, management includes avoiding the precipitating factors, improving maternal milk synthesis by increasing breast stimulation and drainage, improving milk removal by correcting the breast-feeding technique, and increasing the infant's daily milk intake by increasing the frequency and duration of breast-feeding. A small percentage of neonates will require complementary feeds. Metoclopramide and domperidone 10 to 20 mg four times a day are effective galactagogues when

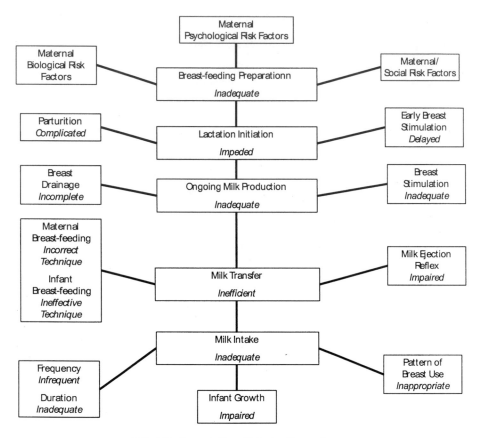

FIG. 5.6. Neonatal insufficient milk syndrome.

increased prolactin stimulation is required (119). Mothers may need support and reassurance that partial breast-feeding or mixed feeding is still beneficial (10).

Maternal Hyperlactation Syndrome

Hyperlactation may result in a characteristic clustering of maternal and infant symptoms and signs. Milk stasis, blocked ducts, deep radiating breast pain, lactiferous ductal colic, inflammatory mastitis, infectious mastitis, and breast abscess are common problems. Clinical experience has shown that most mothers experiencing any or all these symptoms have a high rate of milk synthesis and have large, thriving infants, or else they have started to wean and are not draining their breasts regularly. These symptoms and signs are all consequences of a rapid rate of milk synthesis combined with milk retention resulting from incomplete breast drainage. They represent the clinical spectrum of the maternal hyperlactation syndrome (114,120) (Fig.

- inadequate maternal milk synthesis
- ineffective milk removal
- inadequate milk intake by the infant

Risk factors known to interfere with milk synthesis include

- absence of mammogenesis or absence of breast growth during pregnancy,
- previous breast surgery (i.e., reduction, mammoplasty),
- anatomically unusually shaped breast,
- Endocrinopathies/relative infertility,
- pituitary dysfunction due to obstetrical hemorrhage or severe hypotension (Sheehan syndrome),
- delay in initiating breast-feeding (more than 12-24 hours) and/or infrequent breast stimulation and drainage (i.e. maternal/infant separation),
- absence of postpartum breast enlargement/engorgement), and
- absence of colostrum.

Risk factors known to interfere with milk removal include

- maternal technical difficulties with positioning and latch due to lack of skill, perineum or abdominal pain, or sedation, and
- infant technical difficulties due to suckling/swallowing or breathing disorders such as prematurity, micrognathia, cleft palate, or cardiac or respiratory complications.

Risk factors known to interfere with milk intake include

- infrequent feeds associated with long sleep periods (>4 hours),
- passive, sleepy baby, and
- restricted access to breast (i.e., one breast per feed or abrupt removal from breast).

Any mother whose infant has lost >7% of birth weight at hospital discharge or who has one of the above risk factors resulting in breast-feeding difficulties may benefit from delayed hospital discharge, requires assistance with breast-feeding, should be given the handout "Signs That Your Baby Is Breast-feeding Well," and should be seen by the physician within 48 hours of discharge. **All other mother/infant pairs should be reviewed at 1 week to ensure successful breast-feeding and adequate infant weight gain.**

FIG. 5.7. Causes of breast-feeding malnutrition.

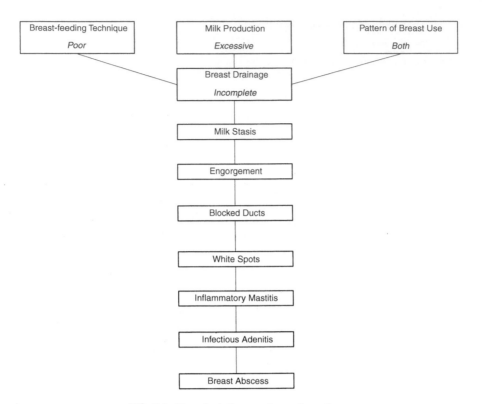

FIG. 5.8. Hyperlactation syndrome in mothers.

5.8). The pathophysiology is analogous to the renal system; retention of urine, due to incomplete bladder emptying, may result in lower and upper urinary tract disease, including bladder distension, spasms, ureteric colic, and hydronephrosis. This problem may become complicated with ascending urinary tract infections, including trigonitis, urethritis, cystitis, pyelonephritis, and renal abscess.

Lactation problems occur when a mother with a high milk output switches her infant from one breast to the other before the first side has been adequately drained. A strong milk-ejection reflex causes a rapid letdown of a large volume of pooled milk, and the infant quickly becomes satiated before all the lactiferous ducts are drained. Incomplete drainage may be aggravated by poor position and latch or by impaired infant suckling (121). When this occurs repeatedly, some of the ducts and lobules constantly remain full.

White Spot

A small white spot may be visible on the nipple; such a spot represents edematous epithelium blocking the nipple pore and milk flow. In some situations, duct obstruction is due to a small granule of casein milk precipitate (122). Lactiferous duct outlet obstruction can cause increased retrograde pressure. Mothers may complain of sharp, ''knife-like'' cramps or shooting pains deep in the breast, often between feeds, because of ductal cramping or colic because of myoepithelium smooth-muscle contractions.

Milk Stasis

A firm, lumpy, slightly tender quadrant in the breast may be felt because of milk stasis. Over time, if this area is not drained, cytokines from the milk may seep into the interstitial tissue, causing it to become inflamed and erythematous, signifying an inflammatory mastitis (123,124).

Acute Mastitis

It was recognized in 1940 that when a breach occurs in the mucous membrane, such as a cracked nipple, superficial skin infections could lead to a deeper cellulitis, adenitis and mastitis, or flushed breast, as it was referred to by Duncan et al. (125). Livingstone et al. found that 50% to 60% of sore, cracked nipples were contaminated with *Staphylococcus aureus* or other microorganisms (126). Subsequent study showed that 25% of mothers with infected, sore nipples developed mastitis if they were not treated aggressively with systemic antibiotic (127). A high rate of milk synthesis combined with continuous poor drainage of a segment of the breast may result in the stagnant milk becoming secondarily infected with common skin pathogens via an ascending lactiferous duct infection and leads to acute mastitis. Infectious mastitis also may be caused by a blood-borne infection; however, that is uncommon and more likely in nonpuerperal mastitis (128). Puerperal mastitis is said to affect 1.4% to 8.9% of nursing mothers presenting with general malaise, chills or sweats, and fever (129). Half of the affected patients may not have fever or systemic symptoms, however, but only localized symptoms and signs of inflammation.

Chronic Mastitis

Chronic mastitis, as in chronic urinary tract infections, may be due to *reinfection* or a *relapsed* infection. Reinfection occurs sporadically because of exposure to a new pathogen, commonly transmitted from the infant. A relapsed infection occurs shortly after completion of therapy; it signifies inadequate primary treatment and failed eradication of the pathogen. An underlying cause, such as a nidus of infection deep in the breast tissue, should be considered. It is hypothesized that lactiferous duct infections may lead to stricture formation, duct dilation, and impaired drainage. The residual milk remains infected.

Breast Abscess

Inadequately treated mastitis and ongoing milk retention can develop into a breast abscess. A high fever with chills and general malaise, associated with a firm, well-demarcated, tender, fluctuating mass, usually with erythema of the skin, indicates abscess formation, although, in some rare instances, systemic symptoms may be absent. Ultrasonography of the breast and needle aspiration under local anesthesia are useful diagnostic techniques for identifying collections of fluid or pus and distinguishing mastitis from a galactocele or inflammatory breast cancer (130–132).

Management Goals

Maternal hyperlactation syndrome can be prevented by decreasing the rate of milk synthesis and preventing milk retention by improving milk removal and breast drainage.

Decreased Rate of Milk Synthesis

Reducing breast stimulation and drainage can decrease the rate of milk synthesis. Decreasing the frequency and duration of breast-feeding reduces prolactin surges, and milk synthesis remains blocked via central inhibitory factors. Decreasing the frequency of breast drainage results in milk retention in the lactiferous ducts, and inhibitor peptides collect and block ongoing milk production via a local negative feedback mechanism. In practical terms, the infant should remain at one breast per feed until he or she is full and spontaneously releases the breast. In this way, the volume of milk ingested is less, but the fat content and calorific value increases as the feed progresses (71). A higher fat intake often satiates the infant for a longer period and decreases the hunger drive. The interval between feeds is lengthened and milk synthesis declines, whereas the second breast remains full longer, and local inhibitor further reduces milk synthesis in that breast. In a small number of mothers, unilateral breast-feeding may result in an overdrainage and can contribute to the ongoing high rate of milk synthesis. In these cases, bilateral breast-feeding and incomplete drainage may result in a decline in overall milk synthesis.

Decreased Milk Retention

Regular breast-feeding facilitates milk removal and breast drainage. When positioned and latched correctly, the infant is usually effective at removing milk and draining each segment. The modified cradle position allows the mother to cup the breast with her hand and apply firm pressure over the outer quadrant and compress retained milk toward the nipple while the infant suckles. If the milk is flowing rapidly, the mother should stop compressing the breast. Switching breast-feeding positions and using the under-the-arm hold allows thorough drainage of all segments and prevents milk stasis. Breast-feeding should start on the fullest breast and the infant should remain on this breast until all areas feel soft. As the pressure in the duct is relieved, breast pain and discomfort lessen.

Removal of Obstruction

If a small white dot on the nipple becomes visible, indicating a blocked nipple pore and outlet obstruction, gentle abrasion or a sterile needle can be used to remove the epithelium skin and relieve the obstruction. Occasionally, a small calculus or granule will pop out suddenly, relieving the obstruction. On firm compressing, a thick stream of milk will often gush out, indicating patency. Occasionally, breast-feeding is ineffective at removing the thickened inspissated milk, and manual or mechanical expression may therefore be necessary. The mother should be shown how to compress her breast firmly using a cupped hand, squeezing gently toward the nipple while pumping to dislodge the milk or calculus. If the breast expression fails to relieve the obstructed segment, a technique known as *manual stripping* can be used (133). This involves cupping the breast between the finger and thumb and applying firm, steady pressure over the tender section, starting from the periphery over the rib cage and drawing the fingers and thumb slowly together toward the nipple, stripping out thickened milk or pus. This procedure should be repeated several times. The skin must be well lubricated before attempting to do this. Analgesia may be necessary, but even with mastitis, the discomfort lessens as the procedure continues. The intraductal pressure is relieved as milk or pus is slowly extruded. Mothers must be taught this technique and instructed to repeat the procedure every few hours, standing in the shower, using soapy fingers, until the breast feels softer and milk is flowing freely. If a breast abscess has formed, incision and drainage under local or general anesthesia is required. Repeat needle aspiration may not be adequate. The incision should be radial, not circumferential, to minimize duct severance. A large drain should be inserted and daily irrigations continued until the cavity closes. It is important that the dressings be applied in a manner such that the infant can continue to breast-feed or the mother should use an efficient breast pump. Regular drainage prevents further milk stasis and maintains lactation.

Treating Infection

Correct breast-feeding techniques and improved drainage of milk are the *sine qua non* of treatment, but antibiotic therapy may be necessary. Inflammatory mastitis occurs within 12 to 24 hours of milk blockage, leading to an infectious mastitis within 24 to 48 hours. Under normal conditions, the milk leukocyte count is less than 10^6 mL of milk, and the bacterial count is less than 10^3 bacteria per milliliter. Within 48 hours of breast symptoms, the leukocyte count increases to more than 10^6 mL of milk, but the bacterial count remains low. This is considered noninfectious inflammation of the breast, and improved milk drainage will resolve the situation quickly. Infectious mastitis is defined as having a bacterial count of more than 10^6 mL of milk. In clinical practice, treatment is empirical. Breast pain and erythema associated with flu-like systemic symptoms and a fever are highly suggestive of infectious mastitis and require antibiotic therapy. Common bacterial pathogens include *Staphylococcus aureus, Escherichia coli, group A β-haemolytic Streptococcus* with occasional *Streptococcus faecalis*, and *Klebsiella pneumonia*. In contrast, nonpuerperal breast infections are mixed infections with a major anaerobic component. Antibiotics of choice include penicillinase-resistant penicillins such as dicloxacillin or erythromycin, cephalosporins, sulfonamides, and clindamycin. A 10- to 14-day course is required. The breast milk excretion of these antibiotics is minimal, and continuation of breast-feeling is considered safe. Clinical improvement is usually seen within 24 to 48 hours, the erythema subsides, the fever decreases, and breast pain improves. A persistent fluctuant mass may indicate abscess formation. The segment of breast must be drained adequately, and long-term antibiotic therapy may be warranted (134).

Prevention of Recurrence

Excessive milk retention can be prevented by correct breast-feeding techniques, ensuring a proper latch, regular drainage, and not skipping feeds. Sleeping through the night, returning to work, the introduction of breast milk substitutes such as bottles of formula, the introduction of table foods, and weaning are all typical periods when breast-feeds may be missed. The resultant "breast confusion" can lead to inadequate drainage and milk retention. Mothers with a high milk output should become skilled at palpating their breasts for lumps, and the bra should be removed before feeding if it is practical to do so. Areas of breast lumpiness or caking that persist after breast-feeding may indicate milk stasis or a blocked duct. Thorough expression of this residual milk should relieve the situation and prevent secondary complications.

Supportive Measures

Mastitis is an inflammatory process that can be complicated by infection and produce systemic symptoms in an already exhausted mother. Home help and bed rest is advisable, and analgesia such as acetaminophen plain or combined with codeine may be necessary. Hot compresses applied to the breast, before breast-feeding or milk expression, encourage blood flow and smooth-muscle relaxation, which in turn helps milk transfer. Cold compresses after feeds may decrease inflammation and edema.

Anecdotal cases of maternal toxic shock syndrome have been reported, and in rare circumstances, *Staphylococcus* toxins can be ingested by the infant. Continuation of breast-feeding is always recommended (135). Weaning may lead to increased milk stasis and abscess formation. If a mother chooses to wean abruptly or if clinically indicated, a lactation suppressant such as bromocriptine 2.5 mg twice daily for 14 days may be used with caution, although the potential for side effects, including nausea, headache, postural hypotension, and stroke, occur in rare circumstances (136). Cabergoline is considered safer.

Sore Nipples

Sore nipples, particularly during the first few days of breast-feeding, are a common symptom experienced by an estimated 80% of breast-feeding mothers. It is generally accepted that transient nipple soreness is within normal limits. Factors such as frequency and duration of breast-feeding, skin or hair color, and nipple preparation do not seem to make a difference in preventing tenderness. Increasing or persistent discomfort is pathological and requires careful evaluation. Detailed studies of infant suckling at the breast have illustrated how tongue friction or gum compression, resulting from inappropriate latch, can cause trauma and result in superficial skin abrasions and painful nipples (99,137). In many cases, repositioning can have a dramatic effect and instantaneously remove the pain and discomfort (131,138–140).

A small percentage of women have naturally sensitive nipples, which remain uncomfortable throughout the duration of breast-feeding, despite careful technique. They experience sensitive nipples, even in their nonlactating state. When nipple pain, excoriations, dermatitis, or ulceration continue despite careful maternal breast-feeding technique, a detailed history and physical examination are required to elucidate secondary causes of sore nipples.

Nipple Trauma

To suckle correctly, an infant must grasp sufficient breast tissue to form a teat, draw it to the back of the pharynx, and initiate suckling in a coordinated manner using rhythmic jaw compressions and a grooved, undulating tongue. Many maternal nipple and infant oral anatomic anomalies can interfere with effective latch and suckle, resulting in nipple trauma and pain. Clinical findings such as maternal inelastic, flat, pseudoinverted or inverted nipples and infant cleft lip and palate are easily identified. More subtle findings may include infant retrognathia, which refers to a small or posterior positioned mandible, or the Pierre-Robin malformation, which combines severe micrognathia, or a posterior tongue with a relative ineffective activity of the muscles that protract the tongue and ankyloglossia (132,141).

Management includes using a semiupright breast-feeding position, which allows gravity to aid in jaw extension and minimizes the degree of overbite and friction. Continuous support and shaping of the breast throughout the feed with hand support of the infant's head and shoulders stabilize the neck and jaw muscles. Heat and gentle manipulation of the nipple may elongate it sufficiently to enable a correct latch. If clinically indicated, frenectomy can release a tethered tongue (142). Over a period of a few weeks, an hypoplastic mandible rapidly elongates, the facial muscles strengthen, the nipple tissue becomes more distensible, the latch improves, and nipple trauma and pain resolve.

Chapped Nipples

Dry, cracked nipples may be chapped due to loss of the moisture barrier in the stratum corneum because of constant wet and dry exposure combined with nipple friction. Management goals include avoiding further trauma by modifying breast-feeding technique, avoiding excessive drying, and restoring the moisture barrier. Moist wound healing allows the epithelium cells to migrate inward and heal the cracks and ulcers (143). Moisturizers and emollients such as USP modified anhydrous lanolin applied to the nipples and areola after each feed are cheap and effective. A mild corticosteroid ointment may help to decrease the inflammation. In most situations, breast-feeding should continue during therapy; if repositioning fails to modify or relieve the pain and discomfort, it may be advisable to stop breast-feeding for 48 to 72 hours to allow healing to occur. The breasts should be emptied every 3 to 4 hours, and an alternative feeding method should be used. It is inappropriate to try to mask the pain by numbing with ice or using strong analgesia or nipple shields because to do so will fail to correct the underlying cause and may lead to further nipple trauma.

Impetigo of the Nipple

Staphylococcus aureus is frequently found distributed over the skin. Natural barriers, such as the stratum corneum, skin dryness, rapid cell turnover, and acid pH of 5 to 6, of the infant's skin usually prevent infection. For disease to result, preexisting tissue injury or inflammation is of major importance in pathogenesis. As in other clinical situations, when there is a break in the integument of the skin surface, there is a predisposition to a secondary infection because of bacterial or fungal contamination, which may lead to a delay in wound healing. Sore nipples associated with skin breakage, including cracks, fissures, and ulceration, have a high chance of being contaminated with microorganisms. The clinical findings on the nipple and areolar of local erythema, excoriations, purulent exudates, and tenderness are suspicious of impetigo vulgaris due to coagulase-positive *S. aureus* and group A β-hemolytic streptococcus. Livingstone et al. showed that mothers with young infants who complained of moderate to severe nipple pain and who had cracks, fissures, ulcers, or exudates had a 64% chance of having positive skin cultures and a 54% chance of having *S. aureus* infection. In some clinical situations, a blocked nipple pore appears white and on culturing is found to be contaminated with *S. aureus*. Most cases of cellulitis, mastitis, and breast abscess involve an ascending lactiferous duct infection with *S. aureus* or β-hemolytic streptococcus; it is therefore important to diagnose impetigo on the nipple by culturing the nipple. Management follows the standard treatment for impetigo, including careful washing with soap and water of the nipples to remove crusting and the use of appropriate antibiotics. Topical antibiotic ointments such as fusidic acid (Fuccidin) or mupirocin (Bactroban) may be effective in conjunction with systemic penicillinase-resistant antibiotics, such as dicloxacillin, a cephalosporin, or erythromycin in penicillin-allergic patients (127). Treatment should continue for 7 to 10 days until the skin is fully healed. The source of the infection is often from the infant's oropharyngeal or ophthalmic flora. In persistent or recurrent infections, it may be necessary to treat the infant as well.

Candidiasis

Candidiasis is commonly caused by *Candida albicans* and less frequently by other *Candida* species. It may be a primary or secondary skin infection. *C. albicans* is endogenous to the gastrointestinal tract and mucocutaneous areas. Normal skin does not harbor *C. albicans*; however, almost any skin damage caused by trauma or environmental changes may lead to rapid colonization by *C. albicans*. Isolation of the organism from a diseased skin may not be the cause of the disease but may be coincidental. *C. albicans* can be a secondary invader in preexisting pathological conditions and may give rise to further pathology. Candidiasis should be suspected when persistent nipple symptoms, such as a burning sensation on light touch and severe nipple pain during feeds, are combined with minimal objective findings on the nipple. Typical signs include a superficial erythema on the nipple and areola or a dry, flaky dermatitis with clear demarcated edges over the areola. A high incidence of oral mucocutaneous candidiasis has been noted in the newborn following vaginal delivery in the presence of maternal candidal vulvovaginitis. Clinical examination of the infant is mandatory because *C. albicans* is passed from the infant's oral pharynx to the mother's nipple, which, being a warm, moist, frequently macerated epidermis, is easily colonized and possibly infected when the integument is broken. In the presence of characteristic and chronic nipple pain and dermatitis, the nipples should be cultured or skin scraping directly observed microscopically to determine the presence of fungal infection (144,145).

The treatment of cutaneous candidiasis includes careful hygiene, removal of excessive moisture, and topical therapy with broad-spectrum antifungal agents such as nystatin, clotrimazole, miconazole or 2% ketoconazole. The creams should be applied to the nipple and areola before and after each breast-feed for 10 to 14 days. In addition, other sites of candidiasis in both mother and infant, including maternal vulvovaginitis, intertrigo, or infant diaper dermatitis, should be treated simultaneously with a topical antifungal cream. Oral thrush in the infant should be treated aggressively with an oral antifungal solution such as nystatin suspension 100,000 U/g. After each feed, the oral cavity should be carefully painted and then 0.5 mL of nystatin suspension inserted into the mouth by dropper for 14 days. Oral fluconazole 3 mg/kg daily for 14 days or oral ketoconazole 5 mg/kg daily for 7 days was recently approved for use of oropharyngeal candidiasis in newborns (146). Gentian violet 0.5% to 1% aqueous solution is cheap and effective if used sparingly under medical supervision. Daily painting of the infant's mouth and mother's nipples for about 5 to 7 days is usually sufficient. Excessive use may cause oral ulceration (147). Failure to eradicate fungal infections is usually due to user, not medication failure. Occasionally, more serious underlying medical conditions such as diabetes or immunodeficiencies may exist. In resistant cases, systemic antifungal agents are required, such as single-dose fluconazole 150 mg. Anecdotal evidence suggests that fluconazole 400 mg per day or ketoconazole 200 mg per day may be used with caution in severe cases of deep or systemic candidiasis. In addition, topical corticosteroids may reduce nipple pruritus and erythema (148). Foreign objects contaminated with yeast, including soothers and rubber nipples, should be avoided or sterilized, if possible, to prevent reinfection. Lay literature is full of nonpharmacologic treatments for candidiasis with little evidence to support them. The health care provider is cautioned against recommending regimens that are complicated. In an otherwise healthy person, the immune defense mechanism can control the growth of candida, assuming the skin integument is intact and remains dry.

Contact Dermatitis

Contact dermatitis in the nipple is an eczematous reaction to an external material applied, worn, or inadvertently transferred to the skin. It may be an allergic or an irritant response. Patients may complain of dry, pruritic, or burning nipples with signs of inflammation, erythema, and edema or excoriations, desquamation, or chronic plaque formation. Management includes careful avoidance of all irritants such as creams, preservatives, detergents, and fragrances. Topical nonfluoridated steroid ointments and emollients applied thinly to the nipple and areola after each feed are effective. Chronic dermatitis is often positive for *S. aureus,* which may require oral antibiotic therapy.

Paget Disease

Paget disease is an intraepidermal carcinoma for which the most common site is the nipple and areola. It usually presents as unilateral erythema and scaling of the nipple and areola and looks eczematous. Unfortunately, the condition is usually part of an intraductal carcinoma, and treatment necessitates cessation of breast-feeding.

Vasospasm or Raynaud Phenomenon

Vasospasm, or Raynaud phenomenon, of the nipple manifests as a blanching of the nipple tip and severe pain and discomfort radiating through the breast after and between feeds. It is often associated with excoriated and infected nipples. There may be a concomitant history of cold-induced vasospasm of the fingers (Raynaud phenomenon). Repetitive trauma to the nipple from incorrect latch or retrognathia, combined with local inflammation or infection and air cooling, can trigger a characteristic painful vasospastic response for which management is often frustrating because resolution is slow. Correcting the latch and alternating breast-feeding positions throughout the feed will prevent ongoing nipple trauma. Avoiding air exposure and applying warm dry heat to the nipples after feeds may help. Standard pharmacologic therapy for Raynaud phenomenon can be effective in reducing the vasospasms. Local infections should be treated aggressively and breast-feeding stopped for several days if necessary to allow healing to occur.

Psoriasis

Psoriasis may present as a pink, flaky plaque over the areola as a result of skin trauma. There is usually an existing psoriatic history. Standard treatment includes fluorinated steroid ointments and keratolytic agents, which should be applied after feeds and then washed off carefully before feedings.

For many years, the medical and nursing literature has recommended a variety of management approaches for sore nipples, ranging from topical application of cold tea bags, carrots and vitamin E, to lanolin, masse cream, antiseptics, alcohol preparations, and air drying (149). The efficacy of each of these modalities has not been proven, however; in fact, the latter is now thought to be detrimental by abstracting water from the skin and precipitating protein, which leaves the skin less pliable and more prone to fissuring. Health care professionals are cautioned against using nontraditional adjunct management modalities for sore nipples because of the risk of iatrogenic disease.

Induced Lactation and Relactation

Given the growing understanding of the value of breast-feeding in terms of nutrition and nurturing, women are seeking information about breast-feeding and adoption. Induced lactation in the nonpregnant woman has been described for many years in both scientific and lay publications and includes the first reports by Hippocrates (150). In several cultures, breast-feeding adopted children has been described as routine (151). Reports concentrate primarily on the issue of the novelty of breast-feeding an adopted child and include few case studies (152–158). The exceptions are the works by Auerbach et al., who studied 240 women who attempted to breast-feed adopted children (155); Livingstone and Armstrong (159); and Nemba, who studied 37 women in Papua, New Guinea (160). Nemba used a simple protocol combining a high degree of motivation with medication, support, and encouragement. Eighty-nine percent of women successfully breast-fed, but a clear definition of breast-feeding was lacking. There are several anecdotally described methods of inducing lactation and preparing for breast-feeding, some of which can be started before the arrival of the infant. Direct nipple stimulation has been described as the most important component of inducing lactation and preparing to breast-feed (161, 162). It not only stretches and readies the skin, but it also triggers the release of prolactin, which is thought to help stimulate the glandular development of the breasts and facilitate milk production (163). Nipple stimulation can be performed by hand or by such mechanical means as an electric breast pump. Hand stimulation has the advantage of being easy and portable, but mechanical pumping stimulates greater milk production in lactating women (164).

A variety of pharmacological lactotrophs and galactagogues have been used to induce lactation. Estrogen and progesterone are used to promote mammogenesis by stimulating alveoli and lactiferous duct proliferation. They inhibit milk synthesis by blocking the action of prolactin on the mammary glands and therefore are used in preparation for breast-feeding only (39,165). Galactagogues such as phenothiazine, sulpiride, and domperidone also have been described (166–170). They are dopamine antagonists and block the inhibition of prolactin, which is a potent lactotroph. Metoclopramide and chlorpromazine are commonly used galactagogues but have many potential side effects, including sedation, extrapyramidal symptoms, and tardive dyskinesia. Domperidone has little effect on the central nervous system and has fewer side effects. Oxytocin is the hormone responsible for milk ejection. It stimulates the contraction of myoepithelial cells around the mammary alveoli and causes milk ejection. It does not directly effect milk synthesis (93). Some researchers believe that hormones used to promote lactation are harmful to the child and do not advise their use (171,172). Drug excretion in breast milk is very limited and in combination with low milk production probably does not pose a risk to the infant. Relactation is often more successful than induced lactation (173).

CONCLUSION

As the prevalence of breast-feeding continues to increase, health professionals will be expected to take a leadership role in the promotion, protection, and support of breast-feeding by providing appropriate guidance, diagnosis, and breast-feeding management throughout the full course of lactation.

REFERENCES

1. Livingstone V. Breastfeeding kinetics: a problem-solving approach to breastfeeding difficulties. Behavioural and metabolic aspects of breastfeeding. *World Rev Nutr Diet* 1995;78:28–54.
2. Livingstone V. Prenatal lactation assessment, *J SOGC* 1994;16:2351–2359.
3. O'Camp P, Fadden PR, Gielen AC, et al. Prenatal factors associated with breastfeeding duration: recommendations for prenatal interventions. *Birth* 1992;19:195–201.
4. Akre J, ed. Infant-feeding–the physiological basics. *Bull World Health Org* 1989;67(Suppl):1–108
5. Cunningham AS, Jelliffe DB, Jelliffe EGP. *Breastfeeding, growth and illness: an annotated bibliography.* New York: UNICEF, 1992:448–480.
6. Dewey KG, Peerson JM, Brown KH, et al. Growth of breast-fed infants deviates from current reference data: a pooled analysis of US, Canadian and European data sets. *Pediatrics* 1995;(3 Pt 1):495–503.
7. Pisacane A, De Vizia B, Valiante A, et al. Iron status in breast-fed infants. *J Pediatr* 1995;127:429–431.
8. Beaudry M, Dufour R, Marcoux S. Relation between infant feeding and infections during the first six months of life. *J Pediatr* 1995;126:191–197.
9. Dewy KG, Heinig MJ, Nommsen-Rivers LA. Differences in morbidity between breast-fed and formula-fed infants. *J Pediatr* 1995;126(5 Pt 1):696–702.
10. Saarinen UM, Kajosaari M. Breastfeeding as prophylaxis against atopic disease: prospective follow-up study until 17 years old. *Lancet* 1995;346:1065–1069.
11. Baumgartner C. Psychomotor and social development of breastfed and bottlefed babies during their first year of life. *Acta Paediatr Hung* 1984;25:409–417.
12. Davies DW, Bell PA. Infant feeding practices and occlusal outcomes: a longitudinal study. *J Can Dent Assoc* 1991;57:593–594.
13. Mitchell EA, Taylor BJ, Ford RP, et al. Four modifiable and other major risk factors for cot death: the New Zealand study. *J Pediatr Child Health* 1992;28:53–58.
14. Campbell SB, Taylor PM. Bonding and attachment: theoretical issues. *Semin Perinatol* 1979;3:3–13.

15. Widstrom AM, Wahlberg V, Matthiesen S, et al. Short-term effects of suckling and touch of the nipple on maternal behavior. *Early Hum Dev* 1990;21:153–163.
16. Diaz S, Rodriguez G, Marshall G, et al. Lactational amenorrhea and the recovery of ovulation and fertility in fully nursing Chilian mothers. *Contraception* 1988;38:37–51.
17. Family Health International. Breastfeeding as a family planning method. *Lancet* 1988;2:1204–1205.
18. Yang C. History of lactation and breast cancer risk. *Am J Epidemiol* 1993;138:1050–1056.
19. Hirose K, Tajima K, Hamajima N, et al. A large-scale, hospital-based case–control study of risk factors of breast cancer according to menopausal status. *Jpn J Cancer Res* 1995;86:146–154.
20. Kalkwarf HJ, Specker BL. Bone mineral loss during lactation and recovery after weaning. *Obstet Gynecol* 1995;86:26–32.
21. Whitemore AS, Harris R, Intyre J, and the Collaboratine Ovarian Cancer Group. Characteristics relating to ovarian cancer risk: collaboratine analysis of 12 US case–control studies. *Am J Epidemiol* 1992;136:1184–1203.
22. Walker M. A fresh look at the risks of artificial infant feeding. *Journal of Human Lactation* 1993; 9:97–107.
23. Frank JW, Newman J. Breast-feeding in a polluted world: uncertain risks, clear benefits [Review]. *Can Med Assoc J* 1993;149:33–37.
24. Lucas A, Morley R, Cole TJ, et al. Breastmilk and subsequent intelligence quotient in children born preterm. *Lancet* 1992;339:261–264.
25. Pollock JI. Long term associations with infant feeding in a clinically advantaged population of babies. *Dev Med Child Neurol* 1994;36:429–440.
26. Lanting CI, Fidler V, Huisman M, et al. Neurological differences between 9-year-old children fed breast-milk or formula-milk as babies. *Lancet* 1994;344:1319–1322.
27. Chandra R. Food allergy: 1992 and beyond. *Nutr Res* 1992;12:93–99.
28. Halken S, Host A, Klansen LG, et al. Effects of an allergy prevention programme on incidence of atopic symptoms in infancy: a prospective study of 159 "high-risk" infants. *Allergy* 1992;47: 545–553.
29. Kajosaari M, Saarinen UM. Prophylaxis of atopic disease by six months' total solid food elimination: evaluation of 135 exclusively breast-fed infants of atopic families. *Acta Paediatr Scand* 1983;72: 411–414.
30. Howie PW, Forsyth JS, Ogston SA, et al. Protective effect of breastfeeding against infection. *BMJ* 1990;300:11–16.
31. Fallot ME, Boyd JL III, Oski F. Breastfeeding reduces incidence of hospital admissions for infections in infants. *Pediatrics* 1980;65:1121–1124.
32. Koletzko SP, Sherman P, Corey M, et al. Role of infant feeding practices in development of Crohn's disease in childhood *BMJ* 1989;298:1617–1618.
33. Scott FW. Cow milk and insulin-dependent diabetes mellitus: is there a relationship? *Am J Clin Nutr* 1990;51:489–491.
34. Karjalainen J, Martin JM, Knip M, et al. A bovine albumin peptide as a possible trigger of insulin-dependent diabetes mellitus. *N Engl J Med* 1992;327:302–307.
35. Renfrew M, Fisher C, Arms S. *Breastfeeding: getting breastfeeding right for you.* Berkley, California: Celestial Arts, 1990:15–19.
36. *The art of successful breastfeeding: a mother's guide* [Video]. Vancouver: University of British Columbia, V5Z 1M1, Canada, 1995.
37. Neifert MR, Seacat JM, Jobe WE. Lactation failure due to insufficient glandular development of the breast. *Pediatrics* 1985;76:823–828.
38. Neifert M, DeMarzo S, Seacat J, et al. The influence of breast surgery, breast appearance, and pregnancy-induced breast changes on lactation sufficiency as measured by infant weight gain. *Birth* 1990;17:32–38.
39. Rillema JA. Development of the mammary gland and lactation. *Trends Endocrinol Metab* 1994;5: 1469–1540.
40. Friesen HG, Cowden EA. Lactation and galactorrhea. In: DeGroot, LJ, ed. *Endocrinology,* 2nd ed. Vol 1. Philadelphia: WB Saunders, 1989:2074–2089.
41. Heyman SJ. Modeling the impact of breastfeeding by HIV infected women on child survival. *Am J Public Health* 1990;80:1305–1309.
42. Lin HH, Kao JH, Hsu HY, et al. Absence of infection in breast-fed infants born to hepatitis C virus-infecteed mothers. *J Pediatr* 1995;126:589–591.

43. Hansen B, Moore L. Recreational drug use by the breastfeeding woman. Part I: illicit drugs. *Journal of Human Lactation* 1989;5:178–180.
44. Fulton B. Recreational drug use by the breastfeeding woman. Part II: illicit drugs. *Journal of Human Lactation* 1990;6:15–16.
45. Bottorff JL, Moore JM. Mothers' perceptions of breast milk. *J Obstet Gynecol Neonatal Nurs* 1990; 19:518–527.
46. Brownlee A. *Breastfeeding, weaning, and nutrition: the behavioural issues.* Behavioural issues in child survival program. Monograph 4. Malibu, CA: International Health and Development Associates, 1990:1–93.
47. Mclorg PA, Bryant CA. Influence of social network members and health care professionals on infant feeding practices of economically disadvantaged mothers. *Med Anthropol* 1989;10:265–278.
48. Alexander JM, Grant AM, Campbell MJ. Randomized controlled trial of breast shells and Hoffman's exercises for inverted and non-protractile nipples. *BMJ* 1992;304:1030–1032.
49. Kesaree N. Treatment of inverted nipples using a disposable syringe. *Journal of Human Lactation* 1993;9:27–29.
50. Righard L, Alade MO. Effect of delivery room routines on success of first breast-feed. *Lancet* 1990;336:1105–1107.
51. Widstrom AJ, Ransjo-Aruidson AB, Christensson K, et al. Gastric suction in healthy newborn infants. *Acta Paediatr Scand* 1987;76:566–572.
52. Woolridge M, Creasley V, Spisornkosol S. The initiation of lactation: the effect of early versus delayed contact for suckling on milk intake in the first week postpartum. *Early Hum Dev* 1985; 12:269–278.
53. Howie PW, McNeilly AS, McArdle T, et al. The relationship between suckling-induced prolactin response and lactogenesis. *J Clin Endocrinol Metab* 1980;50:670–673.
54. Klaus MH. The frequency of suckling: a neglected but essential ingredient of breastfeeding. *Obstet Gynecol Clin North Am* 1987;14:623–633.
55. Yamauchi Y, Yamanouchi I. Breastfeeding frequency during the first 24 hours after birth in full-term neonates. *Pediatrics* 1990;86:171–175.
56. Keefe MR. The impact of infant rooming-in on maternal sleep at night. *J Obstet Gynecol Neonatal Nurse* 1988;17:122–126.
57. Yamauchi Y, Yamanouchi I. The relationship between room-in/not rooming-in and breastfeeding variables. *Acta Paediatr Scand* 1990;79:1017–1022.
58. Elander G, Lindberg T. Short mother-infant separation during first week of life influences the duration of breastfeeding. *Acta Paediatr Scand* 1984;73:237–240.
59. Royal College of Midwives. *Successful breastfeeding.* New York: Churchill Livingstone, 1991: 25–33.
60. Moon JL, Humenick SS. Breast engorgement: contributing variables and variables amenable to nursing intervention. *J Obstet Gynecol Neonatal Nurse* 1989;18:309–315.
61. Newman J. Breastfeeding problems associated with the early introduction of bottle and pacifiers. *Journal of Human Lactation* 1990;6:59–63.
62. Shrago L. Glucose supplementation of the breastfed infant during the first three days of life. *Journal of Human Lactation* 1987;32:82–86.
63. Woolridge MW. *Baby-controlled breastfeeding: biocultural implications in breastfeeding. In: Stuart-Macadam P, Dettwyler K, eds. Biocultural perspectives.* New York: Aldine De Gruyter, 1995:217–222.
64. Hanson LA, Hahn-Zoric M, Berndes M, et al. Breastfeeding: overview and breast milk immunology. *Acta Paediatr Jpn* 1994;36:557–561.
65. Fitzsimmons SP, Evans MK, Pearce CL, et al. Immunoglobulin A subclasses in infants' saliva and in saliva and milk from their mothers. *J Pediatr* 1994;124:566–573.
66. Saunders S, Carroll J. Post partum breastfeeding support: impact on duration. *J Am Diet Assoc* 1988;88:213–215.
67. Neville MC, Keller R, Seacat J, et al. Studies in human lactation: milk volumes in lactating women during the onset of lactation and full lactation. *Am J Clin Nutr* 1988;48:1375–1386.
68. Hartmann PE, Prosser CG. Physiological bases of longitudinal changes in human milk yield and composition. *Fed Proc* 1984;43:2448–2453.
69. Woolridge MW, Baum JD, Drewett RF. Individual patterns of milk intake during breastfeeding. *Early Hum Dev* 1982;7:265–272.

70. Prentice A, Addey C, Wilde CJ. Evidence for local feedback control of human milk secretion. *Biochem Soc Trans* 1989;17:122–124.
71. Woolridge MW, Ingrim J, Baum JD. Do changes in pattern of breast usage alter the baby's nutrient intake. *Lancet* 1990;336:395–397.
72. McNeilly AS, Robinson IC, Houston MJ, et al. Release of oxytoxin and prolactin in response to suckling. *BMJ* 1983;286:257–259.
73. WHO/UNICEF. *Protecting, promoting and supporting breastfeeding: the special role of maternity services.* Geneva: World Health Organization, 1989.
74. Lawrence R. *Breastfeeding: a guide for the medical profession,* 5th ed. St. Louis: CV Mosby, 1999: 35–56.
75. Djiane J, Houdebine LM, Kelly P. Prolactin-like activity of anti-prolactin receptor antibodies on casein and DNA synthesis in the mammary gland. *Proc Natl Acad Sci USA* 1981;78:7445–7448.
76. Pestell RG, Best JD, Alford FP. Lymphocytic hypophysitis: the clinical spectrum of the disorder and evidence for an autoimmune pathogenesis. *Clin Endocrinol* 1990;33:457–466.
77. Imura, H, ed. *The pituitary gland.* New York: Raven Press, 1994:1–28.
78. Livingstone VH, Gout PW, Crickmer SD, et al. Serum lactogens possessed normal bioactivity in patients with lactation insufficiencies. *Clin Endocrinol* 1994;41:193–198.
79. Neifert MR, McDonough SL, Neville MC. Failure of lactogenesis associated with placental retention. *Am J Obstet Gynaecol* 1981;140:477–478.
80. Kelly PA, Djiane J, Pastel-Vinay MC, et al. The prolactin/growth hormone receptor family. *Endocr Rev* 1991;12:235–251.
81. De Carvalho M, Robertson S, Friedman A, et al. Effect of frequent breastfeeding on early milk production and infant weight gain. *Paediatrics* 1983;72:307–311.
82. Livingstone VH. Liberty bottle or liability bottle? A formula for failure. *Can Fam Physician* 1988; 34:1143–1146.
83. Aono T, Shioji T, Shoda T, et al. The initiation of human lactation and prolactin response to suckling. *J Clin Endocrinol Metab* 1977;44:1101–1106.
84. Harris, L, Morris SF, Friebery A. Is breastfeeding possible after reduction mammoplasty? *Plast Reconstr Surg* 1992;89:836–839.
85. Synderman RK. Reduction mammoplasty. In: Gallager HS, ed. *The breast.* St. Louis: Mosby, 1978.
86. Widdice L. The effects of breast reduction and breast augmentation surgery on lactation: an annotated bibliography. *Journal of Human Lactation* 1993;9:161–167.
87. Newton M, Newton N. Postpartum engorgement of the breast. *Am J Obstet Gynecol* 1951;61: 664–667.
88. Bocar D, Shargo L. *Eingorgement.* Oklahoma City: Lactation Consultant Services, 1990.
89. Lennon I, Lewis BR. Effect of complementary feeds on lactation failure. *Breastfeeding Review* 1987;11:24–26.
90. Henrickson M. A policy for supplementation/complementary feedings for breastfed newborn infants. *Journal of Human Lactation* 1990;63:11–13.
91. Human Milk Banking Association of North America, Inc. *Recommendations for collection, storage, and handling of a mother's milk for her own infant in a hospital setting.* West Hartford, CT: HMBANA, 1993.
92. Drewett RF, Woolridge MW. Milk taken by human babies from the first and second breast. *Physiol Behav* 1981;26:327–329.
93. Newton M, Newton N. The let-down reflex on human lactation. *J Pediatr* 1948;33:698–704.
94. Neifert MR, Seacat JM. How to help patients breastfeed successfully. *Contemp Obstet Gynecol* 1986;29:85–103.
95. Woolridge MW. The "anatomy" of infant sucking. *Midwifery* 1986;2:164–171.
96. Righard L, Alade MO. Sucking technique and its effect on success of breastfeeding. *Birth* 1992; 19:185–189.
97. Bullock F, Woolridge MW, Baum JD. Development of co-ordination of sucking, swallowing, and breathing: ultrasound study of term and preterm infants. *Dev Med Child Neurol* 1990;32:669–678.
98. Wolfe LS, Glass RP. *Feeding and swallowing disorders in infancy: assessment and management.* Tucson, AZ: Therapy Skill Builders, 1992:23–54.
99. Blass EM, Teicher M. Suckling. *Science* 1980;210:15–22.
100. McBride MC, Danner SC. Sucking disorders in neurologically impaired infants: Assessment and facilitation of breastfeeding. *Clin Perinatol* 1987;14:109–131.

101. Palmer MM, Crawley K, Blanco IA. Neonatal oral motor assessment scale: a reliability study. *J Perinatol* 1993;8:28–35.
102. Notestine GE. The importance of the identification of ankyloglossia (Short Lingual Frenulum) as a cause of breastfeeding problems. *Journal of Human Lactation* 1990;6:113–115.
103. Ankyloglossia (tongue tie). *Journal of Human Lactation* 1990;6:101–155.
104. Daly SC, Di Rosso A, Owens RA, et al. Degree of breast emptying explains changes in the fat content, but no fatty acid composition, of human milk. *Exp Physiol* 1993;78:741–755.
105. Nysenbaum AN, Smart JL, Sucking behaviour and milk intake of neonates in relation to milk fat content. *Early Hum Dev* 1982;6:205–213.
106. Baronowski T, Bee DE, Rassin RK, et al. Social supports, social influence, ethnicity, and breastfeeding decision. *Soc Sci Med* 1983;17:1559–1611.
107. Stuart-Macadam P. Biocultural perspectives on breastfeeding. In: Stuart-Macadam P, Dettwyler KA, eds. *Breastfeeding biocultural perspectives*. New York: Aldine De Gruyter, 1995;1–37.
108. Livingstone V. In hospital lactation assessment. *J SOGC* 1996;18:45–54.
109. Dewey KG, Heinig MJ, Nommsen LA, et al. Growth of breastfed and formula fed infants from 0 to 18 months: the DARLING study. *Pediatrics* 1992;89:1035–1040.
110. Livingstone V. Problem-solving formula for failure to thrive in breastfed infants. *Can Fam Physician* 1990;36:1541–1545.
111. Page-Goertz S. Discharge planning for the breastfeeding dyad. *Pediatr Nurs* 1989;15:543–544.
112. Lawrence RA. *Breastfeeding: a guide for the medical profession,* 5th ed. St. Louis: Mosby,1999: 215–277.
113. Meintz Maher S. *An overview of solutions to breastfeeding and sucking problems.* Franklin Park, IL: La Leche League International, 1988.
114. Daly S. The short-term synthesis and infant regulated removal of milk in lactating women. *Exp Physiol* 1986;78:209–220.
115. Freed LM, Neville MC, Hamosh P, et al. Diurnal and within-food variations in activity and triglyceride content of human milk. *J Pediatr Gastroenterol Nutr* 1986;6:938–942.
116. Meier PP, Lysakowski Y, Engstrom JL, et al. The accuracy of test weighing for preterm infants. *J Pediatr Gastroenterol Nutr* 1990;10:62–65.
117. Whitfield M, Kay R, Stevens S. Validity of routine clinical test weighing as a measure of intake of breast-fed infants. *Arch Dis Child* 1981;56:919–921.
118. Woolridge MW, Butte N, Dewey KG. Methods for the measurement of milk volume intake of the breast-fed infant. In: Jensen RG, Neville MC, eds. *Human lactation: milk components and methodologies.* New York: Plenum Press, 1985:5–21.
119. Hofmeyr GJ, Van Iddekinge B, Blott JA. Domperodone: secretion in breast milk and effects on puerperal prolactin levels. *Br J Obstet Gynaecol* 1985;92:141–144.
120. Livingstone V. Too much of a good thing: maternal and infant hyperlactation syndromes. *Can Fam Physician* 1996;42:89–99.
121. Fetherston C. Risk factors for lactation mastitis. *Journal of Human Lactation* 1998;14:101–109.
122. Hoyle D. Blocked ducts. *New generation* 1992;1:16–17.
123. Thomson AC, Espersen T, Maigaard S. Course and treatment of milk stasis, non-infectious inflammation of the breast and infectious mastitis in nursing women. *Am J Obstet Gynecol* 1984;149: 492–495.
124. Filteau SM, Lietz G, Mulokozi G. Milk cytokines and subclinical breast inflammation in Tanzanian women: effects of dietary red palm oil or sunflower oil supplementation. *Immunology* 1999;97: 595–600.
125. Walsh A. Acute mastitis. *Lancet* 1949;2:635–639.
126. Livingstone V, Willis C, Berkowitz J. *Staphylococcus aureus* and sore nipples. *Can Fam Physician* 1996;42:654–659.
127. Livingstone V, Stringer LJ. The treatment of *Staphyloccocus aureus* infected sore nipples: a randomized comparative study. *Journal of Human Lactation* 1999;15:241–246
128. Walter AP, Edmiston E, Krepel J, et al. A prospective study of the microflora of nonpuerperal breast abscess. *Arch Surg* 1988;123:908–911.
129. Riordan J, Nichols F. A descriptive study of lactation mastitis in long term breastfeeding women. *Journal of Human Lactation* 1990;6:53–58.
130. Hayes R, Michell M, Nunnerly HB. Acute inflammation of the breast: the role of breast ultrasound in diagnosis and management. *Clin Radiol* 1991;44:253–256.

131. Engin G, Acunas B. Granulmatous mastitis: gray-scale and color Doppler sonographic findings. *J Clin Ultrasound* 1999;27:101–106.
132. Dahlbeck SW, Donnelly JF, Theriault RL. Differentiating inflammatory breast cancer from acute mastitis. *Am Fam Physician* 1995;52:929–934.
133. Bertrand H, Rosenblood LK. Stripping out pus in lactational mastitis: a means of preventing breast abscess. *Can Med Assoc J* 1991;145:299–306.
134. Inch S, Von Xylander S, Savage F. *Mastitis causes and management.* Geneva: Department of Child and Adolescent Health and Development, World Health Organization, 2000:1–45.
135. Arsenault G. Toxic shock syndrome associated with mastitis. *Can Fam Physician* 1992;38:399–402.
136. Herings RM, Stricker BH. Bromocriptine and suppression of postpartum lactation. *Pharm World Sci* 1995;17:133–137.
137. Shrago LC. The breastfeeding dyad: early assessment, documentation, and intervention: NAACOG's clinical issues in prenatal and women's health nursing. *Breastfeeding* 1992;3:583–597.
138. Woolridge MW. Aetioogy of sore nipples. *Midwifery* 1986;2:172–176.
139. de Carvalho M, Robertson S, Klaus MH. Does duration and frequency of early breastfeeding effect nipple pain? *Birth* 1984;11:81–84.
140. Gunther M. Sore nipples: causes and prevention. *Lancet* 1945;2:347–355.
141. Coulter Danner L. Breastfeeding the infant with a cleft defect: NAACOG's Clinical Issues in Perinatal and Woman's Health Nursing. *Breastfeeding* 1995;3:634–639.
142. Marmet C, Shell E, Marmet R. Neonatal frenotomy may be necessary to correct breastfeeding problems. *Journal of Human Lactation* 1990;6:117–121.
143. Sharp D. Moist wound healing for sore or cracked nipples. *Breastfeeding Abstracts* 1992;12:19–20.
144. Lesher J. Fungal diseases of the skin. In: Ravel R, ed. *Conn's Current Therapy.* Philadelphia: WB Saunders, 1996:790–791.
145. Tanguay KE, Mcbean M, Jean E. Nipple candidiasis among breastfeeding mothers: case control study of predisposing factors. *Can Fam Physician* 1994;40:1407–1413.
146. Utter AR. Gentian violet treatment for thrush: can its use cause breastfeeding problems? *Journal of Human Lactation* 1990;6:178–180.
147. Pharmagram Letter, Pfizer Canada Inc, Kirkland, Quebec, H8J 2M5, 1996.
148. Huggins KE, Billen SF. Twenty cases of persistent sore nipples: collaboration between lactation consultant and dermatologist. *Journal of Human Lactation* 1993;9:155–160.
149. Auerbach KG, Riordan J, Countryman BA. The breastfeeding process. In: Auerbach KG, Riodan J, eds. *Breast and human lactation.* Boston: Jones and Bartlett Publishers, 1993:232–233.
150. Jelliffee DB, Jelliffee EFP. Non-puerperal induced lactation [Letter]. *Paediatrics* 1972;50:170–171.
151. Mead M. *Sex and temperament in three primitive societies.* New York: Dell, 1963:186–187.
152. Melinda CM, Melinda L. The family physician and adoption. *Am Fam Physician* 1985;31:109–118.
153. Mobbs GA, Babbage NG. Breastfeeding adopted children. *Med J Aust* 1971;2:436–437.
154. Cohen R. Breastfeeding without pregnancy [Letter]. *Pediatrics* 1971;48:996–997.
155. Anonymous. Can adoptive mothers breastfeed? [Editorial]. *Lancet* 1985;1:2–7.
156. Auerbach KG, Avery JL. Induced lactation: a study of adoptive nursing by 240 women. *Am J Dis Child* 1981;135:340–343.
157. Eregie CO. Non-puerperal lactation in nutritional rehabilitation: case report. *East Afr Med J* 1997; 74:59–60.
158. Newton M. Breastfeeding by adoptive mothers. *JAMA* 1970;212;11.
159. Livingstone V, Armstrong C. Breastfeeding and adoption: a retrospective qualitative survey. *Journal SOGC* 1999;21:1161–1167.
160. Nemba K. Induced lactation: a study of 37 non-puerperal mothers. *J Trop Pediatr* 1994;40:240–241
161. Illingworth RS. Non-puerperal lactation. *Midwives Chron* 1972;85:188.
162. Cheales-Siebenaler NJ. Induced lactation in an adoptive mother. *Journal of Human Lactation* 1999; 15:41–43.
163. Walter M, Auerbach K. Breast pumps and other technologies. *Breastfeeding and human lactation.* Boston: Jones & Bartlett Publishers, 1993:279–332.
164. Sutherland A, Auerbach KG. *Relactation and induced lactation (Unit 1).* Lactation Consultant Series. Garden City Park, NY: Avery Publishing Group, 1985.
165. Infant feeding: the physiological basics. *Sci J WHO* 1989;67:19–40.
166. Sousa PLR, Barros FC, Pinheiro GNM, et al. Re-establishment of lactation with metoclopramide. *J Trop Pediatr* 1975;21:214–215.

167. Weichert CE. Prolactin cycling and the management of breastfeeding failure. *Adv Pediatr* 1980; 27:391–407.
168. Aono T, Aki T, Voile K, et al. Effect of sulpride on poor puerperal lactation. *Am J Obstet Gynaecol* 1982;143:927–932.
169. Petraglia F, De Leo V, Sardelli S, et al. Domperidone in defective and insufficient lactation. *Eur J Obstet Gynaecol Reprod Biol* 1985;19:281–287.
170. MacDonald TM. Metoclopramide, domperidone and dopamine in man: actions and interactions. *Eur J Clin Pharmacol* 1991;40:225–230.
171. Auerbach KG. Extraordinary breast feeding: relactation/induced lactation. *Trop Paediatr* 1981;27: 52–55.
172. Thearle MJ, Weissenberger R. Induced lactation in adoptive mothers. *Aust N Z J Obstet Gynaecol* 1984;24:283–286.
173. Phillips V. Relactation in mothers of children over 12 months. *J Trop Pediatr* 1993;39:45–48.

6

Managing the Patient with a Breast Mass

Odysseus Argy, Kevin S. Hughes, and Constance A. Roche

Awareness of breast cancer has been heightened not only because it is the most frequently occurring cancer in women (1) but also because of extensive media coverage. This awareness contributes to the increased anxiety experienced by patients who have a breast mass that could be malignant. Detection of a breast mass in a patient is also a source of anxiety for the clinician who must consider a confusing array of variables. These variables include, but are not limited to, risk factors, clinical findings, indications for mammography, the implications of any findings, the role of ultrasound and fine needle aspiration (FNA), the need for referral, the patient's anxiety and wishes, and the risk of liability.

The clinical approach to identifying a breast mass can be simplified by understanding the likelihood of finding a particular pathology in a patient, defining the options available for making the diagnosis, and tailoring the evaluation to the patient's needs. This chapter delineates the optimal approach for individual patients by reviewing and integrating the risk factors, history, physical findings, differential diagnosis, tests such as FNA and mammography, patient preferences, and methods of documentation. We also review the experience of the Breast Center at the Lahey Clinic Medical Center (Burlington, MA) to describe some of the expected results of this approach.

WHAT A MASS CAN REPRESENT

Cancer must be included in the differential diagnosis of any breast mass, but certain patient populations are more at risk for the development of cancer than other groups (2). Breast masses in premenopausal women are more common than in postmenopausal women, but breast cancer occurs far more frequently in the latter group. Generally, a breast mass represents either a benign condition, such as a cyst, fibroadenoma, or fibrocystic changes, or a malignant condition such as infiltrating carcinoma or carcinoma *in situ*.

Cysts occur as the result of lobular involution with age and are therefore uncommon in young women and more likely to occur in women who are approaching menopause (3). Cysts are found less often in women who have reached menopause, although hormone replacement therapy may predispose some of these women to the development of cysts.

Cysts present as a mass that can be clinically identical to a fibroadenoma or a carcinoma. They contain nonbloody fluid and disappear completely when aspirated. When the material drained from a cyst is bloody, the mass does not completely disappear after drainage, recurs rapidly, or accumulates again more than twice when followed up over 4 to 6 weeks; then, a suspicion of cancer is raised, and the patient should be referred to a surgeon. Rather than using ultrasound to confirm a suspected cyst, most surgeons aspirate the cyst because the procedure is both diagnostic and therapeutic. Because no mass should ever be assumed to be a cyst, regardless of the age or risk factors of a patient, any mass that has developed in a postmenopausal woman should be considered malignant until proven otherwise.

Fibroadenomas, which are hyperplastic lobules that develop most often in women in the third and fourth decades of life, are usually solitary and discrete and respond to estrogen and progesterone (4). In women under 25 years of age who present with a new mass, fibroadenoma is the most common diagnosis. Breast cancer is rare in this age group, and cysts are uncommon (5).

The term *fibrocystic change* is used to describe any nonspecific finding in the breast that is not a cyst, a fibroadenoma, or a cancer. The term is a frequently used diagnosis that does not define any specific pathology.

The most commonly found carcinoma of the breast is infiltrating ductal carcinoma, which constitutes 70% of all breast cancers (6). There are many less common histologic types, but infiltrating lobular carcinoma, which represents about 6% of all breast cancers, is of particular interest because this variant tends to present as a poorly defined mass without mammographic findings and is therefore easy to miss.

HISTORY

Risk Factors

Clinicians should be aware of the factors that may increase the risk of breast cancer in any woman, but especially in a woman with a breast lump. Risk factors include histologic and hereditary factors as well as those related to menstrual and reproductive history.

The histologic risk factors are the easiest to quantify. Atypical hyperplasia (ductal or lobular) and lobular carcinoma *in situ* (LCIS) are the two most significant ones. *Atypical hyperplasia* is defined as an overgrowth of epithelial cells with cytologic atypia. Women with this diagnosis on a previous breast biopsy have a risk of developing breast cancer that is about four times greater than that of the general population (relative risk, 4) (7). Stated another way, this represents an absolute risk of 12% over the next 15 years following biopsy. The long-term risk has been reported to revert to normal after 10 years, but this is controversial (8,9).

Despite its name, LCIS is not a cancer but a marker of risk. Women with LCIS have a risk of developing breast cancer estimated to be about 25% to 30% over the 30 years following the biopsy (10–12).

Either of these diagnoses increases the likelihood that a new mass may be cancerous. A woman with atypical hyperplasia or LCIS who presents with a mass should be referred to a specialist for evaluation.

To assess hereditary risk, a thorough family history is necessary. This should include the history of cancer in immediate family members as well as grandparents, aunts, uncles, and first cousins. The paternal and maternal sides are equally important because cancer susceptibility genes are autosomal and therefore can be transmitted by either parent. Even though the focus of the history of cancer in the family is on breast and ovarian cancer, the occurrence of other cancers may also suggest a hereditary syndrome. In a woman whose family history suggests that she has a hereditary predisposition, aggressive evaluation of any breast lump is indicated and referral to a specialist is warranted.

Although most breast cancers are sporadic, about 5% to 10% are the result of hereditary predisposition (13). In a typical family with hereditary cancer, many family members are affected, diagnosis is likely to be at a relatively young age, and there are more likely to be some patients with more than one primary cancer. Awareness of these characteristics provides an index of suspicion to identify patients with such syndromes. Not all families with hereditary cancer, however, have all these features. For example, if the patient's mother had breast cancer at age 30 (a strikingly young age), the patient's risk is higher, even though other family members have not been affected.

Several hereditary cancer syndromes have been identified in which carriers are at increased risk for breast cancer. The most common and most important are hereditary breast cancer syndrome and hereditary breast or ovarian cancer syndrome. In a typical family with hereditary breast cancer syndrome, many family members have breast cancer, diagnosis is likely at a young age, and bilateral disease is likely to occur. This syndrome is most often the result of a mutation in the *BRCA1* or *BRCA2* gene. If ovarian cancer is also present in the family, the syndrome is referred to as the *hereditary breast and ovarian cancer syndrome*, and is also likely to be the result of a mutation in *BRCA1* or *BRCA2* (14–16).

Other less common hereditary cancer syndromes may indicate a predisposition to breast cancer. Cowden syndrome is characterized by hamartomatous lesions of the oral cavity and skin as well as a predisposition to both benign and malignant conditions of the breast and thyroid. This syndrome is associated with germline mutations in the *PTEN* gene (17). Li–Fraumeni syndrome is characterized by very early onset breast cancer, soft-tissue sarcomas, brain tumors, leukemias, and other cancers and is associated with mutations in the *p53* gene (18).

Hereditary nonpolyposis colorectal cancer syndrome (HNPCC) is a syndrome in which numerous relatives develop colon cancer, commonly at an early age. Persons with this syndrome are also at increased risk for other cancers, including cancer of the endometrium, stomach, ovary, urogenital tract, and possibly breast cancer. HNPCC is likely the result of a mutation in one of several genes: *hMLH1*, *hMSH2*, *hPMS1*, and *hPMS2* (19,20).

In summary, if a patient has many relatives with cancer, if the cancers occurred at a young age, and if any family member had multiple primary cancers, the possibility of a hereditary cancer syndrome must be considered. If multiple breast cancers or breast and ovarian cancers have developed, the likelihood of hereditary breast cancer syndrome or hereditary breast and ovarian cancer syndrome should be considered. If colon and endometrial and breast cancer have occurred, HNPCC should be considered. If benign or malignant thyroid abnormalities, colon polyps, and breast cancer have been diagnosed, Cowden syndrome is likely. If family members have sarcomas, hematologic malignancies, and brain tumors, the Li–Fraumeni syndrome may be present. If a patient has the characteristics of any hereditary cancer syndrome, management of a breast mass is best left to the specialist.

Other risk factors that must be recorded include the age of onset of menarche and menopause, age at the birth of the first child, and the number of previous breast biopsies. In large populations, these factors may be useful in differentiating subtle differences in risk (21). In individual patients, however, these factors have little use in decision making about the management of a mass (22).

History of the Mass

In the context of this chapter, a patient is defined as having a breast mass if she or one of her health care providers have, or believe they have, felt a mass. The time of the first detection of the mass should be documented. If it was first detected by the clinician, a note should be made in the record about whether the patient was also able to palpate it after it was identified. If the patient detected the mass, the clinician should document when it was first discovered, its size and softness or hardness, any change in size over time, and fluctuations with the menstrual cycle. The presence or absence of nipple discharge and its character are important. The pertinent positive and negative aspects of the history determine the index of suspicion for a malignant process.

The likelihood of a carcinoma increases when the patient reports that the mass is enlarging or becoming harder or that it was initially difficult to detect but is now more obvious. Although the history that a mass changes in size with the menstrual cycle and remains stable from cycle to cycle is consistent with fibrocystic changes, the surrounding normal breast tissue still can fluctuate with the menstrual cycle, causing a carcinoma to be confused with a benign process.

Breast pain should be distinguished from a breast mass. Patients often refer to a tender point in the breast as a lump. Cyclic breast pain associated with the menstrual cycle is a common symptom, but it is seldom a sign of breast cancer. The patient must clarify whether there is a palpable mass versus a place that is sensitive to touch. Patients often equate a mass becoming more sensitive over time with a mass becoming larger. It is important for the patient to distinguish the attributes of pain from the attributes of the mass.

PHYSICAL EXAMINATION

About one third of patients under age 40 who present with a self-detected breast mass have a dominant mass confirmed on examination by a surgeon (23). This ratio of perceived-to-confirmed breast masses is similar in patients over the age of 40 years. Although this appears to be a low rate of confirmation, the failure to identify a dominant mass is related to many factors. The breast, in general, is not smooth and consistent to palpation because the mixture of breast tissue and fat changes with age and the individual and is variously described as thickened, ridged, or lumpy. The breast examination, whether done by the patient or the examiner, is further complicated by the fact that breast tissue also undergoes cyclic hormonal changes with time, and some areas become thicker or thinner relative to surrounding structures. As a result, women often perceive normal variations and areas of thickening as a mass or lump.

The clinical breast examination should be performed systematically and thoroughly. The examination involves inspection, palpation of all breast tissue, comparison of both breasts for symmetry visually and by palpation, and examination of the axillae and supraclavicular areas.

Inspection

A visual inspection should be performed with the patient seated, and her arms raised, with attention to skin changes such as erythema, dimpling, obvious masses, peau d'orange, or asymmetry. Dimpling occurs when the supporting ligaments of the breast are tethered or contracted. Even when dimpling is not apparent while the patient is sitting, it sometimes can be elicited during the examination by pushing the skin together over a mass. If the skin is not tethered to the mass, the skin bulges. If there is foreshortening of the ligaments of the breast by a cancer, however, the skin dimples. Although a large benign mass can displace ligaments and produce this sign, any dimpling over the mass significantly raises the level of suspicion for cancer. Extensive dimpling without palpation represents peau d'orange and is highly suspicious.

Changes in the nipples are also important because the nipple lesion of Paget's disease, which is an underlying *in situ* or invasive breast cancer, may accompany a breast mass. New nipple inversion may also be a significant finding, whereas longstanding inversion has little clinical significance.

Any inflammatory skin changes in a woman over age 40 that do not resolve promptly with appropriate antibiotics and conservative therapy raise the suspicion of inflammatory breast cancer. This is a rare but particularly aggressive malignancy that is frequently assumed to be mastitis. This assumption may result in a delayed diagnosis.

Palpation

All breast tissue should be palpated first with the patient seated and then with the patient lying down with her arms extended over her head. Changing the positions of the arm changes the tension of the breast over the chest wall and pectoral musculature, allowing greater differentiation between breast tissue and the underlying structures.

Several characteristics of the breast mass should be evaluated by the clinician. Features suggestive of a benign lesion include the presence of a smooth firm mass that is separate, or dominant, compared with surrounding tissue. In contrast, a malignant lesion is typically an irregular hard mass that may or may not be clearly demarcated from the surrounding tissue. Tenderness suggests an inflammatory or hormonal process rather than one that is neoplastic, but tenderness does not exclude the possibility of malignancy.

If the patient reports discharge in addition to the mass, the nipple should be squeezed to produce the discharge. Nipple discharge, which is uncommon, usually suggests a benign process such as duct ectasia or papilloma, but the risk of carcinoma increases when nipple discharge occurs in association with a mass (24). The nipples should not be squeezed routinely because useful findings are unlikely in the absence of a history of discharge.

When the patient presents with a mass, the examiner should methodically and thoroughly examine all other areas of the breast first, before assessing the area of the mass. This helps to avoid missing other significant findings that may be overlooked by focusing too intently on the mass.

Examination of Nodal Basins

The muscles surrounding the axilla should be relaxed when palpating for nodes, which can best be accomplished with the patient sitting and her arm comfortably supported by the examiner. The clinician pushes his or her fingertips high into the axilla and then drags them down over the ribs to about the level of the nipple. Enlarged lymph nodes "pop" as they slide from under the fingers. The axillae should be examined for asymmetry. Enlarged nodes and their characteristics (mobile or fixed, isolated or matted, soft or firm or hard) should be noted. An attempt should be made to reproduce any findings with the patient lying down, and her arm extended to 80 or 90 degrees.

Appropriate documentation of the history and breast examination is an important component of good medical care and also decreases the risk of litigation. Precise documentation may prevent uncertainty as to what was and what was not found during the examination. Drawing the breast and regional node area is an ideal way to document the pertinent negative and positive findings and locations. The location of the palpable mass can be identified on the sketch by drawing a circle around the area of the mass. A specific note should be made if no masses were identified in each nodal basin examined and in each breast. If the patient palpated a mass that the examiner cannot detect, she should be asked to demonstrate the mass. If she cannot locate the mass during the examination, this also should be documented. In addition, if no mass is present, an arrow, not a circle, can be used to illustrate the breast area in question; drawing a circle suggests that a mass was found by the examiner.

CLINICAL WORKUP

The most important aspect of the internist's evaluation is the determination of whether the breast mass can be followed in the office or the patient should be referred to a surgeon or breast center. In addition to a history and physical examination, the diagnostic studies to evaluate a breast mass include mammography, ultrasound, and FNA. Generally, mammography is not performed in women under age 25 because cancer is rare in that age group and dense breast tissue limits the diagnostic accuracy of the technique (25). Screening mammography is particularly effective for identifying small, nonpalpable lesions representing carcinoma *in situ* and early stage invasive cancers and usually is initiated at age 40 in the absence of risk factors (26). In contrast, diagnostic mammography in the presence of a mass fails to reveal a significant number (9%–22%) of palpable cancers (27), particularly in women under age 50 (28). Thus, whereas mammography is useful for evaluating a palpable mass, a negative mammogram in this setting should not lead the clinician to conclude that the mass is benign. If a patient is to be referred to a surgeon or breast center, it is preferable to have the mammogram performed, if indicated, before the referral and available at the time of the consultation.

Mammography

When a patient over the age of 30 has felt a mass, but none is found by the clinician, and there is no family history of breast cancer, a mammogram should be performed (if one has not been done in the last year.) If the family history has revealed any risk factors for breast cancer, the age limit for doing a mammogram drops to 25. If the mammogram is negative and the patient is anxious, a referral should be made to a surgeon. If the mammogram is negative and the patient is not anxious, reevaluation in 2 months is recommended. If at that time there is still no evidence of a mass, the patient can be followed by the clinician until both are satisfied that the examination is within normal limits.

If the patient is over age 30 and a significant mass is palpated, a mammogram should be performed (if one has not been done in the last 6 months), and the patient should then be referred to a surgeon. When a patient is referred to a surgeon or breast center, regardless of whether a mass is found by the examiner, the most recent mammogram should accompany her for review.

Ultrasonography

Ultrasonography is being used with greater frequency and efficacy to evaluate breast masses, particularly those that are not suspicious (29). Even though the primary care physician can use mammography to evaluate a mass, we believe that it is more efficient and cost-effective if the consulting surgeon orders the ultrasound because surgeons often aspirate a suspected cyst without the use of ultrasonography. If fluid is aspirated and the lump disappears then an ultrasound is unnecessary. In addition, if a palpable mass is sufficiently suspicious and obtaining more information via ultrasound is likely, the intervention of the surgeon is required regardless of the ultrasonographic findings. If no palpable mass is found by the internist, but the patient believes that a mass is present, it is perilous to depend on ultrasonography to determine whether a surgical consult is needed.

Cyst Aspiration or Fine Needle Aspiration

If the internist aspirates a cyst, the procedure must be performed to the standards of a surgeon who is familiar with this procedure. Performing FNA for cytology on a solid mass is best done by the surgeon because the yield from the procedure correlates directly with the experience of the physician.

Possible Outcomes of the Workup Performed by the Primary Care Provider

If no significant risk factors (i.e., no family history or history of LCIS or atypical hyperplasia) are identified, a mass that is clinically benign (consistent with a fibroadenoma or cyst) in a young woman can be followed up over time. The patient can be reevaluated 2 months later at a similar time in her menstrual cycle, when there is the least influence of hormonal activity (usually about 1 week after the start of menstruation). If there is no change in the examination and the patient is comfortable with monitoring the mass, continued observation is warranted.

In several other situations, follow-up for 2 to 3 months is an option in place of immediate referral: First, if the patient palpated a mass, but at the time of the examination, the mass was not palpable by either the clinician or the patient, and a mammogram, if appropriate, was negative; second, when the patient palpated a mass and the clinician did not, but the patient still believes the mass is present, and an appropriate mammogram was negative; and third, when the patient palpated a mass and the clinician palpated normal thickening of the breast tissue, and the patient agrees they are both feeling the same thing, and a mammogram, if appropriate, was negative.

If the patient is not referred to a surgeon or breast center, the patient must understand and approve of this decision. The patient should be instructed to call before the scheduled follow-up examination if the mass becomes consistently palpable or more prominent. The patient's chief complaint, the clinical findings, the mutually agreed decision, and instructions should be documented in the chart.

If significant risk factors (significant family history or history of LCIS or atypical hyperplasia) are present, patients with previous documentation of the risk factors should be under the care of a surgeon, a breast center, or risk assessment clinic. If risk factors are identified at the time of the patient's initial visit with the clinician, and the patient or the clinician believes that a mass has been palpated, the patient should be referred to a surgeon.

SURGICAL WORKUP

On referral, it is the responsibility of the surgeon to decide whether a mass can be followed or warrants an invasive procedure, such as an excisional biopsy or aspiration. Indications for removal of a mass include the inability to confirm that it is benign by noninvasive or minimally invasive means or if the patient will not be comfortable until the mass is excised.

The noninvasive approach consists of a physical examination, mammography, and ultrasonography. The invasive options consist of cyst aspiration, FNA, office core biopsy, and open surgical biopsy.

The surgeon uses the noninvasive tools to determine the necessity for an invasive procedure and which invasive procedure should be performed. It also may be necessary to use several invasive procedures sequentially to arrive at a decision. The surgeon's evaluation of a mass may identify a cyst, a fibroadenoma that necessitates a biopsy or a return visit, a breast mass that necessitates a biopsy or a return visit, or breast cancer.

Cyst

When an abnormality is palpable, the first priority is to determine if it is a cyst. A surgeon may aspirate a mass suspected of being a cyst, even if it has been defined as a simple cyst by ultrasonography. A palpable cyst can make the physical examination of the breast more difficult, hide small otherwise palpable cancers, and produce blind spots on the mammogram. In addition, most women do not want a palpable lump to remain in their breast. For this reason, it is not cost-effective to perform ultrasonography before attempting aspiration on a palpable mass that is likely to be a cyst. During aspiration, if nonbloody fluid is aspirated, and the mass disappears, the patient should be reexamined in 2 to 3 months and instructed to call sooner if the mass recurs or other masses develop. If fluid cannot be aspirated, and the mass is solid, the workup continues. The next step is to determine whether the solid mass is a fibroadenoma.

Fibroadenoma: Biopsy Required

If the mass is consistent with a fibroadenoma by physical examination, the surgeon then determines whether excision is necessary. Removal may be recommended if the mass is obvious, large, causes patient discomfort, or if the patient wishes to have it removed. Most patients do not want to feel an obvious mass in their breast each time they shower and do not want their significant other to find the mass during intimacy. If removal of the mass is planned, no further workup is necessary.

Fibroadenoma: Return Visit Required

If the mass is consistent with a fibroadenoma by physical examination, and removal is not recommended because it is small, difficult to locate, or if the patient prefers to avoid surgery, further workup may be required to confirm the clinical impression. Ultrasonography confirms the smooth borders of a fibroadenoma, making removal less critical, or it identifies abnormalities that are inconsistent with a fibroadenoma, making histologic diagnosis necessary. If the surgeon, with or without the benefit of additional testing, is confident that the mass is a fibroadenoma, the patient is reexamined in 3 months and instructed to call sooner if the mass enlarges or hardens or other masses develop. Patients should continue to undergo periodic examinations until the surgeon and the patient are convinced that the condition is benign.

Breast Mass: Return Visit Required

If a mass is not a cyst or a fibroadenoma and is of extremely low suspicion by physical examination and mammography (i.e., no significant mammographic findings are present, and the mass does not feel suspicious), it can be followed up if the patient is reassured and comfortable with such a plan. The patient must be informed that there is no guarantee that the mass is benign and must realize that she is an active participant in the decision to try to forego surgery. The patient is scheduled to be reexamined at 3-month intervals and instructed to call sooner if the mass changes, enlarges, or hardens or other masses develop. Patients continue to return for periodic revisits until the surgeon and the patient are both comfortable that the condition is benign. If the patient becomes uncomfortable with the plan to follow up a mass, removal is advised.

Some surgeons use the triple test during breast mass evaluation to determine whether it is sufficiently suspicious to warrant an invasive study to establish a definitive diagnosis. The triple test combines clinical findings with mammography and FNA. If the clinical examination is benign, the mammogram is not suspicious, and FNA cytology is negative for malignancy, then the negative predictive value is 100% (30). Surgeons who apply the triple test believe that patients who satisfy those criteria can be safely observed without the need for performing an open biopsy. At the Lahey Clinic, we prefer to use FNA selectively, so we do not routinely use the triple test.

Breast Mass: Biopsy Required

If the mass is not a cyst or a fibroadenoma and is the least bit suspicious by physical examination or mammography, it requires further evaluation. If the mass is likely to be benign but is of such a nature that it is likely to be removed anyway, a further noninvasive workup is not cost-effective. In this case, scheduling surgery is the most efficient and cost-effective approach. Otherwise, performing ultrasonography may be useful; if the results are negative, the surgeon and patient may be sufficiently comfortable that the lesion is benign and amenable to follow-up. On the other hand, if the ultrasound reveals an unexpected finding, excision then can be planned. If the mass remains at all suspicious after physical examination, mammography, and other diagnostic methods, it should be excised.

Breast Cancer: Fine Needle Aspiration Diagnostic of Cancer

If breast cancer is strongly suspected, a FNA can often confirm that impression. In experienced hands, finding tumor cells on FNA is diagnostic of breast cancer when the mass or mammogram is highly suspicious. The FNA diagnosis may be used to begin therapeutic intervention, either for immediate definitive surgery or for preoperative chemotherapy. If the mass or the mammogram is highly suspicious, and the FNA is negative, cancer cannot be ruled out and further evaluation is needed. The rate of false-negative FNA precludes the use of this test to abrogate the need for excision of a suspicious mass.

THE LAHEY EXPERIENCE

We recently evaluated the data from the Breast Center at the Lahey Clinic in which 2,200 patients with 2,222 breast conditions, including abnormal mammogram, breast mass, or discharge, were reviewed. Each woman was examined, her x-rays and ultrasound studies were reviewed with a radiologist, additional mammogram and ultrasound examinations were undertaken as needed, and cyst aspiration or FNA was performed as appropriate. At the end of the visit, each woman was categorized in only one of the six previously described categories.

Of the 2,222 conditions, 1,215 were breast masses. The results of follow-up and excision of these masses are shown in Fig. 6.1; 764 masses (63%) were clinically benign and had follow-up. During the follow-up period, which ranged from 3 months to 2.5 years, 59 (7.7%) of the 764 clinically benign masses changed in a manner that required intervention, revealing 52 benign lesions, three atypical hyperplasias, two LCIS, and two invasive cancers. The overall malignancy rate for these masses that were followed up clinically was 2 of 764 (0.3%).

Even though ideally no cancers should be missed when masses are followed up, the cancer rate in patients with low-risk masses should be compared with the cancer rate in patients with low-risk lesions on mammography, but no palpable mass, who also have follow-up. The rate of ductal carcinoma *in situ* (DCIS) or invasive cancer among patients with Breast Imaging Reporting and Data System III mammograms (6-month mammogram recommended) has been reported to range from 2% to 8% (31). In our series, when we recommended that 6-month mammography be performed in 237 patients without masses, six patients (2.5%) were found later to have cancer.

Forty-eight (3.9%) of the 1,215 breast masses were classified as fibroadenomas and 127 (10.5%) were believed to be cysts. About half of the fibroadenomas underwent histologic evaluation at a later point, and all were benign. Thirteen of the cysts that had follow-up underwent biopsy at a later time, revealing one case of DCIS and one invasive cancer, for a total cancer rate of 1.6% (2 of 127).

Of the 1,213 patients 274 (22.5%) had moderately or highly suspicious masses, and 49 were found to have carcinoma by FNA. (Establishing the diagnosis of cancer preoperatively allowed the patient and surgeon to plan definitive therapy, including

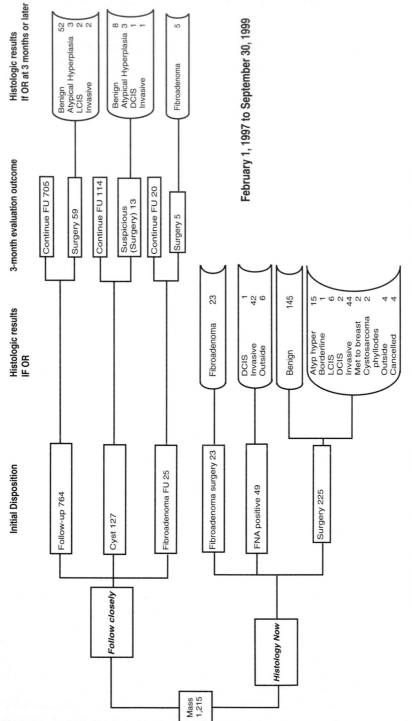

FIG. 6.1. Categorization and clinical outcomes of women seen at the Lahey Clinic Breast Center.

Initial Disposition

Histologic results IF OR

3-month evaluation outcome

Histologic results If OR at 3 months or later

February 1, 1997 to September 30, 1999

Mass 1,215

Follow closely

Histology Now

Follow-up 764
Cyst 127
Fibroadenoma FU 25

Fibroadenoma surgery 23
FNA positive 49
Surgery 225

Fibroadenoma 23

DCIS 1
Invasive 42
Outside 6

Benign 145

Atyp hyper 15
Borderline 1
LCIS 6
DCIS 2
Invasive 44
Met to breast 2
Cystosarcoma 2
phyllodes
Outside 4
Cancelled 4

Continue FU 705
Surgery 59
Continue FU 114
Suspicious (Surgery) 13
Continue FU 20
Surgery 5

Benign 52
Atypical Hyperplasia 3
LCIS 2
Invasive 2

Benign 8
Atypical Hyperplasia 3
DCIS 1
Invasive 1

Fibroadenoma 5

options for surgical and adjuvant chemotherapeutic management, without unnecessary delays incurred by waiting for pathology after biopsy). The remaining 225 patients with moderately suspicious masses underwent excision. Of the 225 moderately suspicious masses, 145 (64.4%) were benign, and 48 (21.3%) revealed either invasive carcinoma, DCIS, or metastasis to the breast.

These data indicate that, in the context of a breast center where the surgeon works closely with the radiologists and selectively uses the diagnostic modalities available, there is a significant fraction of patients with breast masses who can be followed up clinically with a low likelihood of subsequent malignancy being discovered.

CONCLUSION

It is important to maintain the perspective that any breast mass can represent carcinoma and that risk increases with advancing patient age. The responsibility of the primary care provider is to determine which patients require referral to a surgeon or breast center. The finding of a breast mass by the patient or her provider does not automatically demand referral as long as the recommended guidelines outlined in this chapter are followed and the patient is comfortable with an appropriate follow-up plan. When the decision to refer is made, the most recent mammogram should accompany the patient to the surgical examination. Other diagnostic studies besides mammogram should be deferred to allow the most cost-effective and efficient evaluation by the surgeon.

REFERENCES

1. Greenlee RT, Murray T, Bolden S, et al. Cancer statistics 2000. *CA Cancer J Clin* 2000;50:7–33.
2. Armstrong K, Eisen A, Weber B. Assessing the risk of breast cancer. *N Engl J Med* 2000;342: 564–571.
3. Hughes LE, Bundred NJ. Breast macrocysts. *World J Surg* 1989;13:711–714.
4. Greenberg R, Skornick Y, Kaplan O. Management of fibroadenomas. *J Gen Intern Med* 1998;13: 640–645.
5. Donegan WL. Evaluation of a palpable breast mass. *N Engl J Med* 1992;327:937–942.
6. Berg JW, Hutter RVP. Breast cancer. *Cancer* 1995;75:257–269.
7. Page DL, DuPont WD, Rogers LW, et al. Atypical hyperplastic lesions of the female breast: a long-term follow-up study. *Cancer* 1985;55:2698–2708.
8. Marshall LM, Hunter DJ, Connolly JL, et al. Risk of breast cancer associated with atypical hyperplasia of lobular and ductal types. *Cancer Epidemiol Biomarkers Prev* 1997;6:297–301.
9. DuPont WD, Page DL. Relative risk of breast cancer varies with time since diagnosis of atypical hyperplasia. *Hum Pathol* 1989;20:723–725.
10. Fisher ER, Costantino J, Fisher B, et al. Pathologic findings from the National Surgical Adjuvant Breast Project (NSABP) Protocol B-17: five-year observations concerning lobular carcinoma *in situ*. *Cancer* 1996;78:1403–1416.
11. Mackarem G, Yacoub LK, Lee AKC, et al. Effects of screening on detection of lobular carcinoma in situ of the breast: nonspecificity of mammography and physical examination. *Breast Dis* 1994; 7:339–345.
12. Kinne DW. Lobular carcinoma *in situ*. *Surg Oncol Clin North Am* 1993;2:65–73.
13. Cannon-Albright LA, Skolnick MH. The genetics of familial breast cancer. *Semin Oncol* 1996;23: 1–5.
14. Burke W, Daly M, Garber J, et al. Recommendations for follow-up care of individuals with an inherited predisposition to cancer. II. BRCA and BRCA2. *JAMA* 1997;277:997–1003.

15. Hoskins KF, Stopfer JE, Calzone KA, et al. Assessment and counseling for women with a family history of breast cancer. a guide for clinicians. *JAMA* 1995;273:577–585.
16. Greene MH. Genetics of breast cancer. *Mayo Clin Proc* 1997;72:54–65.
17. Liaw D, Marsh DJ, Li J, et al. Germline mutations of the PTEN gene in Cowden disease, an inherited breast and thyroid cancer syndrome. *Nat Genet* 1997;16:64–67.
18. Hisada M, Garber JE, Fung CY, et al. Multiple primary cancers in families with Li-Fraumeni syndrome. *J Nat Cancer Inst* 1998;90:606–611.
19. Green SE, Bradburn DM, Varma JS, et al. Hereditary non-polyposis colorectal cancer. *Int J Colorect Dis* 1998;13:3–12.
20. Marra G, Boland CR. Hereditary nonpolyposis colorectal cancer: the syndrome, the genes, and historical perspectives. *J Natl Cancer Inst* 1995;87:1114–1125.
21. Gail MH, Brinton LA, Byar DP, et al. Projecting individualized probabilities of developing breast cancer for white females who are being examined annually. *J Natl Cancer Inst* 1989;81:1879–1886.
22. Mackarem G, Roche CA, Hughes, KS. The effectiveness of the Gail Model in estimating risk for development of breast cancer in women under 40 years of age. *Breast J* 2001;7:34–39.
23. Morrow M, Wong S, Venta L. The evaluation of breast masses in women younger than forty years of age. *Surgery* 1998;124:634–641.
24. Murad TM, Contesso G, Mouriesse H. Nipple discharge from the breast. *Ann Surg* 1982;195:259–264.
25. Ford K, Marcus E, Lum B. Breast cancer screening, diagnosis and treatment. *Disease-a-Month* 1999; 45:333–405.
26. Kopans DB. Updated results of the trials of screening mammography. *Surg Oncol Clin North Am* 1997;6:233–263.
27. Scott S, Morrow M. Breast cancer: making the diagnosis. *Surg Clin North Am*1999;7:991–1005.
28. Young JO, Sadowsky NL, Young JW, et al. Mammography of women with suspicious breast lumps. *Arch Surg* 1986;121:807–809.
29. Lister D, Evans AJ, Burrell HC, Blamey RW, et al. The accuracy of breast ultrasound in the evaluation of clinically benign, discrete, symptomatic breast lumps. *Clin Radiol* 1998;53:490–492.
30. Kaufman Z, Shpitz B, Shapiro M, et al. Triple approach in the diagnosis of dominant breast masses: combined physical examination, mammography, and fine needle aspiration. *J Surg Oncol* 1994;56: 254–257.
31. Knutzen AM, Gisvold JJ. Likelihood of malignant disease for various categories of mammographically detected, nonpalpable breast lesions. *Mayo Clin Proc* 1993;68:454–460.

7

The Epidemiology of Breast Cancer

Thomas A. Sellers and Dawn M. Grabrick

Of the various diseases that affect the breast, cancer represents a significant problem from clinical and public health perspectives. Surveys of American women have found it to be the most significant health concern, despite the fact that cardiovascular disease exacts a far greater burden. Breast cancer is the most commonly diagnosed cancer among women in the United States and the world. An estimated 1 in 8 women in the United States will develop the disease in their lifetime (1). Breast cancer is a leading cause of female cancer deaths in the United States, second only to lung cancer. Although incidence rates have leveled off and age-adjusted mortality rates have decreased in recent years (2), breast cancer remains a public health burden. In 1998 alone, it is projected that 178,800 new cases of female breast cancer and 43,500 deaths due to breast cancer will have occurred in the United States (1). The purpose of this chapter is to review some of the major epidemiologic risk factors for the disease. It is important to emphasize, however, that, despite literally hundreds of studies, established risk factors are estimated to account for no more than 47% of breast cancer cases (3). Thus, all women are at risk of the disease, and appropriate screening should be provided regardless of risk factors.

DESCRIPTIVE EPIDEMIOLOGY

Breast cancer incidence exhibits wide geographic variation, as shown in Table 7.1 (4). The highest age-standardized rates are observed in North America and northern Europe, and the lowest rates are observed in Asia and Africa. Rates have been intermediate in areas of southern Europe and South America. In more recent years, some of the differences in incidence rates have been decreasing, one example being between the United States and Japan (5). A number of reasons have been proposed to explain geographic variation in incidence rates, including differences in body weight; some aspect of diet; endogenous hormone levels; and reproductive factors such as age at menarche, menstrual cycle length, parity, and lactation (5).

Breast cancer risk has been observed to change quite markedly following migration, especially if migration occurs at a young age (6). In general, migrants to the United States from low-risk countries and their second- and third-generation offspring are observed to have incidence rates approaching those of the United States, although the speed at which incidence rates change has varied by ethnic group and study (5).

The incidence of breast cancer increases with age (Fig. 7.1). In the United States,

TABLE 7.1. *Worldwide age-standardized female breast cancer incidence rates and standard errors (per 100,000)*

	Incidence	Standard error
Africa		
Mali, Bamako	10.2	1.15
Central and South America		
Goiania, Brazil	40.4	1.79
Costa Rica	28.8	0.76
North America		
Canada	76.8	0.30
Los Angeles, CA, USA: Chinese	36.8	2.34
San Francisco, CA, USA: Hispanic white	70.8	2.56
San Francisco, CA, USA: Japanese	68.4	6.01
US, SEER: White	90.7	0.39
US, SEER: Black	79.3	1.11
Asia		
Qidong, China	11.2	0.60
Bombay, India	28.2	0.48
All Jews, Israel	77.4	0.87
Osaka, Japan	24.3	0.28
Kangwha, Korea	7.1	1.51
Europe		
Finland	65.0	0.56
Somme, France	68.2	2.07
Eastern States, Germany	48.2	0.45
Florence, Italy	67.0	1.36
Cracow, Poland	44.0	1.31
Basque Country, Spain	45.8	0.90
Zurich, Switzerland	65.7	1.24
England and Wales, UK	68.8	0.26
Oceania		
New South Wales, Australia	67.2	0.62
Hawaii, USA: White	96.5	3.43
Hawaii, USA: Filipino	57.4	3.61

SEER, surveillance, epidemiology, and end results.
Adapted from Parkin D, Whelan S, Ferlay J, et al. Cancer incidence in five continents. VII. Lyon: IARC Scientific Publications, 1997, with permission.

observed incidence rates are lower among African Americans than among whites, but mortality from breast cancer is higher among African Americans. The rate of increase in breast cancer incidence with age slows down around 50 years of age, corresponding to the average age at menopause (7). This phenomenon is one of many indications that female reproductive hormones are involved in the etiology of breast cancer.

→

FIG. 7.1. Female breast cancer: Age-specific incidence and mortality rates by race, United States, 1993–1997. Rates are per 100,000 and are age-adjusted to the 1970 U.S. standard population (plotted on log scale). (From Ries LAG, Eisner MP, Kosary CL, et al. *SEER Cancer Statistics Review 1973–1997*. Bethesda, MD: National Cancer Institute, 2000:119–120, with permission.)

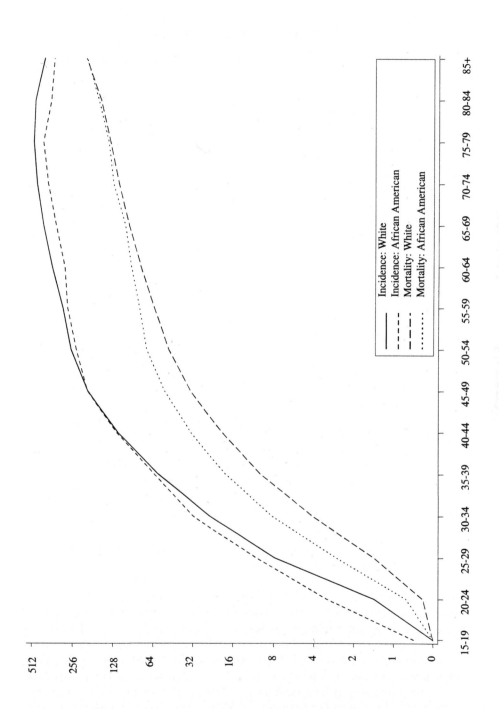

	Incidence: White
	Incidence: African American
	Mortality: White
	Mortality: African American

HORMONAL RISK FACTORS

Breast cancer has long been known to be a hormonally associated malignancy. The 100-fold difference in rates between men and women and the influence of menopause on the rate of age-specific increases are but two examples of evidence. The etiologic role of estrogens in the pathogenesis of breast cancer is widely accepted and well documented. Estrogens appear to influence risk either through receptor-mediated events or by direct estrogen-mediated genotoxicity (8). The other major ovarian hormone, progesterone, may be involved in the development of breast cancer as well (7). The contribution of other hormones, such as prolactin and androgens, has been studied much less extensively.

The following sections review the epidemiologic data on both endogenous correlates of reproductive hormone exposure and exogenous sources of hormones, specifically, oral contraceptives and hormone replacement therapy (HRT). The section concludes with a discussion of epidemiologic studies of measured serum hormone levels and breast cancer.

Age at Menarche

Epidemiologic studies have consistently shown an association between age at menarche and breast cancer risk. A 2- to 3-year delay in the onset of menstruation has been observed to decrease the relative risk (RR) of breast cancer by 10% to 20% (9). Although breast cancer risk decreases with increasing age at menarche, a smooth gradient of risk is not always seen (10). Studies have shown late age at menarche to be associated with decreased risk of both premenopausal and postmenopausal breast cancers (9). It is thought the increased breast cancer risk associated with an early age at menarche may simply be due to the longer duration of ovarian activity (11).

Women with an early age at menarche tend to establish regular ovulatory cycles more quickly than women with a later age at menarche (11). Because women with irregular cycles frequently experience anovulatory cycles, a delay in menstrual cycle regularization is associated with a reduced cumulative exposure to ovulatory cycles (12, 13). It has been hypothesized that irregular cycles are associated with a decreased risk of breast cancer, but epidemiologic studies have yielded inconsistent results (14).

A shorter menstrual cycle length is associated with greater exposure to estrogen and progesterone together (14). Women with longer cycles spend relatively less time in the luteal phase, when mitotic activity in the breast is thought to peak (15), and therefore might be expected to have a lower risk of breast cancer (16). A 1993 review of reproductive factors and breast cancer indicated fairly consistent findings with regard to a shorter cycle length between 20 and 39 years of age being associated with an increased risk of breast cancer (9). More recent studies have not always supported this conclusion. For example, the Menstruation and Reproductive History Study, begun in 1934 at the University of Minnesota as a prospective study of menstrual cycle variability, found little evidence for an association of median cycle length with breast cancer, except for possibly an increased risk among women who had cycles of extreme length ($\leq$26 or $\geq$34 days) at ages 25 to 29 years (17). A large population-based case–control study observed, if anything, a slightly reduced risk of breast cancer associated with shorter cycles, although misclassification may have occurred because women reporting monthly cycles were automatically classified as having 28-day cycles (10).

In summary, while other characteristics of the menstrual cycle have not been conclusively linked to breast cancer, early age at menarche is well-established as a factor associated with a moderate increase in risk. Over the past century, the average age at menarche among girls in developed countries has decreased from 16 to 13 years (18). This trend may explain some of the increase in breast cancer incidence that occurred over the same time period (19).

Age at Menopause

Around the time of menopause, there is a distinct slowing in the rate of increase in age-specific breast cancer incidence rates. A later age at menopause has long been known to be associated with a higher risk of breast cancer (9). After menopause, estrogen levels are low, progesterone is virtually absent, and rates of breast cell proliferation are very low (20). Both early natural menopause and surgically induced menopause have been observed to lower risk. Bilateral oophorectomy may confer greater protection than natural menopause, possibly because of a more marked and sudden decline in levels of endogenous hormones following surgery (21). Bilateral oophorectomy before age 40 has been observed to lower lifetime breast cancer risk by about 50% compared with natural menopause (9). Hysterectomy alone does not appear to reduce risk (9), suggesting the importance of ovarian hormones.

Pregnancy

The association of pregnancy with breast cancer risk has been studied extensively. Pregnancy actually has a dual effect on risk of breast cancer; it offers long-term protection but a short-term increase in risk. This is likely due, at least in part, to the fact that pregnancy is accompanied by both proliferation (in the early stages) and differentiation (in the later stages) of breast epithelial cells. Two observations have been consistently seen in epidemiologic studies. An early age at first birth has been associated with a reduced risk of breast cancer, while nulliparity has been linked to an increased risk of breast cancer after age 40 (9).

An early age at first birth may reduce the risk of breast cancer through the differentiation of breast tissue, making it less susceptible to carcinogens, or through long-lasting changes in the hormonal milieu (9). Evidence from several studies indicates that a first full-term pregnancy after age 30 may be associated with a higher risk of breast cancer than that associated with nulliparity (9). It has been hypothesized that a full-term pregnancy at an early age may reduce the probability of tumor initiation, whereas a later full-term pregnancy may promote the growth of existing tumor cells (22).

The first full-term pregnancy has the greatest effect on risk reduction. The estimated RR of breast cancer for nulliparous versus parous women ranges from about 1.2 to 1.7 (9). Some studies have shown a more favorable hormonal profile among parous versus nulliparous women. For example, a study of 59 nulliparous women and 47 parous women found higher levels of sex hormone–binding globulin (SHBG) and lower levels of free estradiol among the parous women (23). A small measure of additional protection with each subsequent pregnancy has been noted in several, but not all, studies (9).

One might speculate that the influence of nulliparity or a late age at first full-term pregnancy reflects a difficulty becoming pregnant. Studies of infertility and breast cancer have yielded inconsistent results, possibly due in part to the difficulty of classifying women in regards to this variable (9). Non-hormonal reasons for infertility do not appear to increase breast cancer risk (9).

It is unclear whether spontaneous or induced abortion affects breast cancer risk. Epidemiologic studies have shown positive, inverse, and no association (9). Inaccurate reporting of spontaneous or induced abortions has been a concern, and it is unclear whether the accuracy differs between women with and without breast cancer. Biologically, an increased risk of breast cancer might be expected as a result of the rapid rise in free estradiol that occurs during the first trimester, coupled with the incomplete differentiation of mammary gland cells (9), but the available evidence is not particularly striking.

In conclusion, endogenous correlates of reproductive hormonal exposure have been studied quite extensively. Early age at menarche, late age at menopause, nulliparity, and late age at first birth are associated with moderate increases in breast cancer risk, whereas a bilateral oophorectomy before age 40 reduces risk. The evidence is less compelling in regard to characteristics of the menstrual cycle and spontaneous or induced abortion.

Oral Contraceptives

Oral contraceptives were introduced in the United States in 1960 and quickly gained popularity, with almost 52 million prescriptions for oral contraceptives dispensed in 1984 (24). In the United States, 85% of women born between 1945 and 1949 have used oral contraceptives compared with only 43% of women born between 1930 and 1934 (25). Increasingly, women are beginning oral contraceptive use at younger ages and are continuing use for longer periods. Given these facts and the hormonal basis of breast cancer, it is not surprising that the influence of oral contraceptives on breast cancer risk has been studied quite extensively.

A large collaborative reanalysis of 54 studies (53,297 women with breast cancer, 100,239 women without breast cancer) was published in 1996 (25). Eligible studies included all those with at least 100 breast cancer cases and information on the use

TABLE 7.2. *Oral contraceptives and breast cancer: results from the Collaborative Group on Hormonal Factors in Breast Cancer*

	Relative risk	95% CI
Never users	1.00	—
Current users	1.24	1.15–1.33
1–4 yr after stopping	1.16	1.08–1.23
5–9 yr after stopping	1.07	1.02–1.13
10+ yr after stopping	1.01	0.96–1.05

CI, confidence interval.
Adapted from Collaborative Group on Hormonal Factors in Breast Cancer. Breast cancer and hormonal contraceptives: collaborative reanalysis of individual data on 53,297 women with breast cancer and 100,239 women without breast cancer from 54 epidemiological studies. *Lancet* 1996;347:1713–1727, with permission.

of hormonal contraceptives and reproductive history; approximately 90% of the studies worldwide were included. As shown in Table 7.2, it was concluded that any increased risk associated with taking combined oral contraceptives is small and limited to current users or use in the previous ten years. The cancers that were diagnosed in women who had used oral contraceptives were less advanced clinically than were those that were diagnosed in women who had never used oral contraceptives. No conclusion could be made as to whether this was due to an earlier diagnosis of breast cancer in oral contraceptive users, the biologic effects of oral contraceptives, or a combination of reasons.

Not all studies suggest an increased risk of breast cancer associated with oral contraceptive use. In fact, the large Cancer and Steroid Hormone (CASH) Study did not find an elevated risk among either past or current oral contraceptive users (26), nor did they observe any increase in risk in analyses restricted to women with a family history of breast cancer (27).

At one time, the hypothesis was raised that increasing duration of oral contraceptive use before a first full-term pregnancy was more strongly related to breast cancer risk (28). Although some subsequent studies have supported this idea, many others have not, including an updated analysis of the study from which the hypothesis arose (29). An earlier age at first use has been suggested as playing an important role as well, but data from the Collaborative Group on Hormonal Factors in Breast Cancer failed to show a significant trend with decreasing age at first use (25). Some evidence does exist for increasing risk with increasing duration of oral contraceptive use (25); however, it has been difficult to sort out the effects of duration of use from recency of use (29).

Substantial changes in the type and concentration of the estrogen and progestin components of oral contraceptives have occurred since their introduction in 1960, from 150 μg of mestranol to less than 50 μg of ethinyl estradiol and about 10 mg of norethynodrel to 1 mg or less of several progestins (30). Hormone dose has not been shown to be a significant predictor of breast cancer risk (25); however, specific hormone types and dosages have not been easy to measure and analyze given the difficulty of recall and the number of times a woman may switch brands.

Some studies have shown a higher risk of breast cancer associated with oral contraceptive use among women with a family history of breast cancer, whereas others have found little or no such evidence (25). In a recent study of 426 multigenerational families ascertained through breast cancer probands, ever having used oral contraceptives was associated with significantly increased risk of breast cancer among sisters and daughters of probands [RR, 3.3; 95% confidence interval (CI), 1.6–6.7] but not among granddaughters and nieces of probands or among women who married into the families (31). This risk was elevated further when analyses were conducted in high-risk families with multiple cases of breast or ovarian cancer. The elevated risk among women with a first-degree family history was most evident for oral contraceptive use prior to 1975, formulations likely to contain higher doses of estrogen and progestins.

Results are starting to become available on oral contraceptive use and breast cancer in carriers of mutations in the major breast cancer susceptibility genes, *BRCA1* and *BRCA2*. A small study of Ashkenazi Jewish women with breast cancer suggests that oral contraceptive use may increase more greatly the risk of breast cancer in carriers of *BRCA1* or *BRCA2* mutations than in noncarriers (32). Knowledge from further studies should allow more detailed evaluation of the risks and benefits of oral contraceptive use for particular groups of women at increased risk of breast cancer.

Progestin-only contraceptives, such as progestin-only pills (minipills) and the injectable contraceptive depot-medroxyprogesterone acetate (DMPA), have been studied much less extensively, largely because of the relative rarity of these exposures compared with combination oral contraceptives. Progestin-only pills were introduced in the United States in 1973 and contain a lower dose of progestin than do combination oral contraceptives (22). DMPA was licensed in the United States as a contraceptive in 1992 (33). There is some evidence that breast cancer risk may be increased among users of DMPA who are less than 35 years old (34) or among recent users of DMPA (25, 34) or progestin-only oral contraceptives (25), but more data are needed.

In summary, the association of oral contraceptives and risk of breast cancer has been studied extensively. Large increases in risk have been ruled out, but the probability of small increases in risk cannot be excluded, especially among subsets of the population.

Hormone Replacement Therapy

Oral contraceptives are only one source of exogenous hormonal exposure. There is a large body of literature that has examined possible risks of breast cancer associated with HRT. Recently, the Collaborative Group on Hormonal Factors in Breast Cancer conducted a reanalysis of data on HRT and breast cancer from 51 epidemiologic studies, encompassing approximately 90% of the world's epidemiologic data on the topic (35). The risk of breast cancer was estimated to increase by 2.3% (95% CI, 1.1%–3.6%) for each year of use among current users or those who last used HRT less than 5 years ago. Women who used HRT for 5 years or longer had an RR of 1.35 (95% CI, 1.21–1.49) compared with never users. As with oral contraceptives, the cancers diagnosed in women who ever used HRT tended to be less advanced clinically than those diagnosed in women who had never used HRT.

Two large prospective studies provide some evidence for a modifying effect of alcohol on risk. The Nurses' Health Study observed a significantly increased risk of breast cancer with current use of estrogen replacement therapy among alcohol consumers but no association among women who did not consume alcohol (36). In the Iowa Women's Health Study, risk was increased among women who used estrogen replacement therapy and consumed at least 4 g of alcohol per day but not among women who never used estrogen replacement therapy and consumed this amount of alcohol (37). A small study of 12 postmenopausal women receiving estrogens observed that consumption of alcohol (0.7 g/kg of body weight) raised blood levels of estradiol by about 300%, equivalent to the periovulatory peak in the menstrual cycle and lasting 5 hours (38). Epidemiologic studies have not been consistent; however, the Collaborative Group on Hormonal Factors in Breast Cancer did not observe a modifying effect of alcohol (1997).

Studies seem more consistent with regard to a modifying effect of body mass index (BMI) or weight. The effect of current or recent use of HRT appears to be most pronounced among leaner women (35). A smooth gradient of increasing risk with decreasing weight or BMI has been observed, increasing the likelihood that this finding was not due to chance.

The association between HRT and breast cancer does not appear to differ significantly by a family history of breast cancer (35). The influence of HRT among carriers of mutations in the major breast cancer susceptibility genes, *BRCA1* and *BRCA2*, is yet unknown.

Some evidence exists for the breast cancers diagnosed among HRT users having a more favorable histology (39). It also has been observed that women who use estrogen replacement therapy before breast cancer diagnosis have lower mortality from breast cancer (or improved survival) in some (40–44) but not all (45,46) studies. Further research is needed in this area, so that the overall risks and benefits of HRT use can be addressed more thoroughly.

Most studies on HRT and breast cancer have focused largely on unopposed estrogen replacement therapy (without progestins), the form in which HRT was initially prescribed. The use of estrogen replacement therapy gained considerable popularity in the United States during the 1960s and 1970s, reaching its peak in 1975, when 28 million prescriptions were filled for noncontraceptive use of estrogens (47). With the discovery of an increased risk of endometrial cancer associated with use of unopposed estrogen, HRT use decreased until combined HRT was introduced (48).

Our knowledge of combined HRT is now increasing as the number of long-term users of these formulations increases. Recent studies indicate that combined estrogen–progestin formulations may increase breast cancer risk more than formulations containing estrogen alone (49–51). Among women in the Breast Cancer Detection Demonstration Project (a nationwide breast cancer screening program) who recently used HRT, the RR increased by 0.01 (95% CI, 0.002–0.03) with each year of estrogen-only use and by 0.08 (95% CI, 0.02–0.16) with each year of estrogen–progestin use (49). When analyses were stratified on BMI, the increased risk was limited to women with a BMI less than or equal to 24.4 kg/m² (49). A population-based case–control study in Los Angeles County, California, observed an odds ratio of 1.24 (95% CI, 1.07–1.45) for every 5 years of estrogen–progestin use; no increase in risk was seen for women who took unopposed estrogens for up to 15 years (50). An updated analysis in a Swedish cohort found a 70% increased risk of breast cancer associated with 6 or more years of current or recent use of estrogen–progestin replacement therapy (51). These epidemiologic data are backed by the observation that peak mitotic activity in breast tissue occurs in the mid-to-late luteal phase of the menstrual cycle, when progesterone levels are at their maximum (7). Additional research on combined HRT and breast cancer can be expected in the near future.

In summary, it appears that if HRT increases risk of breast cancer, the magnitude is probably small. Moreover, the extensive literature suggests that short-term (<5 years) duration is safe. Women without an intact uterus should probably avoid combination therapy. Any decision regarding HRT should balance possible breast cancer risks against the benefits of decreased risk of osteoporosis, stroke, and total mortality.

Serum Hormones

Because many of the well-established risk factors for breast cancer appear to influence hormones, one might predict that levels of serum hormones would be related to risk. Studies of premenopausal women have been difficult to interpret because of the large variation in hormone levels over the menstrual cycle and, not surprisingly, have yielded inconsistent results (52). Data from studies of postmenopausal women, however, have been able to shed some light on the issue. Based on the results of prospective studies, endogenous estradiol does appear to be associated with postmenopausal breast cancer (52). Summarizing six such studies, the overall mean concentration of estradiol in the blood was 15% higher (95% CI, 6%–24%; $p = 0.0003$) among 329 women who subsequently developed breast cancer compared with 1,105 women who remained cancer free (52).

Whereas most estradiol is bound to serum albumin, a significant percentage is bound to SHBG, levels of which may be affected by many factors, including obesity (11). Serum levels of SHBG are a determinant of the proportion of estradiol available to enter breast epithelial cells (53). As would be predicted, studies have largely shown serum concentrations of SHBG to be lower among breast cancer cases than controls (53).

Other hormones have been examined, but the results have been less conclusive. In addition to estradiol, postmenopausal women who develop breast cancer appear to have relatively high serum levels of testosterone, dehydroepiandrosterone sulphate, and androstenedione; however, serum concentrations of these four hormones are known to be correlated (53). Although several studies of progesterone or its major urinary metabolite, pregnanediol, have found lower levels in breast cancer cases than in controls (54), at least one study found this relationship reversed when analyses were restricted to matched pairs in which both subjects showed evidence of luteal activity (55). The Nurses' Health Study recently found an increased risk of postmenopausal breast cancer associated with high plasma prolactin levels after controlling for a number of variables, including plasma estrogen and androgen levels and time of day of the blood draw (56). Previous studies of prolactin and breast cancer have shown inconsistent results.

Several limitations of studies of serum hormone levels must be considered. The method used to measure hormone levels has varied (52). In some studies, collection was not performed on a fixed day of the cycle (for studies of premenopausal women), nor was it done in a comparable manner for cases and controls (11). Studies often rely on one blood sample, which may not be representative of a woman's average hormone levels (53). In addition, case–control studies are limited by the fact that hormone levels in women with breast cancer could be affected by the presence of the cancer or by its treatment.

In summary, the study of serum hormone levels and breast cancer has been a challenging area, especially among premenopausal women. Beyond the challenges already mentioned, one cannot be certain that what is detected in the blood or urine is representative of the hormonal milieu in breast tissue. Nonetheless, studies of serum hormones appear to support the role of reproductive factors in breast cancer.

ANTHROPOMETRIC RISK FACTORS

The previous sections highlighting the importance of hormonal factors raise questions about other potential influences on circulating levels of estrogens. One area of considerable interest is body weight and body mass. The rationale for such studies includes the fact that for postmenopausal women the predominant source of circulating estrogens is aromatization of androgens in adipose tissue.

Most studies suggest that body mass is positively but weakly associated with postmenopausal breast cancer (57). The evidence supporting such an association is stronger, and more consistent, from case–control studies than from prospective studies. For example, more than 20 published studies have observed postmenopausal breast cancer patients to have higher weight or higher BMI than controls. The prospective studies, although fewer in number but larger in size, have found weaker associations. Recent results (58) from a large case–control study (5,031 cases, 5,255 controls) provide a useful perspective on the associated risks. In this study, women in the upper quintile of body weight (>173 pounds) or BMI (>29.45 kg/ m^2) were at 60% to 80% greater risk of breast cancer than peers in the lowest quintiles (<125 pounds, <21.9 kg/m^2). There was clear evidence of a dose–response relationship between body mass and breast cancer risk (Fig. 7.2).

Curiously, body mass is inversely associated with premenopausal breast cancer (59). This apparent anomaly has focused research on weight change between adoles-

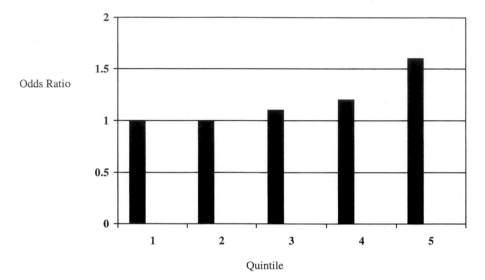

FIG. 7.2. Association of body mass and breast cancer risk. [Adapted from Trentham-Dietz A, Newcomb PA, Egan KM, et al. Weight change and risk of postmenopausal breast cancer (United States). *Cancer Causes Control* 2000,:533–542, with permission.]

cence and adulthood. Body mass in early adulthood (ages 18–21 years) has also been inversely associated with breast cancer (60). Body mass (61) and relative weight (62,63) at even younger ages (8–16 years) appears to be inversely associated with both premenopausal and postmenopausal breast cancer. Weight gain since early adulthood also appears to be positively associated with postmenopausal breast cancer. In a large prospective cohort study conducted in Iowa, weight gain between the ages of 18 and 50 years was examined in relation to subsequent breast cancer occurrence (60). Weight gain was associated with increased risk, regardless of body mass at age 18 years. For example, low body mass at age 18 and high weight gain were associated with a 1.9-fold increased risk, whereas weight gain among the heaviest women at age 18 increased risk 1.6-fold. In the prospective Nurses' Health Study, based on 1,000 premenopausal cases and 1,517 postmenopausal cases, weight gain from age 18 was associated with decreased risk of premenopausal cancer but increased risk of postmenopausal breast cancer (64), especially among women who had never used estrogen replacement therapy. The largest study to date on the subject, a case–control study involving more than 5,000 cases, observed that each 5 kg (about 11 pounds) increased risk by 8% (58). Early adolescence, in particular, may be the most critical time for the effects of rapid weight gain (and growth in general) on breast carcinogenesis. Thus, control of weight gain appears to be one area that should be effectively targeted as a means to minimize breast cancer risk.

Relatively strong evidence from both case–control and cohort studies shows a modest, positive association between body height and risk of both premenopausal and postmenopausal breast cancer (65). Adult height may, in part, reflect the influence of nutritional factors during early childhood and adolescence on growth, with taller adult height reflecting more adequate availability of food and energy and greater exposure to growth-related hormones. Whereas adult height is determined largely by genetic factors in most societies in which food shortages are not an issue, there may still be some residual effect of nutritional status. This is demonstrated, in part, by the dramatic increases in height (66) and acceleration in growth rate (67) over the past few decades in Japan, as more food, especially, more fatty, Western-style dishes, have become widely available. Cross-cultural comparisons also demonstrate a positive association of height and breast cancer rates, internationally (68), and, in one within-country study, among counties in Norway (69).

It is becoming increasingly evident that body mass and body weight have limitations as markers of breast cancer risk. In particular, abdominal adiposity appears to be more biologically active than peripheral fat distribution. Abdominal adiposity is correlated with circulating levels of estrogens and is inversely associated with SHBG (thereby resulting in an increase in bioavailable estrogens). Measurement of central versus peripheral fat distribution can be measured quite reliably in epidemiologic studies through a ratio of the circumferences of the waist and hips (70). In general, women with a high waist-to-hip ratio (WHR) (i.e., apple shaped) are at elevated risk of postmenopausal breast cancer compared with women with low WHR (pear shaped). This has been demonstrated in both retrospective and prospective studies and is independent of overall levels of obesity. The few studies on premenopausal women do not indicate any association. In the Iowa Women's Health Study, a high WHR was associated with an approximate 50% increase in risk after adjustment for age and body mass (71). Subsequent analyses suggest that this effect is primarily among women with a family history of breast cancer (72).

DIET AND NUTRITION

The previous section on anthropometric factors and breast cancer raises obvious questions about the role of energy and other dietary factors. Indeed, there has been a substantial public interest in the role of dietary factors, especially dietary fat, in the etiology of breast cancer. An expert report commissioned by the World Cancer Research Fund and the American Institute for Cancer Research provides the most extensive and current review of the scientific evidence linking diet to breast cancer (73). Most of this section is based on that report.

A logical starting point for this section is dietary fat. Because fat is calorically dense, diets high in fat favor energy imbalance and the development of obesity. As reviewed in the previous section, this indirectly links high fat diets with postmenopausal breast cancer risk. Considerable scientific efforts have sought a direct relation between fat content of the diet and risk of the disease, however. Evidence for such an association is supported by animal studies that clearly demonstrate that dietary fat accelerates mammary tumorigenesis (74), independent of the effect of calories. Cross-cultural comparisons also show a strong linear correlation (0.7 – 0.9) of breast cancer mortality with per capita consumption of dietary fat (75). Despite the indication from such studies that dietary fat intake may influence breast cancer risk, evidence has not been forthcoming from analytic epidemiologic studies conducted within a particular country. Although there is some support for an association in case–control studies (76), results from seven prospective cohort studies have been null. Hunter and colleagues published a pooled analysis of more than 335,000 women and nearly 5,000 breast cancer cases (77) and found no association of dietary fat intake in adulthood and risk of breast cancer. The energy-adjusted RR for the highest quintile of fat intake was 1.1 (0.9 – 1.2). When analyses were conducted of women with fat intake less than 20% of calories, no beneficial effect of low intake was observed. It is important to consider, however, that fewer than 2% of the women in the meta-analysis had fat intakes less than 20% of calories, and only 6% had fat intakes between 20% to 25% of calories. Animal studies suggest a plateau effect of calories at about 20% (75). If this phenomenon can be extended to humans, it may explain why a clear association of fat with risk has not been observed in human studies because most Western populations take substantially above 20% of calories from fat.

The basis for the apparent inconsistency between prospective and retrospective study designs is the subject of considerable scientific debate. Some investigators suggest that the lack of association with dietary fat intake and subsequent occurrence of breast cancer is not surprising given the measurement error attendant with dietary assessment (78). Despite the lack of consistency in the literature on dietary fat and etiology, a number of studies have been conducted to explore whether dietary fat restriction will improve survival for women with the disease. A recent meta-analysis of the relevant literature suggests that dietary fat reductions can lead to a 7.4% decrease in serum estradiol among premenopausal women and a 23.0% decrease among postmenopausal women (79). Thus, although there is no strong evidence to implicate dietary fat and breast cancer risk, insufficient data exist to rule out such a possibility. Because there are other health benefits with low fat diets, it remains a prudent recommendation for patients.

The emerging literature on types of fat (monounsaturated, polyunsaturated) does not shed light on the fat–breast cancer controversy because findings tend to be mixed. It is worth noting, however, that breast cancer rates tend to be low in Mediterranean countries, where use of olive oil is common. Three case–control studies suggest that high consumption of olive oil is associated with significantly lower risks. It is not clear whether this is related to monounsaturated fat, vitamin E, or other constituents. Vegetable fat, fish oils (omega-6 and omega-3 fatty acids), and cholesterol have not been adequately studied (73).

Diets high in fat are often also high in animal products, especially meat. Although such data have been collected, there has been relatively little emphasis on protein and meat consumption as possible risk factors. Meats are an excellent source of heterocyclic amines, which are formed in meats cooked at high temperatures such as well-done meats, and are known mutagens in mammary carcinogenesis. Recently, a strong positive association between doneness levels in meat and postmenopausal breast cancer risk was found in a case–control study nested in the Iowa Women's

Health Study. Women who consumed hamburger, beef steak, and bacon at a well-done level had a 4.6-fold (95% CI, 1.4–16) greater risk of breast cancer compared with women who usually consumed these meats at a rare or medium-done level (80).

Most published studies of diet and breast cancer have sought the identification of factors that increase risk of disease. A recent trend has involved efforts to identify factors that may decrease risk.

A large amount of data exists to show that fruits and vegetables may be protective (73). Almost all the published epidemiologic data show either decreased risk with higher intakes or no association. The evidence is more abundant for vegetables, particularly green vegetables, than for fruits.

Considerable research has been done to isolate the possible protective components of fruits and vegetables. Vitamin and mineral intakes, for example, have been frequently studied. It seems unlikely, however, that the fat-soluble vitamins (retinol, Vitamin E) are related to risk. High intakes of carotenoids may decrease risk, but more research is needed, especially to resolve whether it is specific carotenoids or some other component of carotenoid-containing foods. Among the water-soluble vitamins, vitamin C may be protective, but the evidence is insufficient. Two prospective studies have now shown that diets low in folate increase risk of breast cancer, but the effect appears to be limited to women who consume alcohol. It may also be relevant that diets high in plant compounds tend to be high in fiber, and some evidence exists that high fiber lowers risk (81). Despite the biologic plausibility, there is limited evidence that vitamin D or selenium lowers risk. Finally, it must be recognized that the active ingredients in fruits and vegetables may not be vitamins or minerals but other bioactive compounds, such as isoflavones and lignans. Scientific interest in these compounds is heightened by their action as phytoestrogens. Metabolic conversion in the gut leads to hormone-like compounds, with roughly 0.1% of the activity of conjugated steroidal estrogens. The hypothesis is that these phytoestrogens may bind to the estrogen receptor without eliciting a major response and yet block the binding of more potent estrogens. In fact, phytoestrogens are structurally similar to tamoxifen, which is an established and effective treatment agent. Epidemiologic evidence is currently quite limited at this time.

OTHER LIFESTYLE FACTORS

Cigarette Smoking

The data linking cigarette smoking with breast cancer are conflicting. The last published review article on the topic concluded that there was little evidence to suggest that cigarette smoking materially increased risk (82). Most early studies focused on the hypothesis that smoking may reduce risk, motivated by a report from MacMahon and colleagues (83), that urinary estrogen levels of smokers during the luteal phase of the menstrual cycle were reduced compared with never smokers. With the exception of a few early case–control studies that used biased control groups, most published studies described a weak positive association between smoking and breast cancer risk. Studies with at least 500 cases reported since the publication of that review have failed to clarify the issue. Field et al. (84) included 1,617 cases and 1,617 controls in New York State and observed no association with smoking status or exposure level. A multicenter, population-based study of 6,888 cases and 9,529 controls found a similar lack of association (85). One large European study found no consistent association between cigarette smoking and breast cancer risk (86), and a population-based case–control study of women under age 55 years found a modest inverse association among the youngest patients (87). Conversely, Calle et al. (88) found that current smoking was associated with significantly increased risk of fatal breast cancer in a cohort study of more than 600,000 women. In summary, little evidence exists that smoking reduces the risk of breast cancer, with some of the larger, more recent studies finding a modest increase in risk. Given the known and considerable risks of cardiovascular and other diseases, there are numerous other reasons to avoid the use of tobacco products.

Alcohol Consumption

The potential association of alcohol use with risk of breast cancer has been examined in more than 50 epidemiologic studies. Many of the studies have been small, however, and the corresponding increases in risk have been generally low, the ability to examine risks associated with low or moderate intakes has been limited, and differences across some studies have been notable. Perhaps the best data on this topic come from a pooled analysis of six prospective cohort studies, representing more than 300,000 women and 4,335 cases of invasive breast cancer (89). The prevalence of alcohol use ranged from 45% to 78%, with reported intakes as high as 60 g or more (about four drinks) per day. The RRs of breast cancer, adjusted for other breast cancer risk factors, are presented in Table 7.3. A linear increase in risk

TABLE 7.3. *Results of pooled analysis of six prospective studies of alcohol use and risk of breast cancer*

Intake[a]	No. of cases	Relative risk	95% CI
None	1,462	1.00	—
>0 to 1.5	680	1.07	0.96–1.19
1.5 to <5.0	882	0.99	0.90–1.10
5.0 to <15.0	727	1.06	0.96–1.17
15.0 to <30.0	360	1.16	0.98–1.38
30.0 to <60.0	194	1.41	1.18–1.69
≥60.0	30	1.31	0.86–1.98

CI, confidence interval.
[a] Grams per day.
Adapted from Smith-Warner SA, Spiegelman D, Yaun SS, et al. Alcohol and breast cancer in women: a pooled analysis of cohort studies. *JAMA* 1998; 279:535–540, with permission.

with increasing intake was observed up to 60 g or more per day, after which no further increase in risk was observed. Although the linear trend was highly statistically significant ($p < 0.001$), the point estimates of risk were not statistically significant at intakes less than 30 g daily. The data do not suggest, however, that alcohol is protective at low levels. When sources of alcohol were considered, risks associated with intakes of 10 g daily were 11%, 5%, and 5% for liquor, beer, and wine, respectively.

It has been postulated that any risk associated with use of alcohol must be through effects on levels of circulating hormones. Unfortunately, few studies have been conducted in this area, and the results are not entirely consistent (90). The literature does suggest that alcohol-associated increases in serum estradiol, if any, are probably modest. A possible exception, but a potentially important one, is women who use HRT. In a small study of 12 women, Ginsburg and colleagues (38) noted a 300% increase in plasma estradiol in women on HRT on consumption of 0.7 g of alcohol per kilogram of body weight. This has been observed in some, but not all, prospective epidemiologic studies. For example, in the Iowa Women's Health Study, Gapstur and colleagues (91) reported that any elevation in risk associated with use of alcohol was restricted to the subset of women who were current or former users of HRT.

The association of alcohol and risk of breast cancer also may occur through mechanisms other than via effects on estrogen levels. For example, alcohol is metabolized to acetaldehyde, which is a known chemical carcinogen. Indirect evidence for this hypothesis comes through epidemiologic studies of diet, alcohol, and breast cancer. In particular, three prospective cohort studies (92–94) have reported significant interactions between alcohol and low folate intakes. Folate, an essential B vitamin, is critically important to the integrity of DNA; low levels are associated with hypomethylation of DNA and strand breaks. Importantly, it appears that adequate levels of folate (i.e., meeting the minimum recommended dietary allowance of 400 µg per day) are sufficient to offset the risks associated with alcohol consumption. As seen in Fig. 7.3, at folate intakes above the median in the Iowa Women's Health Study, no differences were found in the incidence of breast cancer across intake levels of alcohol.

In summary, alcohol is one of the most consistent risk factors for breast cancer, albeit modest in magnitude. Given the high prevalence of alcohol use, even modest RRs could translate into a significant public health impact. Although data are limited, there is some suggestion that women who use alcohol are more likely than nondrinkers to present with regional disease (than local) at the time of diagnosis (95). Before one considers a recommendation that alcohol be avoided to minimize risk of breast cancer, it is important to be cognizant of the literature demonstrating favorable cardiovascular benefit and reduction in osteoporosis from modest use of alcohol, especially red wine, which is high in the antioxidant resveratrol. Women on HRT who use alcohol should be especially vigilant about early detection, and for all women, it would appear to be advisable to ensure an adequate daily intake of folate or folate-containing foods.

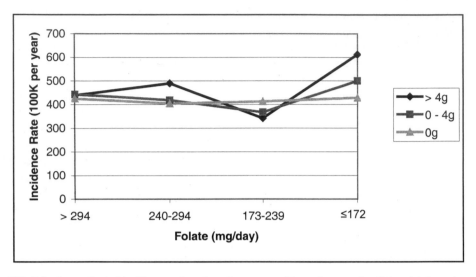

FIG. 7.3. Age-adjusted incidence rates of postmenopausal breast cancer by dietary folate and alcohol use in the Iowa Women's Health Study.

Exercise and Physical Activity

The potential health benefits of exercise have long been recognized. In the *Dialogues*, Timeus tells Socrates "Concerning the manner by which the body and mind are to be preserved, moderate exercise reduces to order, according to their affinities, the particles and affections that are wandering about the body." It is therefore not surprising that exercise has been hypothesized to reduce risk of breast cancer. In fact, numerous studies and published reviews have appeared in the literature on this topic. Because exercise is a modifiable factor that can influence risk, demonstrable evidence for such an effect is highly desirable.

The last published review on the subject appeared in 1998 (87). At that time, seven of nine studies suggested that occupational physical activity reduced risk of breast cancer; in five of these seven studies, the results were statistically significant. Comparatively speaking, more studies have examined recreational physical activity. Of 16 investigations, 11 included in that review observed lower risks of breast cancer among the most active women; however, the estimated risk reductions varied considerably, from a low of 12% to a high of 60%. Moreover, dose–response relationships were not always evident, and apparent benefits were sometimes limited to specific subgroups. In particular, there is some evidence that the benefits are greatest for women who are lean, parous, and premenopausal (96). Recently, Rockhill and colleagues (97) reported results from the Nurses' Health Study cohort. After 16 years of follow-up, more than 3,100 cases of breast cancer were reported. Women who engaged in moderate or vigorous physical activity for 7 or more hours per week had 18% lower risk of breast cancer than women who engaged in such activities for less than 1 hour per week. In the Iowa Women's Health Study of postmenopausal breast cancer, the most active women had only an 8% lower risk (98), which was consistent with the null hypothesis of no benefit. Interest recently shifted to activity levels during adolescence. Rockhill and colleagues (99) found no association between strenuous activity at least twice per week during high school or between 18 and 22 years of age in the Nurses' Health Study II. This level of activity may not be sufficient for a beneficial effect, however. Mittendorf and colleagues (100) examined self-reported physical activity in a large case–control study (6,888 cases and 9,539 controls) of women aged 17 to 74 years. They observed that women who reported any strenuous physical activity between the ages of 14 and 22 years had only a 5% reduction in risk; however, those who reported vigorous exercise at least once per day had a 50% risk reduction (95% CI, 40%–70%). A subsequent report (101) based on the same data set revealed that the beneficial effect was limited to women who either lost weight or gained little weight since the age of 18 years.

The biologic basis that may underlie any beneficial effect of regular physical activity is not firmly established. As reviewed by McTiernan and colleagues (102), however, a number of plausible mechanisms may be invoked, including effects on immune function (increased number or activity of macrophages, lymphokine-activated killer cells and their regulating cytokines), menstrual cycle (delayed onset of menses, longer menstrual cycle, a decreased number of cycles, decreased estrogen production), obesity (decreased body fat leads to decreased levels of estrogens from fat stores), bioavailable estrogens (increased SHBG), and metabolic profiles (decreased circulating insulin and glucose, possible effects on insulin-like growth factor I and its corresponding binding proteins).

Despite the relatively large number of studies that have been conducted on the topic, questions remain. Given the complexity of the topic, this uncertainty is not surprising. Questions exist regarding the types of activity—occupational, recreational, and household—and their relative importance. The components of activity—frequency, intensity, and duration—have not been adequately studied. The biologic basis of any observed beneficial effect is not firmly established, and more work is needed regarding the association of physical activity at various periods in life. Regardless, an inverse association of activity with risk of breast cancer has been observed for premenopausal, perimenopausal, and postmenopausal breast cancer. When one also considers the additional benefits of exercise on bone density, weight control, and heart disease, the promotion of regular physical activity to patients should be encouraged.

Mammographic Breast Density

The risk factors discussed so far (except serum hormone levels) can be readily determined through patient interview or self-completed questionnaire. The magnitude of breast cancer risk associated with reproductive history, hormone use, anthropometrics, and diet is relatively small. Conversely, the risks associated with high levels of mammographically dense tissue are second in magnitude only to inherited mutations in *BRCA1* or *BRCA2*. As this section describes, however, many traditional epidemiologic risk factors are associated with mammographic breast density. Thus, considerable research has focussed on the question of whether epidemiologic risk factors exert their influence on breast density.

The breast consists of three main tissues: fat, fibrous, and ductal. On the mammogram, fat is radiographically translucent, but the ductal and fibrous tissues have the same density (103). Most visible density on the mammogram is due to the fibroglandular tissue consisting of the functional elements or parenchyma and supporting elements or stroma. The parenchyma generally refers to the ducts, epithelial cells, and intralobular connective tissue surrounding the ducts; the stroma depicts the dense collagenous interlobular connective tissue, which contains blood vessels, nerves, lymphatics, and some adipose tissue (103).

The earliest studies that attempted to characterize differences in the patterns of breast tissues were conducted by Wolfe and colleagues (104), who proposed a categorical classification system of four patterns: N1, P1, P2, and DY. The N1 characterized a fatty breast with only very small amounts of dysplasia (areas of increased density) and no visible duct formation. The P1, P2, and DY categories capture elements of ductal pattern and increasing levels of density: less than 25%, 25% to 50%, and greater than 50%, respectively. Although early studies showed striking associations with breast cancer occurrence, a criticism of the Wolfe classification has been interreader consistency (105). Thus, most subsequent studies have attempted to quantify the percentage of total breast area or volume using computer-assisted techniques (106,107). Details of the various approaches are beyond the scope of this chapter. Suffice it to say that both subjective and objective measures of breast density have been used to study the association of breast density to breast cancer. Whether defined by the parenchymal pattern or measures of percent breast density, the radiographic appearance of the breast has been shown to be a major risk factor for breast cancer (105,108). Results from previous studies were summarized in a review article (109). Although the study designs, methods, and cut-points varied, the results are similar, with an approximate fivefold increased risk for women in the highest compared to the lowest quintiles of density (Fig. 7.4). Early studies have been criticized because of the potential for masking bias. In this scenario, prevalent cancers would be more likely to be missed in dense breasts and then come to attention later, resulting in a spurious estimate of high risk. Similarly, many early studies suffered from misclassification of breast density and inadequate control of potential confounders. In studies where these issues were addressed, the risk estimates for breast density are consistently and strongly associated with breast cancer (105).

The biologic basis for the excess risk associated with increased mammographic

---

FIG. 7.4. Mammographic breast density and breast cancer risk. *Relative risk of highest versus lowest categories of density. (Adapted from Boyd NF, Lockwood GA, Byng JW, et al. Mammographic densities and breast cancer risk. *Cancer Epidemiol Biomarkers Prev* 1998;7:1133–1144, with permission.)

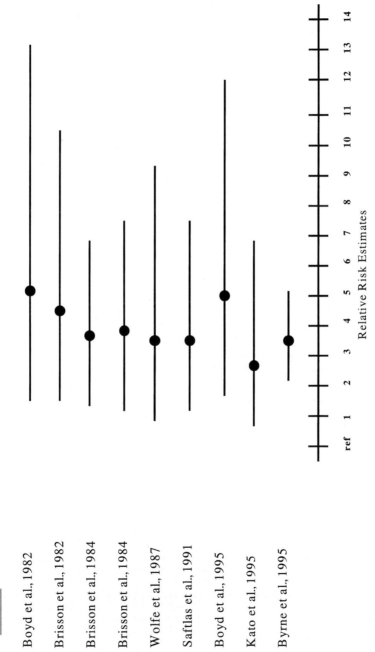

breast density remains unknown; however, several characteristics associated with mammographic breast density are also risk factors for breast cancer (105). There appears to be a hormonal influence on percent density, as evidenced by the positive associations with late age at menopause, late age at first birth, and nulliparity. In addition, use of HRT is associated with increased percent density (110). Curiously, although body mass and abdominal adiposity are associated with increased risk of breast cancer, they are inversely associated with percent density. This implies that any influence of obesity on risk is unlikely to be through an effect on breast density. Finally, recent studies suggest that a significant proportion of the variability may be genetically determined (111, 112). In summary, mammographic breast density is a major risk factor for breast cancer. Because of the natural involution of breast tissue with age, evaluation of the risk of a particular patient needs to be made with regard to levels relative to other women of the same age.

SUMMARY AND CONCLUSIONS

Breast cancer is a major medical and public health problem. This chapter describes the magnitude of the problem and summarizes the results of epidemiologic investigations to identify risk factors for the disease. Often epidemiologic research has been the impetus for correlative laboratory investigations, which in turn can substantiate or refute initial observations and hypotheses. When biologic mechanisms are known, these were also included. As shown in Table 7.4, a large number of established risk factors for breast cancer have been identified. Some, such as family history and inherited mutations in *BRCA1* and *BRCA2* are discussed elsewhere in this book. Space considerations precluded the opportunity to review all risk factors, including hypotheses of viral etiologies, pesticides, benign breast diseases, and others.

Although many of the risk factors listed in Table 7.4 are unalterable, reflecting

TABLE 7.4. *Summary of risk factors for breast cancer by strength of evidence*

Established risk factors	Possible risk factors	Suspected risk factors
Age	Short menstrual cycle	Infertility
Family history	Oral contraceptives	Abortions
Early age at menarche	Hormone replacement therapy	Low fiber intake
Late age menopause	Low SHBG	Low folate intake
Nulliparity	Abdominal obesity	
Late age at first pregnancy	Dietary fat	
Obesity (postmenopausal breast cancer)	Low fruit and vegetable intake	
Alcohol consumption	Cigarette smoking	
Mammographic breast density	Physical inactivity	
Oophorectomy (protective)		
High levels of estrogen		
Height		

SHBG, sex hormone-binding globulin.

the contribution of genetics and unavoidable exposures, a number of others are modifiable and should be targets for intervention. It is also important to emphasize that the established epidemiologic risk factors confer neither large increases in risk nor account for all of the variability in the incidence of the disease. Rather, most exposures confer modest increases in risk, and many of the causes of breast cancer remain to be discovered. Collectively, however, the patterns of disease in populations begin to help unravel the underlying biology. Effective control of the disease is predicated on this essential knowledge.

REFERENCES

1. Landis SH, Murray T, Bolden S, et al. Cancer statistics, 1998 [published errata appear in *CA Cancer J Clin* 1998;48:192 and 1998;48:329]. *CA Cancer J Clin* 1998;48:6–29.
2. Chu KC, Tarone RE, Kessler LG, et al. Recent trends in U.S. breast cancer incidence, survival, and mortality rates. *J Natl Cancer Inst* 1996;88:1571–1579.
3. Madigan MP, Ziegler RG, Benichou J, et al. Proportion of breast cancer cases in the United States explained by well-established risk factors. *J Natl Cancer Inst* 1995;87:1681–1685.
4. Parkin D, Whelan S, Ferlay J, et al. *Cancer incidence in five continents.* VII. Lyon: IARC Scientific Publications, 1997.
5. Kelsey JL, Bernstein L. Epidemiology and prevention of breast cancer. *Annu Rev Public Health1996; 17:47–67.*
6. Parkin DM. Epidemiology of cancer: global patterns and trends. *Toxicol Lett* 1998;102–103: 227–234.
7. Pike MC, Spicer DV, Dahmoush L, et al. Estrogens, progestogens, normal breast cell proliferation, and breast cancer risk. *Epidemiol Rev* 1993;15:17–35.
8. Liehr JG. Dual role of oestrogens as hormones and pro-carcinogens: tumour initiation by metabolic activation of oestrogens. *Eur J Cancer Prev* 1997;6:3–10.
9. Kelsey JL, Gammon MD, John EM. Reproductive factors and breast cancer. *Epidemiol Rev* 1993; 15:36–47.
10. Titus-Ernstoff L, Longnecker MP, Newcomb PA, et al. Menstrual factors in relation to breast cancer risk. *Cancer Epidemiol Biomarkers Prev* 1998;7:783–789.
11. Bernstein L, Ross RK. Endogenous hormones and breast cancer risk. *Epidemiol Rev* 1993;15:48–65.
12. MacMahon B, Trichopoulos D, Brown J, et al. Age at menarche, probability of ovulation and breast cancer risk. *Int J Cancer* 1982;29:13–16.
13. Apter D, Vihko R. Early menarche, a risk factor for breast cancer, indicates early onset of ovulatory cycles. *J Clin Endocrinol Metab* 1983;57: 82–86.
14. Kelsey JL. Breast cancer epidemiology: summary and future directions. *Epidemiol Rev* 1993;15: 256–263.
15. Potten CS, Watson RJ, Williams GT, et al. The effect of age and menstrual cycle upon proliferative activity of the normal human breast. *Br J Cancer* 1988;58:163–170.
16. Henderson BE, Ross RK, Judd HL, et al. Do regular ovulatory cycles increase breast cancer risk? *Cancer* 1985;56:1206–1208.
17. Whelan EA, Sandler DP, Root JL, et al. Menstrual cycle patterns and risk of breast cancer. *Am J Epidemiol* 1994;140:1081–1990.
18. Van Wieringen J. Secular growth changes in human growth: a comprehensive treatise. In: Faulkner F, Tanner J, eds. New York: Plenum Press, 1986:307–331.
19. King SE, Schottenfeld D. The epidemic of breast cancer in the U.S.—determining the factors. *Oncology* 1996;10:453–472.
20. Meyer JS, Connor RE. Cell proliferation in fibrocystic disease and postmenopause breast ducts measured by thymidine labeling. *Cancer* 1982;50:746–751.
21. Brinton LA, Schairer C, Hoover RN, et al. Menstrual factors and risk of breast cancer. *Cancer Invest* 1988;6:245–254.
22. Prentice RL, Thomas DB. On the epidemiology of oral contraceptives and disease. *Adv Cancer Res* 1987;49:285–401.

23. Bernstein L, Pike MC, Ross RK, et al. Estrogen and sex hormone-binding globulin levels in nulliparous and parous women. *J Natl Cancer Inst* 1985;74:741–745.
24. Piper JM, Kennedy DL. Oral contraceptives in the United States: trends in content and potency. *Int J Epidemiol* 1987;16:215–221.
25. Collaborative Group on Hormonal Factors in Breast Cancer. Breast cancer and hormonal contraceptives: collaborative reanalysis of individual data on 53,297 women with breast cancer and 100,239 women without breast cancer from 54 epidemiological studies. *Lancet* 1996;347:1713–1727.
26. Cancer and Steroid Hormone Study. Oral-contraceptive use and the risk of breast cancer. *N Engl J Med* 1986;315:407–411.
27. Murray PP, Stadel BV, Schlesselman JJ. Oral contraceptive use in women with a family history of breast cancer. *Obstet Gynecol* 1989;73:977–983.
28. Pike MC, Henderson BE, Casagrande JT, et al. Oral contraceptive use and early abortion as risk factors for breast cancer in young women. *Br J Cancer* 1981;43:72–76.
29. International Agency for Research on Cancer. IARC Monographs on the Evaluation of Carcinogenic Risks to Humans, Vol 72. *Hormonal contraception and post-menopausal hormonal therapy.* Lyon: World Health Organization, 1999.
30. Mishell DR Jr. Oral steroid contraceptives. In: Lobo RA, Michell DR Jr, Paulson RJ, et al., eds. *Textbook of infertility, contraception, and reproductive endocrinology.* Malden, MA: Blackwell Science, 1997:800–826.
31. Grabrick DM, Hartmann LC, Cerhan JR, et al. Risk of breast cancer with oral contraceptive use in women with a family history of breast cancer. *JAMA* 2000;284:1791–1798.
32. Ursin G, Henderson BE, Haile RW, et al. Does oral contraceptive use increase the risk of breast cancer in women with BRCA1/BRCA2 mutations more than in other women? *Cancer Res* 1997; 57:3678–3681.
33. Stone R. Depo-Provera: controversial contraceptive wins approval from FDA panel [news]. *Science* 1992;256:1754.
34. Skegg DC, Noonan EA, Paul C, et al. Depot medroxyprogesterone acetate and breast cancer: a pooled analysis of the World Health Organization and New Zealand studies. *JAMA* 1995;273: 799–804.
35. Collaborative Group on Hormonal Factors in Breast Cancer. Breast cancer and hormone replacement therapy: collaborative reanalysis of data from 51 epidemiological studies of 52,705 women with breast cancer and 108,411 women without breast cancer. *Lancet* 1997;350:1047–1059.
36. Colditz G, Stampfer MJ, Willett WC, et al. Prospective study of estrogen replacement therapy and risk of breast cancer in postmenopausal women. *JAMA* 1990;264:2648–2653.
37. Gapstur SM, Potter JD, Sellers TA, et al. Increased risk of breast cancer with alcohol consumption in postmenopausal women. *Am J Epidemiol* 1992;136:1221–1231.
38. Ginsburg ES, Mello NK, Mendelson JH, et al. Effects of alcohol ingestion on estrogens in postmenopausal women. *JAMA* 1996;276:1747–1751.
39. Gapstur SM, Morrow M, Sellers TA. Hormone replacement therapy and risk of breast cancer with a favorable histology: results of the Iowa Women's Health Study. *JAMA* 1999;281:2091–2097.
40. Grodstein F, Stampfer MJ, Colditz GA, et al. Postmenopausal hormone therapy and mortality. *N Engl J Med* 1997;336:1769–1775.
41. Willis DB, Calle EE, Miracle-McMahill HL, et al. Estrogen replacement therapy and risk of fatal breast cancer in a prospective cohort of postmenopausal women in the United States. *Cancer Causes Control* 1996;7:449–457.
42. Sturgeon SR, Schairer C, Brinton LA, et al. Evidence of a healthy estrogen user survivor effect. *Epidemiology* 1995;6:227–231.
43. Henderson BE, Paganini-Hill A, Ross RK. Decreased mortality in users of estrogen replacement therapy. *Arch Intern Med* 1991;151:75–78.
44. Bergkvist L, Adami HO, Persson I, et al. The risk of breast cancer after estrogen and estrogen-progestin replacement. *N Engl J Med* 1989;321:293–297.
45. Strickland DM, Gambrell RD Jr, Butzin CA, et al. The relationship between breast cancer survival and prior postmenopausal estrogen use. *Obstet Gynecol* 1992;80:400–404.
46. Ewertz M, Gillanders S, Meyer L, et al. Survival of breast cancer patients in relation to factors which affect the risk of developing breast cancer. *Int J Cancer* 1991;49:526–530.
47. Kennedy D, Baum C, Forbes M. Noncontraceptive estrogens and progestins: use patterns over time. *Obstet Gynecol* 1985;65:441–446.

48. Hemminki E, Kennedy DL, Baum C, et al. Prescribing of noncontraceptive estrogens and progestins in the United States, 1974–86. *Am J Public Health* 1988;78:1479–481.
49. Schairer C, Lubin J, Troisi R, et al. Menopausal estrogen and estrogen-progestin replacement therapy and breast cancer risk. *JAMA* 2000;283:485–491.
50. Ross RK, Paganini-Hill A, Wan PC, et al. Effect of hormone replacement therapy on breast cancer risk: estrogen versus estrogen plus progestin. *J Natl Cancer Inst* 2000;92:328–332.
51. Persson I, Weiderpass E, Bergkvist L, et al. Risks of breast and endometrial cancer after estrogen and estrogen-progestin replacement. *Cancer Causes Control* 1999;10:253–260.
52. Thomas HV, Reeves GK, Key TJ. Endogenous estrogen and postmenopausal breast cancer: a quantitative review. *Cancer Causes Control* 1997;8:922–928.
53. Key TJ. Serum oestradiol and breast cancer risk. *Endocr Relat Cancer* 1999;6:175–180.
54. Key TJ, Pike MC. The role of oestrogens and progestagens in the epidemiology and prevention of breast cancer. *Eur J Cancer Clin Oncol 1988;24:29–43.*
55. Bernstein L, Yuan JM, Ross RK, et al. Serum hormone levels in pre-menopausal Chinese women in Shanghai and white women in Los Angeles: results from two breast cancer case-control studies. *Cancer Causes Control* 1990;1:51–58.
56. Hankinson SE, Willett WC, Michaud DS, et al. Plasma prolactin levels and subsequent risk of breast cancer in postmenopausal women. *J Natl Cancer Inst* 1999;91:629–634.
57. Hunter DJ, Willett WC. Diet, body build, and breast cancer. *Annu Rev Nutr* 1994;14:393–418.
58. Trentham-Dietz A, Newcomb PA, Egan KM, et al. Weight change and risk of postmenopausal breast cancer (United States). *Cancer Causes Control* 2000;11:533–542.
59. Ursin G, Longnecker MP, Haile RW, et al. A meta-analysis of body mass index and risk of premeno-pausal breast cancer. *Epidemiology* 1995;6:137–141.
60. Barnes-Josiah D, Potter JD, Sellers TA, et al. Early body size and subsequent weight gain as predictors of breast cancer incidence (Iowa, United States). *Cancer Causes Control* 1995;6:112–118.
61. Le Marchand L, Kolonel LN, Earle ME, et al. Body size at different periods of life and breast cancer risk. *Am J Epidemiol* 1988;28:137–152.
62. Hislop TG, Coldman AJ, Elwood JM, et al. Childhood and recent eating patterns and risk of breast cancer. *Cancer Detect Prev* 1986;9:47–58.
63. Brinton LA, Swanson CA. Height and weight at various ages and risk of breast cancer. *Ann Epide-miol* 1992;2:597–609.
64. Huang Z, Fasco MJ, Figge HL, et al. Expression of cytochromes P450 in human breast tissue and tumors. *Drug Metab Dispos* 1996;24:899–905.
65. Hunter DJ, Willett WC. Nutrition and breast cancer. *Cancer Causes Control* 1996;7:56–68.
66. Kondo S, Takahashi E, Kato K, et al. Secular trends in height and weight of Japanese pupils. *Tohoku J Exp Med* 1978;126:203–213.
67. Tsuzaki S, Matsuo N, Ogata T, et al. Lack of linkage between height and weight and age at menarche during the secular shift in growth of Japanese children. *Ann Hum Biol* 1989;16:429–436.
68. Micozzi MS. Cross-cultural correlations of childhood growth and adult breast cancer. *Am J Phys Anthropol* 1987;73:525–537.
69. Vatten LJ, Kvikstad A, Nymoen EH. Incidence and mortality of breast cancer related to body height and living conditions during childhood and adolescence. *Eur J Cancer* 1992;28:128–131.
70. Weaver TW, Kushi LH, McGovern PG, et al. Validation study of self-reported measures of fat distribution. *Int J Obes Relat Metab Disord* 1996;20:644–650.
71. Folsom AR, Kaye SA, Prineas RJ, et al. Increased incidence of carcinoma of the breast associated with abdominal adiposity in postmenopausal women. *Am J Epidemiol* 1990;31:794–803.
72. Sellers TA, Kushi LH, Potter JD, et al. Effect of family history, body-fat distribution, and reproduc-tive factors on the risk of postmenopausal breast cancer. *N Engl J Med* 1992;326:1323–1329.
73. Potter JD. *Food, nutrition and the prevention of cancer: a global perspective.* Washington: American Institute for Cancer Research, 1997:252–287.
74. Freedman LS, Clifford C, Messina M. Analysis of dietary fat, calories, body weight, and the develop-ment of mammary tumors in rats and mice: a review. *Cancer Res 1990;50:5710–5719.*
75. Carroll KK. Experimental evidence of dietary factors and hormone-dependent cancers. *Cancer Res* 1975;35:3374–3383.
76. Howe GR, Hirohata T, Hislop TG, et al. Dietary factors and risk of breast cancer: combined analysis of 12 case–control studies. *J Natl Cancer Inst* 1990;82:561–569.
77. Hunter DJ, Spiegelman D, Adami H-O, et al. Cohort studies of fat intake and the risk of breast cancer - a pooled analysis. *N Engl J Med* 1996;334:356–361.

78. Prentice RL. Measurement error and results from analytic epidemiology: dietary fat and breast cancer. *J Natl Cancer Inst* 1996;88:1738–1747.
79. Wu AH, Pike MC, Stram DO. Meta-analysis: dietary fat intake, serum estrogen levels, and the risk of breast cancer. *J Natl Cancer Inst* 1999;91:529–534.
80. Zheng W, Anderson KE, Kushi, LH, et al. A prospective cohort study of intake of calcium, vitamin D, and other micronutrients in relation to incidence of rectal cancer among postmenopausal women. *Cancer Epidemiol Biomarkers Prev* 1998;7:221–225.
81. Baghurst PA, Rohan TE. High-fiber diets and reduced risk of breast cancer. *Int J Cancer* 1994;56: 173–176.
82. Palmer JR, Rosenberg L. Cigarette smoking and the risk of breast cancer. *Epidemiol Rev* 1993;15: 145–156.
83. MacMahon B, Trichopoulos D, Cole P, et al. Cigarette smoking and urinary estrogens. *N Engl J Med* 1982;307:1062–1065.
84. Field NA, Baptiste MS, Nasca PC, et al. Cigarette smoking and breast cancer. *Int J Epidemiol* 1992;21:842–848.
85. Baron JA, Newcomb PA, Longnecker MP, et al. Cigarette smoking and breast cancer. *Cancer Epidemiol Biomarkers Prev* 1996;3:399–403.
86. Braga C, Negri E, La Vecchia C, et al. Cigarette smoking and the risk of breast cancer. *Eur J Cancer Prev* 1996;5:159–164.
87. Gammon MD, John EM, Britton JA. Recreational and occupational physical activities and risk of breast cancer. *J Natl Cancer Inst* 1998;90:100–117.
88. Calle EE, Miracle-McMahill HL, Thun MJ, et al. Cigarette smoking and risk of fatal breast cancer. *Am J Epidemiol* 1994;39:1001–1007.
89. Smith-Warner SA, Spiegelman D, Yaun SS, et al. Alcohol and breast cancer in women: a pooled analysis of cohort studies. *JAMA* 1998;279:535–540.
90. Purohit V. Moderate alcohol consumption and estrogen levels in postmenopausal women: a review. *Alcohol Clin Exp Res* 1998;22:994–997.
91. Gapstur SM, Potter JD, Drinkard C, et al. Synergist effect between alcohol and estrogen replacement therapy on risk of breast cancer differs by estrogen/progesterone receptor status in the Iowa Women's Health Study. *Cancer Epidemiol Biomarkers Prev* 1995;5:313–318.
92. Zhang S, Hunter DJ, Hankinson SE, et al. A prospective study of folate intake and the risk of breast cancer. *JAMA* 1999;281:1632–1637.
93. Rohan TE, Jain MG, Howe GR, et al. Dietary folate consumption and breast cancer risk. *J Natl Cancer Inst* 2000;92:266–269.
94. Sellers TA, Kushi LH, Cerhan JR, et al. Dietary folate intake, alcohol, and risk of breast cancer in a prospective study of postmenopausal women. *Epidemiology* 2001;12:420–428.
95. Vaeth PA, Satariano WA. Alcohol consumption and breast cancer stage at diagnosis. *Alcohol Clin Exp Res* 1998;22:928–934.
96. Friedenreich CM, Thune I, Brinton LA., et al. Epidemiologic issues related to the association between physical activity and breast cancer. *Cancer* 1998;83:600–610.
97. Rockhill B, Willett WC, Hunter DJ, et al. A prospective study of recreational physical activity and breast cancer risk. *Arch Intern Med* 1999;159:2290–2296.
98. Moore DB, Folsom AR, Mink PJ, et al. Physical activity and incidence of postmenopausal breast cancer. *Epidemiology* 2000;11:292–296.
99. Rockhill B, Willett WC, Hunter DJ, et al. Physical activity and breast cancer risk in a cohort of young women. *J Natl Cancer Inst* 1998;90:1155–1160.
100. Mittendorf R, Longnecker MP, Newcomb PA, et al. Strenuous physical activity in young adulthood and risk of breast cancer (United States). *Cancer Causes Control* 1995;6:347–353.
101. Shoff SM, Newcomb PA, Trentham-Dietz A, et al. Early-life physical activity and postmenopausal breast cancer: effect of body size and weight change. *Cancer Epidemiol Biomarkers Prev* 2000;9: 591–595.
102. McTiernan A, Ulrich C, Slate S, et al. Physical activity and cancer etiology: associations and mechanisms. *Cancer Causes Control* 1998;9:487–509.
103. Egan R. *Breast imaging: diagnosis and morphology of breast diseases*. Philadelphia: WB Saunders, 1988:30–58.
104. Wolfe JN. Risk for breast cancer development determined by mammographic parenchymal pattern. *Cancer* 1976;37:1486–1492.

105. Oza AM, Boyd NF. Mammographic parenchymal patterns: a maker of breast cancer risk. *Epidemiol Rev* 1993;15:196–208.
106. Boyd NF, Byng JW, Jong RA, et al. Quantitative classification of mammographic densities and breast cancer risk: results from the Canadian National Breast Screening Study. *J Natl Cancer Inst* 1995;87:670–675.
107. Byng JW, Boyd NF, Fishell E, et al. Automated analysis of mammographic densities. *Phys Med Biol* 1996;41:909–923.
108. Saftlas AF, Szkle M. Mammographic parenchymal patterns and breast cancer risk. *Epidemiol Rev* 1987;9:146–174.
109. Boyd NF, Lockwood GA, Byng JW, et al. Mammographic densities and breast cancer risk. *Cancer Epidemiol Biomarkers Prev* 1998;7:1133–1144.
110. Kaufman Z, Garstin WI, Hayes R, et al. The mammographic parenchymal patterns of women on hormonal replacement therapy. *Clin Radiol* 1991;43:389–392.
111. Pankow JS, Vachon CM, Kuni CC, et al. Genetic analysis of mammographic breast density in adult women: evidence of a gene effect. *J Natl Cancer Inst* 1997;89:549–556.
112. Vachon CM, Kuni CC, Anderson K, et al. Association of mammographically-defined percent breast density with epidemiologic risk factors for breast cancer. *Cancer Causes Control* 2000; 11:653–662.
113. Ries LAG, Eisner MP, Kosary CL, et al. *SEER Cancer Statistics Review 1973–1997.* Bethesda, MD: National Cancer Institute, 2000:119–120.

8

Principles of Breast Cancer Screening

Ismail Jatoi

Among physicians, there is a deep-rooted belief that the early detection of cancer is beneficial. Thus, cancer screening is generally assumed to be an effective means of reducing mortality. This assumption is not necessarily correct, however. Consider, as an example, the case of lung cancer screening. For years, many physicians assumed that screening for lung cancer by sputum cytology or chest radiographs was beneficial. Eventually, clinical trials proved that these assumptions were wrong (1). As a result, lung cancer screening with sputum cytology and chest radiographs is not routinely recommended today. This example illustrates the need to study carefully the merits of cancer screening before drawing any conclusions concerning its effectiveness.

A few investigators have steadfastly maintained that breast cancer is a systemic disease at inception and that screening should therefore have little impact on reducing mortality (2,3). Proponents of this paradigm have long argued that the early detection and timely extirpation of the primary breast tumor should not alter the natural history of the disease. Indeed, a prominent physician has argued that we are missing the forest (the systemic problem) because our efforts are primarily directed at the tree (the breast tumor) (4). Most clinicians, however, do not accept this view. For many years, the prevailing view has been that the cancer begins as a cell or clone of cells that multiply and grow in size (5). At some point during the growth of this breast mass, metastasis occurs, and the resulting metastatic deposits lead to the death of the patient. Thus, most physicians strongly believe that the early detection and treatment of breast cancer (before the onset of symptoms) should significantly reduce mortality. Therefore, considerable interest has focused on screening as a means of reducing breast cancer mortality.

Three screening methods for breast cancer are commonly used: mammography and clinical breast examination (CBE) by trained personnel and breast self-examination (BSE) (6). Various studies have examined the effectiveness of screening in reducing breast cancer mortality, and this chapter reviews many of these studies (Table 8.1). It is also important to note that breast-screening programs target large, healthy (asymptomatic) populations, and very few of these women are actually found to have breast cancer. Thus, the potential benefit of screening must be weighed against its potential for harm. The risks and benefits of breast cancer screening are discussed here.

TABLE 8.1. *Evidence of benefit for the three screening modalities*

Screening modality	Randomized controlled trials to assess benefit		Significant reduction in breast cancer mortality
Mammography	HIP	Gothenburg	25% in women aged 50 yr and older
	Malmo	Edinburgh	(7–9 yr of follow-up)
	Two-country	CNBSS I	18% in women aged 40–49 yr
	Stockholm	CNBSS II	(>12 yr of follow-up)
Breast self-examination	St. Petersburg, Russia		No proven benefit
	Shanghai, China		
Clinical breast examination	Mumbai, India		Results not yet available

HIP, Health Insurance Plan; CNBSS, Canada National Breast Screening Study.

THEORETICAL CONSIDERATIONS

Cancer therapy has generally been directed toward patients who have symptoms; however, proponents of screening have long argued that the asymptomatic period in the natural history of cancer represents a "window of opportunity" for treatment (7). The *total preclinical phase* (TPCP) refers to the period from the initiation of cancer to the onset of symptoms (8). Generally, the beginning of the TPCP is not known. The *detectable preclinical phase* (DPCP) is a component of the TPCP, and this term refers to the period when the cancer is detectable with a screening test (8). The starting point of the DPCP depends on the screening test used. A screening test that detects cancer very early in its natural history will be associated with a longer DPCP compared with a test that detects it later. The *sensitivity* of a screening test refers to the proportion of patients with a disease who have a positive result (true-positive rate); the *specificity* of a test refers to the proportion of patients without the disease who have a negative result (true-negative rate) (9). A longer DPCP is associated with a more sensitive screening test.

Prevalence refers to the total number of persons who have a disease at a particular time; *incidence* refers to the number of persons who develop a disease over a specific period (10). In any screening program, the first screening round is referred to as the *prevalent screen*, and the cancers detected are known as the *prevalent cancers*. The number of cancers detected during the prevalent screen depends on the DPCP (i.e., a longer DPCP is associated with a greater number of prevalent cases). Following the prevalent screen, the subsequent screening rounds are known as the *incident screens*, and the cancers detected are referred to as the *incident cancers*. Cancers diagnosed between screening sessions generally present as symptomatic cases and are referred to as *interval cancers* (11). Anderson et al. showed that, as a group, the prevalent cancers generally have a more favorable tumor biology and better prognosis than cancers detected at the incident screens (10). The interval cancers generally have the worst prognosis (11).

Cole and Morrison argued that before screening for any cancer is initiated, three conditions must be met (8). First, there must be effective treatment for the cancer, and the treatment must be more effective in screen-detected cases than in clinically detected cases. Obviously, if there is no available treatment for the cancer, screening will provide no survival advantage. Additionally, if treatment is equally effective in screen-detected and clinically detected cases, then, again, screening will provide no survival advantage. Second, there should be a high prevalence among persons who undergo screening. A high prevalence is necessary to justify the expense of a screening program. Third, the cancer should have serious consequences (i.e., a high mortality rate or significant morbidity).

Many investigators believe that breast cancer meets the three conditions outlined by Cole and Morrison. Numerous studies have been undertaken to determine the effectiveness of breast cancer screening in reducing mortality. Before discussing the breast cancer screening studies, we must first consider the biases inherent in those studies. Three biases merit particular attention: lead time, length, and selection.

Lead-time Bias

Screening detects cancers "early," but this alone does not justify screening. Screening can only be justified if it prevents or delays the time of death from cancer. *Survival* refers to the period from diagnosis of cancer to death. "Lead-time bias" refers to the interval between the diagnosis of cancer by screening and by usual clinical detection (12). As screening advances the time of breast cancer diagnosis, patients with screen-detected cancers will appear to have better survival rates than those with clinically detected cancers, even if screening does nothing to delay death. As a result of lead-time bias, screening may appear to prolong life, when it simply extends the period over which the cancer is observed. The effect of lead-time bias is illustrated in Fig. 8.1.

Length Bias

Slower growing cancers exist for a longer period in the preclinical phase and are more likely to be detected by screening. In contrast, faster growing tumors exist for a shorter period in the preclinical phase and are more likely to be detected in the intervals between screening sessions. This phenomenon is termed *length bias* (13). Indeed, we now know that there are differences in the biologic properties of the mammographically detected (screen-detected) breast cancers and those detected clinically. When histologic differentiation, tumor necrosis, mitotic counts, estrogen and progesterone receptors, histological type, DNA ploidy, and S-phase fraction are compared, the mammographically detected cancers are generally found to have a more favorable tumor biology (14).

Selection Bias

Women who are health conscious are more likely to volunteer for periodic breast cancer screening. In general, these women are more likely to eat nutritional foods,

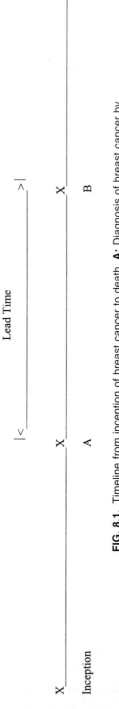

Lead Time

X — Inception

X — A

X — B

X — Death (C)

FIG. 8.1. Timeline from inception of breast cancer to death. **A:** Diagnosis of breast cancer by mammography. **B:** Diagnosis of breast cancer by palpation. A–C: "Survival" for mammographically detected cancers. B–C: "survival" for cancers detected by palpation. A–B: Lead-time bias.

exercise regularly, and maintain a healthy lifestyle. As a result, volunteers have a lower mortality rate from all causes than women who do not volunteer for breast cancer screening. This is sometimes referred to as the *healthy-screenee effect* (15). Thus, studies that compare volunteers for breast cancer screening with nonvoluntary controls are subject to a selection bias. The lower mortality of women who undergo screening might not necessarily be due to screening but to other factors associated with healthy volunteers. The effect of selection bias was suggested in a case–control study from the United Kingdom. Moss et al. compared volunteers and nonvolunteers for breast cancer screening (16). Women from two separate communities were compared. In one community, women had the opportunity to undergo periodic screening (screening district), whereas in the other community, no screening program was available (comparison district). These authors found that breast cancer mortality was higher among the nonvolunteers of the screening district compared with women in the comparison district. This difference in mortality was attributed to selection bias.

Various studies examined the efficacy of breast cancer screening: case–control, retrospective, and prospective; however, the best way to exclude the biases discussed here is to conduct randomized prospective clinical trials with all-cause mortality as the endpoint. Unfortunately, clinical trials that use all-cause mortality as the endpoint require huge numbers of subjects and are therefore not practical. Thus, the breast cancer screening trials have used cause-specific (breast cancer) mortality as a surrogate endpoint. These randomized prospective trials are discussed in the following sections.

MAMMOGRAPHIC SCREENING

The distinction between *diagnostic* mammography and *screening* mammography is important (17). Diagnostic mammography is used to evaluate patients with breast symptoms (such as a breast lump). In contrast, screening mammography targets asymptomatic women. In this chapter, we consider the merits of screening mammography. Diagnostic mammography is discussed in other chapters of this book.

The concept of mammographic screening for asymptomatic women has evolved over many years (18). Salomon, a surgeon, is credited with initiating mammography in 1913, using gross mastectomy specimens (19). Subsequently, in 1930, Warren reported on the use of mammography in patients (20). The concept of mammographic screening for asymptomatic women was proposed by Gershon-Cohen et al. in the 1950s (21). In the 1950s and 1960s, Gershon-Cohen et al. and Egan published reports indicating that mammography could detect impalpable cancers in asymptomatic women (22,23). Soon after, randomized prospective trials were initiated to determine the effectiveness of mammographic screening in reducing mortality from breast cancer.

Eight randomized prospective trials have examined the effectiveness of screening mammography (24). These are the Health Insurance Plan (HIP) trial of New York, Swedish Two County, Gothenburg, Stockholm, Malmo, Edinburgh, the Canadian National Breast Screening Study I (CNBSS I), and the CNBSS II. A total of 500,000 women were enrolled in these eight trials, and approximately 170,000 were below the age of 50 at the start of the trials.

The design of these trials differed considerably (Table 8.2). Four trials evaluated the effectiveness of screening with mammography and CBE, whereas the other four trials evaluated the effectiveness of screening with mammography alone. In some trials, mammographic screening was undertaken with one view per breast, whereas others included two views per breast. The screening interval in these trials ranged from 12 to 33 months, and the ages of the women enrolled in these studies ranged from 40 to 74 years. Additionally, the randomization method varied (i.e., cluster or individual).

Health Insurance Plan Trial

The HIP trial was initiated in New York in 1963 and involved 60,696 women between the ages of 40 and 64 at entry (25). Women were randomized either to undergo periodic screening or to receive usual medical care. Screening consisted of mammography and CBE. Analysis of the cancers detected by screening in the HIP trial revealed the following: 45% were detected by CBE alone, 33% by mammography alone, and 22% by mammography and CBE. Thus, any reduction in breast cancer mortality in the screened group cannot necessarily be attributed to mammography alone. A mortality reduction in the study group may also mean that screening by CBE is an effective screening modality.

At 10-year follow-up, the HIP trial demonstrated a 29% reduction in breast cancer mortality in the screened group compared with the control group (25). This result also can be described in terms of a relative risk (RR) reduction (RR of 1.0 indicates no difference between the screened and control groups). Thus, after 10 years of follow-up, the RR of death from breast cancer in the study group was 0.71 [95% confidence interval (CI), 0.55–0.93). The CI does not cross 1.0, indicating that the result is statistically significant.

There has been considerable interest in comparing the effect of screening in women who were below and above age 50 years at the start of the trials (26). If these two subsets are examined separately, differences emerge. In the HIP trial, at 10 years follow-up, the RR of death from breast cancer for women below the age of 50 in the screened group was 0.77 (95% CI, 0.50–1.16) whereas for those above age 50, it was 0.68 (95% CI, 0.49–0.96). Thus, there was no significant benefit to screening women below age 50, but for those over age 50, periodic screening significantly reduced breast cancer mortality. With further follow-up to 18 years, however, the benefit of screening younger women in the HIP trial begins to approach statistical significance, with RR of death from breast cancer of 0.77 (95% CI, 0.53–1.11) compared with controls (27). This trend is seen in other studies as well and is further discussed in the following sections.

Swedish Trials

Four randomized prospective trials on breast cancer screening were conducted in Sweden: the two-county (Kopparberg and Ostergotland), Malmo, Stockholm, and

TABLE 8.2. *Characteristics of the randomized controlled trials of mammographic screening*

Trial	Entry years	Age at entry (yr)	Screening method	Randomization	Screening frequency	No. of women
HIP	1963–1969	40–64	2-view MM and PE	Individual	Annually 4 rounds	60,696
Malmo	1976–1986	45–69	1-or 2-view MM	Cluster: birth cohort	18–20 mo, 5 rounds	41,478
Two-county	1977–1985	40–74	1-view MM	Cluster: geographic	24–33 mo, 4 rounds	133,065
Stockholm	1981–1985	40–64	1-view MM	Cluster: birth cohort	28 mo, 2 rounds	59,176
Gothenburg	1982–1988	40–59	2-view MM	Individual (age <50 yr) Cluster (age >50 yr)	18 mo, 4 rounds	49,553
Edinburgh	1978–1985	45–64	1- or 2-view MM and PE	Cluster: physician	24 mo, 4 rounds	54,671
CNBSS I	1980–1987	40–49	2-view MM and PE	Individual: volunteer	Annually, 5 rounds	50,430
CNBSS II	1980–1987	50–59	2-view MM and PE vs. PE	Individual: volunteer	Annually, 5 rounds	39,405

HIP, Health Insurance Plan; MM, mammography; CNBSS, Canada National Breast Screening Study; PE, physical examination.

Gothenburg trials (28). These trials were initiated between 1976 and 1982 and enrolled approximately 283, 000 women between the ages of 40 and 74. In these trials, women were randomized either to undergo periodic screening with mammography alone or to receive usual care. CBE was used as a screening modality in the HIP, Edinburgh, and Canadian trials, but it was not used in any of the Swedish trials.

In 1993, Nystrom et al. published an overview of the four Swedish trials, based on 5 to 13 years of follow-up (28). For women of all ages, a significant reduction in breast cancer mortality was seen in the screened group, with RR of 0.76 (95% CI, 0.66–0.87). For women aged 40 to 49 at the start of the trials, however, there was an insignificant reduction in breast cancer mortality in the study group, RR 0.87 (95% CI, 0.63–1.20). In 1996, another overview was conducted, with an additional 4 years of follow-up (29). In that overview, the benefit of screening for women aged 40 to 49 at the start of the Swedish trials approached statistical significance, with RR 0.77 (95% CI, 0.59–1.01). A further follow-up overview of the Swedish trials was reported in 1997 by Hendrick et al. (30). In that study, the RR of death from breast cancer in the screened group was 0.71 (95% CI, 0.57–0.89) for women between the ages of 40 to 49 at the start of the trials. Thus, with long-term follow-up, a statistically significant benefit to screening younger women finally emerges in the Swedish trials.

Edinburgh Trial

The Edinburgh randomized trial of breast cancer screening recruited 44,288 women between the ages of 45 and 64 from 1978 and 1981 (31). This initial recruitment included 11,391 women between the ages of 45 and 49 at entry (cohort 1). Subsequently, an additional 10,383 women were recruited in two cohorts during the periods 1982 to 1983 (cohort 2) and 1984 to 1985 (cohort 3) (32). Thus, the Edinburgh trial included a total of 54,671 women who were between the ages of 45 and 64 at the start of the study.

The design of the trial was similar to that of the HIP trial. Women were randomized either to undergo periodic screening with mammography and CBE or to receive usual care. For women of all ages, after 10 years of follow-up, the RR of death from breast cancer in the screened group was 0.82 (95% CI, 0.61–1.11). For women below age 50 at entry, the RR was 0.78 (95% CI, 0.46–1.31). Recently, Alexander et al. reported the results of 14 years of follow-up for all women enrolled in the Edinburgh trial (33). The RR of death in the screened group, when compared with the control group, was 0.87 (95% CI, 0.70–1.06). After adjusting for the socioeconomic status of the general medical practices from which the participants in the study were recruited, the rate ratio was 0.79 (95% CI, 0.60–1.02).

Canadian Trials

The CNBSS consisted of two separate randomized prospective trials (CNBSS I and CNBSS II), both initiated in 1980 (34,35). The CNBSS I was specifically designed to assess the efficacy of screening women below age 50 and included 50,430 women between the ages of 40 and 49 at the start of this study. Women were randomized either to undergo periodic screening or to receive usual care. Screening consisted of annual mammography and CBE. After an average follow-up of 7 years, there was an insignificant excess in breast cancer mortality in the screened group, RR 1.36 (95% CI, 0.84–2.21). This insignificant excess in mortality persisted even after 10.5 years of follow-up, RR 1.14 (95% CI, 0.83–1.56).

The CNBSS II examined the efficacy of screening women who were between the ages of 50 and 59 at the start of the trial. The design of the CNBSS II study was different from that of the CNBSS I. Women were randomized to undergo either screening with annual mammography and CBE (study group) or CBE alone (control group). Surprisingly, after 7 years of follow-up, breast cancer mortality in the two groups was nearly identical, with the RR of death in the study group 0.97 (95% CI, 0.62–1.52). Similar results were reported after 13 years' follow-up; the number of breast cancer deaths in the study and control groups was 107 and 105, respectively, and the cumulative rate ratio was 1.02 (95% CI, 078–1.33) (36). These results might be interpreted to mean that screening mammography does nothing to reduce breast cancer mortality beyond that which can be achieved by screening with CBE alone. The potential use of CBE as a screening method is discussed later in this chapter.

OVERVIEWS (META-ANALYSES) OF THE MAMMOGRAPHIC SCREENING TRIALS

As indicated, the eight mammographic screening trials produced varying results. Several investigators published overviews (meta-analyses) incorporating the results of these eight trials. Most of these meta-analyses focused on the group of women between the ages of 40 and 49 years at the start of these trials. In 1995, Kerlikowske et al. published a meta-analysis of the eight randomized controlled trials and four case–control studies on mammographic screening (37). This meta-analysis showed that, for women between the ages of 50 and 74 at the start of the studies, a significant reduction in breast cancer mortality was evident in the screened group after 7 to 9 years' follow-up, the RR 0.74 (95% CI, 0.66–0.83). Longer follow-up did not alter the magnitude of this benefit. In contrast, for women between the ages of 40 and 49 at the start of these studies, the duration of follow-up did affect the risk of death from breast cancer. For these younger women, the RR of death from breast cancer in the screened group was 1.02 (95% CI, 0.73–1.27) after 7 to 9 years' follow-up and 0.83 (95% CI, 0.65–1.06) after 10 to 12 years of follow-up.

That same year, Smart et al. reported a meta-analysis of all published and presented data on the eight mammographic screening trials (38). For women in the screened group between the ages of 40 and 49 at the start of the trials, the RR of death from breast cancer was 0.84 (95% CI, 0.69–1.02).

In 1996, an updated meta-analysis of the eight mammographic screening trials was reported in Falun, Sweden (29). In that study, the RR of death from breast cancer in the screened group for women aged 40 to 49 years at entry was 0.85 (95%

CI, 0.71–1.01) compared with controls. The following year, Hendrick et al. published a meta-analysis of the eight mammographic screening trials, with average follow-up time of 12.7 years (30). For women aged 40 to 49 at the start of the screening trials, a significant reduction in breast cancer mortality was seen in the screened group, the RR being 0.82 (95% CI, 0.71–0.95). Thus, a statistically significant benefit of screening younger women emerges after long-term follow-up.

The individual clinical trials and the meta-analyses therefore suggest that the impact of screening differs between younger and older women. For women who are over age 50 at the start of the screening trials, a significant reduction in breast cancer mortality is apparent after 7 to 9 years of follow-up, and longer follow-up does not change the magnitude of this benefit. In contrast, for women below age 50 at the start of the screening trials, the benefit of screening emerges gradually, with a significant reduction in breast cancer mortality appearing after 12 or more years of follow-up.

Gotzsche and Olsen have recently challenged the studies indicating that mammographic screening is effective in reducing breast cancer mortality (39). They scrutinized data from the eight randomized controlled trials on mammographic screening and argued that most of these trials were flawed (with the exception of the Canadian trials and the Malmo trial in Sweden). Gotzsche and Olsen reported discrepancies in the number of women randomized to the screened and control arms of the studies and also differences in the mean ages of women in the two arms of the studies. In their meta-analysis, only trials were included that they believed were adequately randomized, and they found that mammographic screening had no effect on breast cancer mortality (pooled RR 1.04, 95% CI, 0.84–1.27). As expected, this study has generated intense controversy, and several investigators have challenged these results (40,41).

EFFECT OF AGE ON MAMMOGRAPHIC SCREENING

Historically, clinical studies that support common sense views are generally well received, whereas studies that fail to support such views are often severely criticized. Some results of the mammographic screening trials are counterintuitive and have generated considerable controversy. Most of the controversy centers on whether mammographic screening for women between the ages of 40 and 49 is beneficial. In recent years, several medical organizations have fueled this controversy by issuing guidelines on mammographic screening that are at odds with one another (42). Despite opposition from several medical groups, mammographic screening for younger women is now generally accepted in the United States. This is not the case in Europe, however. Indeed, for more than a decade, the United States has stood alone among the major industrialized countries in encouraging mammographic screening for women between the ages of 40 and 49. There are several possible reasons for the difference between the American and European positions on this issue (43). For instance, the ''fee for service'' health care system in the United States may encourage the use of mammographic screening for younger women.

Additionally, the medicolegal climate in the United States also may contribute to the greater willingness of American physicians to recommend mammographic screening for women below age 50. Despite the widespread use of mammographic screening for younger women in the United States, the U.S. breast cancer mortality rates continue to mirror those of many industrialized countries that do not recommend screening for this age group (44).

Why does it take longer to see a benefit for women who are below age 50 at the start of the mammographic screening trials? There are several possible explanations (45). One possibility is that screening may detect very slow-growing (*indolent*) tumors in younger women. Thus, a reduction in breast cancer mortality may take longer to appear in younger women. Kerlikowske argued, however, that if this is the case, then detecting these slow-growing tumors after age 50 perhaps could provide the same reduction in risk of breast cancer deaths (46). Alternatively, screening might not be very effective in younger women. Indeed, the delayed benefit of screening younger women actually might be attributed to screening these women after the age of 50. This possibility was studied by de Koning et al. using a computer simulation model known as MISCAN (Microsimulation Screening Analysis) (47). Their study suggested that most of the reduction in breast cancer mortality for women who were between the ages of 40 and 49 at the start of the screening trials was, in fact, the result of screening these women beyond the age of 50.

Another important question is why the effect of mammographic screening is different for women below and above age 50. Some investigators have argued that there is no rational basis for the abrupt change in the effectiveness of mammographic screening at age 50 (48). Yet age 50 corresponds approximately to the age of the menopause, and the biology and epidemiology of breast cancer differ in premenopausal and postmenopausal women (49). For example, there is a steep rise in breast cancer incidence until about age 50, followed by a less rapid increase after that age (50). Additionally, obesity is associated with a lower risk of premenopausal breast cancer and a higher risk of postmenopausal cancer (51). The menopause also appears to have an effect on the primary breast tumor. For instance, premenopausal women have a lower proportion of estrogen receptor–positive tumors and a higher labeling index than do postmenopausal women (52). Thus, the results of the mammographic screening trials are consistent with the results of other studies showing differences in the biology and epidemiology of premenopausal and postmenopausal breast cancers.

Why might mammographic screening be less effective in premenopausal women than in postmenopausal women? This question, of course, remains wide open to speculation, but several possibilities should be considered. As screening advances the time of breast cancer diagnosis and allows for the early initiation of therapy, one might speculate that postmenopausal women benefit more from early therapy than do premenopausal women. Another possibility is that the sensitivity of mammography might be lower in premenopausal women, making it less effective as a screening test. Finally, Tabar et al. suggested that tumors of premenopausal women grow more rapidly than those of postmenopausal women (53). In fact, the incidence of interval cancers (diagnosed between screening sessions) appears to be greater in premenopausal than in postmenopausal women. Thus, Tabar et al. suggest that reducing the interval between screening sessions (from 2 years to 1 year) may improve the efficacy of mammographic screening for younger women.

The effectiveness of mammographic screening for women aged 40 to 49 remains one of the most hotly debated issues in medicine. As a result of this controversy, another randomized prospective trial was initiated in the United Kingdom (54). Women in this trial will be aged 40 to 41 at entry and randomized either to undergo periodic screening or receive usual care (no screening). Women randomized to the screening arm of the study will be offered mammographic screening at the first visit and annually thereafter for 7 or 8 years. On reaching the age of 50, women in both the screening and control arms of the study will be offered regular screening. In this trial, the study group will consist of 65,000 women, and the control group will contain 135,000 women.

Much interest centers on the optimal age for initiation of mammographic screening (40 versus 50); the upper age limit for screening has received less attention. Although organizations in the United States generally recommend mammographic screening for women aged 70 and older, little data support these recommendations (55). Analysis of data from the Swedish trials might be interpreted to mean that mammographic screening for women over age 70 is not effective (56); however, meaningful conclusions cannot be drawn because few women over age 70 were included in these trials. Because a woman's risk of developing breast cancer increases with age, the efficacy of mammographic screening for older women remains an important issue. Using a mathematical model (the Markov model), Kerlikowske et al. studied the effect of mammographic screening in older women (57). Their analysis suggests that mammographic screening after age 69 is moderately cost-effective and results in a small gain in life expectancy for women with high bone mineral density (BMD) but is more costly in those with low BMD. These investigators calculated that, to prevent one death, either 1,064 women with high BMD or 7,143 women with low BMD would need to be screened routinely from ages 69 to 79 years. Clearly, the risks and benefits of mammographic screening should be weighed carefully before recommending mammographic screening for older women. The risks of screening are discussed later in this chapter.

SCREENING BY CLINICAL BREAST EXAMINATION

CBE can be used either for screening (detecting cancers in asymptomatic women) or diagnosis (evaluating breast complaints). Screening by CBE differs from screening by BSE in that it requires the use of trained personnel. Since the advent of mammographic screening, the role of CBE as a screening modality has diminished. Indeed, there is evidence to suggest that the increased use of mammographic screening in the United States generally has been accompanied by a decline in the use of CBE as a screening modality (58). In Europe, many breast cancer screening programs have abandoned CBE entirely, relying only on mammography (59). Yet several influential medical organizations, such as the American College of Radiology, the National Cancer Institute, and the American Cancer Society, continue to recommend screening with CBE in addition to mammography (60). It is also important to note that about 5% to 10% of all breast cancers are detectable by CBE but not by mammography (60). Although the impact of screening by CBE on breast cancer mortality has not been fully elucidated, it seems premature to abandon screening by CBE. Furthermore, screening programs should train their personnel to perform proper CBE.

CBE readily detects cancers larger than 1 cm (61). Additionally, in the U.S. Breast Cancer Detection and Demonstration Project (BCDDP), 39% of mammographically detected cancers smaller than 1 cm also were detectable by CBE (62). Mittra et al. suggested that careful screening by CBE would fail to detect *in situ* cancers and 22% of the mammographically detected invasive cancers smaller than 1 cm (61). They argued that this advantage of mammography over CBE is not likely to be clinically significant.

To date, there are no data from randomized prospective trials to compare screening by CBE with no screening. Four of the eight mammographic screening trials also included CBE as a screening modality: HIP, Edinburgh, and the Canadian NBSS I and II (26,31,34,35). The results of these four trials suggest that screening with CBE can effectively detect breast cancers. Barton et al. calculated that screening by CBE has a sensitivity of approximately 54% and a specificity of about 94% (63).

In the HIP trial, women were randomized to screening with mammography and CBE or no screening (27). This study was conducted during the early years of the development of mammography, and a disproportionally large number of cancers were detected by CBE. Overall, in the HIP trial, 67% of the cancers in the screened population were detected by CBE. Of these, 45% were detected by CBE alone and 22% by CBE and mammography. Only 33% of the cancers were detected by mammography alone. In the HIP trial, age seemed to influence the effectiveness of CBE in detecting breast cancer. For women aged 50 to 59 years, 40% of the cancers were detected by CBE alone and 42% by mammography alone; however, for women aged 40 to 49, CBE was much more effective in detecting tumors than mammography, with 61% of cancers detected by CBE alone and 19% by mammography alone. Thus, CBE might have contributed much to the reduction in breast cancer mortality observed in the screened group of the HIP trial.

In the Edinburgh trial, women were randomized to screening with mammography and CBE or no screening (31). In that study, 74% of the cancers in the screened group were detected by CBE, with 3% detected by CBE alone and 71% by mammography and CBE. Mammography alone detected 26% of the cancers in the screened population. Thus, the Edinburgh trial also suggests that screening by CBE is effective in detecting cancers.

In the CNBSS I, women aged 40 to 49 were randomized to screening with mammography and CBE or to no screening (34). The results of the CNBSS I are consistent with those of other trials showing no benefit to screening younger women during the first 7 to 9 years of follow-up. In the CNBSS II, women aged 50 to 59 at entry were randomized to either screening with CBE alone or CBE and mammography (35). Whereas other trials showed a benefit to mammographic screening for this age group, the CNBSS II found that it provided no survival advantage. This result might be interpreted to mean that mammographic screening contributes nothing to breast cancer mortality reduction beyond that achievable with screening with CBE alone. In the CNBSS, CBE detected 59% of the cancers in women aged 40 to 49. Of these, 32% were detected by CBE alone and 27% by CBE and mammography. For women aged 50 to 59, 44% of the cancers were detected by CBE, with 18% detected by CBE alone and 26% detected by CBE and mammography. The results of the CNBSS are therefore consistent with those of the HIP trial, indicating that screening by CBE is more effective in detecting cancers of younger women.

Although screening by CBE is effective in detecting breast cancer, its impact on breast cancer mortality is not known. If screening by CBE could reduce breast cancer mortality, it might be particularly useful in some developing countries, where mammographic screening is often not affordable and breast cancer mortality rates are rising. Thus, a randomized controlled trial was initiated in Mumbai, India, under the direction of Dr. Indraneel Mittra to determine the impact of screening by CBE on breast cancer mortality (6). The trial will enroll 70,000 women who will be equally divided between study and control groups. The study group will be taught BSE and will receive annual CBE by trained personnel for 5 years; the control group will receive usual care. The total follow-up period in this trial will be 10 years.

Mittra et al. argued that there is a need for a clinical trial, where women would be randomized to either receive screening with mammography or CBE (61). They argued that there is now compelling evidence to indicate that screening with CBE is an effective screening modality and that a direct comparison with screening mammography is therefore warranted.

SCREENING BY BREAST SELF-EXAMINATION

Screening by BSE has been advocated since the early part of the twentieth century (64). Today, it is widely promoted by various medical societies, breast cancer advocacy groups, and the media as an effective screening tool (generally in conjunction with screening mammography). Many hospitals and clinics throughout the United States sponsor classes where women are taught BSE techniques. BSE is a very appealing screening method. It is inexpensive, self-generated, and nonintrusive. Its efficacy in reducing breast cancer mortality has not yet been proven, however.

Two randomized controlled trials have examined the effect of screening by BSE on breast cancer mortality. The first of these was the World Health Organization trial of BSE undertaken in St. Petersburg, Russia (65). Women in this study were recruited from 1985 to 1989. There were 57,712 women from 14 randomly selected outpatient hospitals who were taught BSE. Another 64,759 women from another 14 outpatient hospitals served as controls. Semiglazov et al. reported the preliminary results of this trial in 1992 (65). The number of breast cancers detected in the two arms of the study was nearly identical (190 cases in the BSE group and 192 in the control group), and there was no significant difference in mortality between the two groups. Additionally, no significant differences were found between the two groups with respect to the size of the primary tumor or incidence of nodal metastasis. Of note, the BSE-trained group had a higher number of excisional biopsies for benign lesions, the RR being 1.5 in the BSE group compared with controls (95% CI, 1.1–1.9). Semiglazov et al reported a further update of this study in 1999 and again found no significant difference in the death rates between the BSE and control groups (66).

Another BSE trial was initiated in Shanghai, China, between 1989 and 1991 (67). In that trial, 267,040 women were randomly assigned on the basis of work sites (520 textile factories) to receive either intensive BSE instruction (study group) or sessions on the prevention of low back pain (control group). After 5 years' follow-up, the number of breast cancer cases and the rate of breast cancer mortality were nearly identical in the two groups. Yet there was more than a twofold increase in the number of breast biopsies in the BSE group compared with the control group.

Screening by BSE is not without risk. There is evidence that it can generate considerable anxiety among women. Furthermore, false-positive and false-negative results may incur considerable costs and risks. Indeed, the two randomized trials mentioned already indicate that women who practice screening with BSE are much more likely to undergo unnecessary breast biopsies. Longer follow-up of the St. Petersburg and Shanghai trials eventually may show that screening by BSE can effectively reduce breast cancer mortality. It is surprising, however, that a downstaging of tumors has not been observed in either trial as a result of screening by BSE.

POTENTIAL HAZARDS OF SCREENING

Clearly, breast cancer screening has advantages. The randomized controlled trials discussed earlier in this chapter indicate that mammographic screening can reduce breast cancer mortality by about 25% in postmenopausal women. Additionally, screen-detected cancers are generally smaller than those detected clinically. Thus, screen-detected cancers are more amenable to treatment with conservative surgery (i.e., lumpectomy, quadrantectomy, or segmental resection) than cancers detected clinically.

Certain hazards are associated with breast cancer screening. Five potentially harmful consequences of screening merit consideration: lead time, false-positives, radiation exposure, overdiagnosis, and cost (Table 8.3).

TABLE 8.3. *Potential hazards of screening*

Lead time	Advanced notice of a cancer diagnosis without tangible gain
Radiation exposure (mammography)	Possible increased risk of breast cancer in patients susceptible to the effects of low-dose radiation
False-positives	Results in unnecessary breast biopsies
Overdiagnosis	Adverse financial/emotional consequences of being falsely labeled as a cancer patient
Cost	Costs of breast cancer screening may divert resources away from more mundane health care needs

Lead Time

Screening advances the time of breast cancer diagnosis, but this does not benefit all women. The randomized controlled trials indicate that mammographic screening in postmenopausal women reduces breast cancer mortality by about 25%. Thus, for most women, advancing the time of breast cancer diagnosis by mammographic screening does not change the outcome. As a result of screening, many women are simply given advanced notice of a cancer diagnosis with no tangible gain. This "lead time" effect of screening (in the absence of any tangible benefit) may have an adverse impact on quality of life.

False-Positives

False-positives are cases that are reported as suspicious or malignant on screening that, on further evaluation (such as a breast biopsy), prove benign. False-positives have an adverse effect on quality of life and result in additional health care expenditures. For screening mammography, the false-positive rate is much greater in the United States than in Europe, perhaps because of the fear of litigation in the United States, resulting in a greater unwillingness of American radiologists to commit themselves to a benign diagnosis. In the American BCDDP, for example, mammographic screening had a positive predictive value of only 10% (68). Thus, for every cancer found, nine women had a false-positive result on mammographic screening. In contrast, the positive predictive value for mammographic screening in Europe during the same period ranged from 30% to 60% (69).

A study from northern California found that the positive predictive value of the first screening mammogram declines steadily from about 19% for women over age 70 to about 4% for women aged 40 to 49 (70). Elmore et al. calculated that, after ten mammograms, a woman has about a 49% cumulative risk of a false-positive result (71). For women between the ages of 40 to 49, the cumulative risk is about 56%, whereas for those aged 50 to 79, the cumulative risk of a false-positive result after ten mammograms is about 47%.

Evidence from the CNBSS II suggests that there are fewer false-positives associated with screening by CBE (61). In that study, women aged 50 to 59 were randomized to either screening with CBE or screening with mammography and CBE. No significant difference was found in the mortality between the two arms of the study. The rate of biopsy of benign breast lumps was three times higher with combined screening, however, compared with screening with CBE alone.

One study found that women are generally aware that mammographic screening can produce false-positive results (72). The study also indicated that most women consider false-positives an acceptable consequence of mammographic screening and are willing to tolerate such results. Indeed, the survey found that 63% of all women thought that 500 or more false-positives per life saved was reasonable, and 37% were willing to tolerate as many as 10,000 false-positives per life saved.

Radiation Exposure

Bailar was one of the first to suggest that low-dose radiation exposure from mammographic screening might induce breast cancer (73). More recently, Beemsterboer et al. developed a computer simulation model to estimate breast cancer deaths caused from exposure to low-dose radiation and the number of lives saved as a result of screening mammography (74). These estimates were based on data from the Swedish mammographic screening trials and the Netherlands breast cancer screening program. In their model, the ratio between the number of breast cancer deaths prevented with those induced as a result of mammographic screening for women aged 50 to 69 was 242:1, assuming a 2-year screening interval and a mean glandular dose of 4 mGy to each breast from a two-view mammogram. When mammographic screening was expanded to include women aged 40 to 49, the ratio was 97:1. Thus, according to this model, the potential hazards of low-dose radiation are greatly increased if mammographic screening is initiated below age 50.

Swift et al. called attention to the potential hazards of mammographic screening in carriers of the gene for ataxia–telangiectasia (AT) (75). These carriers are at increased risk for developing breast cancer after exposure to relatively low doses of radiation. Approximately 1.4% of all individuals are heterozygote carriers of the gene for AT, so the population potentially at risk from the harmful effects of low-dose radiation is large. Identifying these persons before mammographic screening would be a huge, expensive undertaking and is probably not feasible. The amount of radiation required to induce breast cancer in a heterozygote carrier of the gene for AT is not clear. Some investigators speculate that a total dose of 20 mGy would be required (75,76). If so, a carrier of the AT gene who undergoes mammographic screening every 2 years might accumulate a hazardous dose of ionizing radiation over a 10-year period, assuming a mean glandular dose of 4 mGy to each breast from a two-view mammogram.

Women who carry mutations in the BRCA1 and BRCA2 genes have an increased risk of developing breast cancer. The task force of the Cancer Genetics Studies Consortium recommends that carriers of the BRCA1 and BRCA2 gene mutations begin annual mammographic screening between the ages of 25 and 35 years (77). This recommendation did not consider, however, the potential hazards of low-dose radiation associated with screening mammography. The BRCA1 and BRCA2 genes are required for DNA repair, and recent studies suggest that women who carry mutations in these genes might be very sensitive to the effects of low doses of radiation (78). Thus, Vaidya and Baum warned of the potential hazards of mammographic screening in women who carry mutations in the BRCA1 and BRCA2 genes (79). Clearly, additional studies are required to determine the optimal method of cancer surveillance for carriers of breast cancer predisposing genes.

Overdiagnosis

In recent years, the incidence of breast cancer in the United States has increased, largely because of ''overdiagnosis'' of breast cancer by mammographic screening.

Peeters and colleagues defined overdiagnosis as "a histologically established diagnosis of intraductal or invasive cancer that would never have developed into a clinically manifest tumor during the patient's normal life expectancy if no screening examination had been carried out" (80). Indeed, the increase in breast cancer incidence has generally paralleled the increase in use of mammographic screening.

To understand how screening might overdiagnose invasive breast cancer, consider the following hypothetical situation. A 65-year-old woman with severe coronary artery disease undergoes routine mammographic screening. As a result of that screening, an occult (nonpalpable) invasive breast cancer is discovered. This cancer is treated with surgery, radiotherapy, and tamoxifen. One year later, this patient dies of a myocardial infarction (MI). Because mammographic screening advances the time of breast cancer diagnosis by about 2 to 4 years, this patient's breast cancer probably would not have been discovered without screening. She probably would have died of a MI, never knowing that she had breast cancer and would have been spared the treatments resulting from her cancer diagnosis. This example illustrates how screening might unmask invasive cancers that would not have become clinically symptomatic or pose a threat to a woman's normal life expectancy.

An even greater problem associated with mammographic screening is the overdiagnosis of noninvasive (*in situ*) cancers (81). Since the advent of mammographic screening, the incidence of ductal carcinoma *in situ* (DCIS) has increased dramatically. DCIS is rarely palpable and therefore seldom detected by clinical examination. Most cases of DCIS are diagnosed by mammographic screening. Indeed, before the advent of mammographic screening, DCIS accounted for only 1% to 2% of all breast cancer cases in the United States (82). In recent years, DCIS has accounted for more than 12% of all breast cancer cases and about 30% of those discovered mammographically (83).

Many clinicians have long assumed that DCIS is a preinvasive cancer that, untreated, invariably progresses to invasive breast cancer. This assumption was based on two observations. First, after simple excision of DCIS, recurrences often occur, many of which are invasive breast cancers. Second, DCIS often is adjacent to invasive breast cancer, suggesting that DCIS was the precursor to the invasive tumor. Evidence now suggests, however, that most cases of DCIS would not progress to manifest breast cancers clinically during a woman's lifetime. Nielsen et al. reported the results of 110 medicolegal autopsies performed at the Fredericksburg Hospital in Copenhagen, Denmark (84). These autopsies were performed on women who had died of accidents. DCIS was found incidentally in 15% of these women, a prevalence four to five times greater than the number of overt cancers expected to develop over a 20-year period. Additionally, in two separate studies, Rosen et al. and Page et al. retrospectively reviewed benign breast biopsies and found numerous instances where the initial pathologist overlooked DCIS (85,86). In both studies, only about 25% developed clinically manifest invasive breast cancers after 15 to 18 years' follow-up. Finally, in women with a previous diagnosis of breast cancer, Alpers and Wellings found DCIS in about 48% of contralateral breasts at autopsy (87), but only about 12.5% of these women would be expected to develop contralateral breast cancer over a 20-year period. Together, these studies suggest that perhaps only one of every four or five cases of DCIS detected mammographically would progress to a clinically manifest breast cancer during a woman's lifetime.

The diagnosis of DCIS by mammographic screening can have a devastating effect on quality of life. Women diagnosed with DCIS often face the same challenges that confront patients diagnosed with invasive cancer, including denial of insurance coverage or coverage with inflated premiums and the denial of life insurance (88, 89). Additionally, despite evidence that conservative surgery is appropriate for patients with DCIS, many women often are treated with total mastectomy (90). Thus, women diagnosed with DCIS may face severe financial and emotional hardships that adversely affect their quality of life. This problem is particularly disheartening considering that most cases of mammographically detected DCIS would not have progressed to a clinically manifest cancer. This hazard of mammographic screening has thus far received little attention.

Schwartz et al. recently conducted a survey of 497 women aged 18 to 97 who did not report a family history of breast cancer (72). Few of these women were aware that mammographic screening could detect nonprogressive breast cancers, and most never heard of DCIS; however, 60% indicated they would like to consider this information before deciding on whether to undergo screening. This study emphasizes the need for obtaining informed consent before screening. The risks and benefits of screening should be discussed with each woman before screening so she can make an informed decision.

Cost

Health care resources are often limited, particularly in developing countries. Ideally, these resources should be distributed equitably across a wide range of health care programs to obtain the maximum benefit. Again, it is important to emphasize that women who are invited to participate in breast cancer screening programs are not "patients" and most do not become patients. Yet breast cancer screening programs often use expensive technology. Resources directed toward maintaining breast cancer screening programs could lower resources available for more pressing and mundane health care programs, adversely affecting the health of an entire community. To put this matter into perspective, Kattlove et al. estimated, in 1995, the cost of potentially saving one life over a 10-year period with mammographic screening (91). For women aged 40 to 49, the estimated cost was $1,480,000; however, for women aged 50 to 59, the estimated cost was $183,000, and for women aged 60 to 69, it was $146,000. If health care resources are limited, these figures should be considered when deciding how best to appropriate scarce resources.

CONCLUSION

More is known about screening for breast cancer than for any other type of cancer. In this chapter, the three most commonly used breast cancer screening methods were discussed. These are mammography, CBE using trained personnel, and BSE. Randomized controlled trials indicate that mammographic screening in postmenopausal women can reduce breast cancer mortality by about 25%; however, its effect in premenopausal women is disputed. To date, no data are available from randomized prospective trials comparing the effect of screening by CBE with no screening on breast cancer mortality. Several mammographic screening trials also incorporated CBE as a screening modality. Evidence from these trials suggests that CBE might be an effective screening tool, and a large randomized prospective study has been initiated in India to study this possibility further. Thus far, data from two large randomized prospective trials indicate that screening with BSE has no impact on breast cancer mortality.

In the lay media, considerable emphasis is given to the potential benefits of breast cancer screening, and little attention is paid to its potential risks. Women who volunteer for breast cancer screening are generally healthy, and few derive any tangible gain from screening. Many women seem to be poorly informed about the impact of screening on their risk of dying of breast cancer. Black et al. surveyed 200 women between the ages of 40 and 50 with no history of breast cancer and found that these women overestimated their probability of dying of breast cancer by more than 20-fold and the effectiveness of screening in reducing mortality by sixfold (92). Thus, a more balanced presentation about breast cancer risk and the effectiveness of screening is warranted. Not only should the potential for benefit should be discussed with each woman prior to screening, but the potential risks should be outlined as well.

ACKNOWLEDGMENT

The opinions or assertions contained herein are the private views of the authors and should not be construed as reflecting the views of the Departments of the Army, Air Force, or Defense.

REFERENCES

1. Eddy DM. Screening for lung cancer. *Ann Intern Med* 1989;111:232–237.
2. MacDonald I. Biological predeterminism in human cancer. *Surg Gynecol Obstet*1951;92:443–452.
3. Black MM, Speer FD. Biological variability of breast carcinoma in relation to diagnosis and therapy. *NY State J Med* 1953;53:1560–1563.
4. Devitt JE. Breast cancer: have we missed the forest because of the tree? *Lancet* 1994;344:734–735.
5. Haagensen CD. *Diseases of the breast*. Philadelphia: WB Saunders, 1956.
6. Jatoi I. Breast cancer screening. *Am J Surg* 1999;177:518–524.
7. Jatoi I. Breast cancer: a systemic or local disease? *Am J Clin Oncol* 1997;20:536–539.
8. Cole P, Morrison AS. Basic issues in population screening for cancer. *J Natl Cancer Inst* 1980;64: 1263–1272.
9. Nielsen C, Lang RS. Principles of screening. *Med Clin North Am* 1999;83:1323–1337.
10. Anderson TJ, Lamb J, Alexander F, et al. Comparative pathology of prevalent and incident cancers detected by breast cancer screening: Edinburgh Breast Screening Project. *Lancet* 1986;1:519–523.
11. Gilliland FD, Joste N, Stauber PM, et al. Biologic characteristics of interval and screen-detected breast cancer. *J Natl Cancer Inst* 2000;92:743–749.
12. Xu JL, Prorok PC. Non-parametric estimation of the post-lead-time survival distribution of screen-detected cancer cases. *Stat Med* 1995;14:2715–2725.

13. Black WC, Welch HG. Advances in diagnostic imaging and overestimation of disease prevalence and the benefits of therapy. *N Engl J Med* 1993;328:1237–1243.
14. Klemi PJ, Joensuu H, Toikkanen S, et al. Aggressiveness of breast cancers found with and without screening. *BMJ* 1992;304:467–469.
15. Schmidt JG. The epidemiology of mass breast cancer screening—a plea for a valid measure of benefit. *J Clin Epidemiol* 1990;43:215–225.
16. Moss SM, Summerley ME, Thomas BJ, et al. A case–control evaluation of the effect of breast cancer screening in the United Kingdom trial of early detection of breast cancer. *J Epidemiol Comm Health* 1992;46:362–364.
17. Monsees BS, Destouet JM. A screening mammography program: staying alive and making it work. *Radiol Clin North Am* 1992;30:211–219.
18. Hurley SF, Kaldor JM. The benefits and risks of mammographic screening for breast cancer. *Epidemiol Rev* 1992;14:101–130/
19. Salomon A. Beitrage zur pathologie und klinik der mammacrcinome. *Arch f klin Chir* 1913;101: 573–668.
20. Warren SL. A roentgenologic study of the breast. *Am J Roentgenol* 1930;24:113–124.
21. Gershon-Cohen J, Ingleby H, Moore L. Can mass x-ray surveys be used in detection of early cancer of the breast? *JAMA* 1956;161:1069–1071.
22. Gershon-Cohen J, Hermel MB, Berger SM. Detection of breast cancer by periodic x-ray examinations. *JAMA* 1961;176:1114–1116.
23. Egan RL. Mammography, an aid to diagnosis of breast carcinoma. *JAMA* 1962;182:839–843.
24. Fletcher SW, Black W, Harris R, et al. Report of the international workshop on screening for breast cancer. *J Natl Cancer Inst* 1993;85:1644–1656.
25. Shapiro S, Venet W, Strax P, et al. Ten to fourteen year effect of screening on breast cancer mortality. *J Natl Cancer Inst* 1982;69:349–355.
26. Eddy DM, Hasselblad V, McGivney W, et al. The value of mammography screening in women under age 50 years. *JAMA* 1988;259:1512–1519.
27. Shapiro S, Venet W, Strax P, et al. *Periodic screening for breast cancer: the Health Insurance Plan Project and Its Sequelae, 1963–1986.* Baltimore: Johns Hopkins University Press, 1988.
28. Nystrom L, Rutqvist LE, Wall S, et al. Breast cancer screening with mammography: overview of Swedish randomized trials. *Lancet* 1993;341:973–978.
29. Breast cancer screening with mammography in women aged 40–49 years: report of the Organizing Committee and Collaborators, Falun Meeting, Falun, Sweden (21 and 22 March 1996). *Int J Cancer* 1996;68:693–699.
30. Hendrick RE, Smith RA, Rutlege JH, et al. Benefit of screening mammography in women aged 40-49: a new meta-analysis of randomized controlled trials. *Monogr Natl Cancer Inst* 1997;22:87–92.
31. Alexander FE, Anderson TJ, Brown H, et al. The Edinburgh randomised trial of breast cancer screening: results after 10 years of follow-up. *Br J Cancer* 1994;70:542–548.
32. Alexander FE. The Edinburgh Randomized Trial of Breast Cancer Screening. *Monogr Natl Cancer Inst* 1997;22:31–35.
33. Alexander FE, Anderson TJ, Brown HK, et al. *Lancet* 1999;353:1903–1908.
34. Miller AB, Baines CJ, To T, et al. Canadian national breast screening study I.Breast cancer detection and death rates among women aged 40 to 49 years. *Can Med Assoc J* 1992;147:1459–1476.
35. Miller AB, Baines CJ, To T, et al. Canadian national breast screening study II. Breast cancer detection and death rates among women aged 50 to 59 years. *Can Med Assoc J* 1992;147:1477–1488.
36. Miller AB, To T, Baines CJ, Wall C. Canadian national breast screening study-2: 13-year results of a randomized trial in women aged 50-59 years. *J Natl Cancer Inst* 2000;92:1490–1499.
37. Kerlikowske K, Grady D, Rubin SM, et al. Efficacy of screening mammography. A met-analysis. *JAMA* 1995;273:149–154.
38. Smart CR, Hendrick RE, Rutledge JH III, et al. Benefit of mammography screening in women ages 40 to 49 years: current evidence from randomized controlled trials. *Cancer* 1995;75:1619–1625.
39. Gotzsche PC, Olsen O. Is screening for breast cancer with mammography justifiable? *Lancet* 2000; 355:129–134.
40. Duffy SW, Tabar L. Screening mammography re-evaluated. *Lancet* 2000;355:747–748.
41. Dean PB. Final comment. The articles by Gotzsche and Olsen are not official Cochrane reviews and lack scientific merit. *Lakartidningen* 2000;97:3106.
42. Jatoi I. The case against mammographic screening for women in their forties. In: Jatoi I, ed. *Breast cancer screening.* Austin, TX: Landes Biosciences, 1997:35–49.

43. Jatoi I, Baum M. American and European recommendations for screening mammography in younger women: a cultural divide? *BMJ* 1993;307:1481–1483.
44. Davis DL, Love SM. Mammographic screening. *JAMA* 1994;271:152–153.
45. Fletcher SW. Breast cancer screening among women in their forties: an overview of the issues. *Monogr Natl Cancer Inst* 1997;22:5–9.
46. Kerlikowske K. Efficacy of screening mammography among women aged 40 to 49 years and 40 to 69 years: comparison of relative and absolute benefit. *Monogr Natl Cancer Inst* 1997;22:79–86.
47. de Koning HJ, Boer R, Warmerdam PG, et al. Quantitative interpretations of age-specific mortality reductions from the Swedish breast cancer screening trials. *J Natl Cancer Inst* 1995;87:1217–1223.
48. Kopans DB. The case in favor of mammographic screening for women in their forties. In: Jatoi I, ed. *Breast cancer screening.* Austin, TX: Landes Biosciences 1997:9–34.
49. Elwood JM, Cox B, Richardson AK. The effectiveness of breast cancer screening by mammography in younger women. *Online J Curr Clin Trials* 25 Feb 1993 (Doc No. 32).
50. Clemmensen J. Carcinoma of the breast: results from statistical research. *Br J Radiol* 1948;21:583.
51. Willett W. *Nutritional epidemiology.* New York: Oxford University Press, 1990.
52. Henderson IC. Biologic variations of tumors. *Cancer* 1992;69:1888–1895.
53. Tabar L, Fagerberg G, Day NE, et al. What is the optimum interval between mammographic screening examinations? An analysis based on the latest results of the Swedish two-county breast cancer screening trial. *Br J Cancer* 1987;55:547–551.
54. Breast cancer screening in women under 50. *Lancet* 1991;337:1575–76.
55. Leitch AM, Dodd GD, Constanza M, et al. American Cancer Society guidelines for the early detection of breast cancer: update 1997. *CA Cancer J Clin* 1997;47:150–153.
56. Larsson LG, Nystrom L, Wall S, et al. The Swedish randomized mammography screening trials. *J Med Screen* 1996;3:129–132.
57. Kerlikowske K, Salzmann P, Phillips KA, et al. Continuing screening mammography in women aged 70 to 79 years: impact on life expectancy and cost-effectiveness. *JAMA* 1999;282:2156–2163.
58. Burns RB, Freund KM, Ash AS, et al. As mammography use increases, are some providers omitting clinical breast examination? *Arch Intern Med* 1996;156:741–744.
59. Paci E, Alexander FE. Study design of randomized controlled clinical trials of breast cancer screening. *Monogr Natl Cancer Inst* 1997;22:21–25.
60. Bobo JK, Lee NC, Thames SF. Findings from 752081 clinical breast examinations reported to a National Screening Program from 1995 through 1998. *J Natl Cancer Inst* 2000;92: 971–976.
61. Mittra I, Baum M, Thornton H, et al. Is clinical breast examination an acceptable alternative to mammographic screening? *BMJ* 2000;321:1071–1073.
62. Report of the Working Group to review the National Cancer Institute-American Cancer Society breast cancer detection demonstration projects. *J Natl Cancer Inst* 1979;62:639–709.
63. Barton MB, Harris R, Fletcher SW. Does this patient have breast cancer? The screening clinical breast examination: should it be done? How? *JAMA* 1999;282:1270–1280.
64. Adair FE. Clinical manifestations of early cancer of the breast—with a discussion on the subject of biopsy. *N Engl J Med* 1933;208:1250–1255.
65. Semiglazov VF, Moiseyenko VM, Bavli JL, et al. The role of breast self-examination in early breast cancer detection (results of the 5-years USSR/WHO randomized study in Leningrad). *Eur J Epidemiol* 1992;8:498–502.
66. Semiglazov VF, Moiseyenko VM, Manikhas AG, et al. Interim results of a prospective randomized study of self-examination for early detection of breast cancer (in Russian). *Vopr Onkol* 1999;45: 265–271.
67. Thomas DB, Gao DL, Self SG, et al. Randomized trial of breast self-examination in Shanghai: methodology and preliminary results. *J Natl Cancer Inst* 1997;89:355–365.
68. Baker LH. Breast cancer detection demonstration project: 5-year summary report. *CA J Cancer J Clin* 1982;42:1–35.
69. Reidy J, Hoskins O. Controversy over mammography screening. *BMJ* 1988;297:932–933.
70. Kerlikowske K, Grady D, Barclay J, et al. Positive predictive value of screening mammography by age and family history of breast cancer. *JAMA* 1993;270:2444–2450.
71. Elmore JG, Barton MB, Moceri VM, et al. Ten-year risk of false positive screening mammograms and clinical breast examinations. *N Engl J Med* 1998;338:1089–1096.
72. Schwartz LM, Woloshin S, Sox HC, et al. US women's attitudes to false positive mammography results and detection of ductal carcinoma *in situ*: cross sectional survey. *BMJ* 2000;320:1635–1640.
73. Bailar JC. Mammography: a contrary view. *Ann Intern Med* 1976;84:77–84.

74. Beemsterboer PM, Warmerdam PG, Boer R, et al. Radiation risk of mammography related to benefit in screening programmes: a favourable balance? *J Med Screen* 1998;5:81–87.
75. Swift M, Morrell D, Massey RB, et al.Incidence of cancer in 161 families affected by ataxia-telangiectasia. *N Engl J Med* 1991;325:1831–1836.
76. Werneke U. Ataxia telangiectasia and risk of breast cancer. *Lancet* 1997; 350: 739–740.
77. Burke W, Daly M, Garber J, et al. for the Cancer Genetics Studies Consortium. Recommendations for follow-up care of individuals with an inherited predisposition to cancer, II: BRCA1 and BRCA2. *JAMA* 1997;277:997–1003.
78. Kinzler KW, Vogelstein B. Gatekeepers and caretakers. *Nature* 1997;386:761–63.
79. Vaidya JS, Baum M. Benefits and risks of screening mammography in women with BRCA1 and BRCA2 mutations. *JAMA* 1997;278:290.
80. Peeters PHM, Verbeek ALM, Straatman H, et al. Evaluation of overdiagnosis of breast cancer in screening with mammography: results of the Nijmegen programme. *Int J Epidemiol* 1989;18: 295–299.
81. Jatoi I, Baum M. Mammographically detected ductal carcinoma *in situ*: are we overdiagnosing breast cancer? *Surgery* 1995;118:118–120.
82. Moore MM. Treatment of ductal carcinoma *in situ* of the breast. *Semin Surg Oncol*1991;7:267–70.
83. Ernster VL, Barclay J, Kerlikowske K, et al. Incidence of and treatment for ductal carcinoma *in situ* of the breast. *JAMA* 1996;275:913–918.
84. Nielsen M, Thomsen JL, Primdahl S, et al. Breast cancer and atypia among young and middle aged women: a study of 110 medicolegal autopsies. *Br J Cancer* 1987;56:814–819.
85. Rosen PR, Braun DW Jr, Kinne DE. The clinical significance of pre-invasive breast carcinoma. *Cancer* 1980;46: 919–925.
86. Page DL, Dupont WD, Rogers LW, et al. Intraductal carcinoma of the breast: followup after biopsy only. *Cancer* 1982;49:751–758.
87. Alpers CE, Wellings SR. The prevalence of carcinoma *in situ* in normal and cancer-associated breasts. *Hum Pathol* 1985;16:796–807.
88. Herold AH, Roetzheim RG. Cancer survivors. *Prim Care* 1992;19:779–791.
89. Berkman BJ, Sampson SE. Psychosocial effects of cancer economics on patients and their families. *Cancer* 1993;72:2846–2849.
90. Winchester DP, Menck HR, Osteen RT, et al. Treatment trends for ductal carcinoma in situ of the breast. *Ann Surg Oncol* 1995;2:207–213.
91. Kattlove H, Liberati A, Keeler E, et al. Benefits and costs of screening and treatment for early breast cancer: development of a basic benefit package. *JAMA* 1995;273:142–148.
92. Black WC, Nease RF, Tosteson AN. Perceptions of breast cancer risk and screening effectiveness in women younger than 50 years of age. *J Natl Cancer Inst* 1995;87:720–731.

9

Breast Imaging

Lawrence W. Bassett and Anne Christine Hoyt

Mammography is the primary imaging modality for breast cancer screening and diagnosis. In the last decade, improvements in the technical quality of mammography and mammography reporting systems rank among the most important advances in breast imaging. Improvements in the overall quality of mammography are related to the efforts of programs established both by professional societies and government agencies. Introduction of the American College of Radiology (ACR) Mammography Accreditation Program in 1987 (1) and the Mammography Quality Standards Act in 1994 (2) is among the most significant of these efforts. In addition, the ACR Breast Imaging Reporting and Data System (BI-RADS) (3) has improved the communication of mammography results, monitoring and tracking of patients, and quality assurance activities, such as the medical audit. Because of its importance and widespread use, the BI-RADS standardized lexicon should be understood by referring physicians and will be used in this chapter.

Ultrasonography is the most important adjunctive imaging modality for the diagnosis of breast cancer. Like mammography, ultrasonography also has undergone significant technical improvements that have extended its contributions to breast imaging. Other imaging modalities undergoing technologic development and clinical trials include digital mammography, magnetic resonance imaging (MRI), and radionuclide imaging. Advances in biopsy techniques led to the widespread use of stereotactic and ultrasound-guided breast core needle biopsy (CNB).

TYPES OF MAMMOGRAPHY

Mammography can be divided into two basic types: screening and diagnostic. *Screening mammography* is an examination of an asymptomatic woman to detect clinically occult breast cancer (4). The standard screening examination includes two views of the breast, sometimes called the *standard views*: a mediolateral oblique (MLO) (Fig. 9.1A,B) and a craniocaudal (CC) (Fig. 9.1C,D) (5). The effectiveness of screening mammography for mortality reduction from breast cancer has been confirmed by evaluations of randomized clinical trials (6). Whereas there is general agreement that screening mammography reduces mortality from breast cancer in women over 50 years of age, there has been considerable debate over the effectiveness of screening mammography for women aged 40 to 49 (7). Based on evidence of benefit from meta-analysis of randomized controlled studies (8), the American Cancer Society and most major professional medical societies continue to recom-

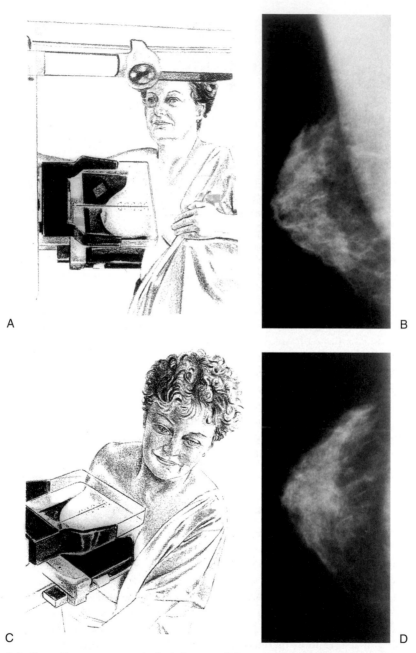

FIG. 9.1. Screening mammography includes a mediolateral oblique (MLO) and a craniocaudal (CC) view of each breast. **A:** Patient positioning for the right MLO view. **B:** Right MLO mammogram. **C:** Patient positioning for the right CC view. **D:** Right CC mammogram.

mend mammography screening for women aged 40 to 49. Two recent trials also support mammography screening for women under the age of 50. The 14-year follow-up of the Edinburgh trial showed a mortality reduction of 21% for women aged 45 to 49 who were screened with mammography (9). The 16-year follow-up of the UK Trial of Early Detection of Breast Cancer showed 27% decreased mortality in women screened with mammography compared with a control group, and equally reduced mortality rates were seen in women who began screening with mammography at age 45 or 46 (10). Furthermore, no mortality reduction was associated with a third group who participated in regular breast self-examination.

Diagnostic mammography, sometimes called *consultative* or *problem-solving mammography*, is indicated when there are clinical findings such as a palpable lump, localized pain, nipple discharge, or an abnormal screening mammogram that requires additional workup (11). The diagnostic examination involves a complete workup tailored to a symptomatic patient or one with abnormal findings on a screening examination. To correlate the clinical and imaging findings, a radiopaque marker (''BB'') often is placed over the area of clinical concern prior to performing the mammograms (Fig. 9.2). The diagnostic workup may include additional views of the breast using spot compression and magnification devices, correlative clinical breast examination, and ultrasonography. With some exceptions, a radiologist should be on site during the performance of diagnostic mammography.

Diagnostic mammography should be performed when a biopsy is being considered

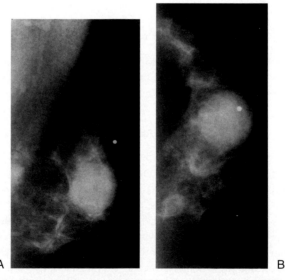

A   B

FIG. 9.2. Diagnostic mammography. The radiologic technologist placed a radiopaque BB directly over the palpable abnormality prior to obtaining the mammograms.**A:** Left mediolateral oblique view with BB in place. **B:** Left craniocaudal view with BB. Ultrasonography revealed a simple cyst, which was aspirated. The other densities in the mammograms proved to be normal fibroglandular tissue.

for a palpable lump in a woman over 30 years of age. The purpose of mammography prior to the biopsy is to define better the nature of the clinical abnormality and to find unexpected lesions, including multifocal carcinoma or intraductal component of an invasive carcinoma. The diagnostic mammogram could also reveal that the finding is benign and does not require a biopsy. An example of the latter would be a typical area of palpable fat necrosis after trauma; however, a negative workup should not defer the biopsy of a clinically suspicious finding (4).

MAMMOGRAPHY REPORT

Over the years, many radiologists and training programs developed their own terminology and methods for reporting mammograms. Referring physicians often complained that the terminology was confusing, conclusions were equivocal, and recommendations were unclear. ACR BI-RADS was a direct response to complaints from referring physicians about these problems (3). BI-RADS included standardized descriptors and final assessments and linked them directly to recommended management protocols. In its development, there was input from the American College of Surgeons, the College of American Pathologists, the American Medical Association, the National Cancer Institute, the Centers for Disease Control and Prevention, the Food and Drug Administration, and the American Cancer Society. The BI-RADS report includes four components: (a) reason for the examination, (b) overall breast tissue composition, (c) description of findings with standardized terms, and (d) overall assessment category.

Reason for the Examination.

Examples include screening mammography, palpable mass (diagnostic mammography), additional workup of a mammographically detected abnormality, or 6-month follow-up of a probably benign finding.

Breast Tissue Composition

Because the sensitivity of mammography is directly related to the relative amounts of fat and fibroglandular content, it is important for the referring physician to be aware of the overall breast tissue composition for the individual woman. The breast tissue can range from almost all radiolucent fat to extremely radiodense tissue. Because breast cancers are radiodense, fat (dark gray to black on mammograms) provides an excellent background in which to detect small cancers. Dense tissue (white on mammograms) can obscure breast cancers. The four categories of breast tissue composition are (a) when the breast is almost entirely fat (Fig. 9.3A), (b) there are scattered islands of fibroglandular densities (Fig. 9.3B), (c) the breast tissue is heterogeneously dense (this may lower the sensitivity of mammography), and (Fig. 9.3C), (d) the breast tissue is extremely dense (which lowers the sensitivity of mammography) (Fig 9.3D).

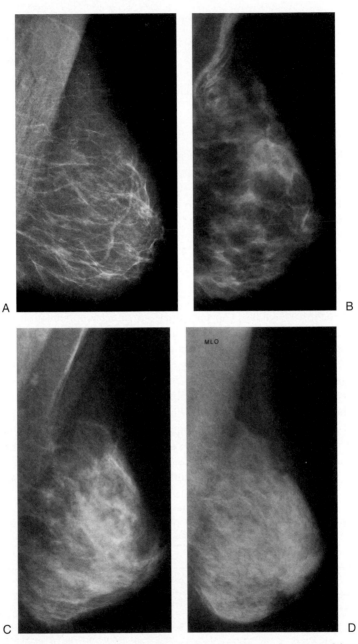

FIG. 9.3. Left mediolateral oblique mammograms demonstrating the four types of tissue composition. **A:** Almost entirely fat. **B:** Scattered fibroglandular densities. **C:** Heterogeneously dense. **D:** Extremely dense.

Description of Findings

Normal and abnormal findings are described using a standard lexicon. The descriptors reflect the probability of malignancy. Masses and calcifications are the most common abnormalities found on mammograms, and the BI-RADS descriptors of these abnormalities are found later in this chapter

Assessment Category

The BI-RADS report ends with an overall assessment (impression or conclusion) and associated recommendations for management. The examination is placed into one of six categories, after which the most important findings can be succinctly summarized. The six assessment categories are shown in Table 9.1.

The category called *incomplete, need additional imaging evaluation* (BI-RADS category 0) is reserved for cases that require further workup before a final assessment can be made. The further workup usually involves additional mammographic views or breast ultrasonography. This incomplete evaluation category usually is limited to screening because diagnostic mammography implies a complete workup. Once the workup is complete, the examination is placed into one of five *final assessment* categories, each of which has a specific management recommendation (Table 9.1). *Negative* (BI-RADS category 1) means that there is nothing in the mammograms to comment on. *Benign* (category 2) means the examination is negative except for typically benign findings. *Probably benign* (category 3) is used for a finding that has a high probability of benignity for which a short-term follow-up is recommended. *Suspicious* (category 4) includes abnormalities that do not have definite morphology of cancer but have enough probability of being malignant to urge a biopsy. *Highly suggestive of malignancy* (category 5) indicates such classic findings of cancer that some surgeons would proceed to definitive surgical treatment with a frozen section to verify malignancy.

Assigning an assessment category number (0–5) to each mammography report

TABLE 9.1. *American College of Radiology Breast Imaging Reporting and Data System (ACR BI-RADS) final assessment categories*

Category	Assessment	Description
0	Incomplete	Need additional imaging evaluation.
1	Negative	There is nothing to comment on.
2	Benign finding	This is also a negative mammogram, but the interpreter may wish to describe a finding.
3	Probably benign	Very high probability of being benign, short-term follow-up recommended to establish stability.
4	Suspicious	Not characteristic of cancer but has reasonable probability of being malignant; biopsy should be considered.
5	Highly suggestive of malignancy	High probability of being cancer; appropriate action should be taken.

provides a user-friendly mechanism for tracking and monitoring mammography patients that does not require an understanding of medical terminology. Thus, office staff supervised by a health care professional can verify that mammography recommendations are carried out.

The assignment of the final assessment to each examination also facilitates outcome analyses, such as the medical audit of a mammography practice or a community screening project. The medical audit is a quality assurance activity to determine the effectiveness of mammography by comparing the mammography interpretation to the outcome of biopsy or follow-up (12). For this purpose, the mammography examination must be categorized as *positive* or *negative* for cancer, and the outcome is based on the results of biopsies or clinical follow-up that verifies whether or not cancer was present. The use of the BI-RADS system eliminates uncertainty concerning mammography interpretations: If the final assessment is negative (category 1), benign (category 2), or probably benign (category 3), the interpretation is categorized as *negative*. If the final assessment is suspicious (category 4) or highly suggestive of malignancy (category 5), the interpretation is considered *positive*.

MAMMOGRAPHY IMAGING BASICS

Understanding the Labels on a Mammogram

Standardized labels are now used on mammograms. This standardization is important because mammograms are frequently transferred from one facility to another. There are minimal requirements under the Mammography Quality Standards Act, and additional guidelines are recommended by the American College of Radiology (Fig. 9.4). Required items include an identification label and the "laterality/view" marker. The identification label indicates the facility and location where the examination was performed (at a minimum, the city, state, and zip code), the first and last name of the patient, and a unique patient identification number, such as the medical record number or date of birth. The laterality (i.e., right or left) and view (e.g., MLO or CC) marker should be near the axilla to facilitate orientation. Additional required labels are related to quality control issues such as the cassette number (the film is inside the cassette when the mammogram is performed), the mammography machine number, and the radiologic technologist who performed the examination. One recommended additional label is a date sticker that can be easily read with overhead light.

Describing the Location of an Abnormality

The location of mammographic (and clinical) abnormalities in the right or left breast is identified by the appropriate quadrant or clock-face descriptor (Fig. 9.5). The depth in the breast can be described as the anterior, middle, or posterior third. Abnormalities located under the nipple are described as *subareolar,* and those deeper in the breast at the level of the nipple are described as *retroareolar.* Obviously, to determine the three-dimensional location of a mammographically identified abnor-

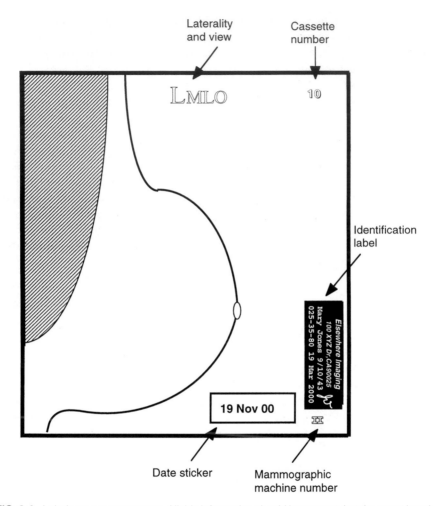

FIG. 9.4. Labels on a mammogram. All this information should be present, but the exact location of labels may vary; however, laterality and view should always be near the axilla.

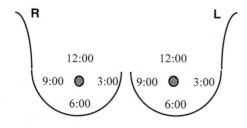

FIG. 9.5. Clock-face method for localizing breast lesions. Note that the 3:00 and 9:00 positions are different for right and left breasts.

mality, at least two views are needed. Typically, the MLO and CC views are available and are used to estimate the location of the finding. A true 90-degree lateral view is obtained if the exact location is required.

For orientation purposes, the laterality and view markers are always placed near the axilla. Hence, medial (inner) and lateral (outer) hemispheres can be identified on the CC view, and upper (superior) and lower (inferior) hemispheres can be identified on the MLO view based on the location of the laterality and view marker.

Masses

A *mass* is defined as a space-occupying lesion that is seen on at least two mammographic projections. Masses are described by their shape and margins (Fig. 9.6). The *shape* can be round, oval, lobulated, or irregular. Oval and round masses are usually benign. An irregular shape suggests a greater likelihood of malignancy. The *margins* of masses are the most important indicator of the likelihood of malignancy (13). The margins can be described as circumscribed, microlobulated, obscured (partially hidden by adjacent tissue), indistinct (ill-defined), or spiculated. *Circumscribed* mar-

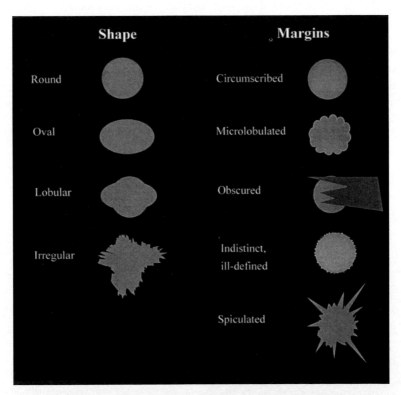

FIG. 9.6. A mass is described by its shape and its margins.

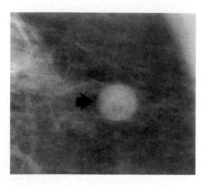

FIG. 9.7. A round mass (*arrow*) located near the axilla showed circumscribed margins and was stable for many years. There is a central radiolucency. The mass represents a benign intramammary lymph node.

gins (Figs. 9.7 and 9.8) favor a benign etiology, and the likelihood of malignancy for a circumscribed mass is very low, probably less than 2% (14–16). Additional workup may be necessary to verify that the margins are completely circumscribed. This workup usually involves additional projections of the mass and magnification spot-compression views. Ultrasonography is used to establish whether a solitary circumscribed mass is cystic or solid. If the mass is a simple cyst, no further workup is needed. If it is solid, the shape and margins should be carefully evaluated, as should as any clinical findings. A solitary, nonpalpable, completely circumscribed solid mass is often managed with a 6-month follow-up to establish that it is stable (not growing). If stable, continued mammographic surveillance is recommended for at least 2 years (17). The presence of multiple circumscribed masses is even stronger evidence of benignity, indicating multiple cysts, fibroadenomas, or benign intramammary lymph nodes (18), and follow-up in 1 year is often sufficient. If one of the masses is "dominant," biopsy is indicated. Dominant masses would include those that are significantly larger, not as well circumscribed, growing, or palpable. *Micro-*

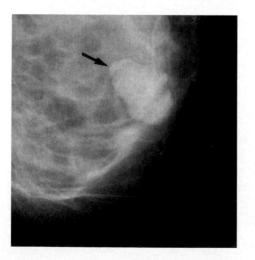

FIG. 9.8. Circumscribed margins. This lobular mass (*arrow*) has circumscribed margins. Biopsy revealed fibroadenoma.

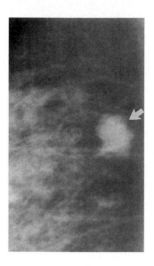

FIG. 9.9. Microlobulated margins (*arrow*) of a colloid carcinoma.

lobulated margins increase the likelihood of malignancy (Fig. 9.9). If the mass is directly adjacent to fibroglandular tissue of similar density, the margin may be *obscured* (Fig. 9.10), and additional imaging should be done in an attempt to show the margins as completely as possible. The finding of *indistinct* margins is suspicious for malignancy (Fig. 9.11). A mass with *spiculated* margins (Fig. 9.12) has lines radiating from its border, and this finding is highly suggestive of malignancy. An area of spicules without any associated mass is called an *architectural distortion* (Fig. 9.13).

The *density* of a mass compared with normal fibroglandular tissue provides another clue as to its etiology. In general, benign masses tend to be lower in density than carcinomas; however, the density of a mass is not always a reliable sign as to whether it is benign or malignant (19).

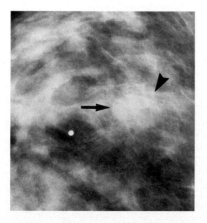

FIG. 9.10. Obscured margins. Part of this palpable mass was circumscribed (*arrow*), but the remainder was obscured by adjacent fibroglandular tissue (*arrowhead*). The radiopaque metal BB had been placed over the palpable abnormality before the mammograms were performed. Biopsy revealed invasive ductal carcinoma.

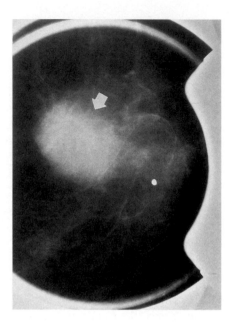

FIG. 9.11. Indistinct margins (*arrow*) of this mass make it suspicious for malignancy. Biopsy revealed invasive ductal carcinoma.

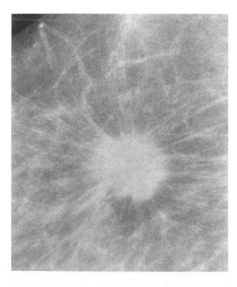

FIG. 9.12. Spiculated margins. The spicules emanating from the borders of this mass place it in the category "highly suggestive of malignancy." Biopsy of the mass confirmed the diagnosis of invasive ductal carcinoma.

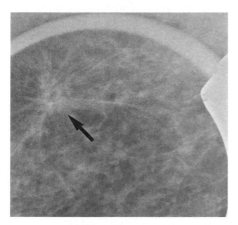

FIG. 9.13. A localized area of spicules without an associated mass (*arrow*) is referred to as an architectural distortion. The differential diagnosis is previous biopsy (postsurgical scar), radial scar, and carcinoma. In this case, there was no history of previous surgery and biopsy revealed invasive ductal carcinoma.

Calcifications

Calcifications are divided into three general types: typically benign, intermediate concern, and higher probability of malignancy (Fig. 9.14) (12,20). *Typically benign* calcifications usually can be identified by their mammographic features and include

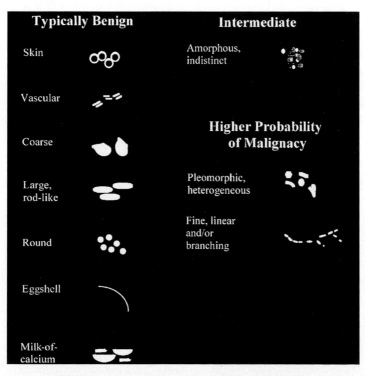

FIG. 9.14. Terminology used to describe calcifications.

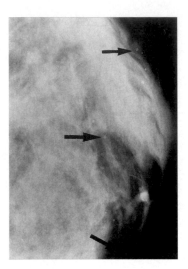

FIG. 9.15. Skin or dermal calcifications (*arrows*) are characterized by radiolucent centers. A location near the skin is another clue to their etiology.

skin (Fig. 9.15), vascular (Fig. 9.16), coarse (Fig. 9.17), large rod-like (Fig. 9.18), round, egg-shell (Fig. 9.19), and milk-of-calcium (Fig. 9.20) types. *Intermediate concern* calcifications can be described as *amorphous* or *indistinct* (Fig. 9.21). These are often round or flake-shaped calcifications that are small or hazy in appearance so that a more specific morphologic classification cannot be made. *Higher probability of malignancy* calcifications can be described as *pleomorphic* or *heterogeneous* (Fig. 9.22) or *fine, linear,* and *branching* (casting) (Fig. 9.23).

Calcifications are also characterized by their distribution: *grouped* or *clustered* calcifications show more than five in a small area (<2 cc) and can be benign or malignant (Figs. 9.21 and 9.22). *Linear* calcifications are in a line and may have

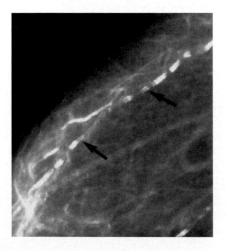

FIG. 9.16. Vascular calcifications frequently have a "railroad track" configuration (*arrows*) reflecting location in the vessel wall.

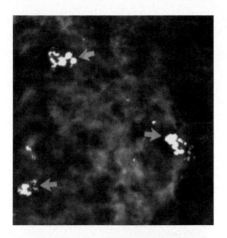

FIG. 9.17. Coarse calcifications (*arrows*) of degenerating fibroadenomas.

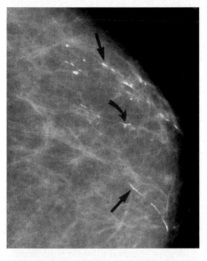

FIG. 9.18. These solid, rod-like calcifications (*arrows*) represent calcified secretions within the ducts of a postmenopausal woman with duct ectasia. Branching configurations (*curved arrow*) can occur but are less common than in ductal carcinoma *in situ*.

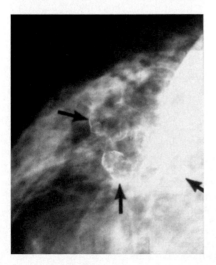

FIG. 9.19. "Eggshell" or "rim" calcifications (*arrows*) are present on the border of several lipid cysts in this case of postsurgical fat necrosis.

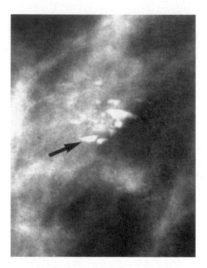

FIG. 9.20. A 90-degree lateral mammogram shows layering of calcifications (*arrow*) at the bottom of tiny fluid-filled cysts. This benign finding is also referred to as "milk-of-calcium" or "tea cup" calcifications.

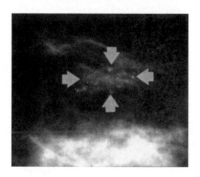

FIG. 9.21. A group of numerous amorphous intermediate calcifications (*arrows*) was barely visible in this mammogram. Biopsy revealed sclerosing adenosis.

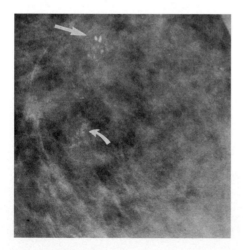

FIG. 9.22. The cluster of pleomorphic and heterogeneous calcifications (*arrow*) has a higher probability of malignancy and the cluster of amorphous and indistinct calcifications (*curved arrow*) is of intermediate concern. Biopsy revealed low-grade intraductal carcinoma at both sites.

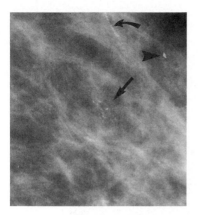

FIG. 9.23. The linear, branching calcifications (*arrow*) in a line with branching points were a manifestation intraductal comedocarcinoma. Incidentally, there is also an artifact simulating a calcification (*arrowhead*), and there are vascular calcifications (*curved arrow*).

small branch points (Fig. 9.23). When linear calcifications are in a line and branch; their distribution is described as duct-like and is suspicious for malignancy. *Segmental* calcifications are distributed in a duct and its branches (Fig. 9.24), which raises the possibility of multifocal carcinoma in a lobe or segment of the breast. *Regional* calcifications are in a larger volume of breast tissue, and not necessarily in a ductal distribution. *Diffuse or scattered* calcifications are distributed randomly through the breast and are almost always benign.

Indirect and Secondary Signs of Malignancy

Other significant findings that can be described in the BI-RADS report include indirect or subtle signs of malignancy, such as new or evolving densities, bilaterally

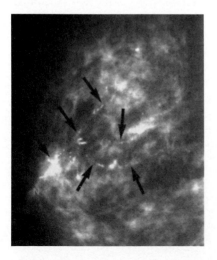

FIG. 9.24. These extensive calcifications (*arrows*) are in a segmental distribution relative to the nipple (*N*), suggesting deposits in a duct and its branches. This raises the possibility of multifocal cancer in a lobe or segment of the breast. Biopsy revealed intraductal carcinoma.

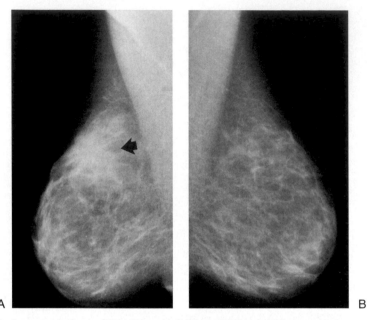

A   B

FIG. 9.25. Asymmetric tissue. Right (**A**) and left (**B**) mediolateral oblique mammograms demonstrate a region of asymmetric tissue (*arrow*) in the right breast. Biopsy revealed ductal carcinoma *in situ*.

asymmetric fibroglandular tissues (Fig. 9.25), and architectural distortion (Fig. 9.13) (21,22). Secondary signs of malignancy include skin thickening, nipple retraction, and axillary node enlargement.

New or evolving densities are identified through comparison with prior examinations and require additional workup, which may include additional views, ultrasound, and possibly biopsy. Asymmetrically distributed fibroglandular tissue may be normal fibroglandular tissue in an asymmetric distribution or the sign of an underlying malignancy. Architectural distortion is described as radiating spicules without a central mass and may be difficult to perceive. Both benign and malignant entities, including surgical scar, carcinoma, and radial scar, may result in architectural distortion (Fig. 9.13). Skin thickening also can be seen with benign and malignant conditions including post radiation change, mastitis, inflammatory breast carcinoma, lymphatic obstruction, and fluid-overload states, such as congestive heart failure and renal failure. New skin or nipple retraction is often a sign of an underlying malignancy. Axillary lymph node enlargement can result from metastatic disease or inflammatory conditions.

POTENTIAL ADVERSE CONSEQUENCES

Referring health care providers should be aware of the possible adverse consequences of mammography, the likelihood of each, and procedures to lower their likelihood. Potential adverse consequences of mammography include excessive biopsies, inadequate communication of results, anxiety associated with a return visit for more views, pain and discomfort, false reassurance, and delay in diagnosis (4).

In the process of detecting as many early breast cancers as possible, a certain number of biopsies will be done for benign mammographic abnormalities. The positive predictive value of biopsies done for mammographic abnormalities (number of cancers detected/number of biopsies) can vary significantly from one facility to another. The recommended positive biopsy rate for experienced interpreting physicians is 25% to 40%. The average in U.S. facilities is close to 20% (23).

Failing to communicate mammography results has been a relatively a common problem (24). The failure to communicate results can lead to delay in diagnosis and treatment of breast cancer. The failure to communicate results in a *timely fashion* can lead to unnecessary anxiety in women. In addition to the formal report to the referring health care provider, women are notified of their results by the mammography facility. The Mammography Quality Standards Act requires that this notification be direct (no intermediary), in writing, and in lay language.

Substantial anxiety can be generated when a woman has to return for additional or repeat mammographic views. These extra views should be done as soon as feasible to reduce anxiety. Staff should be supportive and available to answer any questions.

When properly performed, mammography may be uncomfortable and sometimes painful. If women have unnecessary pain and severe discomfort, they may not return for future screening examinations. Therefore, mammography should be performed using proper breast compression, so women will feel as little pain and discomfort as possible. Routine mammography should not be done when the breasts are tender or in the week before menstruation for women who have breast pain associated with menses (25–27).

False reassurance occurs when a woman ignores a palpable abnormality because of a previous negative screening mammogram. Delay in diagnosis occurs when a clinical finding is not acted on because mammograms turn out to be negative. Referring health care providers should inform women that a negative mammogram should not delay the clinical evaluation of a breast lump or other suspicious clinical finding, including a possible biopsy. A lump or other abnormal clinical finding that develops after a negative screening examination should be evaluated as soon as possible and not delayed until the next screening examination.

FALSE-NEGATIVE MAMMOGRAMS

A false-negative mammogram is one that is interpreted as negative, but cancer is diagnosed within a predetermined time, usually 1 to 2 years. The 1995 Physician Insurers Association of America study disclosed that failure to diagnose breast cancer had become the leading cause for malpractice cases lost by physicians (28). Causes for false-negative mammograms include dense breast tissue, suboptimal technical quality, errors in interpretation, and failure of communication (29). The most common cause of a false-negative mammogram is dense fibroglandular tissue (30). For this reason, in the standardized report, breast tissue densities are conveniently divided into four categories based on tissue density: (a) almost entirely fat; (b) scattered fibroglandular densities; (c) heterogeneously dense; and (d) extremely dense, which lowers the sensitivity of mammography. The sensitivity of mammography decreases with increasing tissue density.

The use of proper technical factors is particularly crucial in detecting breast cancer, especially in evaluating a woman with dense breast tissue. Suboptimal positioning and underexposure increase the risk of a false-negative mammogram. Using dedicated equipment, adequate compression and proper exposure can optimize the mammographic examination.

Pitfalls in the interpretation of mammograms include failure to recognize indirect signs of malignancy, misinterpreting circumscribed carcinomas as benign, satisfaction of search, and failure to take clinical findings into account. For palpable masses, a BB should be placed over the mass prior to mammography. Ultrasonography is an important adjunct to mammography when the mammographic examination is equivocal or negative.

BREAST ULTRASOUND

Breast ultrasound is an essential adjunct to mammography for the workup and diagnosis of palpable and mammographically detected abnormalities. Historically, breast ultrasound was used to differentiate solid and cystic masses (31). In the past decade, advances in ultrasound technology have led to high-resolution ultrasound equipment and to the identification of sonographic features to help differentiate benign and malignant solid masses (32,33). In addition to lesion characterization, breast ultrasound is used to guide interventional breast procedures, including cyst aspiration, CNB, fine needle aspiration, and ultrasound-guided preoperative needle localization.

Anatomy

Familiarity with the sonographic anatomy of the breast is essential in understanding breast ultrasound. Breast ultrasound reveals the anatomic structures from the skin surface to the chest wall (Fig. 9.26). Normal skin measures less than 3 mm and

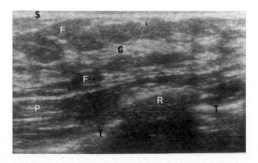

FIG. 9.26. Ultrasound anatomy. The skin (S) is represented by horizontal echogenic lines. Below this there is a layer of hypoechoic subcutaneous fat (F). This is followed by alternating bands of fibroglandular tissue (G) and fat. The retromammary fat lies on the chest wall. The pectoral muscle (P), ribs (R) and thoracic cavity (T) are deep to retromammary fat.

is composed of two parallel echogenic (white) lines separated by a thin, hypoechoic (dark) band. Just deep to the skin lies the subcutaneous fat followed by the interwoven bands of fibroglandular tissue and breast fat. Both subcutaneous and breast fat are mildly hypoechoic (gray), whereas the fibroglandular tissue is hyperechoic (white). Deep to the fibroglandular tissue is the retroglandular fat, which lies against the chest wall. The chest wall is composed of the more superficial band of the pectoralis muscle, the ribs laying deep to the pectoralis muscle, and the parietal pleura. The pectoralis muscle, ribs, and pleura have characteristic sonographic features that are easily and reliably identified.

Cystic Masses

Breast ultrasound can reliably identify cystic masses. The two types of cystic masses are *simple* and *complex*. The sonographic features of a simple cyst are a round or oval shaped, anechoic (black with no internal echoes) mass with smooth margins, an imperceptible wall, and increased posterior acoustic echoes (Fig. 9.27) (31). The latter feature means it appears as if a flashlight is shining through the back of the cyst. Because cysts develop within the terminal duct lobular unit of the breast, it is not uncommon to see clusters of cysts or coalescing cysts. Simple cysts need no further workup unless aspiration is indicated. Indications for cyst aspiration include a painful cyst, a large cystic that compromises mammographic imaging, patient anxiety, or a debris-filled or complex cyst.

A *complex cyst* is defined as a cyst with a solid component. Usually, the solid component is described as a mural nodule or an intracystic mass. A cyst with a solid component is suspicious for a malignancy such as a papillary carcinoma or a necrotic infiltrating ductal carcinoma. The diagnostic evaluation of a complex cyst may include complete surgical excision, CNB of the solid component, or ultrasound-guided partial aspiration for cytologic analysis.

It is not uncommon to identify a ''cyst'' filled with fine internal echoes, such as a debris-filled cyst. These cystic masses do not fulfill the criteria for a simple cyst,

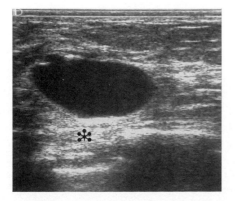

FIG. 9.27. Simple cyst. Ultrasound features are a round or oval, anechoic (black with no internal echoes) mass with smooth margins, an imperceptible wall, and increased posterior acoustic echoes.

and further evaluation may be needed. If a debris-filled cyst is suspected, ultrasound-guided aspiration can be performed to verify its cystic nature, to exclude a solid mass, and to confirm complete resolution of the mass after aspiration.

Solid Masses

Criteria differentiating benign and malignant solid masses have evolved. Recent studies have generated new interest in the use of sonography to distinguish benign and malignant solid breast masses (33). Although no single or combination of sonographic features is 100% diagnostic of benignity, careful use of established criteria can help differentiate benign and malignant solid masses and avoid biopsy of certain solid masses. Mass shape, margins, width relative to height, echogenicity, and posterior echoes are the minimum preliminary characteristics that should be assessed in all solid masses.

Typically benign sonographic features of solid masses include an ellipsoid or oval shape, width greater than anteroposterior diameter, three or fewer lobulations, circumscribed margins, a pseudocapsule, echogenicity hyperechoic to fat (whiter than fat), and, most importantly, *absence* of any malignant feature (Fig. 9.28).

Malignant sonographic features of solid masses include an irregular or angular shape; more than three lobulations; ill-defined, spiculated, or microlobulated margins; width greater than anteroposterior diameter ("taller than wide"); markedly hypoechoic (dark) echogenicity; posterior shadowing (black shadows posterior to the mass) and duct extension; branch pattern or punctate calcifications (Fig. 9.29).

Indeterminate sonographic features of solid masses include maximum diameter, echo texture, echogenicity equal to fat, and normal or increased posterior acoustic echoes.

In conclusion, the results of benign versus malignant ultrasound features of solid masses are encouraging. These features have potential for decreasing the number of biopsies performed for benign solid masses. Studies have also shown interobserver variability from one ultrasound interpreter to another in the evaluation for these features and in making a final diagnosis (34). Furthermore, there appears to be

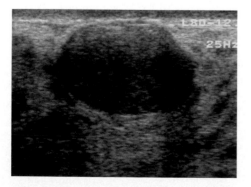

FIG. 9.28. Typical sonographic features of a benign solid mass. This mass is wider than tall, oval with circumscribed margins and has one gentle lobulation. Biopsy revealed fibroadenoma.

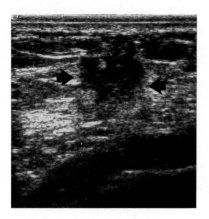

FIG. 9.29. Typical sonographic features of a malignant solid mass. The mass is taller than wide and manifests an irregular shape with irregular margins and posterior shadowing. Biopsy revealed carcinoma.

overlap in these features, and some malignant masses may have features suggesting they are benign, which could lead to false-negative interpretations of malignant solid masses. Therefore, at this time, these sonographic diagnostic criteria should not be generally applied as the sole criteria in determining whether to perform a biopsy of a solid mass. Additional investigations are needed to explore issues of reproducibility of specific criteria in a variety of practices and among different interpreters.

Once a solid mass is identified, appropriate action should be taken. Solid masses with any suspicious mammographic or sonographic feature should undergo biopsy. An incidentally identified, nonpalpable solid mass that demonstrates benign mammographic and sonographic features may be managed with a 6-month follow-up. Any *palpable* or *growing* benign-appearing solid mass warrants at least a needle biopsy.

CORE NEEDLE BIOPSY

Several tissue sampling techniques are available to the patient who requires tissue diagnosis. In the past, biopsy alternatives included excisional biopsy or fine needle aspiration cytology (FNAC). Medical and technological advances have led to a third, less invasive technique, CNB of the breast. CNB is a desirable alternative to excisional biopsy because it is less costly, results in less morbidity, and leaves minimal to no scar. CNB of the breast overcomes some of the limitations of FNAC because insufficient samples are less frequent, the interpretation can be performed by a pathologist without special training in cytopathology, it can usually differentiate invasive from *in situ* carcinoma, and it can more completely characterize a lesion (35,36).

Appropriate CNB techniques use a large-bore, 11- to 14-gauge needle in combination with imaging guidance to sample a clinical or imaging identified abnormality. Imaging guidance can be provided by ultrasound (Fig. 9.30) or mammography (stereotactically guided). Stereotactically guided CNB uses two views acquired at different angles to determine the location of a lesion in the breast. Choice of ultrasound

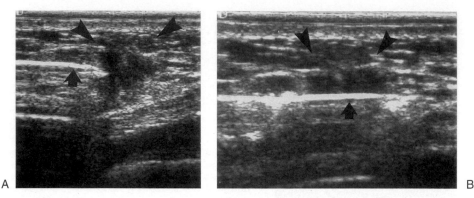

A   B

FIG. 9.30. Ultrasound-guided core needle biopsy. **A:** Prefire image shows the biopsy needle tip at the edge of the mass undergoing biopsy. **B:** Postfire image verifies that the biopsy needle is within the mass.

versus stereotactically guided CNB is based on which modality best demonstrates the abnormality and the location of the abnormality in the breast.

Indications, Relative Contraindications, and Complications

Imaging-guided CNB is indicated for most nonpalpable, mammographically suspicious abnormalities (37). Abnormalities categorized as "probably benign" (BI-RADS 3), "suspicious" (BI-RADS 4), and "highly suggestive of malignancy" (BI-RADS 5) can undergo biopsy. Overuse of the technique for sampling of "probably benign" (BI-RADS 3) abnormalities that would otherwise be managed with a 6-month follow-up, however, can increase the cost of screening with little to no benefit (38). CNB of "highly suggestive of malignancy" (BI-RADS 5) lesions can expedite surgical planning by avoiding the need to perform intraoperative frozen-section analysis to verify malignancy prior to definitive surgical treatment.

Stereotactic CNB is contraindicated in patients who exceed the weight limit of the biopsy table or have extremely thin breasts that preclude safely firing the biopsy device. Abnormalities located just under the skin or areola or deep against the chest wall may be inaccessible. Microcalcifications that are widely separated and not clustered or too faint to resolve with the stereotactic unit may be inappropriate for stereotactic CNB. Patients who are unable to cooperate, lie prone or still; who have bleeding disorders; or who are on anticoagulation therapy may not be suitable candidates. The location of the abnormality in the breast of a woman with breast implants dictates whether biopsy is feasible.

CNB of the breast has few complications. Potential complications include neck, back, arm, and shoulder pain related to patient positioning; bleeding; infection; and vasovagal reaction. In patients with normal coagulation profiles and no predisposition to infection, the risk of serious bleeding or infection is minimal.

Appropriate Post Core Biopsy Follow-up

CNB is a sampling technique; hence, appropriate post CNB follow-up to ensure lesion stability is critical in all patients with a benign biopsy result. The rate of false-negative CNB results is not known with certainty, but it is believed to be 2% (39). Several steps can be followed to minimize false-negative biopsy results. First, an adequate number of core samples should be obtained at biopsy to avoid sampling error, and specimen radiography should be performed in all cases where calcifications are sampled to verify that the calcifications are contained within the biopsy core samples. Once the biopsy result is available, radiologic–pathologic concordance or discordance should be assessed. In our practice, any patient with radiologic–pathologic discordance should undergo excisional biopsy of the abnormality. In addition, a number of problem CNB histologic diagnoses may require excisional biopsy. There is consensus that a CNB diagnosis of atypical ductal hyperplasia mandates excisional biopsy. There is still controversy about the need for excisional biopsy after CNB diagnosis of radial scar, papilloma, lobular carcinoma *in situ,* and atypical lobular hyperplasia (40–44).

Finally, appropriate post CNB imaging follow-up of benign diagnoses is essential. This follow-up begins with a 6-month follow-up using the imaging modality that best demonstrated the abnormality prior to biopsy (mammography or ultrasound). This is followed by a second 6-month follow-up and then a 1-year follow-up to establish 2 years of imaging stability in all patients with a benign core biopsy result. Any interval growth or suspicious change on imaging or clinical grounds warrants surgical excision.

OTHER BREAST IMAGING MODALITIES

Digital Mammography

Digital mammography records the image of the breast electronically rather than on film. The digital image can be stored in a computer database and later printed out as a film or displayed on a monitor. Potential advantages of digital mammography include the ability for postprocessing of images to bring out areas of interest, teleradiology for consultation or remote interpretation of transmitted images, and computer-aided detection and diagnosis (45). Digital mammography has the potential to eliminate some problems associated with conventional film-screen mammography, such as storage space requirements and lost films. Because film processing is eliminated, digital images can be viewed within seconds. Digital imaging has already proved useful for stereotactic guidance of needle biopsies. Current problems to be overcome before digital mammography can be widely disseminated include the high cost of the equipment (two to three times the cost of conventional mammography units) and lagging viewing station technology (which makes readouts slow and cumbersome).

Magnetic Resonance Imaging of the Breast

MRI has been applied successfully for the evaluation of silicone breast implants for intracapsular and extracapsular rupture (46). The initial studies to determine the

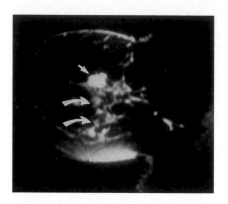

FIG. 9.31. Breast magnetic resonance image. A sagittal image of the right breast after the injection of a paramagnetic contrast agent (gadolinium) shows a contrast-enhancing mass (*arrow*) and enhancement in the adjacent duct system (*curved arrows*). Biopsy revealed a 1.5-cm invasive carcinoma and extensive ductal *carcinoma in situ* in the adjacent duct system.

potential value of MRI for detecting breast cancer were initiated in the 1980s (47). In these studies, MRI was not found to be reliable for the detection or diagnosis of breast cancer. Later investigations using intravenous MR contrast agents, however, showed a high sensitivity for the detection of breast cancer (Fig. 9.31) (48–51). Nonetheless, high cost and low specificity currently limit the use of MRI as a breast cancer screening tool. Another limitation is that MRI may not reliably identify malignant calcifications. Nonetheless, there are several potential roles for contrast-enhanced breast MRI: (a) determining the size and extent of invasive cancers; (b) identifying multifocal and multicentric lesions; (c) evaluating the ipsilateral breast of a woman with unilateral axillary metastases, and (d) identifying recurrent carcinoma in the conservatively treated breast. Multicenter clinical trials are under way to determine the exact role of MRI in evaluation of breast cancer.

Radionuclide Imaging

Another area of active investigation involves radionuclide scanning of the breast after the injection of radionuclide-labeled substances that concentrate in breast tumors. Technetium-99m (Tc99m) methoxyisobutyl isonitrile (MIBI) breast scintigraphy (*scintimammography*) has been under investigation for several years now. Early reports indicated high sensitivity (>90%) and specificity (slightly <90%) (52). Recent reports, however, indicate a relatively low sensitivity for small cancers, those found only by mammography (56%), and those 1 cm or larger (39%) (53,54). Therefore, the role of 99m MIBI breast scintigraphy is yet to be determined. It may be useful in avoiding biopsies of palpable breast masses larger than 1 cm with indeterminate mammographic and ultrasonographic features that will not be removed if the scintigraphic study is negative.

Tumor uptake also has been identified on positron emission tomography after the injection of fluorine-18 2-deoxy-2-fluoro-D-glucose (55). This agent also accumulates in axillary nodes, potentially providing information about nodal status. These methods will require additional studies to determine sensitivity, specificity, and cost-effectiveness.

In addition, Tc99m sulfur colloid is proving useful for identification of sentinel nodes (56). Prior to surgery, the isotope is injected into the breast in the vicinity of a biopsy proven breast cancer. The injected isotope should drain through the same lymphatic chain as the tumor. At surgery, the sentinel nodes draining the site of the cancer are identified using a radioisotope probe. The sentinel nodes are removed and evaluated histologically. If the sentinel nodes are negative for tumor, axillary node dissection and its associated complications may be avoided. Further studies are needed to determine the false-negative rate for sentinel node biopsy in general practice.

REFERENCES

1. McLelland R, Hendrick RE, Zinninger MD, et al. The American College of Radiology mammography accreditation program. *Am J Roentgenol* 1991;157:473–497.
2. *Mammography Quality Standards Act of 1992.* Public Law 102539.
3. American College of Radiology (ACR). *Breast imaging reporting and data system (BI-RADS),* 3rd ed. Reston, VA: ACR, 1998.
4. Bassett LW, Hendrick RE, Bassford TL, et al. *Quality determinants of mammography: clinical practice guideline.* No 13. AHCPR Publication 95-0632. Rockville, MD: Agency for Health Care Policy and Research, Public Health Service, U.S. Department of Health and Human Services, October 1994.
5. American College of Radiology (ACR). *Standards for the performance of screening mammography.* [Adopted by the ACR Council 1990, Revised 1994]. In: ACR Digest of Official Actions. Reston, VA: ACR, 1994.
6. Tabár L, Fagerberg C J, Gad A, et al. Reduction in mortality from breast cancer after mass screening with mammography: randomized trial from the Breast Cancer Screening Working Group of the Swedish National Board of Health and Welfare. *Lancet* 1985;1:829–832.
7. National Institutes of Health Consensus Development Panel. National Institutes of Health Consensus Development Panel: breast cancer screening for women 40–49, January 21–23, 1997. *J Natl Cancer Inst* 1997;39:1015–1026.
8. Smart CR, Hendrick RE, Rutledge JH III, et al. Benefit of mammography screening in women ages 40 to 49 years. Current evidence from randomized controlled trials. *Cancer* 1995;75:1619–1626.
9. Alexander FE, Anderson TJ, Brown HK, et al. 14 years of follow-up from the Edinburgh randomized trial of breast-cancer screening. *Lancet* 1999;353:1903–1908.
10. Moss SM, Coleman DA, Chamberlain TJ, et al. 16-year mortality from breast cancer in the UK Trial of Early Detection of Breast Cancer. *Lancet* 1999;353:1909–1914.
11. American College of Radiology (ACR): *Standards for the performance of diagnostic mammography and problem-solving breast evaluation* [Adopted by the ACR Council 1994]. In: ACR Digest of Official Actions. Reston, VA: ACR, 1994.
12. Linver MN, Osuch JR, Brenner RJ, et al. Mammography medical audit: primer for the mammography quality standards act (MQSA). *Am J Roentgenol* 1995;165:19–25.
13. Gold RH, Montgomery CK, Rambo ON. Significance of margination of benign and malignant infiltrative mammary lesions: roentgenologic-pathologic correlation. *Am J Roentgenol* 1973;118:881–894.
14. Hall FM, Storella JM, Silverstone DZ, et al. Nonpalpable breast lesions: recommendations for biopsy based on suspicion of carcinoma at mammography. *Radiology* 1988;167:353–358.
15. Moskowitz M. The predictive value of certain mammographic signs in screening for breast cancer. *Cancer* 1983;51:1007–1011.
16. Sickles EA. Nonpalpable, circumscribed, noncalcified solid breast masses: likelihood of malignancy based on lesion size and age of patient. *Radiology* 1994;192:439–442.
17. Brenner RJ, Sickles EA. Acceptability of periodic follow-up as an alternative to biopsy for mammographically detected lesions interpreted as probably benign. *Radiology* 1989;171:645–646.
18. Feig SA. Breast masses: mammographic and sonographic evaluation. *Radiol Clin North Am* 1992; 30:67–92.

19. Jackson VP, Dines KA, Bassett LW, et al. Diagnostic importance of radiographic density of non-calcified breast masses: analysis of 91 lesions. *Am J Roentgenol* 1991;157:25–28.
20. Bassett LW. Mammographic analysis of calcifications. *Radiol Clin North Am* 1992;30:93–105.
21. Sickles EA. Mammographic features of 300 consecutive nonpalpable breast cancers. *Am J Roentgenol* 1986;146:661–663.
22. Sickles EA. Mammographic features of "early" breast cancer. *Am J Roentgenol* 1984;143:461–464.
23. Brown ML, Houn F, Sickles EA, et al. Screening mammography in community practice: Positive predictive value of abnormal finding and yield of follow-up diagnostic procedures. *Am J Roentgenol* 1995;165:1373–1377.
24. Robertson CL, Kopans DB. Communication problems after mammographic screening. *Radiology* 1989;172:443–444.
25. Brew MD, Billings JD, Chisholm RJ. Mammography and breast pain. *Australas Radiol* 1989;33:335–336.
26. Jackson VP, Lex AM, Smith DJ. Patient discomfort during screen-film mammography. *Radiology* 1988;168:421–423.
27. Stomper PC, Kopans DB, Sadowsky NL, et al. Is mammography painful? A multicenter patient study. *Arch Intern Med* 1988;148:521–524.
28. Physician Insurer's Association of America. *Breast cancer study 1995*. Washington, DC: Physician Insurers Association of America, 1995.
29. Feig SA, Shaber GS, Patchefsky A, et al. Analysis of clinically occult and mammographically occult breast tumors. *Am J Roentgenol* 1977;128:403–408.
30. Mann BD, Giuliano AE, Bassett LW, et al. Delayed diagnosis of breast cancer as a result of normal mammograms. *Arch Surg* 1983;118:23–24.
31. Hilton SvW, Leopold GR, Olson LK, et al. Realtime breast sonography: Application in 300 consecutive patients. *Am J Roentgenol* 1986;147:479–486.
32. Fornage BD, Lorigan JG, Andry E. Fibroadenoma of the breast: sonographic appearance. *Radiology* 1989;172:671–675.
33. Stavros AT, Thickman D, Rapp CL, et al. Solid breast nodules: use of sonography to distinguish between benign and malignant lesions. *Radiology* 1995;196:123–134.
34. Rahbar G, Sie AC, Hansen GC, et al. Benign versus malignant solid breast masses: US differentiation. *Radiology* 1999;213:889–894.
35. Parker SH, Lovin JD, Jobe WE, et al. Stereotactic breast biopsy with a biopsy gun. *Radiology* 1990;176:741–747.
36. Jackson VP, Bassett LW. Stereotactic fine-needle aspiration biopsy for nonpalpable breast lesions. *Am J Roentgenol* 1990;154:1196–1197.
37. Bassett LW, Winchester DP, Caplan RB, et Al. Stereotactic core-needle biopsy of the breast. *CA Cancer J Clin* 1997;47:171–190.
38. Sickles EA, Parker SH. Appropriate role of core breast biopsy in the management of probably benign lesions. *Radiology* 1993;188:315.
39. Lee CH, Philpotts LE, Horvath LJ, et al. Follow up of breast lesions diagnosed as benign with stereotactic core-needle biopsy: frequency of mammographic change and false negative rate. *Radiology* 1999;212:189–194.
40. Brem RF, Behrndt VS, Sanow L, et al. Atypical ductal hyperplasia: histologic underestimation of carcinoma in tissue harvested from impalpable breast lesions using 11-G stereotactically guided directional vacuum-assisted biopsy. *Am J Roentgenol* 1999;172:1405–1407.
41. Jackman RJ, Nowels W, Rodriguex-Soto J, et al. Stereotactic, automated, large-core needle biopsy of nonpalpable breast lesions: false-negative rates and histologic underestimation rates after long-term follow up. *Radiology* 1999;210:799–805.
42. Liberman L, Bracero N, Vuolo MA, et al. Percutaneous large-core biopsy of papillary breast lesions. *Am J Roentgenol* 1999;172:331–337.
43. Liberman L, Sama M, Susnik, et al. Lobular carcinoma in situ at percutaneous breast biopsy: surgical biopsy findings. *Am J Roentgenol* 1999;173:291–299.
44. Philpotts LE, Shaheen NA, Carter D, et al. Comparison of rebiopsy rates after stereotactic core needle biopsy of the breast with 11-G vacuum suction probe vs. 14-G automatic gun. *Am J Roentgenol* 1999;172:683–687.
45. Shtern F. Digital mammography and related technologies: a perspective from the National Cancer Institute. *Radiology* 1992;183:629–630.

46. Gorczyca DP, Sinha S, Ahn CY, et al. Silicone breast implants in vivo: MR imaging. *Radiology* 1992;185:407–410.
47. El Yousef SJ, O'Connell DM, Duchesneau RH, et al. Benign and malignant breast disease: magnetic resonance and radiofrequency pulse sequences. *Am J Roentgenol* 1985;145:1–8.
48. Harms SE, Flamig DP, Evans WP, et al. MR imaging of the breast: current status and future potential. *Am J Roentgenol* 1994;163:1039–1047.
49. Heywang SH, Wolf A, Pruss E, et al. MR imaging of the breast with Gd-DTPA: use and limitations. *Radiology* 1989;171:95–103.
50. Heywang-Kobrunner SH, Schlegel A, et al. Contrast-enhanced MRI of the breast after limited surgery and radiation therapy. *J Comput Assist Tomogr* 1993;17:891–900.
51. Orel SG, Schnall MD, LiVolsi VA, et al. Suspicious breast lesions: MR imaging with radiographic-pathologic correlation. *Radiology* 1994;190:485–493.
52. Khalkhali I, Mena I, Jouanne E, et al. Prone scintimammography in patients with suspicion of carcinoma of the breast. *J Am Coll Surg* 1994;178:491–497.
53. Tolmos J, Cutrone JA, Wang B, et al. Scintimammographic analysis of nonpalpable breast lesions previously identified by conventional mammography. *J Natl Cancer Inst* 1998;90:846–849.
54. Prats E, Carril J, Herranz R, et al. Spanish multicenter scintigraphic study of the breast using Tc99m MIBI: report of results. *Rev Esp Med Nucl* 1998;17:338–350.
55. Adler LP, Crowe JP, Al-Kaisi NK, et al. Evaluation of breast masses and axillary lymph nodes with (F-18) 2-Deoxy-2-fluoro-D-glucose PET. *Radiology* 1993;187:743–750.
56. Winchester DJ, Sener SF, Winchester DP, et al. Sentinel lymphadenectomy for breast cancer: experience with 180 consecutive patients: efficacy of filtered technetium 99m sulphur colloid with overnight migration time. *J Am Coll Surg* 1999;188:597–603.

10

Special Diagnostic Techniques for Breast Cancer

Laura E. Witherspoon and R. Phillip Burns

In addition to history and physical examination, several diagnostic techniques are available to the surgeon evaluating breast abnormalities. The choice of technique depends on whether the abnormality is identified as a palpable mass or as a nonpalpable abnormality that is visualized on diagnostic mammogram or ultrasound. After pertinent history is obtained, the surgeon completes a thorough breast examination. It is beneficial to have the patient point out specific areas of concern derived from self-breast examination or symptoms. The surgeon reviews all imaging studies and correlates them with the radiologist's interpretation. It is essential that films be available at the time of the patient's office visit, so that radiographic findings can be correlated with the physical examination. Review of radiology reports alone is not optimal; the surgeon must become knowledgeable in interpreting mammograms and ultrasound to select the most appropriate diagnostic workup.

In the past, most primary techniques used for the diagnosis of a breast abnormality involved open surgical biopsy based on palpation of a mass or preoperative needle-wire localization of a nonpalpable mammographic abnormality. Fine needle aspiration (FNA) cytology for palpable masses has been used in some centers, but it depends on the availability of an experienced cytopathologist.

More recently, several diagnostic techniques have been developed that have significantly altered the strategy for evaluating these patients. Image-guided techniques, such as stereotactic core biopsy and ultrasound-guided biopsy, are now more widely available in the evaluation of nonpalpable breast abnormalities (those discovered on mammogram or ultrasound). Introduction of these techniques initiated a shift in initial tissue sampling for diagnosis from the operating room to the office or outpatient setting. Most diagnostic workups for nonpalpable breast abnormalities now can be accomplished using local anesthesia and minimally invasive techniques. Near-complete excision of lesions now can be accomplished by some of these procedures. These techniques, when used by experienced physicians, provide accuracy equivalent to that achieved by open biopsy (1,2).

Patient acceptance of the trend toward office diagnosis of breast problems has been favorable in that these procedures are more cost-effective as well as less threatening to women. Office-based procedures can be scheduled and performed expeditiously without the need for elaborate patient preparation. Patients are often able to drive themselves to and from procedures with minimal time lost from work and other activities. The cost of procedures performed in the office setting is generally less than those performed in the hospital. With smaller-volume biopsies, there is an improved cosmetic result and less alteration of breast architecture due to postoperative scarring, making follow-up more straightforward.

Image-guided biopsy techniques, such as stereotactic core biopsy and ultrasound-guided core biopsy, demand technical and interpretive skills that can be introduced and developed in the setting of an established practice. Physicians need to undergo appropriate training and develop expertise in breast pathophysiology and correlative examination as well as breast imaging and image-guided procedures. These advanced procedures generally are performed by either a surgeon or radiologist or by a collaborative arrangement between the two. Diagnostic procedures of all types are used most appropriately in the setting of comprehensive patient care where the physician performing the procedure is also responsible for the overall evaluation, treatment, and follow-up of the patient.

IMAGE-GUIDED TECHNIQUES

Image-guided techniques are used to evaluate nonpalpable breast abnormalities, such as those discovered by ultrasound or mammogram.

Ultrasound-guided Biopsy

Increased portability, affordability, and improved technical performance of ultrasound systems has led to a far more aggressive use of this modality in the evaluation of nonpalpable breast abnormalities. The decision of whether to use ultrasound versus stereotactic localization versus excisional treatment for breast-tissue analysis of nonpalpable breast lesions requires experience and training in comprehensive breast care.

The basic principles of ultrasound-guided needle aspiration or core biopsy involves precise identification of the area of suspicion under the appropriate ultrasound transducer (usually linear array 7 MHz) followed by real time penetration of the area of concern with the appropriate sampling needle device under ultrasound visualization and guidance. Standard disposable needles, special longer needles with echogenic tips, spring loaded core needles and special suction or cutting needles all can be used in ultrasound-guided breast-tissue sampling. Needles are aligned in the longitudinal plane (parallel to the ultrasound transducer), which allows complete visualization of the needle through the lesion on the image screen during aspiration or biopsy. Commercially available needle guides that attach to the ultrasound transducer head are available; through these guides, needles can be directed to the area of concern using preset angles and positions. With experience, most surgeons will adopt a free-hand needle guidance technique because this provides more flexibility in needle direction and tissue harvest.

Lesions appropriate for aspiration or biopsy with ultrasound guidance initially are approached with FNA. If the lesion is determined to be cystic, aspiration of the fluid with attendant collapse of the cystic structure usually will occur. In situations where lesions are found to be solid, or in cases where incomplete decompression of cystic structures occur, high-suction aspiration may be obtained and smears prepared for cytologic evaluation as in FNA evaluation. In lesions that prove to be solid with fine needle investigation, progression to tissue sampling with a spring-loaded large core needle is usually performed.

Breast Cyst Aspiration

After the lesion is stabilized under the ultrasound probe, the area around the probe is cleansed of gel and prepared with either alcohol or Betadine. Local anesthesia of 1% Xylocaine, usually with epinephrine and sodium bicarbonate, added to relieve local bleeding and discomfort, respectively, is injected under ultrasound guidance. Usually, 2 to 5 mL is injected in the skin and subcutaneous tract up to the lesion, and the same needle is used to penetrate the lesion and aspirate fluid (Fig. 10.1). A 25-gauge needle initially is used to limit discomfort and usually will allow successful aspiration of cysts. Breast cyst fluid may be sufficiently viscous to require the use of a larger needle (20- or 18-gauge) to allow the fluid to traverse the needle lumen. If the lesion is cystic, the fluid is aspirated and, assuming a homogeneous benign-appearing cyst wall, the procedure is terminated at that point. If concern exists

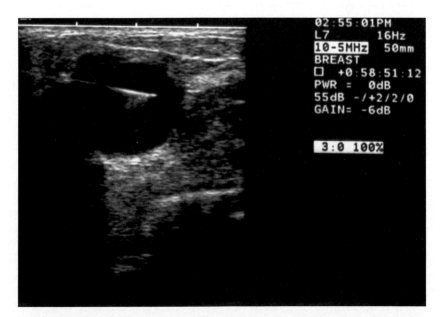

FIG. 10.1. Ultrasound-guided cyst aspiration. Needle tip is seen within cyst cavity.

regarding the ultrasound characteristics of tissue adjacent to an aspirated cyst, passing a 20- or 18-gauge needle through this area under high suction pressure will allow for FNA and slide preparation as in usual FNA assessment. Special needles with increased length and echogenic tips are available, but with experience, standard disposable needles can be used successfully with significant cost saving. In lesions where multicystic or septated lesions exist, moving the ultrasound probe only slightly in a "painting" or "skiing" fashion may allow aspiration of complex cysts through the same needle puncture and tract with less pain to the patient. The disposition of cyst fluid is controversial. Aspiration of a clearly simple cyst seldom requires cytologic evaluation. Fluid removed from complex cysts or cloudy or bloody fluid probably does merit cytologic analysis. Some patients are more satisfied if cytologic analysis is performed on removed fluid regardless of the character of aspirated fluid. If decompression of the cystic lesion does not occur or the lesion is solid with fine needle investigation, additional sampling with a large-core needle biopsy (CNB) may be necessary.

Core Needle Biopsy

If the lesion appears particularly suspicious for malignancy or proves to be solid with FNA, conversion to ultrasound-guided large-CNB is indicated. These large-core (14-gauge down to 12-gauge) needles are available in both disposable units or as disposable needles for use with a reusable spring-loaded gun; the latter is more cost-effective in high-volume practice situations.

A similar preparative technique is used, and 3 to 15 mL of local anesthesia should be injected to obtain adequate patient analgesia. A small incision with a no. 11 blade is sufficient to allow needle entry through the skin. Attached ultrasound-guided or free-hand technique can be used to direct the needle. Before placement of the spring-loaded needle into the breast tissue, it is useful to test-fire the gun to allow the patient to become familiar with the sound of the firing mechanism and to make the procedure less traumatic. The entry point is best made 1 to 2 cm away from the transducer probe to allow better needle, manipulation and positioning in relationship to the lesion (Fig. 10.2). It is possible for the surgeon both to hold the ultrasound probe and manipulate the spring-loaded needle, but stabilizing the ultrasound probe by either a technician or assistant may be useful in allowing improved needle control by the surgeon. The needle is directed to the edge of the suspected area of concern and photodocumentation of the image completed (Fig. 10.3). The patient then is warned that the firing mechanism is to be activated, and the spring-loaded instrument is fired. The path of the needle through or across the lesion of concern can be noted in real time on the ultrasound monitor screen and the position of the needle post fire again photodocumented for reference (Fig. 10.4). The needle is removed from the breast and the biopsy specimen extracted and evaluated. Multiple biopsies can be taken using this procedure. The usual number of biopsies recommended is a minimum of three, with more harvested if either specimen quality is inadequate (soft, fatty tissue or no tissue) for the diagnosis of carcinoma or additional areas of

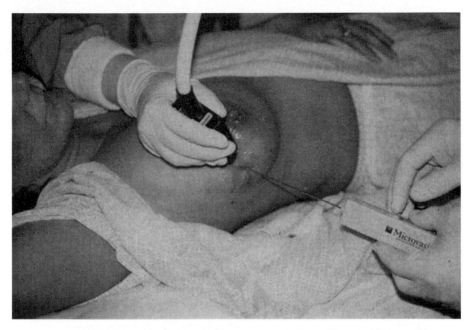

FIG. 10.2. Ultrasound-guided core needle biopsy, skin entry site.

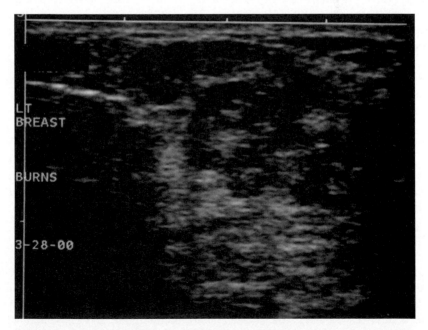

FIG. 10.3. Ultrasound-guided core needle biopsy. Needle is adjacent to solid lesion.

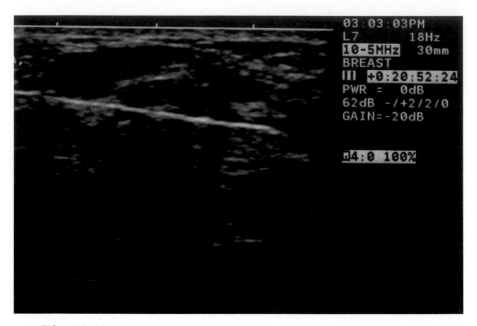

FIG. 10.4. Ultrasound-guided core needle biopsy. Needle is seen traversing lesion.

biopsy deemed desirable based on lesion characteristics or size. If the core of tissue initially sampled appears highly suspicious for carcinoma (firm, solid, gritty), then only one or two specimens might be adequate. It is our empiric experience that patients with malignant lesions tend to experience more pain at biopsy.

Application of an ice pack immediately after performance of the CNB helps to reduce ecchymosis and swelling after a biopsy, thereby reducing postoperative pain. Postbiopsy pain medication is usually unnecessary, but attention must be given to individual patient and surgeon preference.

Routine histologic evaluation is performed on the core specimens, and most pathologists feel confident rendering a definitive diagnosis on this tissue. Appropriate follow-up depends on histopathology, character of the lesion, physical examination, and clinical index of suspicion. Most benign lesions are followed up clinically at 6-month intervals with repeat imaging evaluation (mammogram or ultrasound or both) at 6 to 12 months.

Mammotome Biopsy

The 11-gauge Mammotome device (Ethicon Endo-Surgery, Inc., Cincinnati, OH, USA) excises larger cores of tissue using a vacuum system and a high-speed rotating cutter; this is available for use free-hand under ultrasound guidance. The Mammotome is inserted with the lesion between the ultrasound probe and the open bowl of the needle. Sampling of the lesion proceeds using hand controls on the Mammotome and is observed under ultrasound. The lesion is seen to decrease progressively in size and may be completely resected during the procedure. A marking clip may be deployed through the device for future reference.

Other Ultrasound-guided Techniques

Definitive treatment of breast abscess with ultrasound guided aspiration or drainage with or without subsequent antibiotic treatment has been reported (3). The advantage of percutaneous breast abscess drainage is particularly relevant in lactating women in that such a procedure can allow continuation of breast-feeding during treatment. Patients who sustain breast hematomas or seromas from trauma or postoperatively from open breast biopsy or partial mastectomy are candidates for ultrasound-guided percutaneous drainage, either with needles or ultrasound-guided placement of a closed suction device. The adequacy of drainage can be assessed with sequential ultrasound evaluation in the office. Some centers have used ultrasound-guided FNA cytology of suspicious axillary lymph nodes to document evidence of metastatic breast disease (4). Core biopsy has not been recommended in this circumstance because of possible injury to adjacent major nerve or vascular structures.

Accuracy and Clinical Application

As more confidence is established in ultrasound-guided biopsy and as image quality with ultrasound improves, more patients will be candidates for ultrasound-guided biopsy in facilities where this technology is available. Generally, ultrasound-guided core needle biopsies are cost-effective and require less expenditure of both personnel and material resources than other forms of tissue sampling. In many facilities where both stereotactic and ultrasound-guided biopsies are available, surgeons prefer performance of ultrasound-guided biopsy over the stereotactic modality if the lesion is visible by both modalities. Some researchers have reported that as many as 80% to 90% of mammographic lesions are amenable to ultrasound-guided biopsy (4). In our opinion, this number is lower. The sensitivity of ultrasound-guided biopsy in appropriate patients has been reported to be as high as 100% (5). As this technology is applied to a wider patient population, the sensitivity probably will decrease somewhat as a result of attempted application to smaller lesions that are more difficult to accurately identify. Nonetheless, this is an excellent technologic advance that offers an opportunity for much more expedient and less threatening evaluation for patients with breast disease.

Stereotactic Breast Biopsy

Stereotactic breast biopsy is a method of sampling breast lesions that are visualized mammographically. This recently popularized technique uses digital mammography and triangulation principles to pinpoint the location of the lesion. Using these data, a motorized needle biopsy gun is directed to the appropriate area of concern in the breast to obtain tissue samples. Mass lesions, as well as microcalcifications, may undergo a biopsy, and most locations within the breast can be targeted and interrogated via this technique. Indications for stereotactic breast biopsy are the same as those for open biopsy: lesions suspicious for malignancy by mammographic criteria. This includes nodular lesions, asymmetric densities, stellate lesions, and suspicious calcifications with or without mass. This includes BI-RADS 4 (Breast Imaging Reporting and Data System) and 5 lesions, although controversy still exists as to whether BI-RADS 5 lesions should be sampled rather than excised. Some BI-RADS 3 lesions also are considered appropriate for biopsy, usually based on additional factors beyond the BI-RADS classification (e.g., patient anxiety, family history, surgeon concern). Stereotactic biopsy generally is not indicated for palpable lesions because biopsy can be done on these lesions in a more direct minimally invasive fashion.

When a lesion is considered appropriate for stereotactic biopsy, a discussion is undertaken with the patient regarding biopsy options. The stereotactic method is considered a minimally invasive procedure that samples only the lesion in question. A small incision is required, and the procedure can be performed comfortably with the patient under local anesthesia. No elaborate preparations are needed, and the patient is allowed to drive to and from the procedure alone; some patients return to work after the procedure. The patient may take regular medications (except anticoagulants) and eat breakfast or lunch before the procedure. She is instructed to wear a comfortable two-piece outfit and to disrobe from the waist up for the procedure.

The stereotactic equipment generally is positioned in a fixed location within an office, ambulatory surgery center, comprehensive breast center, or hospital. Mobile units are also available on a lease basis. To maximize patient comfort, a private setting for the facility is preferable. A dedicated mammography technologist is essential to the smooth functioning of the stereotactic unit. The technologist is responsible for maintenance and calibration of this complex equipment and can be helpful in maintaining quality control of the unit in conjunction with a radiation physicist.

Stereotactic Core Needle Biopsy

The two manufacturers of stereotactic tables and equipment are Fisher Mammotest (Denver, CO, USA) and LoRad Stereoguide (Danbury, CT, USA). These units use a prone-position mammography unit connected to computer monitors for visualization of digital mammogram images and a motorized control module for computer directed positioning of the biopsy needle.

Before initiating the procedure, the physician reviews the mammogram with the technologist to assess the best directional approach to the lesion. The procedure

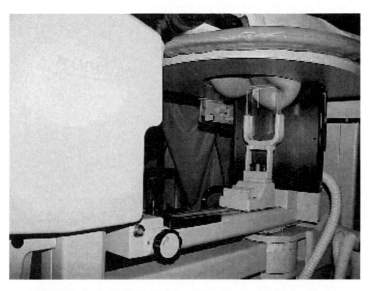

FIG. 10.5. Patient positioned prone for stereotactic breast biopsy.

begins with the patient positioned prone on the procedure table with the breast in a dependent position through an aperture in the table (Fig. 10.5). The breast is placed in directional compression that is considered most optimal for access to the lesion (i.e., craniocaudal, medial to lateral). The LoRad table can accommodate a caudo-cranial approach as well. An initial scout digital image is obtained with the X-ray tube at zero-degrees orientation to the breast (Fig. 10.6). If the lesion is well visualized on this view, stereo images are obtained at + 15-degree and − 15-degree angles (Fig. 10.7). These two images are displayed on the computer monitor, and the central portion of the lesion in each view is marked with a digital marker (targeting "mouse") with additional, offset target sites selected around the central target to provide more biopsy sites (Fig. 10.8). The computer then calculates the coordinates for horizontal, vertical, and depth axes to direct the attached core needle device to the targeted lesion in the breast. This information is digitally communicated to the motorized arm, which carries the large-core biopsy needle (14- or 12-gauge). After skin preparation and infiltration with local anesthesia, a small skin incision is made at the appropriate needle entry site. The needle is manually advanced to the appropriate depth as calibrated by the computer, and repeat stereo images are taken to ensure accurate placement of the needle tip in relationship to the lesion in question (Fig. 10.9). The spring-loaded needle is then fired across the target, and this position is confirmed with repeat stereo images (Fig. 10.10). The needle is removed, and the tissue specimen extracted. The multiple additional offset targets then are harvested in a similar fashion. A total of three to ten core specimens are generally harvested for nodular lesions with six to ten or more specimens if the indication for biopsy

FIG. 10.6. Initial 0° scout image on digital screen.

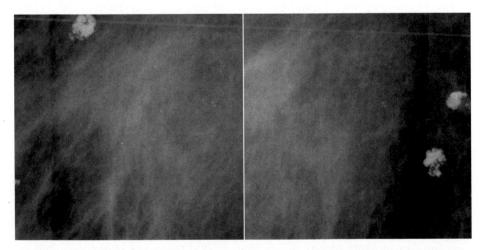

FIG. 10.7. Digital stereotactic images at +15° and −15°.

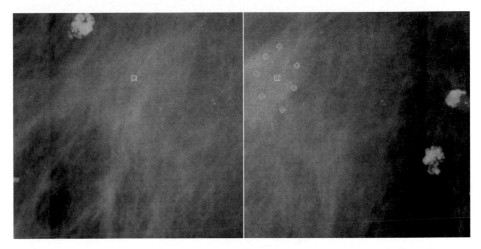

FIG. 10.8. Lesion marked centrally on both stereotactic views with additional offset sites on − 15° view.

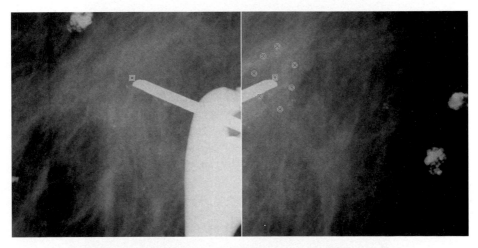

FIG. 10.9. "Pre-fire" stereotactic images after core needle placement.

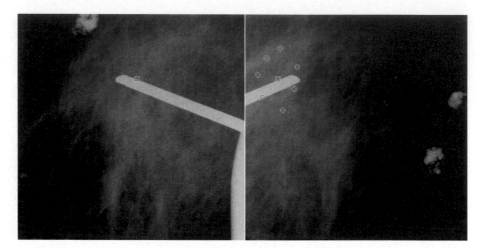

FIG. 10.10. "Post-fire" stereotactic images.

includes calcification. A final zero-degree view of the breast then is obtained to demonstrate the area biopsied. If the biopsy is performed for microcalcifications, a specimen mammogram is taken of the cores to document the presence of calcifications (Fig. 10.11). Tissue specimens are sent for permanent histopathology examina-

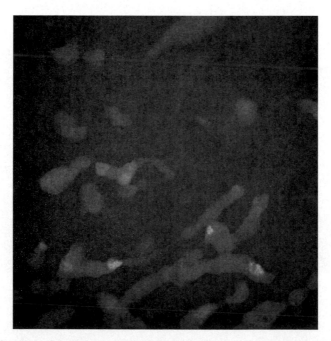

FIG. 10.11. Specimen images obtained after biopsy for microcalcifications.

tion. The breast incision is closed with adhesive strips and covered with a dry dressing. An ice pack is immediately applied to reduce swelling and to improve patient comfort.

Mammotome

The Mammotome biopsy system (Ethicon Endo-Surgery Inc.) is available, which uses different needle technology to sample mammogram detected lesions in conjunction with the same stereotactic table mentioned in the core biopsy section. This is a vacuum-driven needle biopsy device, which uses suction and a rotational cutting blade within the needle to obtain specimens. Needles are available in 14-gauge and larger 11-gauge sizes. Specimens are delivered into a vacuum chamber for extraction allowing circumferential sampling from the central target without having to move the needle in and out of the breast. When a small lesion is completely removed using this device, a small titanium clip is deployed through the needle as a marker for future identification of the biopsy site. The mammotome generally removes a greater volume of tissue than the spring-loaded core needle and, in some circumstances, may result in fewer indeterminate pathology reports (6).

Accuracy and Clinical Application

The ability of stereotactic biopsy to determine the presence of malignancy is equivalent to that of open biopsy (7–10), but the entire lesion is usually not removed. Although a benign lesion usually does not require removal, some patients will require subsequent excision of the area of concern based on patient concern and anxiety or clinical and histopathology findings. This possibility should be discussed with the patient before stereotactic biopsy. Additional technology is being researched and developed using stereotactic principles; various energy sources such as cryoprobes and laser tips ultimately may be used for ablative treatment of breast cancer in a minimally invasive fashion (11).

Excisional Large Core Biopsy

Two systems, ABBI (United Status Surgical Corporation, Norwalk, CT, USA) and Site-Select (Imagyn Medical Technologies Inc., Newport Beach, CA, USA), are available for removal of even larger biopsy specimens using needle biopsy technique. Both use similar stereotactic localization and targeting techniques followed by wire cannula placement through the lesion of concern and larger core cannula excision, which may result in removal of the entire lesion. Indications for performance of the procedure are similar to that for other techniques. For the ABBI procedure, the patient is premedicated with an oral benzodiazepine and an oral narcotic (12). Positioning of the patient and localization of the lesion are accomplished in a similar fashion to that previously described for stereotactic needle biopsy. Cannula size is selected based on the size of the lesion (5, 10, 15, 20 mm), and an appropriate incision is made. A needle is inserted into the area of the lesion and a ''T'' wire marker deployed. An incision that will accommodate the appropriate biopsy cannula is made in the skin, and the biopsy cannula is passed through the incision and breast tissue, cutting through the tissue with an oscillating blade. After the cutting cannula has advanced beyond the needle tip and the ''T'' marker, the distal end of the tissue specimen is transected with a cautery snare and the cannula removed with the tissue specimen inside. The specimen can be marked with sutures for orientation and a specimen radiograph obtained. Hemostasis is achieved with pressure or cautery. Metal clips can be placed at the wound base and wound margins for subsequent identification. The patient is turned supine to accomplish sutured wound closure of the skin incision. Site-Select reportedly removes less normal breast tissue and is manually deployed. It does not use electrocautery and comes in a 15-mm diameter only. These procedures are more invasive than standard stereotactic CNB and thus carry a greater potential for procedure-related complications. There is a potential to resect completely small cancers in an accurate fashion with this method of minimally invasive treatment, but whether this represents adequate treatment remains to be seen.

Needle Localization Excisional Biopsy

The gold standard for definitive tissue diagnosis of a nonpalpable breast lesion identified on mammogram or ultrasound evaluation is needle localization excisional biopsy. This procedure involves identification of an area of suspicion in the breast by mammography or ultrasound image and subsequent image-guided placement of a wire guide into the lesion for identification in the breast at the time of open excisional biopsy (13). This procedure has become increasingly utilized in the last 30 years concomitant with increased early identification of breast lesions by mammography. Nonpalpable lesions not amenable to biopsy by other imaged-guided techniques such as stereotactic CNB, ultrasound CNB, and FNA cytology analysis, are candidates for this procedure. Indications that may preclude other forms of image-guided sampling include difficult locations (axilla, inframammary crease); lesions of very small size; lesions not well localized (diffuse calcifications); radial scar, judgment of the operating surgeon; or insufficient confidence in these techniques by either the patient or surgeon.

The basic technique for needle localization excision involves identification of the suspicious lesion with the appropriate image (stereotactic or ultrasound) and utilization of this image to guide a needle [Kopans (Cook, Inc., Bloomington, IN)] to or through the lesion involved. The barrel of the needle is removed leaving behind a hook wire. Multiple wires may be placed in certain circumstances to improve localization of the lesion within the breast at the time of excision. (It has been particularly useful in our experience to perform such localizations as part of a comprehensive breast program to allow for more direct approach to subsequent excision in terms of localization of incision placement in the breast). Once the hook wire is placed, the patient is taken to the operating room, where the hook wire is used as a guide for localization of suspicious breast tissue and subsequent excision of that tissue. Specimen radiographs are obtained in most cases and in essentially all cases where the indication for biopsy involves calcification. Incision location is determined by the surgeon based on the most direct approach to the lesion, the possible need for additional surgery after diagnosis, and consideration to limit cosmetic alteration. This procedure results in sensitivity of 98% to 99% accuracy (14), which is the standard to which other image guided techniques are compared.

NON–IMAGE-GUIDED TECHNIQUES

The preceding discussion focused on nonpalpable abnormalities of the breast. Evaluation of the patient with a palpable abnormality proceeds somewhat differently. If the area in question clearly represents a discrete palpable mass, then diagnostic biopsy procedures may proceed without the need for any image guidance. In some instances, however, the lesion may feel more "vague," and its exact dimensions are difficult to define. In these cases, the use of image guidance can direct a biopsy effort more accurately and increase the amount of useful information obtained.

In many cases, a dominant palpable mass will have been imaged already by mammogram or ultrasound. If the lesion appears to be a cyst, the initial maneuver should be a FNA to attempt decompression. This procedure is performed either with or without local anesthesia by stabilizing the mass between fingers. Fluid is withdrawn and the patient is reexamined to determine whether the mass has resolved.

In the patient with a solid palpable mass, there are several diagnostic options; the workup of a dominant mass, of course, proceeds independent of whether the mass is visualized on any imaging study. The surgeon may decide to proceed with open excisional biopsy in the operating room as the initial maneuver, depending on a number of factors and on the patient's preference. The surgeon also may elect to proceed with FNA cytology or core biopsy. Results from either FNA or non–image-guided CNB must be concordant with the physical examination and imaging studies that have been reviewed. If discordant results occur, the surgeon should proceed with open breast biopsy because there is a potential for sampling error with these techniques. In addition, a report of "suspicious" or "atypical" cells necessitates open biopsy to obtain a definitive result. Use of these diagnostic techniques should be in the setting of a palpable dominant mass; blind biopsies of apparently normal breast tissue are of no diagnostic benefit (15).

Fine Needle Aspiration

FNA cytology of the breast has been in use for several years, although the degree of use varies among surgeons. Proponents consider FNA a cost-effective means for making the diagnosis of a palpable lesion and that FNA has negligible potential for complications (16). It requires no special or expensive equipment. Those with reservations believe diagnosis by FNA cytology is limited by a lack of confidence in cytology to render definitive treatment (17). Success has been related to a number of factors, including level of interest in the technique, level of training, volume of procedures, ongoing feedback regarding quality of specimens, and immediate microscopic examination of the specimens by experienced cytopathologist (15).

The technique of FNA uses a 22- to 25-gauge needle attached to a 10- to 20-mL syringe. Smaller, 26- to 27-gauge needles may be needed if the lesion is small or contained within the dermis. The syringe may be used freehand or attached to a handle, which facilitates maintenance of high-pressure suction on the syringe. The skin is prepared with alcohol, and the mass is stabilized with the nondominant hand. Local anesthesia may be used. Several passes of the needle through the lesion are made while applying suction to the syringe. Suction should be released prior to bringing the needle out of the skin; the material aspirated should remain within the needle and not be brought up into the barrel of the syringe. The syringe then is detached from the needle and air is drawn into the syringe, which then is used to expel the material onto a glass slide. A smear is made between two glass slides, and these are fixed in absolute alcohol for cytologic examination. Additional passes are made through the lesion, and up to four passes should be made for lesions larger than 1 cm. The number of passes made is also affected by the quality of material retrieved and by patient tolerance.

The results of FNA are assigned to one of five categories: benign, atypical/indeterminate, suspicious/probably malignant, malignant, and unsatisfactory. Any result other than benign is likely to require further workup or open biopsy. Recommendations from the National Cancer Institute Consensus Conference in 1996 (15) regarding quality assurance of this process include maintaining a false-positive rate of less than 1%, regularly assessing the false negative rate, and ensuring concordance of the FNA results with open biopsies (when available). These standards must be maintained to use FNA as a reliable diagnostic technique.

The so-called triple test is advocated by some investigators as a reliable diagnostic algorithm in the evaluation of palpable breast masses (18). When physical examination, imaging studies, and FNA cytology all indicate a benign diagnosis, the diagnosis is reliably benign, and the patient can be assigned to follow-up in 6 months. When the physical examination, imaging studies, and FNA cytology all indicate a malignant diagnosis, the diagnosis is reliably malignant, and plans for definitive therapy can be made. The false-positive and false-negative rates of the triple test approach that of open biopsy with frozen section. "Mixed" results on the triple test (two of three positive or two of three negative) mandate open surgical biopsy (15,18).

Core Needle Biopsy

CNB also is used to evaluate a palpable breast mass. In the past, the Tru-Cut (Baxter International, Inc., Deerfield, IL) biopsy needle was the only core needle available, was somewhat cumbersome to manage, and required the use of two hands to manipulate successfully. More recently developed spring-loaded core needles used in stereotactic and ultrasound-guided breast biopsy techniques are in much more prevalent use. These small hand-held devices contain a disposable 12- to 14-gauge core needle; the core biopsy device can be operated with the dominant hand while stabilizing the lesion with the opposite hand. Local anesthesia is required, and a small incision is made through the skin to allow atraumatic passage of the needle into the lesion. Multiple cores of tissue can be obtained for formal histologic diagnosis rather than cytologic diagnosis alone. This means of obtaining tissue from a palpable breast mass is rapid and extremely well tolerated by the patient; insufficient specimens are uncommon and pathologic evaluation requires no special pathologic expertise. CNB has largely supplanted FNA in our practice in the evaluation of palpable masses. Based on the results of CNB, we can move with confidence to a definitive treatment plan without further invasive workup.

SUMMARY

The evaluation of breast disease is challenging and complicated by the frequently harsh emotional toll even a benign lesion can cause a patient. The identification of symptomatic or self-examination changes are disturbing enough to a woman, but physical examination findings by a physician or diagnostic mammographic or ultrasound image changes of suspicion are even more traumatic. Whereas most breast abnormalities are benign, it is important that all physicians remain diligent in complete assessment and follow-up of breast disease issues to identify breast cancer at its earliest detectable stage. The selection of when and in whom the most appropriate invasive study is indicated requires a combination of education, experience, and careful follow-up. In cases when invasive evaluation is deemed appropriate, the selection of which procedure to use depends on many factors, including the type of lesion (palpable or nonpalpable) and the available technology (ultrasound-guided aspiration or biopsy, stereotactic CNB, needle localization biopsy, FNA or needle core biopsy of palpable lesion, or excisional biopsy). The lack of availability or access to technology representing any of the preceding options may limit the use of that specific procedure but should not limit the ability of the surgeon to define the histopathology involved in an area of suspicious breast change. Whereas the current trend in breast care involves earlier identification of nonpalpable lesions through mammographic and ultrasound images with use of minimally invasive procedures (ultrasound-guided needle aspiration and biopsy or stereotactic needle biopsy), the standard for comparison remains open excision (with or without image localization), which may be the only form of treatment available. Open biopsy procedures are much less frequently performed than in previous years but continue as an important part of the breast evaluation and treatment algorithm.

REFERENCES

1. Israel PZ. The revolution in breast biopsy: where is the surgeon? *Am Surg* 1996;62:93–95.
2. Burns RP. Image-guided breast biopsy. *Am J Surg.* 1997;173:9–11.

3. Staren E. Surgical office-based ultrasound of the breast. *Am Surg* 1995;61:619–627.
4. Staren ED, Fine RE. Breast ultrasound for surgeons. *Am Surg* 1996;62:108–112.
5. Parker SH, Jobe WE, MA Dennis. Ultrasound-guided automated large core breast biopsy. *Radiology* 1993;187, 507–511.
6. Zannis VJ, Aliano KM. The evolving practice pattern of the breast surgeon with disappearance of open biopsy for nonpalpable lesions. *Am J Surg*1998;176:525–528.
7. Parker SH, Burbank F, Jackman RJ. Percutaneous large-core breast biopsy: a multi-institutional study. *Radiology* 1994;193:359–364.
8. Israel PZ, Fine RE. Stereotactic needle biopsy for occult breast lesions: a minimally invasive alternative. *Am Surg* 1995;61:87–91.
9. Roe SM, Mathews JA, Burns RP, et al. Stereotactic and ultrasound core needle breast biopsy performed by surgeons. *Am J Surg* 1997;174:699–704.
10. Janes RH, Bouton MS. Initial 300 consecutive stereotactic core-needle breast biopsies by a surgical group. *Am J Surg* 1994;168:533–537.
11. Robinson DS, Parel JM, Denham DB, et al. Stereotactic uses beyond core biopsy: model development for minimally invasive treatment of breast cancer through interstitial laser hyperthermia. *Am Surg* 1996;62:117–118.
12. Mathews BD, Williams GB. Initial experience with the advanced breast biopsy instrumentation system. *Am J Surg* 1999;177:97–101.
13. Kopans DB, Smith BL. Preoperative imaging-guided needle localization and biopsy of nonpalpable breast lesions. In: Harris JR, ed. *Diseases of the breast,* 1996:139–143.
14. Kaelin CM, Smith TJ, Homer MJ, Taback B, Azurin D. Safety, accuracy, and diagnostic yield of needle localization biopsy of the breast performed using local anesthesia. *J Am Coll Surg.* 1994; 179:267–272.
15. National Cancer Institute-sponsored conference, Bethesda, Maryland, September 9–10, 1996, with representatives of the American Society of Cytopathology, Papanicolaou Society of Cytopathology, American College of Radiology, American College of Obstetricians & Gynecologists, American Academy of Family Physicians, Society of Surgical Oncology, College of American Pathologists, National Consortium of Breast Centers, International Academy of Cytology, American Society of Clinical Pathologists, American Cancer Society, American College of Surgeons, and the American Society for Cytotechnology. The uniform approach to breast fine needle aspiration biopsy: a synopsis. *Breast Journal* 1996;2:357–363.
16. Wanebo ELT, Feldman PS, Wilhelm MC, et al. Fine needle aspiration cytology in lieu of open biopsy in management of primary breast cancer. *Ann Surg*1984;199:5:569–579.
17. Burbank F. Stereotactic breast biopsy: its history, its present, and its future. *Am Surg* 1996;62: 128–150.
18. Hermansen C, Poulsen HS, Jensen J, et al. Diagnostic reliability of combined physical examination, mammography, and fine-needle puncture (''triple-test'' in breast tumors). *Cancer* 1987;60: 1866–1871.

11

Premalignant and Malignant Breast Pathology

Roy A. Jensen, Jean F. Simpson, and David L. Page

This chapter discusses the current status of pathology in the care and management of patients with premalignant and malignant breast disease. Reliably identifiable conditions that are linked to the development of breast cancer, such as proliferative breast disease, and recent concepts and controversies regarding ductal carcinoma *in situ* (DCIS) are discussed. New technology, including sentinel lymph node (SLN) mapping and image guided breast biopsy, are having an impact on the practice of pathology and also are presented. In light of new therapeutic options, prognostic factors for breast cancer are discussed and correlated with traditional aspects of breast pathology.

PATHOLOGY AND SIGNIFICANCE OF PROLIFERATIVE BREAST DISEASE

General Aspects of Breast Cancer Risk

Mild nodularity is present in most breasts, and cysts are present in the breasts of more than half of women in their fifth and sixth decades. There is no known or proven link between breast cancer risk and cysts, fibrosis, nodularity, or pain. This situation, with its acknowledged poor confines of definition, is thus best considered *fibrocystic change.*

Epidemiologists have long concerned themselves with identifying links between certain conditions and the risk of malignancy. Many risk factors for breast cancer have been identified, predominantly related to specifics of menstrual and reproductive history as well as family history of breast cancer. Most of these risk factors indicate a magnitude of cancer risk less than twice that of the general population (1–4) and are correctly not considered determinant premalignant conditions.

Although histologic determinants of breast cancer risk have been accepted (discussed later), it is still not clear whether the incidence of these anatomic markers is more than slightly increased in lumpy or mammographically dense breasts (5–7). These anatomic markers, all of which are hyperplastic epithelial lesions (8), have been associated with an increased cancer risk in several studies. Follow-up studies of women after benign breast biopsy are the most feasible and practical way to evaluate the prognostic clinical significance of various histologic changes. The most that can be asked from such studies, however, is that they will indicate the magnitude of risk for subsequent breast disease, that is, predictability by percentage likelihood, which is not definitive for any single patient. A rough estimate of the correctness of an association between cancer and some predictor is obtained from empirical observations of comparable women. These measures of strength of associations often are expressed as relative risk (RR), which is a complex statement of a fraction divided by a fraction. Thus, the statement that women with atypical hyperplasia (AH) have a four times increased risk of cancer is derived from the following fraction:

$$\frac{\textit{Women with AH developing carcinoma/All women with AH}}{\textit{Women in reference population developing carcinoma/All women in reference population}}$$

Studies carried out in Nashville, Tennessee, over the last 20 years indicated that 70% of women undergoing benign breast biopsy have no increased risk of subsequent carcinoma development (9). These women were characterized as having no well-developed foci of epithelial hyperplasia, previously termed *papillomatosis* or *epitheliosis*. Women with cysts of any size, as well as apocrine change, were included in this "nonproliferative" or "low-risk" group. This is probably the most useful conclusion from these studies because it has been generally believed that any woman undergoing a breast biopsy has some form of breast disease and an increased risk of breast cancer of approximately twice that of the general population. Note that the women in this study underwent biopsy between 1950 and 1968 in the premammography era.

Approximately one quarter of the women who were reviewed had hyperplastic lesions of moderate or greater quantitative characteristic without atypia. These women had a slight elevation risk, which may be best related as in the range of 1.5 to 2 times that of the general population. Most believe that this magnitude of risk elevation is insufficient to alter clinical management practices from those applied to women of similar age. It would seem prudent to encourage such women to follow the yearly mammogram recommendation. Well-developed histologic examples of sclerosing adenosis are also indicative of this slightly elevated risk of invasive cancer (10).

Atypical hyperplastic lesions were found in approximately 4% of otherwise benign biopsies and indicated an RR of subsequent breast carcinoma development four to five times that of the general population (11). Note that this RR of later invasive carcinoma applies to the study group and analogous women of similar age followed up for a similar period. This means that this RR cannot be applied to the risk of breast carcinoma over a lifetime. The absolute risk for perimenopausal women (the age group that most frequently undergoes biopsy), with AH would be 8% to 10% in 10 to 15 years. This magnitude of risk is similar to that for the contralateral breast after invasive carcinoma development and treatment in one breast. The two types of atypia [ductal (ADH) and lobular (ALH) patterns] demonstrated little difference

TABLE 11.1. *Relative risk of invasive carcinoma after diagnosis of atypical lobular hyperplasia (ALH) related to age at biopsy and family history*

	No. of women	No. of cancers	Relative risk[a]	95% CI	p Value
All women with ALH	126	16	4.2	2.6–6.9	<0.000001
No family history	106	11	3.5	1.9–6.2	0.00001
Family history[b]	19	5	8.5	3.5–20	<0.000001
Age 20–30 yr	5	0	0.0	—	0.78
Age 31–45 yr	52	4	2.7	1.0–7.2	0.039
Age 46–55 yr	59	12	6.4	3.6–11	<0.000001
Age 56–65 yr	8	0	0.0	—	0.60
Age >65 yr	2	0	0.0	—	0.80

CI, confidence interval.

[a]Compared with women from Atlanta, Georgia, in the Third National Cancer Society Survey controlled for age and number of years at risk.

[b]History of breast cancer in sister, mother, or daughter.

From Page DL, Dupont WD, Rogers LW, et al. Atypical hyperplastic lesions of the female breast: a long-term follow-up study. *Cancer* 1985;55:2698–2708, with permission.

from each other except in age incidence (Tables 11.1 and 11.2). Each recognized an approximately equal incidence of later carcinoma in each breast, although the risk associated with ALH is greatly reduced in postmenopausal women and showed a slight preference for the ipsilateral breast cancer development (12). Note that Table 11.2 indicates that most of our knowledge about AH relates to women of perimenopausal age and that we really know little about it in younger or older women. These groups (no proliferative disease, proliferative disease without atypia,

TABLE 11.2. *Relative risk of invasive carcinoma after diagnosis of atypical ductal hyperplasia (ADH) related to age at biopsy and family history*

	No. of women	No. of cancers	Relative risk[a]	95% CI	p Value
All women with ADH	150	18	4.3	2.7–6.9	<0.000001
No family history	122	11	3.2	1.8–5.8	0.00004
Family history[b]	28	7	9.7	4.7–20	<0.000001
Age 20–30 yr	14	1	7.0	0.98–50	0.024
Age 31–45 yr	60	7	4.5	2.1–9.4	0.00001
Age 46–55 yr	51	6	3.5	1.6–7.7	<0.001
Age 56–65 yr	10	2	6.5	1.6–26	0.002
Age >65 yr	15	2	5.0	1.2–20	0.012

CI, confidence interval.

[a]Compared with women from Atlanta, Georgia, in the Third National Cancer Society Survey controlled for age and number of years at risk.

[b]History of breast cancer in sister, mother, or daughter.

From Page DL, Dupont WD, Rogers LW, et al. Atypical hyperplastic lesions of the female breast: a long-term follow-up study. *Cancer* 1985;55:2698–2708, with permission.

TABLE 11.3. *Relative risk[a] for invasive breast carcinoma based on histologic examination of breast tissue without carcinoma*

No increased risk
  Nonproliferative disease
  Adenosis, sclerosing or florid[b]
  Apocrine change
  Duct ectasia
  Mild epithelial hyperplasia of usual type
Slightly increased risk (1.5–2 times)
  Hyperplasia of usual type, moderate
    or florid
Moderately increased risk (4–5 times)
  Atypical hyperplasia or borderline
    lesions
  Atypical ductal hyperplasia
  Atypical lobular hyperplasia
High risk (8–10 times)
  Carcinoma *in situ*
  Lobular carcinoma *in situ*
  Ductal carcinoma *in situ* (noncomedo)[c]

[a]Women in each category are compared with women matched for age who have had no breast biopsy. These risks are not lifetime risks.
[b]Jensen et al. (10) indicated that well-developed examples of sclerosing adenosis had a slight increased risk indication.
[c]Only smaller examples of noncomedo ductal carcinoma *in situ* have been consistently assessed as risk indicators after biopsy only.
  Modified from Fitzgibbons PL, Henson DE, Hutter RVP, et al. Benign breast changes and the risk for subsequent breast cancer: an update of the 1985 consensus statement. *Arch Path Lab Med* 1998;122:1053–1055, with permission.

and AH) and their risk implications have been recognized (13), almost without alteration, by a consensus statement (summarized in Table 11.3).

It is evident that the dichotomous approach to malignancy in the breast, that is, determining whether a mass is benign or malignant, is inadequate. Some lesions termed *malignant* have little threat to life, and some benign lesions must be regarded with concern because of their marker status for elevated subsequent risk. As the complexity of diagnostic and therapeutic options in the breast has increased in scope and clarity, so has the anatomic stratification of breast disease (3).

HISTOLOGIC CRITERIA FOR ATYPICAL HYPERPLASIA OF BREAST

The AHs have been histologically defined as having some, but not all, the features of analogous types of carcinoma *in situ* (CIS). They have therefore been named AH of ductal and lobular type in keeping with their close pattern analogies with similarly named types of CIS (11,14). Because their recognition depends on the diagnostic features of CIS, those features, when present in less than fully developed form, serve as the criteria for AH. A study by Tavassoli and Norris (15) used similar histologic

TABLE 11.4. *Histologic criteria for carcinoma* in situ

Noncomedo ductal carcinoma *in situ* (DCIS)	Lobular carcinoma *in situ* (LCIS)
Uniform population of cells throughout entire area (at least two spaces)[a]	Characteristic, uniform cells constitute the entire population of cells in a lobular unit
"Punched-out," neatly rounded, geometric spaces or bulbous, well-formed defined papillary fronds	Filling (no interspersed, intercellular spaces between cells) of all the acini (terminal ductules)
Round, hyperchromatic, monotonous, evenly placed nuclei	Expansion and/or distortion of at least one-half acini in the lobular unit

[a]A space is defined as an area bounded by basement membrane.

criteria and found a similar risk of later cancer. Their criteria for ADH includes an overall size criterion of less than 2 mm in aggregate diameter.

ADH is recognized when some of the qualitative histologic features that characterize noncomedo DCIS are found; however, not all the major features of DCIS are fully present throughout involved spaces (Table 11.4).

Many features, diagnostic and otherwise, of DCIS have been and may be cited in this context; however, some are more specific and sensitive than others. It is those that are present most often and most indicative of DCIS that should be emphasized (16): (a) a uniform population of cells (i.e., not the varied nuclear contours of usual hyperplasia); (b) smooth geometric spaces between cells or micropapillary formations; and (c) hyperchromatic nuclei. To clarify a difficult diagnostic situation, the first criterion should be met in at least two adjacent spaces. Any case having the first or the second criterion, without having both in fully developed form in two spaces, is diagnostic of ADH. The presence of cells reminiscent of DCIS of noncomedo type is mandatory. The third criterion may be regarded as contributory but neither specific nor sufficient for a diagnosis of ADH and may be ignored in an occasional case. A swirling cellular pattern or irregular and slit-like intercellular spaces as seen in usual hyperplasia will deny the diagnosis of ADH. This last feature emphasizes the basic intent of the term *atypical hyperplasia*; that is, it is not the usual pattern of hyperplasia, no matter how exuberant.

Histologic criteria for the diagnosis of lobular carcinoma *in situ* (LCIS) are presented in Table 11.4. When identical cytologic appearances are found in lobular units, but less than half the acini in a lobular unit are filled, distorted, and distended with the uniform population of characteristic cells, then ALH is diagnosed (11,14). Other studies have shown that lesser degrees of involvement indicate a lesser risk (17). The diagnosis of ALH as opposed to LCIS is most often a result of the lesion failing to distend and completely fill the acini (i.e., intercellular spaces are present) of the lobular unit in question. Care must be taken not to misinterpret intracellular lumina as intercellular spaces. Well-fixed and stained histologic preparations are mandatory for the reliable identification of these changes.

The cytology of ALH (and LCIS) is usually quite bland, with round, somewhat lightly stained nuclei and cytoplasm evenly spaced one from another without evident pattern or polarity. Small nucleoli may be present. The uniformity and roundness of the cell population are the major guideposts to a diagnosis of ALH. Within lobular units, the presence of a cell population different from ALH cells is strong evidence against a diagnosis of LCIS and should prompt reserve in the diagnosis of ALH. Occasionally, most cells in usual hyperplasia will be rounded, mimicking the cells of lobular neoplasia. If the pattern is otherwise characteristic of usual hyperplasia, it should be regarded as such. If any lobular unit meets the criteria for LCIS, that diagnosis overrides the presence of ALH (18).

Reliable diagnostic criteria of diagnosis demand that each end of the spectrum be set. The upper end or more developed examples of ALH border on LCIS. The lesser or least developed examples of ALH border on mildly disordered appearances of lobules for which no diagnostic term is proposed. Thus, we do not recognize lobular hyperplasia as a diagnostic term because of imprecision of histologic definition and current lack of clinical relevance. The least developed but diagnostic examples of ALH must have a group of almost identical, characteristic cells, evenly spaced relative to each other, which are definitely increased in number over that normally present in the acinus. This approach assists the diagnosis of ALH when fixation artifact or mammary involution produces a loss of polarity of acinar cells that may mimic ALH (19). Also avoided is the possibility of mistaking similarly altered foci of mild hyperplasia of usual type for ALH. Occasionally, a clear separation of ALH from ADH is difficult. Fortunately, the currently recognized prognostic implications are so similar that it matters little which type of atypia is diagnosed in this situation.

AHs are discovered in about 4% of otherwise benign breast biopsies from the premammography era. Mammographically directed biopsies probably have a higher incidence, approaching 10% (20,21).

There is an elevated risk of subsequent invasive carcinoma after biopsies demonstrating these alterations. The magnitude of this risk has been characterized as *moderate* (11,13,20) because it is intermediate between that recognized by proliferative disease without atypia (slightly increased risk 1.5 to 2 times that of the general population) and that recognized by LCIS (21,22) and small examples of DCIS (16, 23) (9 to 11 times that of the general population).

PATHOLOGY AND SIGNIFICANCE OF DUCTAL CARCINOMA *IN SITU*

The therapy for DCIS is controversial, but it is being increasingly decided by the pathologic evidence. What we know of the natural history of DCIS is that the comedo and noncomedo examples seem quite different. As detailed in several reviews, the information from studies that followed up on patients after biopsy alone indicates a great difference between the small noncomedo examples of DCIS and the larger comedo DCIS lesions. The currently available evidence from cases that have been treated by planned surgical excision without radiation therapy indicates that the noncomedo examples of DCIS can be treated adequately by this modality.

This chapter reviews the histopathology of DCIS and makes the major point that we are currently in a state of transition in our understanding of DCIS. Studies supporting the stratification of DCIS by histologic pattern plus cytology and size will be contrasted to the rapidly disappearing classic posture that all DCIS is biologically similar and treatment options need not be stratified by the different subtypes or varieties of DCIS.

Size or Extent of Ductal Carcinoma *In Situ*

The range of clinical presentations of DCIS is immense, extending from large, palpable masses to the tiniest examples that overlap occasionally with ADH (24, 25) using current criteria. These smaller lesions should be recognized as being almost trivial. Size criteria have been helpful at this low end of the DCIS spectrum because lesions that are in the size range of 2 to 5 mm are regularly circumscribed and usually adequately removed by the initial biopsy procedures. The natural history of these smaller lesions, without attempts at margin assessment, is detailed in papers published in 1978 (23) and 1982 (16).

The larger examples of DCIS, usually with comedo features, are also well known. They have been assumed to be multicentric in the past, but more recent studies with careful three-dimensional reconstruction (26) make it clear that these lesions are continuous in three dimensions in almost all cases. The biologic event underlying this spread or involvement of much of the breast by a histologically similar process is not yet known. The more extensive examples with higher-grade nuclei are often also associated with Paget disease of the nipple (27).

Histologic Type

There is a wide recent acceptance of the heterogeneity of DCIS (28–30). Furthermore, many accept that cytology and histologic pattern (Table 11.5) can be used

TABLE 11.5. *Classification of ductal carcinoma* in situ

Histology	Cytology	Necrosis	Calcification
Comedo[a]	High grade	Extensive	Linear, branched
Intermediate	Intermediate	Limited	Focal, punctate
Noncomedo	Low grade	Absent	Microscopic foci
Cribriform			
Solid			
Micropapillary[b]			

[a] Although different terms are used for this high-grade category, the presence of both advanced nuclear atypia and extensive necrosis are necessary criteria.
[b] Some of these are high grade and may be considered comedo type. When present in pure form, they may be extensive.

together to make assignment into categories more precise, reproducible, and clinically useful.

The close association of nuclear abnormalities and the presence of necrosis identified microscopically have resulted in several classification proposals that are quite parallel despite slightly different terminology. Both the recently proposed Van-Nuys histologic classification (31) and an approach proposed and tested for interobserver variation by Scott et al. (32) use slight modifications of the classification by Lagios et al. first proposed in 1989 (33), although collapsed from four tiers to three. Basically, the systems recognize high-grade categories with necrosis and high-degree nuclear atypia and a low-grade group with orderly nuclei and no necrosis. An intermediate group helps refine the assignment of cases in the "high" and "low" groups by accepting cases with intermediate grade nuclei and limited necrosis (Fig. 11.1).

Some pathologists have used histologic pattern and cytologic grade as separate determinants, but this approach negates the precise identification of the highest and lowest grades of lesions. It is the determination of the highest and lowest grade of lesions by the combined approach that is most likely to determine whether the lesion could be cured by conservation treatment as indicated by the work of Lagios et al. (33). Initially, they separated lesions into four categories, with the top two categories having advanced nuclear atypia and necrosis, separated only by the remnants of a

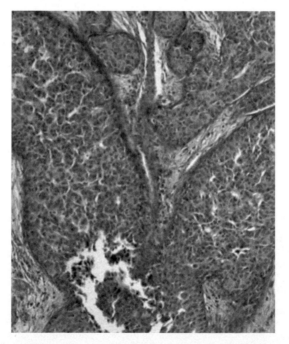

FIG. 11.1. Ductal carcinoma *in situ* (DCIS) intermediate grade with necrosis. This DCIS lesion exhibits grade 2 nuclei and clearly shows an area of necrosis. This level of nuclear atypia and the limited extent of the necrosis are insufficient for a diagnosis of comedo DCIS.

TABLE 11.6. *Ductal carcinoma* in situ *(DCIS) of the breast: effect of grade on recurrence following excision only*

Study	Follow-up (mo)	Recurrence rate (high-grade/comedo) (%)	Recurrence rate (low-intermediate grade/ noncomedo) (%)
Lagios (33)	100	11/36 (30.5)	1/42[a] (2)
Bellamy (35)	60	10/25 (40)	0/6 (0)
Ottesen (40)	63	23/76 (30.6)	3/36 (8.3)
Schwartz (39)	47	10/21 (47.6)	1/51 (2)

[a]The single recurrence was from a patient whose biopsy contained intermediate grade DCIS, no low-grade DCIS cases recurred.

micropapillary or cribriform pattern in one of the categories. On further scrutiny, Schwartz and Lagios (34) combined these two categories. Thus, there seems to be no utility in recognizing minor remnants of cribriform or micropapillary pattern in high-grade lesions because a large percentage of these cases recur after planned wide excision. It is precisely this approach of using pathoanatomic principles to identify clinically useful endpoints that distinguishes the modern approach to histopathology from the historical descriptive approach. It is quite evident that the lower-grade, non-comedo lesions are likely to be smaller and also may be amenable to treatment with low recurrence rates (Table 11.6).

There is a suggestion, as yet only documented in two studies (28,35), that the pure micropapillary pattern of DCIS (not combined with other patterns) may be associated more frequently with quite extensive disease. This is not true if occasional micropapillae are intermixed with the solid and cribriform patterns, a relatively common finding.

Differential Diagnosis

There has been a lack of concordance between different pathologists in determining whether small lesions should be considered AH or CIS. In general, lesions that involve only a few membrane-bound spaces and measure less than 2 to 3 mm in greatest dimension should be regarded as hyperplastic lesions (± atypia) and not as CIS. A greater degree of concordance is seen in larger lesions (33). Even the diagnosis of difficult, smaller, borderline lesions will approach concordance between observers if pathologists agree on the criteria (25).

Clinical Outcome

Several studies assessed the risk of subsequent invasive carcinoma for patients for whom the diagnosis of DCIS was not made at the initial biopsy for small, noncomedo lesions. Approximately one third of these patients developed invasive breast cancer in the same region of the same breast within 10 to 18 years. Attempted wide excision of large, comedo DCIS lesions is notoriously unsuccessful (36,37).

Developing evidence strongly supports the idea that adequate excision of DCIS lesions without radiotherapy (Table 11.6) may lead to cure (38). As noted in other sections of this review, smaller noncomedo examples of DCIS are regularly treated successfully at least with follow-up extending to 7 or 8 years (34,35,39,40). These surgical protocols have involved careful, planned, wide excision. Most cases have been mammographically detected, and a few cases were discovered incidentally have been successfully treated also.

Role of Radiation

What is the role of radiotherapy in reducing local recurrence after wide excision of a localized area of DCIS? Preliminary data (with follow-up of less than 4 years) from a study in the United States (41) suggests that radiotherapy may reduce the rate of disease recurrence within the breast following an adequate excision of a localized area of DCIS. It is not clear from this study whether the benefits of radiotherapy relate to all types of DCIS or whether the benefits will be demonstrable beyond 43 months' follow-up. To determine the optimum treatment for DCIS detected in screening programs, several clinical trials are under way. It is widely accepted that the mammographically detected DCIS lesion should be considered separately from the regularly larger lesions presenting with palpable masses and nipple discharge (42). Whether radiation therapy aids in retarding or negating recurrence in some lesions awaits careful subtype analysis of such cases. The relevance of stratification by histologic pattern has been demonstrated, however, in groups of patients treated by radiotherapy after surgical excision (43).

It appears that small examples of noncomedo DCIS are nonobligate precursor lesions, and only 25% to 30% eventuate in invasive carcinomas if left untreated. They may be regarded as increased risk lesions because their RR of later invasive cancer development is about ten times that of the general population. It is obvious that if adequately removed surgically, small examples of noncomedo DCIS may be regarded as cured. It is by no means guaranteed, however, that carcinoma will not develop elsewhere within these breasts, just that it should be the exception rather than the rule.

Complete embedding of the lesion with accounting for the three-dimensional extent of the disease within the breast is critical for conservative treatment of DCIS. Almost any case of DCIS excised with a 1-cm margin should not recur locally (44). What has not been established is that all cases of DCIS that are amenable to local excision for cure require a 1-cm margin. An Eastern Oncology Cooperative Group Trial (ECOG 5194) is currently accruing patients to determine which DCIS lesions may be cured by local excision alone. Entry criteria include complete submission of the lesion by sequential sectioning, margins clear of DCIS by at least 3 mm, and size of the DCIS 1 cm or less for high-grade DCIS, and 2.5 cm or less for intermediate or low-grade DCIS. Patients are accepted into this trial after central review of their slides.

Conclusions

There is strong evidence that small size and low histologic grade interact to produce lesions that can be easily cured by local excision without radiation therapy. This would certainly be true of lesions that are smaller than 1 cm in largest diameter. The greatest extent of a lesion is most easily determined by careful pathologic–mammographic correlation, which is mandatory in most instances. It is also clear that extensive high-grade comedo lesions are not easily cured and that recurrences are common even after radiation therapy. Precisely which concurrence of histologic grade and size is to be the determinant of therapeutic decision making is an area under investigation currently. It should be understood, however, that local recurrence in this setting is very unlikely to be a life-threatening event and that a woman's desire for breast conservation with a willingness to accept the possibility of local recurrence may be as important with regard to therapeutic decision making as any other consideration.

EVALUATION OF SENTINEL LYMPH NODES

The presence of axillary lymph node metastases remains the single best predictor of overall survival in breast cancer patients. Axillary lymph node status is also the primary determinant for the use of systemic adjuvant therapy, especially for patients with small primary carcinomas. In the early 1990s, intraoperative lymphatic mapping and sentinel lymphadenectomy (SLND) were introduced, with the promise of accurately predicting tumor status of the axillary lymph nodes draining the primary breast carcinoma. SLN mapping with SLND is becoming accepted as an alternative to formal axillary lymph node dissection (45–50), and surgeons are quickly mastering the technical aspects of performing the procedure (51,52). The reported false-negative rates range from 0% in single institution (53) studies to 11.4% in large multi-institution studies. Several studies have used more intensive pathologic evaluation of sentinel nodes to maximize detection of micrometastases (54). Advances in surgical technique and experience are expected to reduce, but not completely eliminate, false-negative results.

Given that the technique is highly accurate and predictive, there are several unresolved issues related to SLN. First, a widely accepted standard method of processing the SLN is not in practice. There is agreement that the SLN should be examined histologically, but there is variability in how many sections need to be examined (55). The recommendations from the College of American Pathologists are given here. Because surgeons may elect to perform a completion axillary dissection on patients with positive sentinel nodes, an intraoperative assessment of the node may help to avoid a second anesthetic procedure. Intraoperative assessment is routine, with imprint cytology preferred over frozen-section analysis (56,57). Touch imprints have been shown to be highly accurate without loss of valuable nodal tissue through cryostat sectioning (58).

The clinical relevance of finding micrometastatic disease in SLNs remains to be determined. Several retrospective studies found that the prognosis of patients with isolated micrometastases to axillary lymph nodes (defined as ≤2 mm in diameter) is the same as that for patients with negative nodes (59–61). Other studies, however, have suggested a significantly worse prognosis for patients with micrometastases detected by serial step sectioning (62) or immunohistochemistry (63–66).

The clinical relevance of micrometastasis, especially those detected only with special techniques, is far from settled (66–68); therefore, until randomized trials confirm the clinical significance of micrometastases found only by immunohistoche-mistry, detection and reporting of micrometastases should be based on hematoxylin and eosin sections. If tumor cells are detected only by immunohistochemistry, the pathology report should reflect that fact. There are insufficient data to recommend changing pathologic tumor stage based only on finding individual cytokeratin-posi-tive cells in axillary lymph nodes.

The following are the current recommendations of the College of American Pa-thologists for examining SLNs:

Sentinel Lymph Node Examination and Reporting

1. SLNs should be sectioned as close to 2 mm as possible and entirely submitted for histologic section, regardless of nodal size.

2. A single microscopic section from each lymph node block is considered suffi-cient for evaluation. Insufficient data exist to recommend routine serial step section-ing of SLNs.

3. Routine cytokeratin staining of histologically negative SLN should not be con-sidered standard until clinical trials demonstrate its clinical significance.

4. For the intraoperative assessment of SLNs, careful gross examination with cytologic evaluation obtained from imprint cytology is preferable to frozen-section examination because the latter method may consume significant amounts of nodal tissue. For staging purposes, immunohistochemical or molecular methods detecting isolated tumor cells within SLNs should not be used to upstage patients, unless verified by H&E sections (at least 0.2 mm).

If immunohistochemical analysis is performed on a lymph node, special care should be given to identify appropriately the source of cytokeratin-positive cells. It is not unusual to have benign glandular inclusions within the lymph node capsule, and these should not be interpreted as metastatic deposits. In addition, benign transport of fragmented epithelial cells has been reported following needle aspiration or core biopsy. These epithelial cells are invariably located within the lymph node sinus and are associated with hemosiderin and macrophages (69).

PATHOLOGIC EVALUATION AND INTERPRETATION OF IMAGE-GUIDED BIOPSIES

Methods to sample breast lesions adequately and with minimal degree of invasiveness are rapidly becoming accepted. Fine needle aspiration (FNA) has long been used to sample palpable lesions, but nonpalpable lesions are increasingly sampled through the use of ultrasound or stereotaxic mammographic guidance (70). In a review of the University of California at Los Angeles Medical Center experience with radiologically guided core biopsy, Nguyen et al. (71) reported excellent sensitivity and specificity. In their review, they present the radiologic assessment according to guidelines of the American College of Radiology Breast Imaging Reporting and Data System (BI-RADS), which relates findings to degree of certainty. This same approach was recently adopted by a National Institutes of Health consensus conference (72) for reporting the results of FNA, that is, diagnoses within the structure of levels of certainty. Nguyen et al. (71) reviewed the advantages and disadvantages of core biopsy, including a discussion of economic factors. When performance of stereotactic core biopsy was limited to examples of BI-RADS category 5 (highly suggestive of malignancy) a surgical procedure was obviated in 42% of patients, resulting in modest cost savings (73).

Sampling of breast lesions can provide more than just a histopathologic diagnosis. Di Loreto et al. (73) showed that characteristics such as presence of estrogen receptor, progesterone receptor, and proliferative activity of the carcinoma detected in the core biopsy are essentially identical to the resected specimen. The impact that these characteristics determined from the core biopsy might have on management is not yet clear.

Since the introduction of core needle biopsy technology, an excisional biopsy has been recommended following a diagnosis of ADH on core biopsy. This has been done to avoid false-negative results and because DCIS has often been found in the excisional specimen. Three studies evaluated follow-up excisional biopsies after a core biopsy of ADH. Gadzala et al. (74) showed a 47% rate of DCIS or invasive carcinoma after a stereotaxic core biopsy diagnosis of ADH, and Moore et al. (75) documented DCIS in one third of excisional biopsy specimens after a core biopsy of ADH. On the other hand, Lin et al. (76) found only two of 18 patients diagnosed with ADH on core biopsy to have DCIS on excisional biopsy, and no cases of invasive carcinoma were found. Patient selection and histologic criteria for atypia may explain differences between these series. With the addition of vacuum assistance and multiple specimens, the diagnosis of ADH may be made more definitively using stereotactic breast biopsy (77). We have found that with the larger needle core biopsies and extensive samples, very limited ADH may not need to be followed by excisional biopsy; however the consideration that a carefully defined ADH may be part of a larger DCIS is extremely important in the resolution of this management decision.

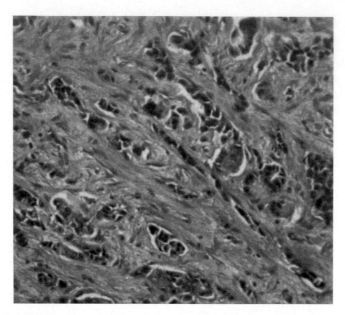

FIG. 11.2. Invasive mammary carcinoma, no special type. This is a typical example of the histologic appearance of most breast cancers diagnosed. There are no features that would qualify it as a so-called special-type cancer (lobular, tubular, mucinous, medullary, etc.), and it represents 70% to 75% of breast cancer cases in most series of unscreened populations. This type of breast cancer is often referred to as an *invasive ductal carcinoma*, but there is actually little or no evidence to suggest that this histologic type of breast arises exclusively from ducts; so we prefer the designation *no special type*.

PROGNOSTIC FACTORS FOR INVASIVE BREAST CANCER

A recent consensus statement from the College of American Pathologists has brought together a multidisciplinary group of clinicians, pathologists, and statisticians to consider prognostic and predictive factors in breast cancer. These have been stratified into categories that reflect the strength of published evidence (78–80).

The factors ranked in category I (factors proven to be of prognostic import and useful in clinical patient management) include tumor, node, metastasis (TNM) staging information, histologic grade (see later discussion), histologic type (Fig. 11.2), mitotic figure counts, and hormone receptor status. Category II (factors that have been extensively studied biologically and clinically but whose importance remains to be validated in statistically robust studies) includes *Her2/neu* status, proliferation markers, *p53* mutation, and lymphatic and vascular channel invasion. Category III included all other factors not sufficiently studied to demonstrate their prognostic value.

Grading of Invasive Mammary Carcinomas

Two general approaches can be taken to solving the problem of predicting outcome for patients with breast cancer. One is to look for new tests and await their verification, and the other is to take tests that are routinely available and find a way to maximize their usefulness by setting uniform and reproducible criteria.

There are many studies from around the world that have validated the utility of histopathologic grading of breast cancers in individual laboratories. Perhaps the best developed of these are from France (81,82), the Netherlands (83–86), and the United Kingdom (87–90). Their predictive power is particularly evident when combined with the more fundamental staging information of tumor size and lymph node status.

Evaluation of these approaches indicates that the counting of mitoses is central to these schemes, as indeed it may be to most grading systems that use nuclear characteristics only. Nuclear grade has not achieved general use, however, and is difficult. Both combined histopathologic schemes of grading used at the Institute Gustave-Roussy in Paris, France, and the University of Nottingham in the United Kingdom carefully measure the mitotic count as an essential part of a tripartite combined grading system along with gland formation and nuclear grade. Indeed, Contesso et al. produced an article in which the midzone or intermediate grade lesions are further stratified (from three to five) to produce useful prognostic information (82).

The basic rationale here is that staging information is mandatory to understanding and predicting the outcome of breast patients and that histopathologic grading has been able in many studies to add significantly to this information. The major question is how much it adds within the groups of node-negative and node-positive patients and how reproducible are the data derived in different laboratories.

Practical Guidelines

Assignment to special types of breast cancer is carried out first, and then cases can be graded (the exception being pure medullary carcinomas, which we believe should be evaluated without being graded). Any case assigned to the medullary or medullary variant category usually would have a combined grade of 3, but obviously, this is inappropriate because their clinical behavior is far better than a high-grade carcinoma of no special type. The other special histologic type that gives inconsistent information by grading is pure invasive lobular carcinoma (Fig. 11.3). Grade does give good information in many of the invasive lobular carcinoma variants because when they are of high grade, prognosis is generally poor.

The combined histologic system modified from Elston and Ellis (90) is currently defined as follows:

1. *Tubule formation:* In cases where definite tubule formation is seen in at least 75% of the tumor area, a score of 1 is given. In cases in which less than 10% of the tumor shows definite tubule formation, then the score of 3 is assigned. The score of 2 is given to the intermediate category. Tubules must be definite, sharply defined, even with a presumption of glycocalyx. Spaces made by dead cells are not accepted.

2. *Nuclear pleomorphism:* In this category, assessment is made of the variability of both the size and shape of the nuclei. If there is little variation and the nuclei

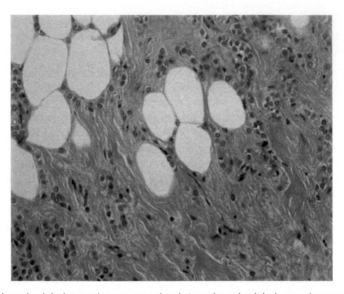

FIG. 11.3. Invasive lobular carcinoma, pure classic type. Invasive lobular carcinomas and lobular variants represent the largest fraction of special-type tumors, and in most series they exhibit a better prognosis. The terms *lobular variant* or *lobular features* are used for tumors that show histology that is similar to the pure example shown above but that also have admixed areas of no special type histology.

appear quite regular, a score of 1 is assigned. Marked variation, particularly when very large and bizarre nuclei are present, scores 3 points. A score of 2 is assigned to nuclei with intermediate features. For both nuclear score 2 and 3, nucleoli are often present, although multiple nucleoli favor a score of 3. Nuclear evaluation is perhaps the most difficult and least reproducible of the categories. In the overall combined score, a decision between nuclear grade 1 and 2 or between 2 and 3 often makes no difference in the final combined histologic grade. For practical implementation of the system, we offer the following general guidelines: In grade I, more than 25% of nuclei with diameter greater than 2 RBC equals 3. More than 25% of nuclei with very large or irregular nucleoli or multiple nucleoli equals 3. More than 25% of nuclei with chromatin clumping and coarseness similar to small cell carcinoma of lung equals 3. In grade II, size, nucleolar prominence or irregularity, chromatin clumping irregularity, and pleomorphism may be separately evaluated and combined to produce a final nuclear grade of 1 to 3 (e.g., 1–3 for size, 1–3 for pleomorphism, 1–3 for chromatin irregularity, and 1–3 for nucleolar irregularity. This approach is offered as a suggestion to foster reproducibility). The resultant total number may be reported as follows: 4 to 6 equals a final nuclear grade of one, 7 to 9 a final grade of 2, and 10 to 12 a final grade of 3.

3. *Mitotic rate:* In this category, excellent histologic preparation is necessary because only structures with the precise features of mitoses should be counted. It

is relatively common to have dark pyknotic nuclei and karyorrhexis that mimic mitoses, and these should not be counted. Perhaps more importantly, apoptotic bodies should not be counted as mitoses. Fewer than ten mitoses per ten high-power fields counts as 1 point, and 20 or more mitoses gives a score of 3. Counting of mitotic figures should be maximized by counting in the area where they are most prevalent, usually at the outer edge of the neoplasm. Ten adjacent fields then are evaluated for mitoses.

Only the invasive carcinoma is evaluated using these three categories.

Combined Grade Reporting and Clinical Implications

The combined histologic grade of 1/3 is given to cases that have combined scores of 3 to 5. The intermediate grade (2/3) is given to cases where the combined score is 6 to 7. The final grade of 3/3, or high combined histologic grade, is given to cases with a combined score of 8 to 9. We hope to develop a cellularity index as well as a reliable way to tie mitoses to a more general reference denominator, such as square millimeters or mitoses per 1,000 cells (91).

It is quite clear that individual medical oncologists and other clinicians involved in the management of breast cancer patients are already using histopathologic criteria of grading to make clinical decisions. Whether they are able to include this in their treatment plans or not demands credibility in their individual pathology services. We trust that this approach will give rigid histopathologic confines of definition and guidelines, so that these assignments can be more uniform (92).

PHYLLODES TUMORS

Phyllodes tumors are relatively rare lesions that histologically resemble the more prevalent fibroadenomas (93). They are most common in women aged 30 to 70 years. Phyllodes tumors are distinguished by hypercellular stromal overgrowth relative to their epithelial component and a prominent leaf-like growth pattern. The majority of these lesions are benign and are easily distinguished as such. However, there are clearly a minor component of phyllodes tumors that behave in a malignant fashion. In addition, most phyllodes tumors designated as malignant in many reported series are more appropriately placed in a borderline category indicating a small, but definite chance of malignant behavior. The behavior of these borderline legions is difficult to predict in an individual patient, but the utility of the borderline designation derives from its ability to alert the surgeon that these lesions need to be completely excised along with a rim of normal breast. There is no indication for lymph node sampling or dissection since phyllodes tumors only rarely metastasize to regional lymph nodes. Malignant phyllodes tumors demonstrate frankly malignant sarcomatous stromal elements, most often fibrosarcomatous areas. In addition, they typically show cellular pleomorphism and mitotic rates over 10 per 10 high power fields. Malignant behavior is particularly likely if liposarcoma, rhabdomyosarcoma, or osteosarcoma elements are present. Diagnosis of benign and borderline tumors is best carried out by evaluating a number of parameters including stromal pleomorphism and cellularity, mitotic rate, and the presence of an infiltrating border. Phyllodes tumors with two of three unfavorable features, but without frankly sarcomatous stroma should be designated as borderline, and any tumor with five to ten mitoses per 10 high power fields should also be included in this category.

REFERENCES

1. Kelsey JL, Berkowitz GS. Breast cancer epidemiology. *Cancer Res* 1988;48:5615–5623.
2. Carter CL, Corle DK, Micozzi MS. A prospective study of the development of breast cancer in 16,692 women with benign breast disease. *Am J Epidemiol* 1988;128:467–477.
3. Page DL, Dupont WD. Anatomic markers of human premalignancy and risk of breast cancer. *Cancer* 1990;66:1326–1335.
4. Page DL, Jensen RA, Simpson JF. Premalignant and malignant disease of the breast: the roles of the pathologist. *Mod Pathol* 1998;11:120–128.
5. Page DL, Winfield A. The dense mammogram. *Am J Roentgenol* 1986;147:487–490(abst).
6. Goodwin PJ, Boyd NF. Mammographic parenchymal pattern and breast cancer risk: a critical appraisal of the evidence. *Am J Epidemiol* 1988;127:1097–1108.
7. Bartow SA, Pathak DR, Black WC, et al. Prevalence of benign, atypical, and malignant breast lesions in populations at different risk for breast cancer. *Cancer* 1987;60:2751–2760.
8. Wellings SR, Jensen HM, Marcum RG. An atlas of subgross pathology of the human breast with special reference to possible precancerous lesions. *J Natl Cancer Inst* 1975;55:231–273.
9. Dupont WD, Page DL. Risk factors for breast cancer in women with proliferative breast disease. *N Engl J Med* 1985;312:146–151.
10. Jensen RA, Page DL, Dupont WD, et al. Invasive breast cancer (IBC) risk in women with sclerosing adenosis (SA). *Cancer* 1989;64:1977–1983.
11. Page DL, Dupont WD, Rogers LW, et al. Atypical hyperplastic lesions of the female breast. A long-term follow-up study. *Cancer* 1985;55:2698–2708.
12. Marshall LM, Hunter DJ, Connolly JL, et al. Risk of breast cancer associated with atypical hyperplasia of lobular and ductal types. *Cancer Epidemiol Biomarkers Prevent* 1997;6:297–301.
13. Fitzgibbons PL, Henson DE, Hutter RVP, et al. Benign breast changes and the risk for subsequent breast cancer: an update of the 1985 consensus statement. *Arch Pathol Lab Med* 1998;122:1053–1055.
14. Page DL, Anderson TJ. *Diagnostic histopathology of the breast.* Edinburgh: Churchill Livingstone, 1987:120–156.
15. Tavassoli FA, Norris HJ. A comparison of the results of long-term follow-up for atypical intraductal hyperplasia and intraducal hyperplasia of the breast. *Cancer* 1990;65:518–529.
16. Page DL, Dupont WD, Rogers LW, et al. Continued local recurrence of carcinoma 15–25 years after a diagnosis of low grade ductal carcinoma in situ of the breast treated only by biopsy. *Cancer* 1995;76:1197–1200.
17. Bodian CA, Perzin KH, Lattes R. Lobular neoplasia: long term risk of breast cancer and relation to other factors. *Cancer* 1996;78:1024–1034.
18. Page DL, Kidd TE Jr, Dupont WD, et al. Lobular neoplasia of the breast: higher risk for subsequent invasive cancer predicted by more extensive disease. *Hum Pathol* 1991;22:1232–1239.
19. Page DL, Dupont WD, Rogers L. Ductal involvement by cells of atypical lobular hyperplasia in the breast. *Hum Pathol* 1988;201–207.
20. Lagios MD, Page DL. *In situ* carcinoma of the breast: ductal carcinoma in situ, Paget's disease, lobular carcinoma in situ. In: Bland K, Copeland EM, eds. *The breast: comprehensive management of benign and malignant diseases.* 2nd ed. Philadelphia: WB Saunders, 1998:261–283.
21. Rosen PP, Lieberman PH, Braun DW Jr, et al. Lobular carcinoma *in situ* of the breast: detailed analysis of 99 patients with average follow-up of 24 years. *Am J Surg Pathol* 1978;2:225–251.
22. Haagensen CD, Lane N, Lattes R, et al. Lobular neoplasia (so-called lobular carcinoma *in situ*) of the breast. *Cancer* 1978;42:737–769.
23. Betsill WL Jr, Rosen PP, Lieberman PH, et al. Intraductal carcinoma: long-term follow-up after treatment by biopsy alone. *JAMA* 1978;239:1863–1867.

24. Page DL, Rogers LW. Combined histologic and cytologic criteria for the diagnosis of mammary atypical ductal hyperplasia. *Hum Pathol* 1992;23:1095–1097.
25. Schnitt SJ, Connolly JL, Tavassoli FA, et al. Interobserver reproducibility in the diagnosis of ductal proliferative breast lesions using standardized criteria. *Am J Surg Pathol* 1996;16:1133–1143.
26. Holland R, Hendriks JHCL, Verbeek ALM, et al. Extent, distribution, and mammographic/histologic correlations of breast ductal carcinoma in situ. *Lancet* 1990;335:519–522.
27. Chaudary MA, Millis R, Lane EB. Paget's disease of the nipple: a ten year review including clinical, pathological, and immunohistochemical findings. *Breast Cancer Res Treat* 1986;8:139–146.
28. Patchefsky AS, Schwartz GF, Finkelstein SD, et al. Heterogeneity of intraductal carcinoma of the breast. *Cancer* 1989;63:731–741.
29. Lennington WJ, Jensen RA, Dalton LW, et al. Ductal carcinoma *in situ* of the breast: heterogeneity of individual lesions. *Cancer* 1994;73:118–124.
30. van Dongen JA, Holland R, Peterse JL, et al. Ductal carcinoma *in situ* of the breast: second EORTC consensus meeting. *Eur J Cancer* 1992;28:626–629(abst).
31. Silverstein MJ, Lagios MD, Craig PH. A prognostic index for ductal carcinoma in situ of the breast. *Cancer* 1996;77:2267–2274.
32. Scott MA, Lagios MD, Axelsson K, et al. Ductal carcinoma *in situ* of the breast: reproducibility of histological subtype analysis. *Hum Pathol* 1997;28:967–973.
33. Lagios MD, Margolin FR, Westdahl PR, et al. Mammographically detected duct carcinoma in situ: frequency of local recurrence following tylectomy and prognostic effect of nuclear grade on local recurrence. *Cancer* 1989;63:618–624.
34. Schwartz GF, Lagios MD, et al. Consensus conference on the classification of ductal carcinoma in situ. *Cancer* 1997;80:1798–1802.
35. Bellamy COC, McDonald C, Salter DM, et al. Noninvasive ductal carcinoma of the breast: the relevance of histologic categorization. *Hum Pathol* 1993;24:16–23.
36. Silverstein MJ, Waisman J, Gamagami P, et al. Intraductal carcinoma of the breast (208 cases): clinical factors influencing treatment choice. *Cancer* 1990;66:102–108.
37. Dean L, Geschickter CF. Comedo carcinoma of the breast. *Arch Surg* 1939;36:225–227.
38. Fechner R. One century of mammary carcinoma *in situ*: what have we learned. *Am J Clin Pathol* 1994;100:654–661.
39. Schwartz GF, Finkel GC, Garcia JC, et al. Subclinical ductal carcinoma *in situ* of the breast: treatment by excision and surveillance alone. *Cancer* 1992;70:2468–2474.
40. Ottesen GL, Graversen HP, Blichert-Toft M, et al. Ductal carcinoma *in situ* of the female breast: short-term results of a prospective nationwide study. *Am J Surg Pathol* 1992;16:1183–1196.
41. Fisher B, Costantino J, Redmond C, et al. Lumpectomy compared with lumpectomy and radiation therapy for the treatment of intraductal breast cancer. *N Eng J Med* 1993;328:1581–1586(abst).
42. Pierce SM, Schnitt S, Harris A. What to do about mammographically detected ductal carcinoma *in situ*. *Cancer* 1992;70:2576–2578.
43. Solin LJ, Yeh I-T, Kurtz J, et al. Ductal carcinoma *in situ* (intraductal carcinoma) of the breast treated with breast-conserving surgery and definitive irradiation. *Cancer* 1993;71:2532–2542.
44. Silverstein MJ, Lagios MD, Groshen S, et al. The influence of margin width on local control of ductal carcinoma *in situ* of the breast. *N Engl J Med* 1999;340:1455–1461.
45. Krag DN, Weaver DL, Alex JC, et al. Surgical resection and radiolocalization of the sentinel lymph node in breast cancer using a gamma probe. *Surg Oncol* 1993;2:335–340.
46. Giuliano AE, Kirgan DM, Guenther JM, et al. Lymphatic mapping and sentinel lymphadenectomy for breast cancer. *Ann Surg* 1994;220:391–401.
47. Ingle JN. Tamoxifen and endometrial cancer: new challenges for an "old" drug. *Gynecol Oncol* 1994;55:161–163.
48. Krag DN, Weaver D, Ashikaga T, et al. The sentinel node in breast cancer: a multicenter validation study. *N Engl J Med* 1998;339:941–946.
49. Veronesi U, Paganelli G, Galimbert V, et al. Sentinel node biopsy to avoid axillary dissection in breast cancer with clinically negative lymph nodes. *Lancet* 1997;349:1864–1867.
50. Weaver DL, Krag DN, Ashikaga T, et al. Pathologic analysis of sentinel and nonsentinel lymph nodes in breast carcinoma: a multicenter study. *Cancer* 2000;88:1099–1107.
51. Morrow M, Rademaker A, Bethke K, et al. Learning sentinel node biopsy: results of a prospective randomized trial of two techniques. *Surgery* 1999;126:714–720.
52. Giuliano AE. See one, do twenty-five, teach one: the implementation of sentinel node dissection in breast cancer. *Ann Surg Oncol* 1999;6:520–521.

53. Giuliano AE, Jones RC, Brennan M, et al. Sentinel lymphadenectomy in breast cancer. *J Clin Oncol* 1997;15:2345–2350.
54. Turner RR, Ollila DW, Stern S, et al. Optimal histopathologic examination of the sentinel lymph node for breast carcinoma staging. *Am J Surg Pathol* 1999;23:263–267.
55. Cibull M. Handling sentinel lymph node biopsy specimens: a work in progress. *Arch Pathol Lab Med* 1999;123:620–621.
56. Motomura K, Inaji H, Komoike Y, et al. Intraoperative sentinel lymph node examination by imprint cytology and frozen sectioning during breast surgery. *Br J Surg* 2000;87:597–601.
57. Ratanawichitrasin A, Biscotti CV, Levy L, et al. Touch imprint cytological analysis of sentinel lymph nodes for detecting axillary metastases in patients with breast cancer. *Br J Surg* 1999;86:1346–1348.
58. Rubio IT, Korourian S, Cowan C, et al. Use of touch preps for intraoperative diagnosis of sentinel lymph node metastases in breast cancer. *Ann Surg Oncol* 1998;5:689–694.
59. Huvos AG, Hutter RVP, Berg JW. Significance of axillary macrometastases and micrometastases in mammary cancer. *Ann Surg* 1971;173:44–46.
60. Clayton F, Hopkins CL. Pathologic correlates of prognosis in lymph node-positive breast carcinomas. *Cancer* 1993;71:1780–1790.
61. Rosen PP, Beattie EJ, Saigo P, et al. Occult axillary lymph node metastases from breast cancers with intramammary lymphatic tumor emboli. *Am J Surg Pathol* 1982;6:639–641.
62. International Breast Cancer Study Group. Prognostic importance of occult axillary lymph micrometastases from breast cancers. *Lancet* 1990;335:1565–1568.
63. Trojani M, de Mascarel I, Bonichon F, et al. Micrometastases to axillary lymph nodes from carcinoma of breast: detection by immunohistochemistry and prognostic significance. *Br J Cancer* 1987;50:303–306.
64. McGuckin MA, Cummings MC, Walsh MD, et al. Occult axillary node metastases in breast cancer: their detection and prognostic significance. *Br J Cancer* 1996;73:88–95.
65. Cote RJ, Peterson HF, Chaiwun B, et al. and the International Breast Cancer Study Group. Role of immunohistochemical detection of lymph-node metastases in management of breast cancer. *Lancet* 1999;354:896–900.
66. Dowlatshahi K, Fan M, Bloom KJ, et al. Occult metastases in the sentinel lymph nodes of patients with early stage breast carcinoma: a preliminary study. *Cancer* 1999;86:990–996.
67. Dowlatshahi K, Fan M, Snider HC, et al. Lymph node micrometastases from breast carcinoma: reviewing the dilemma. *Cancer* 1997;80:1188–1197.
68. Allred DC, Elledge RM. Caution concerning micrometastatic breast carcinoma in sentinel lymph nodes. *Cancer* 1999;86:905–907.
69. Carter BA, Jensen RA, Simpson JF, et al. Benign transport of breast epithelium into axillary lymph nodes after biopsy. *Am J Clin Pathol* 2000;113:259–265.
70. Devia A, Murray KA, Nelson EW. Stereotactic core needle biopsy and the workup of mammographic breast lesions. *Arch Surg* 1997;132:512–516.
71. Nguyen M, McCombs MM, Ghandehari S, et al. An update on core needle biopsy for radiologically detected breast lesions. *Cancer* 1996;78:2340–2345.
72. Abati A, Abele J, Bacus SS, et al. The uniform approach to breast fine needle aspiration biopsy - A synopsis. *Acta Cytol* 1996;40:1120–1126.
73. Di Loreto C, Puglisi F, Rimondi G, et al. Large core biopsy for diagnostic and prognostic evaluation of invasive breast carcinomas. *Eur J Cancer* 1996;32A:1693–1700.
74. Gadzala DE, Cederbom GJ, Bolton JS, et al. Appropriate management of atypical ductal hyperplasia diagnosed by stereotactic core needle breast biopsy. *Ann Surg Oncol* 1997;4:283–286.
75. Moore MM, Hargett CW, Hanks JB, et al. Association of breast cancer with the finding of atypical ductal hyperplasia at core breast biopsy. *Ann Surg* 1997;225:726–731.
76. Lin PH, Clyde JC, Bates DM, et al. Accuracy of stereotactic core-needle breast biopsy in atypical ductal hyperplasia. *Am J Surg* 1998;175:380–382.
77. Jackman RJ, Burbank F, Parker SH, et al. Atypical ductal hyperplasia diagnosed at stereotactic breast biopsy: improved reliability with 14 gauge, directional, vacuum-assisted biopsy. *Radiology* 1997;204:485–488.
78. Fitzgibbons PL, Page DL, Weaver DL, et al. Prognostic factors in breast cancer: College of American Pathologists consensus statement 1999. *Arch Pathol Lab Med* 2000;124:966–978.
79. Fitzgibbons PL, Connolly JL, Page DL. Updated protocol for the examination of specimens from patients with carcinomas of the breast. *Arch Pathol Lab Med* 2000;124:1026–1033.
80. Hammond ME, Fitzgibbons PL, Compton CC, et al. College of American Pathologists Conference

XXXV: solid tumor prognostic factors: which, how, and so what. *Arch Pathol Lab Med* 2000;124: 958–965.

81. Le Doussal V, Tubiana-Hulin M, Friedman S, et al. Prognostic value of histologic grade nuclear components of Scarff-Bloom-Richardson (SBR): an improved score modification based on a multivariate analysis of 1262 invasive ductal breast carcinomas. *Cancer* 1989;64:1914–1921.
82. Contesso G, Mouriesse H, Friedman S, et al. The importance of histologic grade in long-term prognosis of breast cancer: a study of 1,010 patients, uniformly treated at the Institut Gustave-Roussy. *J Clin Oncol* 1987;5:1378–1386.
83. Baak JPA, Van Dop H, Kurver PHJ, et al. The value of morphometry to classic prognosticators in breast cancer. *Cancer* 1985;56:374–382.
84. Baak JPA. Mitosis counting in tumors. *Hum Pathol* 1990;21:683–685.
85. Van Diest P, Risse EKJ, Schipper NW. Comparison of light microscopic grading and morphometric features in cytological breast cancer specimens. *Pathol Res Pract* 1989;185:612–616.
86. Uyterline AM, Schipper NW, Baak JP. Limited prognostic value of cellular DNA content to classical and morphometrical parameters in invasive ductal breast cancer. *Am J Clin Pathol* 1988;89:301–307.
87. Todd JH, Dowle CS, Williams MR. Confirmation of prognostic index in primary breast cancer. *Br J Cancer* 1987;56:489–492.
88. Hitchcock A, Ellis IO, Robertson JFR. An observation of DNA ploidy, histological grade, and immunoreactivity for tumour-related antigens in primary and metastatic breast carcinoma. *J Pathol* 1989;159:129–134.
89. Elston CW. Grading of invasive carcinoma of the breast. In: Page DL, Anderson TJ, eds. *Diagnostic histopathology of the breast.* Edinburgh: Churchill Livingstone, 1987:300–311.
90. Elston CW, Ellis IO. Pathological prognostic factors in breast cancer. I. The value of histologic grade in breast cancer: experience from a large study with long-term follow-up. *Histopathology* 1991;19:403–410.
91. Simpson JF, Dutt PL, Page DL. Expression of mitoses per thousand cells and cell density in breast carcinomas: a proposal. *Hum Pathol* 1992;23:608–611.
92. Henson DE. The histologic grading of neoplasms. *Arch Pathol Lab Med* 1988;112:1091–1096.
93. Page DL, Anderson TJ. *Diagnostic histology of the breast.* Edinburgh: Churchill Livingstone, 1987: 341–350.

12

Management of Ductal Carcinoma *In Situ*

Stephen S. Falkenberry, Blake Cady, and Maureen A. Chung

Few topics in medicine are as controversial or confusing as the appropriate treatment of ductal carcinoma *in situ* (DCIS) of the breast. The exact prevalence of DCIS is unknown, but autopsy studies have shown that 4% to 15% of women without a history of breast cancer will harbor DCIS, whereas 1% to 2% have invasive cancer (1). Formerly an uncommon clinically detected entity accounting for only 1% to 2% of breast cancers, DCIS now accounts for about 25% to 30% of mammographically detected breast cancers and an even higher percentage in populations with high mammographic screening compliance (2). Most cases of DCIS are mammographically detected. The most common mammographic sign of DCIS is the presence of microcalcifications, followed by a mammographic density. The particular pattern of calcifications correlates well with the histologic subtype of DCIS. Nearly all women with linear branching, so-called casting calcifications will have comedo carcinoma *in situ*, with or without invasion. Nonbranching linear calcifications are associated with DCIS in about 80% of cases. Other patterns of microcalcifications, such as granular clustered microcalcifications, tend to be associated with lower-grade non-comedo DCIS (3). Because most lesions are mammographically detected, stereotactic core and needle localization excisional biopsies usually are performed to establish the diagnosis, but only complete excision of the lesion can definitively rule out invasive breast cancer. As recently as the mid-1980s, mastectomy was the treatment of choice for women with DCIS. During a period in which invasive breast cancer was increasingly being treated with breast-conserving surgery (BCS), this paradox became the focus of studies resulting in a trend toward the use of BCS in the treatment of noninvasive breast cancer. Although it is generally agreed that many, if not most, cases of DCIS can be managed with BCS, many questions still remain, including the following:

1. How extensive should resection and therefore margin width be?
2. Which patients (if not all) should receive adjuvant postoperative radiation therapy (RT)? Can a subset of women at such low risk for recurrence be reliably identified to avoid radiation?
3. What role does systemic (i.e., tamoxifen) therapy play in the treatment of local disease (i.e., DCIS)?
4. What is the significance of a diagnosis of DCIS with regard to subsequent risk of invasive breast cancer?

Before addressing these questions, a brief review of our current understanding of DCIS as a distinct entity is appropriate. The biologic behavior of DCIS and its potential as a precursor of invasive carcinoma are unknown; however, DCIS shares many features with invasive carcinoma, suggesting a precursor role in the continuum from normal ductal epithelium to invasive carcinoma. Several small studies of women originally diagnosed with benign breast lesions, but retrospectively determined to have DCIS, show a significant increase in the risk of both ipsilateral tumors in the area of the original lesion and contralateral tumors, suggesting that DCIS is both a precursor and marker lesion (4–6). Eusebi et al. in 1994 reported on 80 cases whose original biopsies were interpreted as benign but that, in retrospect, were actually DCIS; they found that 11.3% ultimately developed invasive carcinoma at a mean 17.5 years of follow-up (7). Page et al. in 1995 reported 32% developed ipsilateral invasive cancer at a mean follow-up of almost 30 years (8).

Simply stated, DCIS is a condition in which the normal ductal epithelium is replaced by cells that have cytologic and molecular features of infiltrating carcinoma. The distinguishing feature of DCIS relative to infiltrating carcinoma is the absence of invasion of the periductal breast stroma. As with infiltrating ductal carcinoma (IDC), DCIS develops in the terminal ductal–lobular unit (TDLU). Relative to the normal TDLU, the epithelium of DCIS demonstrates abnormal proliferation rates that increase with histologic grade (9,10). Relative to normal TDLU epithelium, estrogen receptor (ER) expression is increased in DCIS and, as with IDC, decreases with increasing histologic grade. The percentage of ER positivity for low-grade DCIS ranges from 40% to 98%, whereas that of high-grade DCIS ranges from 14% to 74%. In all studies, ER positivity is consistently higher in low-grade lesions (10–14). In contrast to normal ductal epithelium, and similar to infiltrating carcinoma, DCIS often overexpresses the oncoprotein *Her2-neu*, and this overexpression increases with increasing tumor grade (12,15,16).

Lukas et al. demonstrated *p53* tumor-suppressor gene mutations in 22% of cases of pure DCIS and p53 protein overexpression in 35% of cases of DCIS with concurrent invasive disease. Neither mutation nor overexpression was demonstrated in adjacent normal ductal epithelium. In cases with DCIS and invasion, the *p53* mutations were identical, suggesting a clonal relationship between the components (17). Zolota et al. reported *p53* overexpression in 20% of noncomedo and 78% of comedo carcinoma *in situ* cases (18).

DNA analysis has revealed that nuclear area and volume progressively increase from ductal hyperplasia without atypia to DCIS (19). Similar progression toward aneuploidy also was demonstrated on fluorescent *in situ* hybridization as DCIS grade increases (20). Cellular telomerase activity is important in maintaining chromosomal stability in proliferating cells. Normal breast tissue has essentially no telomerase activity, whereas DCIS and invasive cancer have demonstrable activity in most cases, suggesting an important role in carcinogenesis (21).

Transforming growth factor beta type II receptor (TGF-βRII) expression mediates the inhibition of cell proliferation and tumor progression. Compared with normal breast tissue, TGF-βRII expression is decreased in neoplastic epithelium and is inversely correlated with mitotic count (22).

Cyclin D1, a cell-cycle regulator gene, is not expressed in normal ductal epithelium or hyperplastic epithelium, with or without atypia. Umekita et al. reported cyclin D1 expression in 72% of DCIS cases, 50% of cases with both DCIS and invasion, and 43% with predominately invasive cancers, suggesting an important role in early carcinogenesis (23).

Chromosomal analyses using comparative genomic hybridization reveal consistent chromosomal DNA losses in DCIS and infiltrating carcinoma but other DNA gains in invasive carcinoma, suggesting the presence of protooncogene activation during progression from DCIS to IDC (24). Further evidence that DCIS is a direct precursor of IDC is the finding of genetic similarity between various histologic grades of DCIS and corresponding morphologic types of IDC. Buerger et al. reported a high degree of genetic homology between low-grade DCIS and invasive tubular carcinoma and between high-grade DCIS and grade 3 IDC (25).

These molecular and genetic similarities to invasive cancer suggest that in many cases DCIS is an immediate precursor to invasive cancer, whereas in others, a marker of ductal epithelium predisposed to the development of invasive cancer.

The complexity of the breast ductal architecture must be considered to understand concepts such as multifocality, multicentricity, the importance of margin status, local recurrence, and the role of adjuvant therapy. Rather than simple linear structures coursing from lobules peripherally to the nipple centrally, the ductal system is a complex network in which ducts of one TDLU overlap with the ducts draining other lobular units. What may pathologically appear to be multifocal (separate foci of DCIS within a quadrant) or even multicentric (separate foci involving multiple quadrants) may be, in many cases, extensive involvement of a single complex ductal system (26). Similarly, extensive DCIS throughout a single duct system may explain local recurrences, even with apparently satisfactory surgical margins. The value of local (radiation) and systemic (hormonal) adjuvant therapy in decreasing DCIS recurrence rates is likely attributable to the treatment of this unrecognized, anatomically diffuse disease.

Although the ideal treatment of DCIS remains to be established, several issues must be considered in formulating a treatment plan for each person:

1. Local disease control, minimizing the risk of recurrence of both DCIS and invasive breast cancer in the original tumor area of the ipsilateral breast
2. Treatment morbidity, cost, and convenience
3. Morbidity and mortality of local recurrence when it occurs
4. Likelihood of ultimate breast conservation
5. Prevention of *new* ipsilateral and contralateral *in situ* and invasive lesions

HISTORY OF TREATMENT

As previously stated, prior to the advent of routine mammographic screening, DCIS was diagnosed in women as a palpable breast mass, nipple discharge, or as an incidental finding at the time of biopsy for other lesions, and it accounted for only 1% to 2% of breast cancers. Because of its infrequency and therefore the lack of understanding of this entity, until the early 1980s, treatment of DCIS was mastectomy. Confusion over the biologic nature and histologic classification of DCIS contributed to the reluctance on the part of most surgeons to perform less definitive surgery. Because some surgeons believed that, in most cases, DCIS was unrecognized invasive disease, axillary lymph node dissection was commonly performed at the time of mastectomy. The incidence of lymph node metastasis varied according to the definition of DCIS used. For instance, Haagensen included as DCIS lesions with up to 49% invasive carcinoma; therefore, 38% of these patients had axillary nodal metastasis (27). With recognition of DCIS as a distinct entity and by applying strict pathologic criteria for establishing a diagnosis, it became apparent that DCIS has essentially no metastatic potential and the rare case of lymph node metastasis in all likelihood represents unrecognized invasive disease.

Based on reports of the high frequency with which invasive cancer coexists with DCIS, the existence of "pure" DCIS as a distinct entity was not accepted by many, and most researchers considered mastectomy the only appropriate therapy. In the early 1980s, based on experience with invasive breast cancer and a better understanding of intraductal cancer, the concept of BCS either with or without RT was applied to DCIS.

Silverstein et al., Lagios et al., and others reported on the rarity of lymph node metastasis in pure DCIS. Such reports resulting in omission of axillary dissection from the standard surgical therapy of DCIS, although sentinel lymph node biopsy with enhanced pathologic evaluation and immunohistochemical (IHC) analysis resulted in revisitation of this subject and will be discussed later (28–31).

Although BCS is an accepted form of therapy for many women with DCIS, a great deal of controversy persists over the role of postoperative RT and hormonal adjuvant therapy.

CONTEMPORARY TREATMENT

The contemporary treatment of DCIS must be based not on historical information, but on an understanding of the contemporary status of the disease. In carefully screened populations, up to 30% of mammographically detected (clinically occult) breast cancers are intraductal. Surgery, postoperative RT, and hormonal therapy will be considered in the context of the previously listed treatment considerations. The median diameter of mammographically discovered DCIS is less than 1 cm.

Local Control of Disease

Surgery

Selecting the most appropriate surgical procedure for DCIS requires careful consideration of clinicopathologic features, cosmetic issues, and patient desires. As a general statement, for all women with DCIS, the lowest risk of ipsilateral recurrence results from total mastectomy. Local control is the rule with mastectomy, although most studies report 1% to 2% local recurrence rates because of either residual DCIS or new tumor formation in the 5% of breast tissue that usually remains on the chest wall after total mastectomy (32). Approximately three fourths or more of women with DCIS, depending on the extent of mammographic screening in the population, are candidates for BCS, sometimes followed by RT (to be discussed later). Patients best suited for mastectomy are those with extensive, multifocal or multicentric, high-grade DCIS in whom achieving satisfactory surgical margins in a cosmetically acceptable fashion is not possible. In the Van Nuys experience, women with extensive high-grade DCIS had local recurrence rates of more than 50%, about half of which were invasive, even after receiving postoperative RT (33). Patients with extensive suspicious calcifications by mammography or in whom the extent of DCIS is underestimated by mammography should be counseled regarding the limitations of post-BCS follow-up and the need for mastectomy. It has been suggested that mastectomy-specimen mammography may allow the surgeon the opportunity to re-excise additional skin if necessary in cases where DCIS extends to the skin margins (34). Unlike extensive invasive carcinoma, postmastectomy RT is rarely indicated; therefore, most patients are candidates for immediate reconstruction at the time of mastectomy for DCIS. The most common reconstructive procedures are subpectoral implants or transverse rectus abdominus myocutaneous flaps.

Wide Local Excision

The term *wide local excision* is often used interchangeably with *lumpectomy*, although, in most cases, there is no palpable lump. Furthermore, wide local excision implies achievement of satisfactory surgical margins rather than excision of gross disease only. Because most intraductal cancers are nonpalpable and diagnosed mammographically, wide excision usually requires mammographic needle localization. When the mammographic lesion, usually microcalcifications, is extensive, two or more localization wires are often helpful to bracket the lesion to be excised. Specimen mammography is imperative to confirm lesion excision, and the use of multicolored inks and placement of surgical clips at the specimen margins allow estimation of margin adequacy.

When women with DCIS are analyzed, those treated with excision alone have local recurrence rates ranging from 6% to 43%, depending on the margin status, histologic grade, tumor size, and length of follow-up (Table 12.1). Because of the high risk of local recurrence after excision alone, adjuvant RT is commonly recommended. Women with large lesions, in whom very wide excision is required to achieve adequate surgical margins, resulting in cosmetic deformity, may be candidates for ipsilateral reconstructive procedures such as latissimus flap or breast transposition to correct the surgical defect as an alternative to mastectomy. Posttreatment mammography may be difficult to interpret in this situation and should be considered part of the decision process.

TABLE 12.1. *Local recurrence after excision only*

Trial (ref. no.)	Local recurrence	Comments
NSABP B-06 (31)	43% at 83 mo	
NSABP B-17 (43)	26.8% at 90 mo	50% invasive
		recurrences
Silverstein et al.	21% at 5 yr; 35% at 10-yr actuarial	
Florence	8% at 5 yr; 23% at 10 yr	
Linkoping	22% at 10 yr	
MSKCC	19% at 6 yr	
Lagios	19% at 10-yr actuarial	
Nottingham	6% at 58 mo	
Schwartz et al. (77)	25% at 10-yr actuarial	

MSKCC, Memorial Sloan Kettering Cancer Center; NSABP, National Surgical Adjuvant Breast Project.

Axillary Evaluation

The incidence of axillary lymph node metastasis by standard hematoxylin and eosin (H & E) staining of one level of each node in cases of pure DCIS is essentially nil, and the rare cases of nodal metastasis almost certainly represent unrecognized invasive disease (35). The risk of occult invasion is related to tumor size, histologic grade, and method of detection. Tumor size greater than 25 mm is associated with occult invasion in up to 45% of cases if whole-organ multiple sectioning of breast tissue is performed (36). Comedo-type DCIS is associated with occult invasion in as many as 63% (37). Small, low-grade mammographic lesions rarely are associated with microinvasion, but about 11% of lesions that are palpable (usually comedo) and are associated with nipple discharge or Paget disease, harbor microinvasion (38). The group with the highest risk of harboring occult invasion generally includes younger patients who have palpable, extensive comedo carcinoma and linear branching (casting) calcifications on mammography. In the series by Tabar et al., 76% of the breast cancer mortality in T1A (i.e., < 5 mm) cancers occurred in women with extensive comedo carcinoma, "casting" microcalcifications, and multiple small foci of invasion larger than microinvasive foci (1 mm). The breast cancer mortality in this subset of patients was approximately 40% (39).

In a study by Zarotsky et al., 2 of 14 (14.3%) patients with DCIS and microinvasion had metastases to sentinel lymph nodes when studied by multiple sections of each lymph node, in contrast to nodes studied by traditional single sections (40). In one patient, a micrometastasis was seen in two sentinel nodes by IHC only and in the other patient by H & E in one node. It is our policy at the Breast Health Center at Women & Infants Hospital in Providence, Rhode Island, to perform sentinel lymph node biopsy in patients with extensive DCIS requiring mastectomy to address this possibility in these extensive lesions. Except for these cases (i.e., extensive, high-grade DCIS requiring mastectomy), routine surgical evaluation of axillary lymph nodes in DCIS is not indicated even by sentinel node biopsy. Lymph node metastasis by standard H & E mastectomy in patients with DCIS and microinvasion less than 1 mm is extremely rare.

Axillary nodal metastases have been demonstrated in up to 12% of cases of pure DCIS using enhanced pathologic evaluation with IHC cytokeratin staining, but it is not known whether these cells are truly metastatic DCIS cells and, if so, what is the clinical significance of IHC-only positive nodes (41).

Postoperative Radiation

Most researchers agree that control of local disease is the primary objective in the treatment of DCIS and that postsurgical RT may enhance local control. The European Organization for Research and Treatment of Cancer (EORTC) protocol 10,853 evaluated 1,010 women with DCIS and revealed a local recurrence rate at 4 years of 9% in patients treated with postoperative RT and 16% treated with excision alone (42). The National Surgical Adjuvant Breast Project (NSABP) B-17 randomized 814 patients with DCIS and excision with clear margins to excision alone or with postoperative RT. At 8 years, 27% of those treated with excision alone and 12% receiving RT had recurred locally (43). A major criticism of both EORTC 10853 and NSABP B-17 is the inadequate reporting of significant pathologic information, such as margin status and tumor size. In NSABP B-17, margins were considered ''clear'' if no tumor cells were present at the actual edge of tissue, but tumor could be a few cell layers away. Nearly one fourth of the cases were unavailable for central pathology review. More than 40% of the cases had no tumor size recorded. This lack of pathologic information regarding exact size or width of surgical margin prohibits careful subset analysis for the purpose of defining low-risk patients in whom RT can be safely omitted.

The current literature suggests that the addition of postexcision whole-breast radiation in the treatment of DCIS reduces the local recurrence rate by about 40% to 50%. Approximately 50% of local recurrences after treatment of DCIS with or without radiation are invasive; radiation reduces the risk of both DCIS and invasive recurrences (42,43). Whereas both the EORTC and NSABP B-17 protocols demonstrated that overall radiation is effective in reducing local recurrence rates in women with DCIS, these trials were not designed to identify subgroups of women most likely to benefit from radiotherapy or those in whom the risk of recurrence is sufficiently low to omit radiation. Although there is little doubt that there may be a proportional benefit to radiation, the absolute benefit varies greatly depending on the risk of recurrence after excision only. To make rational recommendations regarding the value of postoperative RT, the risk of local recurrence for each case, with and without RT, should be estimated.

Numerous clinicopathologic factors, such as tumor size, histologic grade, mode of detection (palpable versus mammographic), margin status, presence of tumor necrosis, and patient age, have been evaluated with regard to local recurrence prognostication. Meta-analysis of 30 reported risk factors for local recurrence identified tumor grade (with or without comedo necrosis), size, and margin status as the only significant prognosticators on multivariate analysis, and formed the basis for the Van Nuys Prognostic Index (VNPI) (44).

Lagios and Silverstein reported on 342 patients with DCIS who were treated with lumpectomy alone or lumpectomy and RT with a median follow-up of 82 months. No benefit in local recurrence risk could be demonstrated in patients with surgical margins of 10 mm or more regardless of size or grade. A significant reduction (11%) in local recurrence was seen only in women with high-grade DCIS and inadequate margins (45). Ringberg et al. reported a local recurrence rate of 6% to 10% at a median 63-month follow-up for women with non-high-grade, nondiffuse growth pattern and free margins; the recurrence rate was 31% to 37% for women with extensive disease (46). Cheng et al. demonstrated that size greater than 2.5 cm and involved surgical margins increased the risk of residual DCIS on re-excision. Twenty-four of 35 (68%) patients with tumor size greater than 2.5 cm and 41 of 136 (30%) with close or positive margins had residual disease. Both tumor size and margin status were significantly related to local recurrence on multivariant analysis (47).

In an attempt to identify a group of patients who could safely be treated with excision alone, Silverstein et al. developed the VNPI in 1996. The VNPI consists of the three variables: size, grade, and margin. Each of these variables was scored from 1 to 3, yielding a total VNPI score ranging from 3 to 9 for each patient (Table 12.2)

Based on VNPI scores calculated from prospectively collected pathologic data, patients were retrospectively assigned to risk groups. Risk of recurrence relative to treatment and VNPI score of 394 patients demonstrated 63 recurrences, 30 (48%) of which were invasive. VNPI score correlated inversely with local recurrence risk. Of 116 patients with VNPI scores of 3 or 4 (low risk), 12-year recurrence-free survival and breast cancer–specific survival were 98% and 100%, respectively, with no benefit from postoperative RT. Recurrence-free survival of 245 patients with VNPI scores of 5, 6, or 7 (intermediate risk) was 70% overall, with a 13% statistically significant decrease in local recurrence rate with RT. Those with VNPI scores of 8 or 9 (high risk) had unacceptably high rates (approximately 70%) of local recurrence, even with adjuvant RT (33,44,48). In retrospectively applying the VNPI system to 367 patients with DCIS, deMascarel et al. reported, as in the Van Nuys experience, that local recurrence increased with VNPI score; however, the local recurrence rate for the low-risk group (VNPI 3 or 4) was slightly higher than expected, 4.6% at 71

TABLE 12.2. *Van Nuys Prognostic Index*

Prognostic indicator	1	2	3
Tumor size (mm)	1–15	16–40	>41
Histologic grade	Grade 1 or 2 without necrosis	Grade 1 or 2 with necrosis	Grade 3
Surgical margin width (mm)	>10	1–9	<1

months' median follow-up compared with 2% at 12 years as reported by Silverstein (49).

In 1999, Silverstein et al. reported that margin status is the single most important variable in predicting local recurrence. Regardless of grade and tumor size, of the 133 patients with DCIS excised to 10 mm or more, three recurrences were found after 12 years of follow-up. There was no statistically significant benefit to postoperative RT in this group (50). It has since been pointed out by Silverstein that margin status does not replace the VNPI because the lowest risk of recurrence is in the lowest VNPI group (3–4); one of 150 patients had a recurrence (51). It may be, however, that margin status is a partial surrogate for tumor size and histologic grade. Although it can be stated that patients with margins of 10 mm or larger are at low risk of recurrence, it is not clear whether all patients require a 10-mm margin to achieve comparable local control. Margin status is the most reliably measurable factor in the pathologic evaluation of DCIS and the only factor within control of the surgeon. It is important that margin status be carefully established and recorded; therefore, surgeons must make every effort to achieve adequate margins, which are systematically oriented by use of multicolored inks prior to sending the specimen for pathologic examination (Table 12.3).

TABLE 12.3. *Breast Health Center, Women and Infants Hospital: protocol for breast biopsy and "lumpectomy"*

Specimen handling by surgeon: routine inking	
Superior margin	Green
Medial margin	Red
Lateral margin	Yellow
Inferior margin	Blue
Posterior margin	Black
Anterior margin	Orange
Specimen x-ray (for mammographically-detected lesions):	
Surgeons place medium-sized clips on specimen: "SAM"	
Superior (green)	1 Clip
Anterior (orange)	2 Clips
Medial (red)	3 Clips
Adequate margin	
One centimeter by specimen x-ray for all mammographically-detected suspected cancer or preoperatively proven cancer by FNA or core biopsy.	
One centimeter by gross palpation for all palpable lesions	
Immediate reexcision to achieve adequate margin	
If eccentrically placed lesion by specimen radiograph indicates margin is inadequate, ink reexcision also.	
Pathologist called in all cases	
Pathologists responsible for fixation	
No frozen section on mammographically detected lesions *unless* immediate surgical procedure alteration results from information.	
If necessary, estimation by pathologist of gross or apparent margin.	
Small clip at base of excision of cancers (or suspected cancers) and at medial, lateral, superior, and inferior margin, if possible.	

FNA, fine needle aspiration.

The Van Nuys prospectively acquired data represent the largest reported experi-ence of its kind and challenge dogma regarding the treatment of DCIS. Caution should be used in using this system, however, because of the following concerns about the VNPI reports:

1. Patients were not prospectively randomized to treatment arms, and therefore, therapy selection bias may be an issue.
2. Very detailed and specific (and in many respects unique) pathologic evaluation was carried out by a small number of pathologists using agreed-on classification, size measurement, and margin status assessment systems. This careful pathology assessment may not be widely available.
3. Relative to commonly performed excisions, generous wide excisions (segmental mastectomies) were the norm, with or without reconstruction.
4. No prospective, randomized trials using the VNPI system have been reported to date for validation.

Because of variations in surgical technique, specimen processing, and pathologic interpretation, the VNPI may not be applicable to all other institutions.

Age is a factor in local recurrence risk after a diagnosis of DCIS. Vincini et al. and Van Zee et al. reported that age under 45 years is an independent risk factor for increased local recurrence, possibly because of the greater proportion with high-grade lesions and smaller initial excision volumes relative to older patients (52–54).

The decision to withhold postoperative RT in "low-risk" patients with DCIS must be made with the understanding that a prospective randomized trial addressing this situation has not been performed, but such modification is intuitive, rational, and practical. The Radiation Therapy Oncology Group is conducting such a trial in the near future, and the hope is that it will confirm the safety of this approach as reported in the Van Nuys experience.

Tamoxifen

Tamoxifen therapy appears to decrease both local recurrence of DCIS and the development of new ipsilateral and contralateral intraductal and invasive cancers. Tamoxifen has long been used as adjuvant systemic therapy for invasive breast cancer. NSABP B-14 and a study reported by Cummings et al. in 1993 demonstrated not only a reduction in systemic recurrences but also a decrease in ipsilateral and contralateral intraductal and invasive breast cancers in women taking adjuvant ta-moxifen (55,56). The NSABP-P1 prevention trial showed an approximate 50% de-crease in risk for both invasive ER-positive and intraductal cancers after 5 years of tamoxifen in women at high risk of developing breast cancer by Gail model calcula-tion (57). NSABP B-24 evaluated 1,804 women with DCIS and randomized them to either lumpectomy plus RT or lumpectomy plus RT and tamoxifen for 5 years. Women in the tamoxifen group had fewer overall breast cancer events at 5 years than the placebo group (8.2% versus 13.4%). The combination of RT and tamoxifen resulted in 68% fewer breast cancer events (DCIS and invasive) than those treated with excision only in NSABP-B17 (58). Again, the issue of margin status in this study has been raised because 26% had either positive or unknown margins. It should be pointed out that tamoxifen prevention trials from the Royal Marsden Hospital in London, England, and the European Institute of Oncology in Milan, Italy, failed to demonstrate a significant reduction in breast cancer when tamoxifen was used for prevention. Whereas these studies differ from NSABP P-1 in the number of patients, patient selection, and allowance of estrogen use, further studies are necessary to define the value of tamoxifen as a chemopreventive agent (59,60).

It is not known whether or not the efficacy of tamoxifen in treating DCIS is dependent on ER status. Future studies evaluating the ER status of DCIS are necessary to answer this question; however, *in vitro* studies showed that apoptosis is increased with antiestrogen therapy only in ER-positive DCIS xenografts (61).

Local Recurrence

Local recurrence after treatment of DCIS can have a significant psychological impact. At a minimum, recurrence requires more local therapy, reexcision, or re-excision plus radiotherapy. Mastectomy usually is performed if the original treatment was BCS followed by RT.

About half of local recurrences are invasive (43,62–64) and carry the additional risks of nodal and systemic metastases, often requiring axillary evaluation and systemic therapy in addition to appropriate local therapy. Breast cancer mortality after treatment of DCIS is attributable to these invasive recurrences (62). Most local recurrences occur in the original tumorectomy site (62,65–67). Local recurrence is diagnosed solely by mammography in 85% of cases and in 92% of pure DCIS recurrences (67). Median time to recurrence is approximately 5 years for patients treated with BCS and RT versus 2 years for excision alone (48,67). Preventing local recurrence after a diagnosis of DCIS is an important goal; however, there appears to be little impact of adjuvant RT on survival. While the meta-analysis of the Early Breast Cancer Trialists' Collaborative Group showed an improvement in absolute mortality of 2% with adjuvant breast RT, neither NSABP B-17 or EORTC 10853 showed a significant decrease in mortality with postoperative RT (42,43,68).

Patients initially treated for DCIS with BCS and RT who develop invasive recurrence, usually small and mammographically discovered, have a cause-specific survival of over 80% following mastectomy. Those with pure DCIS recurrences or with mammographically detected lesions rarely develop metastatic disease (62,69). This excellent survival rate is an important issue in counseling patients regarding posttreatment surveillance and adds strength to the appropriateness of BCS for DCIS. Treatment of recurrence is dictated by the size and location of the recurrence, previous treatment, patient preference, and whether the recurrence is purely intraductal or invasive (Table 12.4).

Although salvage mastectomy is standard in patients originally treated with BCS and RT, limited data suggest that further BCS with or without brachytherapy to the tumor bed is an option for women highly motivated to avoid mastectomy who are

TABLE 12.4. *Treatment options for local recurrence after treatment for DCIS*

Original therapy	Type of LR	Treatment options
BCS alone	Pure DCIS	Further BCS alone if non—high-grade, ≥ 1 cm margins
		Further BCS plus RT
		Mastectomy
	Invasive	BCS with SLNB (or ALND) plus RT
		Modified radical mastectomy or total mastectomy with SLN and appropriate systemic therapy
BCS plus RT	Pure DCIS	Total mastectomy
		Wide reexcision plus brachytherapy
		Wide reexcision if non—high-grade and margin ≥ 1 cm
	Invasive	Modified radical mastectomy and appropriate systemic therapy
		Wide local excision with ≥1-cm margins
Mastectomy	Pure DCIS	Wide excision plus radiation
	Invasive	Wide excision plus axillary evaluation, followed by radiation and appropriate systemic therapy

ALND, axillary lymph node dissection; BCS, breast-conserving surgery; DCIS, ductal carcinoma *in situ*; LR, local recurrence; RT, radiation therapy; SLNB, sentinel lymph node biopsy.

willing to accept a higher risk of recurrence. Mullen et al. reported on 19 such patients with an actuarial 5-year failure rate of 20% and no therapy-related complications (70). The long-term effectiveness of this approach remains to be determined.

For women with small, non–high-grade, pure DCIS local recurrences, originally treated with BCS alone, wide reexcision to achieve satisfactory margins, with or without postoperative RT, is an option. Although approximately one third of such patients were treated with further BCS in the NSABP B-17 trial, long-term follow-up on these patients is lacking (43).

In general, invasive recurrence after treatment of DCIS should be treated with salvage mastectomy with surgical evaluation of the axillary lymph nodes if RT was given initially. Limited data exist on the value of sentinel lymph node biopsy in this setting, but it would seem to be a logical procedure. Levels I and II axillary dissection should be considered if sentinel node biopsy is not suitable. BCS with axillary evaluation by sentinel node biopsy, followed by RT, is an option for women originally treated with BCS without RT. Recurrence after mastectomy for DCIS is often invasive and should be treated with wide excision and axillary evaluation, followed by RT.

LIFETIME RISK OF INVASIVE CANCER AND CHEMOPREVENTION

Women who have been diagnosed with DCIS have an increased lifetime risk of developing new invasive carcinoma in both the ipsilateral and contralateral breast. This lifetime risk is approximately 0.5% to 1% per year up to approximately 15 years, after which risk plateaus (71,72).

After completion of therapy for DCIS, it is therefore appropriate to counsel women on this increased lifetime risk and to discuss early detection and preventive strategies. Early detection strategies include regular mammography and clinical examination indefinitely.

Primary preventive strategies include chemoprevention with tamoxifen, based on the results of the NSABP P-1 trial, participation in the STAR Trial (study of tamoxifen and raloxifene), or prophylactic bilateral mastectomy. While promising, questions still remain regarding the long-term benefit of tamoxifen on breast cancer incidence and, even more importantly, on mortality. In the NSABP P-1 trial, only ER-positive tumors were prevented, suggesting that breast cancer mortality may be reduced to a much smaller degree than incidence, if at all (57).

POSTTREATMENT FOLLOW-UP

Women diagnosed with and treated for DCIS are at risk for true local recurrence and new ipsilateral and contralateral breast cancer events. Early detection with optimal outcome requires careful surveillance. A commonly recommended follow-up schedule after treatment for DCIS includes the following:

1. Clinical breast examination by a physician every 4 to 6 months
2. Mammogram of treated breast every 6 months (after BCS) for 2 years and annually thereafter
3. Yearly contralateral mammogram

In view of the fact that nearly 50% of recurrences following RT occur after 4 years, some have suggested continuing ipsilateral mammography every 6 months for up to 5 or 10 years (2). Treatment of recurrences is successful in most cases if detected early.

SPECIAL SITUATIONS

Paget Disease and Ductal Carcinoma *In Situ*

Mammary Paget disease is defined by the presence of characteristic tumor cells in the epidermis of the nipple-areolar complex. Approximately 95% of cases are associated with an underlying DCIS or IDC. The most common clinical manifestation of Paget disease is an eczematoid lesion of the nipple and, less commonly, nipple discharge or a palpable mass.

Historically, mastectomy has been the standard therapy for Paget disease. Fourquet et al., in one of the largest series published on mammary Paget disease, found that all 67 patients treated with modified radical mastectomy had underlying DCIS, and microinvasion was found in 23%. No axillary nodal metastases were identified. At 82 months' follow-up, none had recurred. In their study, 44 patients were treated with BCS with RT, 36 of whom had biopsy only of the primary tumor, followed by RT, eight had complete excision of the nipple–areolar complex with underlying

TABLE 12.5. *Breast Health Center, Women and Infants Hospital: protocol for the management of duct carcinoma* in situ *(DCIS)[a]*

Features specified: Size, grade, necrosis, surgical excision margins, method of detection, microinvasion

Strategy based on the Van Nuys Prognostic Index (VNPI)

The VNPI scoring system. One to three points are awarded for each of three different predictors of local breast recurrence (size, surgical excision margins, and pathologic classification). Scores for each of the predictors are totaled to yield a VNPI score ranging from a low of 3 to a high of 9.

Score	1	2	3
Size (mm)	≤15	16–40	≥41
Margins (mm)	≥10	1–9	<1
Pathologic classification	Non-high grade without necrosis	Non-high grade with necrosis	High grade with or without necrosis

VNPI 3 or 4
  Primary cancer: Excision to 1-cm surgical margins
  Axillary dissection: None
  Adjuvant radiotherapy: None
VNPI 5,6, or 7
  Primary cancer: Excision or reexcision to 1-cm surgical margins
  Axillary dissection: None
  Adjuvant radiotherapy: Selection between observation or radiation therapy depending on excision margin. If 1-cm margin or negative reexcision, no radiation
VNPI 8 or 9
  Primary cancer: Mastectomy with or without reconstruction (implies 1-cm margin cannot be achieved)
  Axillary dissection: None or sentinel node biopsy only
  Adjuvant radiotherapy: None after mastectomy

[a] Includes DCIS with microinvasion (≤1 mm invasive focus).

breast tissue. At 82 months' median follow-up, there were eight local recurrences (22%) in the group receiving RT, two of which were associated with microinvasion. None of the eight treated with nipple–areolar excision prior to RT had recurrence (73). Smaller studies on the treatment of mammary Paget disease with underlying DCIS showed local recurrence rates ranging from 0% to 40% in patients treated with wide excision only and 0% to 22% when treated with RT after excision. Whether treated by mastectomy or BCS with or without RT, mortality in most studies has been 0% to 5% (74–76).

Based on the limited current data, it appears that excision of the nipple–areolar complex with underlying central breast tissue with careful analysis to ensure adequate margins is an acceptable alternative to mastectomy. Some patients may benefit from added RT. Because of the frequent association of Paget disease with invasive carcinoma, evaluation of the axilla, preferably with sentinel node biopsy, should be considered at the time of mastectomy.

Ductal Carcinoma *In Situ* Presenting with Nipple Discharge

When women with DCIS present with spontaneous ipsilateral discharge, the extent of disease is often greater than clinical or mammographic evaluation would indicate. The risk of recurrence after excision alone is significant (77). Bauer et al. reported on 43 women with nipple discharge from DCIS. Discharge cytology was positive in only 16% of those examined, and only 50% had filling defects on ductography; microinvasion was detected in 28%. Multifocal or extensive DCIS was found in 86%, and 84% had residual disease after initial biopsy. Mastectomy was required to achieve adequate excision in 74% (78). It appears that nipple discharge is a predictor of unfavorable disease pattern in women with DCIS and that most will ultimately require mastectomy to achieve local control (Table 12.5).

SUMMARY

Our understanding of the histology, clinical behavior, and optimal treatment of DCIS is rapidly evolving. The preponderance of evidence suggests the following:

1. As mammographic screening compliance improves, more cases of DCIS will be detected. This does not necessarily equate to an increase in actual incidence. If DCIS is a precursor in many cases to invasive cancer, detection of DCIS ultimately should decrease the incidence and mortality of invasive cancer.

2. Prevention of local recurrence (both DCIS and invasive cancer) is an important goal. As with most diseases, however, apportionment of treatment aggressiveness should be based on the risk of the cancer. Although radiation is an effective modality in treating DCIS with inadequate margins, there are subsets of women in whom the morbidity, inconvenience, and cost of radiation far outweighs a small benefit. This subset appears to be women with non–high-grade, small, mammographically detected tumors with adequate (1 cm) surgical margins. This therapy needs to be confirmed by prospective randomized trials, building on the Van Nuys experience. It is quite likely that not all women even require 10-mm margins to achieve satisfactory local control. Local recurrence prevention is an important goal, but it has little to no impact on breast cancer survival, regardless of various therapy options.

3. Preventing new breast cancer events in women identified to be at increased risk by virtue of their DCIS diagnosis may be another important goal. Whether tamoxifen or other selective ER modifiers will provide such long-term risk reduction and reduce breast cancer mortality remains to be determined.

Each patient should be treated in an individualized fashion after careful consideration of personal, clinical, and pathologic factors through a multidisciplinary approach. It is important that each patient be made aware of the limitations in our current understanding of DCIS, so that rational, honest counseling can take place.

REFERENCES

1. Welch HG, Black WC. Using autopsy series to estimate the disease "reservoir" for ductal carcinoma *in situ* of the breast: how much more breast cancer can we find? *Ann Intern Med* 1997;127:1023–1028.

2. Consensus Conference Committee. Consensus on the Classification of Ductal Carcinoma *In-situ*, April 25–28, 1997. *Cancer* 1997;80:1798–1802.
3. Hermann G, Keller RJ, Drossman S, et al. Mammographic pattern of microcalcifications in the preoperative diagnosis of comedo ductal carcinoma in situ: histopathologic correlation. *Can Assoc Radiol J* 1999;50:235–240.
4. Page DL, Dupont WD, Rogers LW, et al. Intraductal carcinoma of the breast: follow-u after biopsy only. *Cancer* 1982;49:751–758.
5. Rosen PP, Braun DW Jr, Kinne D. The clinical significance of pre-invasive breast carcinoma. *Cancer* 1980;46:919–925.
6. Betsill WL Jr, Rosen PP, Lieberman PH, et al. Intraductal carcinoma: long-term follow-up after treatment by biopsy alone. *JAMA* 1978;239:1863–1867.
7. Eusebi V, Feudale E, Foschini MP, et al. Long-term follow-up of *in situ* carcinoma of the breast. *Semin Diagn Pathol* 1994;11:223–235.
8. Page DL, Dupont WD, Rogers LW, et al. Continued local recurrence of carcinoma 15-25 years after a diagnosis of low grade ductal carcinoma *in situ* of the breast treated only by biopsy. *Cancer* 1995; 76:1197–1200.
9. Allred DC, Hilsenbeck SG, Fugua SAW, et al. Cell turnover (proliferation and apoptosis) in normal epithelium and premalignant lesions in the same breasts. *Breast Cancer Res Treat* 1996;
10. Zafrani B, Leroyer A, Fourguet A, et al. Mammographically detected ductal carcinoma in-situ of the breast analyzed with a new classification: a study of 127 cases: correlation with estrogen and progesterone receptors, p53, c-erba B-2 proteins, and proliferative activity. *Semin Diagn Pathol* 1994; 11:208–214.
11. Albonico G, Querzoli P, Fereti S, et al. Mia phenotypes of breast carcinoma in situ defined by image analysis of biological parameters. *Pathol Res Pract* 1996;192:117–123.
12. Berardo M, Hilsenbeck SG, Allred DC. Histological grading of noninvasive breast cancer and its relationship to biological features. *Lab Invest* 1996;74:15A.
13. Helin HJ, Helle MJ, Kallioniemi O-P, et al. Immunohistochemical determination of estrogen and progesterone receptors in human breast carcinoma: correlation with histopathology and DNA flow cytometry. *Cancer* 1989;63:1761–1767.
14. Pollen DN, Snead DRJ, Roberts EC, et al. Oestrogen receptor expression in ductal carcinoma in situ of the breast: relationship to flow cytometric analysis of DNA and expression of the c-er3B-2 oncoprotein. *Br J Cancer* 1993;68:156–161.
15. Bobrow LG, Happerfield LC, Gregory WM, et al. The classification of ductal carcinoma in situ and its association with biological markers. *Semin Diagn Pathol* 1994;11:199–207.
16. Kanthan R, Xiang J, Magliocco AM. P53, ErbB2, and TAG-72 expression in the spectrum of ductal carcinoma *in situ* of the breast classified by the Van Nuys system. *Arch Pathol Lab Med* 2000;124: 234–239.
17. Lukas J, Niu N, Press MF. P53 mutations and expression in breast carcinoma in-situ. *Am J Pathol* 2000;156:183–191.
18. Zolota V, Gerokosta A, Melachrinou M, et al. Microvessel density, proliferating activity, p53 and bcl-2 expression in *in situ* ductal carcinoma of the breast. *Anticancer Res* 1999;19:3269–3274.
19. Ruiz A, Almenar S, Callaghan RC, et al. Benign, preinvasive and invasive ductal breast lesions: a comparative study with quantitative techniques: morphometry, image- and flow cytometry. *Pathol Res Pract* 1999;195:741–746.
20. Visscher D, Jimenez RE, Grayson M III, et al. Histopathologic analysis of chromosome aneuploidy in ductal carcinoma *in situ*. *Hum Pathol* 2000;31:201–207.
21. Shpitz B, Zimlichman S, Zemer R, et al. Telomerase activity in ductal carcinoma *in situ* of the breast. *Breast Cancer Res Treat* 1999;58:65–69
22. Gobbi H, Arteaga CL, Jensen RA, et al. Loss of expression of transforming growth factor beta type II receptor correlates with high tumour grade in human breast *in-situ* and invasive carcinomas. *Histopathology* 2000;36:168–177.
23. Umekita Y, Yoshida H. Cyclin D1 expression in ductal carcinoma *in situ*, atypical ductal hyperplasia and usual ductal hyperplasia: an immunohistochemical study. *Pathol Int* 2000;50:527–530.
24. Aubele M, Mattis A, Zitzelsberger H, et al. Extensive ductal carcinoma *in situ* with small foci of invasive ductal carcinoma: evidence of genetic resemblance by CGH. *Int J Cancer* 2000;85:82–86.
25. Buerger H, Otterbach F, Simon R, et al. Different genetic pathways in the evolution of invasive breast cancer are associated with distinct morphologic subtypes. *J Pathol* 1999;189:521–526.
26. Faverly DRG, Burgers L, Bult P, et al. Three-dimensional imaging of mammary ductal carcinoma *in situ*: clinical implications. *Semin Diagn Pathol* 1994;11:193–198.

27. Haagensen CD. Intraductal carcinoma. In: Haagensen CD, ed. *Diseases of the breast*. Philadelphia: WB Saunders, 1971:586–590.
28. Silverstein MJ, Gierson ED, Waisman JR, et al. Axillary lymph node dissection for T1a breast carcinoma: is it indicated? *Cancer* 1994;73:664–667.
29. Lagios MD, Margolin FR, Westdahl PR, et al. Mammographically detected duct carcinoma *in situ*. *Cancer* 1989;63:618–624.
30. Ashikari R, Hajdu SI, Robbins GF. Intraductal carcinoma of the breast (1960–1969). *Cancer* 1971; 28:1182–1187.
31. Fisher ER, Sass R, Fisher B, et al. Pathologic findings from the National Surgical Adjuvant Breast Project (protocol 6), I. Intraductal carcinoma (DCIS). *Cancer* 1986;57:197–208.
32. Clark L, Ritter E, Glazebrook K, Tyler D. Recurrent ductal carcinoma in-situ after total mastectomy. *J Surg Oncol* 1999;71:182–185.
33. Silverstein MJ, Lagios MD, Craig PH, et al. A prognostic index for ductal carcinoma *in situ* of the breast. *Cancer* 1996;77:2267–2274.
34. Rubio I, Mirza N, Sahin A, et al. Role of specimen radiography in patients treated with skin-sparing mastectomy for ductal carcinoma *in situ* of the breast. *Ann Surg Oncol* 2000;7:544–548.
35. Silverstein MJ, ed. *Ductal carcinoma in situ of the breast*. Baltimore: Williams & Wilkins, 1997: 580.
36. Lagios MD, Westdahl PR, Margolin FR, et al. Duct carcinoma *in situ*: relationship of extent of noninvasive disease to the frequency of occult invasion, multicentricity, lymph node metastases and short-term treatment failures. *Cancer* 1982;50:1309–1314.
37. Patchefsky AS, Schwartz GF, Finkelstein SD, et al. Heterogeneity of intraductal carcinoma of the breast. *Cancer* 1989;63:731–741.
38. Gump FE, Jicha DL, Ozello L. Ductal carcinoma *in situ* (DCIS): a revised concept. *Surgery* 1987; 102:790–795.
39. Tabar L, Chen HH, Duffy SW, et al. A novel method for prediction of long-term outcome of women with T1a, T1b, and 10-14 mm invasive breast cancers: a prospective study. *Lancet* 2000;355: 429–433.
40. Zarotsky J, Hansen N, Brennan M, et al. Lymph node metastasis from ductal carcinoma in-situ with microinvasion. *Cancer* 1999;85:2439–2443.
41. Klauber-Demore N, Tan LK, Liberman L, et al. Sentinel lymph node biopsy: is it indicated in patients with high-risk ductal carcinoma *in situ* and ductal carcinoma *in situ* with microinvasion? *Ann Surg Oncol* 2000;7:636–642.
42. Julien JP, Mijken N, Fentimen IS, et al. Radiotherapy in breast-conserving treatment for ductal carcinoma in situ: first results of the EORTC randomized phase III trial 10853. EORTC Breast Cancer Cooperative Group and EORTC Radiotherapy Group. *Lancet* 2000;12:528–533.
43. Fisher E, Dignam J, Tan-Cheim E, et al. Pathologic findings from the National Surgical Adjuvant Breast Project (NSABP) Eight-Year Update of Protocol B-17. *Cancer* 1999;86:429–438.
44. Silverstein JM, ed. *Ductal carcinoma of the breast*. Baltimore: Williams & Wilkins, 1997:271–284.
45. Lagios MD, Silverstein MJ. Ductal carcinoma *in situ*. The success of breast conservation therapy: a shared experience of two single institutional nonrandomized prospective studies. *Surg Oncol Clin N Am* 1997;6:385–392.
46. Ringberg A, Idvall I, Ferno M, et al. Ipsilateral local recurrence in relation to therapy and morphological characteristics in patients with ductal carcinoma *in situ* of the breast. *Eur J Surg Oncol* 2000;26: 444–451.
47. Cheng L, Al-Kaisi NK, Gorden NH, et al. Relationship between the size and margin status of ductal carcinoma *in situ* of the breast and residual disease. *J Natl Cancer Inst* 1997;89:1356–1360.
48. Silverstein MJ. Prognostic factors and local recurrence in patients with ductal carcinoma *in situ* of the breast. *The Breast* 1998;4:349–362.
49. DeMascarel I, Bonichor F, MarGrogan G, et al. Application of the Van Nuys Prognostic index in a retrospective series of 367 ductal carcinoma *in situ* of the breast examined by serial microscopic sectioning: practical considerations. *Breast Cancer Res Treat* 2000;61:151–159.
50. Silverstein MJ, Lagios MD, Groshen S, et al. The influence of margin width on local control of ductal carcinoma *in situ* of the breast. *N Engl J Med* 1999;340:1455–1461.
51. Silverstein MJ. Not everyone with ductal carcinoma in situ of the breast treated with breast preservation needs post-excision radiation therapy. *The Breast* 2000;9:189–193.
52. VanZee KJ, Liberman L, Samli B, et al. Long term follow-up of women with ductal carcinoma in-situ treated with breast conserving surgery: the effect of age. *Cancer* 1999;86:1757–1767.

53. Vincini FA, Kestin LL, Goldstein NS, et al. Impact of young age on outcome in patients with ductal carcinoma *in situ* treated with breast conserving therapy. *J Clin Oncol* 2000;18:296–306.
54. Goldstein NS, Vincini FA, Kestin LL, et al. Differences in the pathologic features of ductal carcinoma in situ of the breast based on patient age. *Cancer* 2000;88:2553–2560.
55. Fisher B, Constantino J, Redmond C, et al. A randomized clinical trial evaluation tamoxifen in the treatment of patients with node-negative breast cancer who have estrogen receptor-positive tumors. *N Engl J Med* 1989;320:479–484.
56. Cummings F, Gray R, Turmey D, et al. Adjuvant tamoxifen versus placebo in elderly women with node-positive breast cancer: long term follow-up and causes of death. *J Clin Oncol* 1993;11:29–35.
57. Fisher B, Constantino J, Wickerham L, et al. Tamoxifen for prevention of breast cancer: report of the National Surgical Adjuvant Breast and Bowel Project P-1 Study. *J Natl Cancer Inst* 1998;90: 1371–1388.
58. Fisher B, Dignam J, Womark N, et al. Tamoxifen in treatment of intraductal breast cancer: National Surgical Adjuvant Breast and Bowel Project B-24 randomised controlled trial. *Lancet* 1999;353: 1993–2000.
59. Powles T, Eeles R, Ashley S, et al. Interim analysis of the incidence of breast cancer in the Royal Marsden Hospital Tamoxifen randomised chemoprevention trial. *Lancet* 1998;352:98–102.
60. Veronesi U, Maisonnewve P, Costo A, et al. Prevention of breast cancer with tamoxifen: preliminary findings from the Italian randomised trial among hysterectomised women. *Lancet* 1998;352:93–97.
61. Gandhi A, Hollan P, Know W, et al. Effects of a pure antiestrogen on apoptosis and proliferation on human breast ductal carcinoma *in situ*. *Cancer Res* 2000;60:4284–4288.
62. Solin L, Fourquet A, McCormack B, et al. Salvage treatment for local recurrence following breast-conserving surgery and definitive irradiation for ductal carcinoma *in situ* (intraductal carcinoma) of the breast. *Int J Radiat Oncol Biol Phys* 1994;30:3–9.
63. Fisher B, Constantino J, Redmond C, et al. Lumpectomy compared with lumpectomy and radiation therapy for the treatment of intraductal breast cancer. *N Engl J Med* 1993;328:1581–1586.
64. Lagios MD, Margolin FR, Westdahl PR, et al. Mammographically detected duct carcinoma in situ: frequency of local recurrence following tylectomy and prognostic effect of nuclear grade on local recurrence. *Cancer* 1989;63:618–624.
65. Lagios MD. Ductal carcinoma *in situ*: controversies in diagnosis, biology, and treatment. *Breast J* 1995;1:68–78.
66. Silverstein MJ, Cohlan BF, Gierson ED, et al. Duct carcinoma in situ: 227 cases without microinvasion. *Eur J Cancer* 1992;28:630–634.
67. Liberman L, Van Zee K, Dershaw D, et al. Mammographic features of local recurrence in women who have undergone breast-conserving therapy for ductal carcinoma *in-situ*. *AJR Am J Roentgenol* 1997;168:489–493.
68. Early Breast Cancer Trialists' Collaborative Group. Favourable and unfavourable effects on long-term survival of radiotherapy for early breast cancer. *Lancet* 2000;355:1757–1770.
69. Osborne M, Borgen P, Wong G, et al. Salvage mastectomy for local control and regional recurrence after breast-conserving operation and radiation therapy. *Surg Gynecol Obstet* 1992;174:189–194.
70. Mullen E, Deutsch M, Blooner W. Re-excision and reirradiation of local recurrence for salvage of lumpectomy failures. *Proc Am Soc Clin Oncol* 1992;11:60(abst).
71. Singletary SE, Taylor SH, Guinee VF, et al. Occurrence and prognosis of contralateral breast cancer. *J Am Coll Surg* 1994;178:390–396.
72. Anderson DE, Badzioch MD. Bilaterality in familial breast cancer patients. *Cancer* 1985;56: 2092–2098.
73. Fourquet A, Zafrani B, Campana F. Breast conserving treatment of Paget's disease with irradiation. In: Silverstein MJ, ed. *Ductal carcinoma in situ of the breast*. Baltimore: Williams & Wilkins, 1997: 545–549.
74. Stockdale AD, Brierly JD, White WF, et al. Radiotherapy for Paget's disease of the nipple: a conservative alternative. *Lancet* 1989;2:664–666.
75. Lagios M, Westdahl P, Rose M, et al. Paget's disease of the nipple: alternative management in cases without or with minimal extent of underlying breast carcinoma. *Cancer* 1984;54:545–551.
76. Bulens P Vanyutsel L, Pigndeus A, et al. Breast conserving treatment of Paget's disease. *Radiother Oncol* 1990:17:305–309.
77. Schwartz G, Schwarting R, Cornfield D, et al. Subclinical duct carcinoma *in situ* of the breast (DCIS): treatment by local excision and surveillance alone. *Proc Am Soc Clin Oncol* 1996;15:101.
78. Bauer R, Eckhert K, Nomoto T. Ductal carcinoma *in situ*-associated nipple discharge: a clinical marker for locally extensive disease. *Ann Surg Oncol* 1998;5:452–455.

13

Surgery for Primary Invasive Breast Cancer

Ismail Jatoi

In the nineteenth century, German pathologist Rudolf Virchow (Fig. 13.1) studied the morbid anatomy of breast cancer. He undertook a series of postmortem dissections and postulated that breast cancer spreads along fascial planes and lymphatic channels (1). Little importance was given to the hematogenous spread of cancer. Virchow's hypothesis influenced the work of American surgeon William Halsted (Fig. 13.2). In the late nineteenth century, Halsted described the radical mastectomy for the treatment of breast cancer (2). This operation removed the breast, the underlying pectoralis muscles, and the ipsilateral axillary lymph nodes. Thus, in keeping with the postulates of Virchow's hypothesis, the lymphatic channels connecting the breast and axillary lymph nodes were extirpated *en bloc*. Halsted argued that resection of a node-negative breast cancer was curative, believing that such tumors were extirpated before distant spread through the lymphatics occurred. Halsted also maintained that the extent of both the mastectomy and axillary dissection were important determinants of outcome. Therefore, breast cancer recurrence and distant metastases often were attributed to inadequate surgery.

By the early twentieth century, the radical mastectomy had become widely accepted as the standard treatment for breast cancer. The risk of local recurrence was far less with the radical mastectomy than with other contemporary procedures. The radical mastectomy also was credited with improving survival from breast cancer during the early years of the twentieth century (3). This improvement in survival was probably largely attributable to the effect of lead-time bias, however, rather than to any advancement in surgical technique. Indeed, by the turn of the century, patients were seeking medical attention sooner (with smaller tumors).

One important observation was inconsistent with the Halsted paradigm. About 30% of node-negative breast cancer patients die of metastatic disease within 10 years after surgery (4). This finding suggests that the lymphatics are not the only source for the distant spread of cancer. Yet most surgeons in the early twentieth century were not willing to discard the halstedian concept that the distant spread of breast cancer occurs solely through the lymphatics. Some proposed that metastatic spread through the internal mammary and supraclavicular lymph node chains might account for distant relapse in women whose axilla were free of nodal involvement (5,6). Extirpation of these additional nodal chains failed to improve outcome, however, and these more extensive lymphadenectomies were soon abandoned (7,8).

The radical mastectomy remained the cornerstone for the treatment of breast

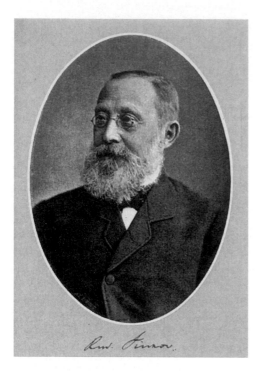

FIG. 13.1. Dr. Rudolf Virchow. (Courtesy of the Pathology Institute, University of Wurzburg.)

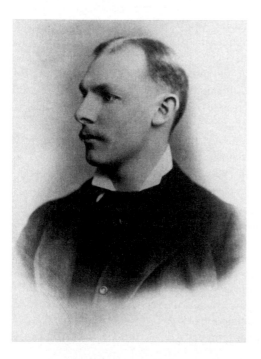

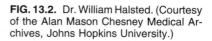

FIG. 13.2. Dr. William Halsted. (Courtesy of the Alan Mason Chesney Medical Archives, Johns Hopkins University.)

cancer for about the first three quarters of the twentieth century. Thereafter, the operation lost favor. By the latter half of the twentieth century, many surgeons regarded the radical mastectomy as too debilitating, and several centers were reporting good outcome with less extensive surgery (9,10). These lesser procedures also included the modified radical mastectomy (which spared the pectoralis muscles) and simple excision of the primary breast tumor. The trend toward less radical surgery was attributable to two important factors (11). First, surgeons during the latter half of the twentieth century were seeing patients with smaller tumors, and these were often amenable to local excision. Second, there were improvements in radiotherapy (RT) techniques, enabling tumoricidal doses to be delivered effectively without significant damage to surrounding tissues. Thus, many surgeons developed an interest in breast-conserving surgery (BCS), undertaken in conjunction with breast RT.

Skepticism concerning the merits of the Halsted radical mastectomy surfaced in 1962, when Bloom et al. reported on the survival of 250 patients with primary breast cancer who received no treatment (12). These patients were diagnosed clinically between the years 1805 and 1933 at the Middlesex Hospital in London, England, and the tissue diagnosis was established at autopsy. The survival rate of these untreated patients was almost identical to Halsted's patients who were treated with the radical mastectomy. This seemed to suggest that surgery contributes little to reducing the risk of death from breast cancer; however, the impact of surgery 100 years ago might have been quite different from what it is today. Patients in the late nineteenth century generally presented with cancers at an advanced stage. In many instances, distant metastases were perhaps already present, and surgery therefore might have had little impact on the natural history of the disease. In contrast, patients seen today generally present with early disease. Thus, in the absence of metastases, local therapy alone could cure some patients.

During the last 25 years, the tenets of the Halsted paradigm were put to the test in several large, randomized prospective trials. These trials examined the effect of various surgical options in the treatment of breast cancer. None of these trials compared surgical treatment with no treatment, and so the true effect of surgery on breast cancer mortality was never established. The results of these trials suggest, however, that the extent of surgery (often in combination with RT) does not affect breast cancer mortality.

The National Surgical Adjuvant Breast Project-04 (NSABP-04) and King's/Cambridge trials randomized patients with clinically node-negative breast cancer to either early or delayed treatment of the axilla (13,14). In the NSABP-04 trial, 1,665 clinically node-negative women received either no initial treatment to the axilla or initial treatment with axillary lymph node dissection (ALND) or RT (13). About 18% of patients who received no initial axillary treatment developed axillary adenopathy and subsequently were treated with ALND. Yet there was no significant difference in breast cancer mortality between patients in the three arms of the trial. In the King's/Cambridge trial, 2,243 women with clinically node-negative breast cancer were randomly assigned to either total mastectomy and immediate RT to the axilla or total mastectomy and careful observation of the axilla (14). In the group assigned to observation, RT was delayed until there was progression or recurrence of the disease in the axilla. No significant difference in breast cancer mortality was found between the two groups, however. The NSABP-04 and King's/Cambridge trials indicated that the delayed treatment of the axilla does not adversely affect breast cancer mortality. This finding suggests that the axillary lymph nodes are not a nidus for the further spread of cancer, a finding that is inconsistent with the Halsted hypothesis.

Halsted also proposed that breast cancer is a locally progressive disease. He had argued that metastases occurred by the contiguous and centrifugal spread of cancer from the primary tumor in the breast. If this were true, then the extent of the mastectomy should influence survival. During the last 25 years, this hypothesis was tested in six large, randomized prospective trials. These were the Milan I, Institute Gustave-Roussy, NSABP-06, U.S. National Cancer Institute, European Organization for Research and Treatment of Cancer (EORTC), and Danish Breast Cancer Group trials (15–20). These trials compared either the radical mastectomy or the modified radical mastectomy with less extensive procedures (variously labeled as segmentectomy, lumpectomy, tylectomy, quadrantectomy, or wide local excision), undertaken in conjunction with an axillary lymph node dissection. All these trials showed that the extent of the mastectomy has no impact on breast cancer mortality.

The NSABP-06 was the largest of these six trials (17). There were 1,843 patients randomized to one of three groups: total mastectomy and axillary dissection (modified radical mastectomy), lumpectomy and axillary dissection, or lumpectomy and axillary dissection followed by breast RT. The NSABP-06 found no difference in survival between patients in the three arms of the study; however, the incidence of local breast tumor recurrence in the lumpectomy plus breast radiation group was significantly lower than that in the lumpectomy group who received no radiation. Thus, RT is generally used today in conjunction with BCS in the treatment of primary breast cancer.

LOCAL RECURRENCES

Local recurrences following total mastectomy may occur on the chest wall; the skin overlying the chest wall; or the axillary, internal mammary, supraclavicular and infraclavicular lymph nodes (21). However, women treated with BCS are also at risk for recurrences in the ipsilateral breast (22). Thus, breast cancer patients treated with BCS have, overall, a greater risk of local recurrence than those treated with total mastectomy. Yet this increased risk of local recurrence does not result in a worse overall survival. Fisher argued that ipsilateral breast tumor recurrences following BCS are indicators of distant disease that is already present (23). He regards such recurrences as markers for poor prognosis but not the cause of the poor prognosis. Studies have shown that, following BCS, women who develop ipsilateral breast tumor recurrences have greater than a threefold increased risk of developing distant metastases compared with those who do not develop such recurrences (24).

Also, patients who develop recurrences in the ipsilateral breast within 3 to 5 years following BCS seem to have a worse prognosis than those who develop such recurrences later (25).

Radiation therapy can reduce the risk of ipsilateral breast tumor recurrences. In the NSABP-06 study, the risk of ipsilateral breast tumor recurrences was about 40% following lumpectomy and about 10% following lumpectomy and RT (17). For patients treated with total mastectomy, the risk of ipsilateral breast tumor recurrences was essentially nil. Ipsilateral breast tumor recurrences are generally treated with salvage mastectomy (total mastectomy), and the 10-year actuarial survival for these patients is about 58% (21). In contrast, local recurrences in the chest wall, ipsilateral axilla, or supraclavicular and infraclavicular fossa carry a worse prognosis. More than 90% of these patients will develop distant metastases, and most will die of this disease within 10 years after recurrence (26).

What factors influence the risk of ipsilateral breast tumor recurrence following BCS? Several investigators have addressed this question. Borger et al. studied 1,026 patients treated at the Netherlands Cancer Institute with BCS and RT (27). Univariate analysis showed that seven factors were associated with an increased risk of ipsilateral breast tumor recurrence: age, residual tumor at reexcision, histologic tumor type, presence of any components of carcinoma *in situ* component, vascular invasion, microscopic margin involvement, and whole-breast radiation dose. Only two factors remained independently significant after proportional hazard regression analysis: age and the presence of vascular invasion. Thus, ipsilateral breast tumor recurrence rates were 6% for patients less than 40 years of age and 8% for patients with tumors showing vascular invasion at 5 years. In the absence of these factors, the risk of ipsilateral breast tumor recurrence after BCS was only about 1% at 5 years.

Turner et al. found that women who carry a *BRCA* mutation (*BRCA1* or *BRCA2*) are more likely to develop ipsilateral breast tumor recurrences following BCS and radiotherapy (28). The median time to ipsilateral breast tumor recurrence was 7.8 years for patients with *BRCA1* or *BRCA2* mutations, compared with 4.7 years for patients without such mutations. The longer time to recurrence in the carriers of these mutations suggests that these were second *de novo* primary tumors. The *BRCA* genes play an important role in DNA repair, and recent studies suggest that persons who carry mutations in these genes might be extremely sensitive to the effects of RT (29). Thus, one might speculate that RT administered following BCS may play a role in the development of *de novo* ipsilateral breast cancers in the carriers of *BRCA* mutations.

SURGICAL OPTIONS

The clinical trials discussed in the preceding sections suggest that permutations in surgical therapy have no impact on breast cancer mortality. As a result, the radical mastectomy is no longer accepted as the standard option for the surgical treatment of primary breast cancer. Although BCS puts the patient at risk for ipsilateral breast tumor recurrence, this risk is reduced with RT. Today, a patient with primary breast cancer is generally presented with three surgical options (Table 13.1). She may elect to undergo a modified radical mastectomy (removal of the breast and axillary lymph nodes). If she chooses this option, she can often avoid RT (although recent studies have shown that, after modified radical mastectomy, node-positive patients also benefit from RT). Patients treated with the modified radical mastectomy also may undergo breast reconstructive surgery, which is discussed later. Alternatively, the patient may choose to undergo a breast-conserving procedure along with an ALND. This is generally considered the preferred surgical option because it results in the best cosmetic and tactile outcome. If a patient elects this option, she will require RT to reduce the risk of ipsilateral breast tumor recurrence.

Various terms are used to describe these breast-conserving procedures, including segmental mastectomy, lumpectomy, tylectomy, wide local excision, and quadrantectomy. Essentially, these terms refer to the extirpation of the breast tumor with various margins of normal breast tissue. The terms *segmental mastectomy* and *lumpectomy* often are used interchangeably. These terms refer to the resection of the breast tumor with enough surrounding normal tissue to result in microscopically tumor-free surgical margins. By definition, tumor cells may approach to within one cell's breadth of the surgical margin. The term *extended tylectomy* was used at the Guy's Hospital in London to describe resection of the breast tumor plus surrounding breast tissue within 3 cm of the tumor mass (30). The microscopic status of the surgical margins was not defined. In the *quadrantectomy*, described by Veronesi et al. at the Tumor Institute of Milan, Italy, the entire quadrant of the breast containing the tumor is removed (15).

After any breast-conserving procedure, RT is administered to eliminate occult tumor foci remaining in the ipsilateral breast. RT to the breast can be initiated 10 to 14 days after surgery. If chemotherapy is also planned, RT is postponed until one or more doses of chemotherapy are administered. RT is discussed in a separate chapter in this book.

TABLE 13.1. *Surgical options for primary invasive breast cancer*

Breast-conserving surgery	Resection of tumor and margin of normal tissue Axillary dissection Radiotherapy always required
Modified radical mastectomy and breast reconstruction	Resection of entire breast Axillary dissection Breast reconstruction Radiotherapy sometimes required
Modified radical mastectomy	Resection of entire breast Axillary dissection Radiotherapy sometimes required

TABLE 13.2. *Factors that may influence surgical treatment of primary breast cancer*

Patient preference
Pregnancy
Previous radiotherapy
Collagen vascular disease
Tumor size in relation to breast size
Multicentric disease

Most patients with primary breast cancer are suitable candidates for breast-conserving procedures, but there are a few contraindications (31) (Table 13.2). These are relative contraindications only, however, and each patient's circumstances should be examined closely (32). For example, pregnant patients are generally advised not to undergo BCS because RT carries substantial risk to the fetus. Yet it is important to remember that several months of chemotherapy are generally given before RT. Thus, if RT is to be administered after delivery, BCS is an option. Patients who have had previous RT to the breasts are also often advised not to undergo BCS. The radiation oncologists will consider the previous dose of radiation administered, however, and many of these patients can be successfully treated with BCS and RT. Additionally, certain coexisting medical problems, such as collagen vascular diseases, may adversely affect the cosmetic results after RT and thereby increase the risk of complications. Collagen vascular disease is an issue only when there is active disease.

Patients with large tumors often are advised to undergo a modified radical mastectomy rather than a breast-conserving procedure. The appropriate tumor size for BCS is poorly defined, however. The various clinical trials used different criteria to recruit patients for BCS. In the Milan trial, BCS was an option only for patients with tumors smaller than 2.5 cm, and those patients underwent excision of the entire quadrant of the breast (quadrantectomy) containing the tumor (15). In the NSABP-06 trial, only patients with tumors smaller than 4 cm were eligible for BCS (lumpectomy), whereas the subsequent NSABP trials accepted patients with tumors as large as 5 cm (17). An important consideration is the size of the tumor in relation to the size of the breast. Today, in some centers, preoperative chemotherapy is used to decrease the size of large tumors, making BCS feasible for more women (33). Thus, a patient with a large tumor and a small breast might be a suitable candidate for BCS if she is prepared to receive preoperative chemotherapy.

Some surgeons argue that BCS should be contraindicated if the tumor is close to or involves the nipple–areola complex. Yet the nipple–areola complex can be easily excised along with the tumor. Although sacrifice of the nipple–areola complex may result in a cosmetic deformity, many women prefer this to losing the entire breast. Thus, the patient's wishes should be considered.

A patient with multicentric cancer (involving more than one quadrant of the breast) is generally not a suitable candidate for BCS. Careful physical examination of the breasts and a preoperative mammogram are helpful in determining the presence of multicentric disease. A patient with a suspicious breast mass should have a mammogram prior to any diagnostic biopsy is done. Mammograms obtained immediately after a breast biopsy are often difficult to interpret due to postbiopsy changes. Thus, if cancer is confirmed with a biopsy, a postbiopsy mammogram might make it difficult to determine whether a patient is a suitable candidate for a breast-conserving operation.

Breast-conserving surgery is a more complex treatment than the modified radical mastectomy. The procedure generally requires two separate incisions, one to remove the primary breast tumor and the other to remove the axillary lymph nodes. In addition, patients treated with BCS require postoperative RT. Nattinger et al. analyzed the U.S. National Surveillance, Epidemiology, and End-Results Tumor Registry and found that, with the increased use of BCS, a greater number of patients were receiving inappropriate surgical treatment for primary breast cancer (34). *Appropriate* surgical therapy was defined as either total mastectomy with ALND (modified radical mastectomy) or BCS with ALND and RT. During the period from 1983 through 1995, the proportion of women undergoing an inappropriate form of modified radical mastectomy remained stable at 2.7%. During this period, however, the proportion receiving an inappropriate form of BCS (omission of RT or ALND or both) increased from 10% in 1989 to 19% at the end of 1995.

Since publication of the results of the NSABP-06 trial, there has been a gradual increase in the use of BCS in the United States. There has also been considerable geographic variation in the acceptance of this procedure, however. Several years ago, Nattinger et al. reported that the frequency of BCS in the various states ranged from 3.5% to 21.2% (35). The highest frequency was reported in the mid-Atlantic (20%) and New England states (17%), and the lowest was in the eastern (5.9%) and western South–Central states (7.3%). A similar geographic variation in the use of BCS was reported in a recent analysis of patients treated within the U.S. Department of Defense (DOD) Healthcare System (36). In the DOD system, physicians rotate through various hospitals in the United States and abroad. Yet geographic variation in the use of BCS persists. Thus, patient preferences in various parts of the United States might differ, resulting in variation in the acceptance of one procedure over another.

By 1990, 18 states had passed legislation requiring physicians to disclose options for the treatment of breast cancer. Nattinger et al. studied the effect of this legislation on the use of BCS (37). They found that such legislation has only a small, transient effect on the rate of use of BCS. Dolan et al. reported that medically indigent women treated in public hospitals are less likely to receive BCS when compared with more affluent patients treated in private hospitals (38). Thus, several complex factors influence the surgical treatment of primary breast cancer.

Breast Reconstructive Surgery

For some patients with primary breast cancer, BCS is not a suitable option. As mentioned previously, these may include some pregnant patients, patients with large or multicentric cancers, some patients who have been previously treated with RT to the breast, and those with active collagen vascular disease. These patients often are advised to undergo modified radical mastectomy (total breast removal and ALND). Most of these patients are good candidates for breast reconstructive surgery, which may be performed either at the time of surgery for primary breast cancer (immediate reconstruction) or later (delayed reconstruction). For several years, there were concerns that immediate reconstructive surgery might mask locoregional recurrences and thereby contribute to a worse outcome (39). Thus, many investigators recommended delayed reconstruction; however, studies suggest that immediate reconstruction does not adversely affect outcome (40,41). Furthermore, immediate reconstruction allows two procedures (the cancer operation and reconstruction) to be performed with the use of one anesthetic and might even be associated with less psychosocial morbidity (42).

Several options are available for breast reconstruction, including the placement of implants or the creation of latissimus dorsi myocutaneous, transverse rectus abdominis myocutaneous (TRAM), and free flaps. A detailed description of these procedures is found in surgical atlases (43,44).

Reconstruction with breast implants is used widely (45). Several methods are now available, including permanent implants, permanent expandable implants, and serial expansion of tissue with an expandable implant followed by implant exchange. Tissue expanders are placed beneath the pectoral muscles and then gradually inflated over several weeks by injecting saline through a subcutaneous port. Once a skin mound is produced that is slightly larger than required, a permanent implant is inserted. Tissue expanders are feasible only for women with small or medium-sized breasts who have not had prior skin radiation. Both silicone gel and saline implants have been used. There have been concerns that silicone gel implants may result in an increased risk of connective tissue disorders. Indeed, this concern has resulted in considerable litigation and debate (46). Several studies, however, failed to demonstrate any association between silicone implants and connective tissue disorders (47, 48).

A breast mound can be refashioned using a myocutaneous flap, where skin and muscle from one anatomic region are transferred to the chest wall, with the vascular pedicle remaining attached. The latissimus dorsi myocutaneous flap is quite popular and is suitable for patients with large breasts or who have been previously treated with RT (49). Thus, it is often used in women who have had RT as part of BCS and who subsequently develop a recurrence requiring salvage mastectomy. Unfortunately, it does not contain sufficient tissue bulk, and so an implant is generally required beneath the flap.

The TRAM has a greater risk of potential complications than does the latissimus dorsi flap (45). It has several advantages as well, however, and is now the most commonly used flap in the United States. The TRAM flap provides sufficient bulk of tissue so that an implant beneath the flap is not necessary. The TRAM flap is useful for patients with a moderate or excessive amount of lower abdominal fat who require additional soft tissue on the chest wall. Thus, it provides not only sufficient tissue for breast reconstruction but also results in an abdominoplasty.

Finally, a breast mound can be refashioned using free flaps; the free TRAM flap is the most popular (50). In a free flap, the skin and underlying muscle are detached from their vascular pedicle, and microvascular techniques are used to reestablish the blood supply once the flap is placed on the chest wall. The free TRAM flap has several advantages over the standard TRAM flap. Less rectus abdominus muscle is required, and the medial contour of the breast generally looks better because a tunnel for the vascular pedicle is not required. Surgeons must have special expertise in performing microvascular procedures.

MANAGEMENT OF THE AXILLA

Since the late nineteenth century, breast cancer surgery has been closely linked to surgery of the axilla. Today, axillary surgery remains an integral part of BCS and the modified radical mastectomy. Nonetheless, surgical management of the axilla is a topic of intense controversy. Axillary lymph node metastases are no longer considered a prerequisite for distant metastases. Thus, the impact of axillary surgery on survival, local control, and staging is frequently debated.

Axillary lymph node dissection refers to the extirpation of lymph nodes in the axilla. The lymph nodes in the axilla are divided into three compartments, based on their anatomic relationship to the pectoralis minor muscle (51). Lymph nodes lateral to the pectoralis minor muscle are classified as level I nodes, those posterior to its lateral and medial borders are classified as level II nodes, and those medial to the muscle are classified as level III nodes. A *complete* ALND refers to the extirpation of lymph nodes from all three compartments. In contrast, a *partial* ALND refers to the extirpation of lymph nodes only from levels I and II, and axillary sampling indicates only resection of the level I nodes.

Metastases to the axillary lymph nodes generally occur in an orderly fashion. Thus, lymph nodes in level I are generally involved first, followed by involvement of nodes in level II and then level III. *Skip metastases* indicate the involvement of lymph nodes at levels II or III but not level I; these occur rarely. Veronesi et al. studied the distribution of nodal metastases in 539 patients who underwent complete ALND (52). Level I nodes were involved in 58% of patients, levels I and II in 22%, and all three levels in 16%. In their series, skip metastases were present in only 4% of cases. Today, most authorities recommend extirpation of lymph nodes from levels I and II (a partial ALND); ten or more nodes are usually removed (53). A partial ALND correctly stages 96% of patients with primary breast cancer as either node-positive or node-negative and rarely gives rise to significant lymphedema of the upper extremity. The 4% false-negative rate associated with a partial ALND is attributable to skip metastases. This false-negative rate can be further reduced with resection of nodes from levels I-III (complete ALND), but this may increase the risk of upper-extremity lymphedema.

The technique of partial ALND is discussed in surgical atlases (54). Essentially, the procedure involves resection of lymph nodes superiorly to the level of the axillary vein, laterally to the latissimus dorsi muscle and medially to the medial border of

TABLE 13.3. *Effects of axillary lymph node dissection (ALND)*

Survival	This issue is controversial, although delayed ALND does not adversely impact on survival.
Local recurrence	ALND reduces risk of 5-yr axillary relapse from 18% to 2%.
Staging	ALND may influence decisions concerning adjuvant therapy and thereby have an impact on survival.

the pectoralis minor muscle. Particular attention should be paid to identifying the long thoracic and thoracodorsal nerves. The long thoracic nerve (nerve of Bell) runs along the lateral aspect of the chest wall and supplies the serratus anterior muscle. Injury to this nerve results in a *winged scapula*. The thoracodorsal nerve accompanies the subscapular artery along the posterior aspect of the axilla and supplies the latissimus dorsi muscle.

What impact does ALND have on survival, local control, and staging in patients with primary breast cancer (Table 13.3)? In recent years, several clinical trials have shed some light on this question. The impact of ALND on the management of patients with primary breast cancer remains a contentious issue.

Survival

For many years, the ALND was considered an important determinant of survival for patients with primary breast cancer. Halsted and his disciples fostered this notion more than 100 years ago, arguing that breast cancer spreads first to the regional lymph nodes and then to distant sites. Subsequently, some investigators provided retrospective data suggesting that the extent of the ALND does influence survival for patients with primary breast cancer. Such data are misleading, however, because there is no accounting for a *stage migration effect*. Consider, as an example, a patient with a 1.5-cm tumor and one metastatic lymph node to the axilla. Surgeon A may perform an extensive lymph node dissection and remove that node. On the other hand, surgeon B may perform a less extensive lymph node dissection and fail to uncover the metastatic node. Thus, if treated by surgeon A, this patient would be diagnosed as having stage II breast cancer. If treated by surgeon B, the same patient would be diagnosed as having stage I disease. When survival rates are compared for any given stage, it may seem that patients treated by surgeon A do better, but this may be attributable to the stage migration effect rather than any therapeutic benefit of the more extensive lymph node dissection.

The best way to determine whether the ALND has any effect on mortality is to compare treatment with ALND and without ALND in a randomized prospective trial. Such a study has never been conducted, although the results of the NSABP-04 and the King's/Cambridge trials, discussed already, indicate that the delayed treatment of the axilla has no effect on breast cancer mortality (13,14). The results of these trials might be interpreted to mean that the axillary lymph nodes are not a nidus for the further spread of cancer. Nonetheless, some investigators argue that the NSABP-04 and King's/Cambridge trials did not include sufficient numbers of patients to detect small differences in survival between those randomized to either early or delayed treatment of the axilla (55). Thus, the effect of ALND on survival remains a contentious issue.

Axillary Relapse

Axillary lymph node metastasis is found in 35% to 40% of patients with palpable breast cancers (56). In many instances, nodal involvement is not clinically evident when the patient first presents with primary breast cancer. Indeed, about 30% of clinically node-negative patients are shown to have nodal involvement following ALND (57). In the absence of ALND, many of these patients eventually would develop clinical evidence of nodal involvement. The NSABP-04 and King's/Cambridge trials provide important information on the effect of axillary treatment in clinically node-negative patients. These trials indicate that radiotherapy and ALND are equally effective in achieving local control of the axilla. In the NSABP-04 trial, clinically node-negative patients with primary breast cancer either received no treatment to the axilla or treatment with ALND or radiotherapy (13). About 18% of the patients who received no initial axillary treatment went on to develop axillary adenopathy within 5 years. In contrast, axillary adenopathy developed in only 2% of patients whose axilla had been treated. Similar results were reported in the King's/ Cambridge trial, where clinically node-negative patients were randomized to receive total mastectomy and RT to the axilla or total mastectomy and observation of the axilla (14). Taken together, these studies suggest that treatment of the axilla (with either ALND or RT) will reduce the 5-year risk of axillary relapse by about 90%.

The importance of axillary treatment on local control is also reported in retrospective studies. Baxter et al. reviewed the records of 112 breast cancer patients who underwent lumpectomy without ALND (58). When these patients first presented with breast cancer, they had no evidence of axillary lymph node involvement on clinical examination. During the subsequent 10-year period, about 28% of these patients developed axillary adenopathy. Axillary adenopathy developed in 10% of patients who presented with tumors 1 cm or less in diameter, in 26% of those who presented with tumors 1.1 to 2.0 cm, and in 33% of those with primary tumors greater than 2.1 cm in diameter.

The extent of the ALND seems to influence the risk of axillary relapse. Graverson et al. reviewed the records of 3,128 patients with primary breast cancer who were clinically node negative at initial presentation (59). The 5-year risk of axillary relapse ranged from 19% when no nodes were removed to 3% when more than five nodes were removed. In the NSABP-04 study, no patient who had more than six nodes removed developed a relapse in the axilla. Thus, an adequate ALND is essential in reducing the risk of relapse in the axilla.

Axillary relapse is generally considered a marker of tumor biology, indicating an increased risk of distant metastasis and death. These relapses are not considered the cause of the poor prognosis. Yet many women are emotionally devastated following axillary relapse. Additionally, axillary relapses can cause significant morbidity. Major vessels and nerves of the axilla sometimes are invaded by the tumor, causing lymphedema or pain. In such instances, the axilla is difficult to manage. Surgical clearance of such axilla often is associated with increased morbidity. Thus, adequate treatment of the axilla at the time of initial diagnosis of primary breast cancer is important.

Staging

For patients with primary breast cancer, clinical assessment of the axilla is notoriously inaccurate. About 30% of patients with palpable axillary nodes prove to be node negative following ALND, and about 30% of clinically node-negative patients prove to have nodal involvement (57). Thus, the ALND traditionally played a vital role in staging patients with primary breast cancer (as either node negative or node positive).

Axillary lymph node status is the single most important prognostic factor in the management of primary breast cancer; however, the prognostic significance of nodal metastasis is poorly understood. For many years, physicians assumed that nodal status was simply a chronological variable. Thus, it was argued that node-positive patients fare worse than node-negative patients because their cancers are discovered later. Evidence now has been found, however, to suggest that nodal status is also a marker of tumor biology. Indeed, a recent study showed that nodal status at initial diagnosis predicts outcome after relapse (60). In that study, patients with four or more involved nodes at initial diagnosis were found to have a significantly worse outcome after relapse compared with node-negative cases, suggesting that nodal metastasis is also a marker of tumor phenotype.

The importance of ALND as a staging procedure was underscored in a study from the Institut Curie in Paris, France (61). In that study, 658 breast cancer patients treated with lumpectomy and breast RT were randomly assigned to either ALND or axillary RT. Adjuvant chemotherapy was administered to a few of these patients, and the decision to administer adjuvant therapy was based on nodal status. Nodal status was not assessed in patients whose axilla were treated with RT, however, and so none of those patients received adjuvant chemotherapy. There was a small but significantly greater overall 5-year survival rate ($p = 0.014$) in the group treated with ALND (96.6%) compared with the group treated with axillary RT (92.6%). Many investigators attribute this small benefit to adjuvant chemotherapy. Therefore, if nodal status will influence the decision to administer adjuvant systemic therapy, the axilla should be managed with ALND and not with RT.

Node-positive patients have a worse prognosis than node-negative patients. Nodal status, however, does not predict response to therapy. Indeed, for both node-negative and node-positive patients, adjuvant systemic therapy reduces the annual odds of relapse and death by approximately 30% and 25%, respectively (62), although the absolute benefit of adjuvant systemic therapy is greater in node-positive patients because their risk of relapse and death is greater. As an example, consider two groups of breast cancer patients: a node-positive group with a 60% risk of death from breast cancer over the next 10 years and a node-negative group with a 20% risk of death. For both groups, the appropriate systemic therapy would reduce the risk of death from breast cancer by about 25%. For this node-positive group, however, the absolute benefit would be 15% (25% of 60% is 15%), whereas for this node-negative group, the absolute benefit would be only 5% (25% of 20% is 5%). Thus, nodal status provides important information not only about prognosis but also about the impact of adjuvant systemic therapy. An older woman with a good-prognosis, node-negative tumor might be less willing to accept the toxicity of systemic therapy compared with a younger woman with a poor-prognosis, node-positive tumor. Some oncologists have proposed that all patients should receive adjuvant chemotherapy, with the addition of tamoxifen for estrogen receptor–positive tumors (63). Such uniform application of systemic therapy might eventually reduce the importance of axillary staging.

SENTINEL LYMPH NODE BIOPSY

The ALND is not without risks. The procedure is associated with wound infections and morbidity of the upper extremity. Wound infection rates between 8% and 19% have been reported, but the reasons for this are poorly understood (64–66). Some investigators speculate that the high rate of axillary wound infection might be due to the dead space beneath devascularized skin flaps or to an altered local immune response from disruption of local lymphatics. The ALND is also associated with significant morbidity of the upper extremity. In one series, the following upper-extremity complications were reported: paresthesia in 70% of patients, pain in 33%, weakness in 25%, arm lymphedema in 10%, and stiffness in 10% (67). Today, more than half the patients with primary breast cancer are node negative. If identified appropriately, these patients could be spared the potential morbidity associated with ALND. In recent years, attention has turned to sentinel lymph node biopsy (SLNB) as a means of achieving this goal.

The sentinel lymph node is the first node to receive lymphatic drainage from a tumor. For any nodal basin, one might assume that, if the sentinel lymph node is free of metastatic tumor, then all other nodes in the basin should be free of tumor as well. Alternatively, involvement of the sentinel lymph node may mean that other nodes in the basin are involved. Thus, the SLNB is a diagnostic test that is useful in determining the status of the regional lymph nodes. This technique allows the surgeon to determine the status of the regional lymph nodes and avoid the morbidity associated with a more extensive lymph node dissection. For patients with primary breast cancer, the absolute contraindications to SLNB include the presence of palpable axillary lymph node metastasis, multifocal breast cancer, or prior breast or axillary surgery that might interfere with lymphatic drainage (68).

The SLNB technique was first described by Cabanas in 1977 as a means of assessing patients with penile carcinoma who might benefit from inguinofemoroiliac dissection (69). Subsequently, Morton et al. demonstrated the feasibility and accuracy of SLNB for nodal staging in melanoma (70). More recently, interest has focused on SLNB as a means of staging patients with primary breast cancer, with the goal of avoiding the morbidity of ALND (71). Once identified, the sentinel node is excised and sent for histopathologic evaluation. Several studies have shown that the SLNB is quite accurate in predicting the status of the axillary lymph nodes (72,73). As yet, however, no data from randomized prospective trials are available that compare long-term outcome of patients treated with SLNB with those treated with ALND. Such trials are now in progress. While awaiting the results of these trials, we should regard ALND, not SLNB, as the standard method of managing the axilla for patients with primary breast cancer (68).

Surgeons can identify the first draining (sentinel) lymph node by injecting isosulfan blue dye or radioactive colloid intradermally around the primary tumor. Recent studies suggest, however, that subareolar injection is as accurate as peritumoral injection (74). In fact, for nonpalpable mammographically detected cancers, subareolar injection might be preferable because it does not require injection under image guidance. There has also been debate as to whether injection with radioactive colloid and blue dye is more accurate than injection with blue dye alone as a means of identifying the sentinel node. Morrow et al. compared the two methods in a randomized trial and found that they were equally effective (75). Thus, the preferences of the surgeon determine which method is used.

Giuliano et al. compared 134 patients with primary breast cancer who received standard ALND with 164 patients who underwent SLNB followed by completion ALND (76). The reported incidence of nodal metastasis was 29% and 42%, respectively. Thus, the reported incidence of node-positive cases is greater with SLNB than with standard ALND. Following ALND, one or two sections of each nonsentinel lymph node are generally examined with routine hematoxylin and eosin (H & E) staining; however, pathologists pay more attention to the sentinel lymph node. These nodes often are evaluated with multiple sectioning, H & E staining, and immunohistochemical staining for cytokeratin. Thus, the SLNB results in a focused histopathologic evaluation of a single lymph node, and the probability of identifying micrometastases is thereby increased. The clinical relevance of these extra cases of micrometastases is poorly understood.

Theoretically, sentinel lymph node–negative patients should not require ALND. The long-term effects of omitting axillary clearance are poorly understood, however. Recent studies suggest that SLNB is associated with a false-negative rate of about 10% compared with 4% following a level I and II ALND (68). The false-negative rate refers to the percentage of patients with nodal metastases who are incorrectly designated as node negative. False-negatives may lead to incorrect decisions concerning adjuvant therapy, thereby affecting outcome. These and other concerns about SLNB will be addressed in several large randomized prospective trials now under way (51). These trials will compare long-term outcome following SLNB or ALND in the management of the axilla. We must await the completion of these trials before accepting SLNB as the standard of care.

CONCLUSION

The modern surgical treatment of breast cancer dates back to the late nineteenth century, with Halsted's description of the radical mastectomy for the treatment of primary breast cancer. During the last 25 years, the results of several randomized prospective trials have shown that the extent of the mastectomy does not influence survival. Thus, the radical mastectomy is no longer routinely used in breast cancer management. BCS with RT is now considered the optimal local therapy. For patients who are not suitable candidates for BCS, the modified radical mastectomy is an acceptable alternative. Patients treated with the modified radical mastectomy should also consider breast reconstructive surgery. Recently, the management of the axilla has been a topic of considerable interest. Attention has turned to SLNB as a possible alternative to the standard axillary lymph node dissection. Large randomized, prospective trials have been initiated to compare long-term outcome for patients with SLNB or axillary lymph node dissection. We await the results of these trials before deciding whether to adopt the SLNB as the standard of care.

ACKNOWLEDGMENT

The opinions or assertions contained herein are the private views of the authors and should not be construed as reflecting the views of the Departments of the Army, Air Force, or Defense.

REFERENCES

1. Virchow R. *Cellular pathology*. Philadelphia: JB Lippincott, 1863.
2. Halsted WS. The results of operations for the cure of cancer of the breast performed at the Johns Hopkins Hospital from June 1889 to January 1894. *Ann Surg* 1894;20:497–455.
3. Margolese RG. Surgical considerations for invasive breast cancer. *Surg Clin North Am* 1999;79: 1031–1046.
4. Bonnadonna G, Valagussa P. The contribution of medicine to the primary treatment of breast cancer. *Cancer Res* 1988;48:2314–2324.
5. Urban JA, Marjoni MA. Significance of internal mammary lymph node metastases in breast cancer. *AJR Am J Roentgenol* 1971;111:130–136.
6. Wagensteen OH. Another look at supraradical operation for breast cancer. *Surgery* 1957;41:857–861.
7. Andreassen M, Dahl-Iversen E, Sorensen B. Extended exeresis of regional lymph nodes at operation for carcinoma of breast and the result of a 5-year follow-up of the first 98 cases with removal of the axillary as well as the supraclavicular glands. *Acta Chir Scand* 1954;107:206–213.
8. Lacour J, Bucalossi P, Cacers E, et al. Radical mastectomy versus radical mastectomy plus internal mammary dissection. *Cancer* 1976;37:206–214.
9. McWhirter R. Simple mastectomy and radiotherapy in treatment of breast cancer. *Br J Radiol* 1955; 28:128–139.
10. Mustakalio S. Conservative treatment of breast carcinoma—review of 25 year follow-up. *Clin Radiol* 1972;23:110–116.
11. Margolese R. Surgical considerations in selecting local therapy. *J Natl Cancer Inst Monogr* 1992; 11:41–48.
12. Bloom HJG, Richardson WW, Harries EJ. Natural history of untreated breast cancer (1805–1933). *BMJ* 1962;2:213–221.
13. Fisher B, Redmond C, Fisher ER, et al. Ten-year results of a randomized clinical trial comparing radical mastectomy and total mastectomy with or without radiation. *N Engl J Med* 1985;312:674–681.

14. Cancer Research Campaign Working Party. Cancer Research Campaign (King's/Cambridge) trial for early breast cancer. *Lancet* 1980;2:55–60.
15. Veronesi U, Saccozzi R, Del Vecchio M, et al. Comparing radical mastectomy with quadrantectomy, axillary dissection and radiotherapy in patients with small cancers of the breast. *N Engl J Med* 1981; 305:6–11.
16. Sarrazin D, Le MG, Arriagada R, et al. Ten year results of a randomized trial comparing a conservative treatment to mastectomy in early breast cancer. *Radiother Oncol* 1989;14:177–184.
17. Fisher B, Bauer M, Margolese R, et al. Five-year results of a randomized clinical trial comparing total mastectomy and segmental mastectomy with or without radiation in the treatment of breast cancer. *N Engl J Med* 1985;312:665–673.
18. Jacobson JA, Danforth DN, Cowan KH, et al. Ten-year results of a comparison of conservation with mastectomy in the treatment of stage I and II breast cancer. *N Engl J Med* 1995;332:907–911.
19. Van Dongan JA, Bartelink H, Fentiman IS, et al. Randomized clinical trial to assess the value of breast conserving therapy in stage I and II breast cancer, EORTC 10801 trial. *J Natl Cancer Inst Mongr* 1992; 11: 15–18.
20. Bilchert-Toft M, Rose C, Anderson JA, et al. Danish randomized trial comparing breast conservative therapy with mastectomy. *J Natl Cancer Inst Monogr* 1992; 11: 19–25.
21. Lonning PE. Treatment of early breast cancer with conservation of the breast: A review. *Acta Oncol* 1991;30:779–792.
22. Fowble B. Ipsilateral breast tumor recurrence following breast-conserving surgery for early-stage invasive breast cancer. *Acta Oncol* 1999;13(Suppl):9–17.
23. Fisher B. Personal contributions to progress in breast cancer research and treatment. *Semin Oncol* 1996;23:414–427.
24. Fisher B, Anderson S, Fisher ER, et al. Significance of ipsilateral breast tumor recurrence after lumpectomy. *Lancet* 1991;338:327–331.
25. Kurtz JM, Spitalier JM, Amalric R, et al. The prognostic significance of late local recurrence after breast-conserving therapy. *Int J Radiat Oncol Biol Phys* 1990;18:87–93.
26. Donegan WL, Perez-Mesa CM, Watson FR. A biostatistical study of locally recurrent breast carcinoma. *Surg Gynecol Obstet* 1966;122:529–540.
27. Borger J, Kemperman H, Hart A, et al. Risk factors in breast-conservation therapy. *J Clin Oncol* 1994;12:653–660.
28. Turner BC, Harrold E, Matloff E, et al. BRCA1/BRCA2 germline mutations in locally recurrent breast cancer patients after lumpectomy and radiation therapy: implications for breast-conserving management in patients with BRCA1/BRCA2 mutations. *J Clin Oncol* 1999;17:3017–3024.
29. Kinzler KW, Vogelstein B. Gatekeepers and caretakers. *Nature* 1997;386:761–763.
30. Atkins H, Hayward JL, Klugman DJ, et al. Treatment of early breast cancer: a report after ten years of a clinical trial. *BMJ* 1972;2:423–420.
31. Winchester D, Cox J. Standards for breast conservation treatment. *CA Cancer J Clin* 1992;42: 134–162.
32. Foster RS, Wood WC. Alternative strategies in the management of primary breast cancer. *Arch Surg* 1998;133:1182–1186.
33. Veronesi U, Bonadonna G, Zurrida S, et al. Conservation surgery after primary chemotherapy in large carcinomas of the breast. *Ann Surg* 1995;222:609–611.
34. Nattinger AB, Hoffmann RG, Kneusel RT, et al. Relation between appropriateness of primary therapy for early-stage breast carcinoma and increased use of breast-conserving surgery. *Lancet* 2000;356: 1148–1153.
35. Nattinger AB, Gottlieb MS, Veum J, et al. Geographic variation in the use of breast-conserving treatment for breast cancer. *N Engl J Med* 1992;326:1147–1149.
36. Kelemen JJ, Poulton T, Swartz MT, et al. Surgical treatment of early-stage breast cancer in the Department of Defense Healthcare System. *J Am Coll Surg* 2001;192:293–297.
37. Nattinger AB, Hoffmann RG, Shapiro R, et al. The effect of legislative requirements on the use of breast-conserving surgery. *N Engl J Med* 1996;335:1035–1040.
38. Dolan J, Granchi TS, Miller CC, et al. Low use of breast conservation surgery in medically indigent populations. *Am J Surg* 1999;178:470–474.
39. Dowden RV, Rosato FE, McGraw JB. Reconstruction of the breast after mastectomy for cancer. *Surg Gynecol Obstet* 1979;149:109–115.
40. Johnson CH, van Heerden JA, Donohue JH, et al. Oncological aspects of immediate breast reconstruction following mastectomy for malignancy. *Arch Surg* 1989;124:819–823.

41. Vinton AL, Traverso W, Zehring RD. Immediate breast reconstruction following mastectomy is as safe as mastectomy alone. *Arch Surg* 1990;125:1303–1308.
42. Dean C, Chetty U, Forrest APM. Effects of immediate breast reconstruction on psychosocial morbidity after mastectomy. *Lancet* 1983;1:459–462.
43. Bostwick J III. *Plastic and reconstructive breast surgery.* St. Louis: Quality Medical Publishing, 2000.
44. Kroll S. *The artistry of breast reconstruction with autologous tissue: art and artistry.* New York: Springer-Verlag, 1999.
45. Corral CJ, Mustoe TA. Special problems in breast cancer therapy: controversy in breast reconstruction. *Surg Clin North Am* 1996;76:309–326.
46. Hulka BS, Kerkvliet NL, Tugwell P. Experience of a scientific panel formed to advise the federal judiciary on silicone breast implants. *N Engl J Med* 2000;342:812–815.
47. Nyren O, Yin L, Josefsson S, et al. Risk of connective tissue disease and related disorders among women with breast implants: a nation-wide retrospective cohort study in Sweden. *BMJ* 1998;316: 417–422.
48. Janowsky EC, Kupper LL, Hulka BS. Meta-analyses of the relation between silicone breast implants and the risk of connective-tissue diseases. *N Engl J Med* 2000; 342:781–790.
49. Schneider WJ, Hill HL Jr, Brown RG. Latissimus dorsi myocutaneous flap for breast reconstruction. *Br J Plast Surg* 1977;30:277–281.
50. Arnez Z, Smith R, Eder R. Breast reconstruction by the free lower transverse rectus abdominis muscular cutaneous flap. *Br J Plast Surg* 1988;41:500–507.
51. Jatoi I. Management of the axilla in primary breast cancer. *Surg Clin North Am* 1999;79:1061– 1073.
52. Veronesi U, Rilke R, Luini A, et al. Distribution of axillary node metastases by level of invasion. *Cancer* 1987;59:682–687.
53. Morrow M. Axillary dissection: when and how radical? *Semin Surg Oncol* 1996;12:321–327.
54. Kaiser LR. *Multidisciplinary atlas of breast surgery.* Philadelphia: Lippincott–Raven, 1997.
55. Harris JR, Osteen RT. Patients with early breast cancer benefit from effective axillary treatment. *Breast Cancer Res Treat* 1985;5:17–21.
56. Epstein RJ. Routine or delayed axillary dissection for primary breast cancer? *Eur J Cancer* 1995; 31A:1570–1573.
57. Sacks NPM, Baum M. Primary management of carcinoma of the breast. *Lancet* 1993;342:1402– 1408.
58. Baxter N, McCready DR, Chapman JA, et al. Clinical behaviour of untreated axillary nodes after local treatment for primary breast cancer. *Ann Surg Oncol* 1996;3:235–240.
59. Graverson HP, Blichert-Toft M, Andersen J, et al. for the Danish Breast Cancer Cooperative Group. Breast cancer: risk of axillary recurrence in node-negative patients following partial dissection of the axilla. *Eur J Surg Oncol* 1988;14:407–412.
60. Jatoi I, Hilsenbeck SG, Clark GM, et al. The significance of axillary lymph node metastasis in primary breast cancer. *J Clin Oncol* 1999;17:2334–2340.
61. Cabanes PA, Salmon RJ, Vilcoq JR, et al. Value of axillary dissection in addition to lumpectomy and radiotherapy in early breast cancer. *Lancet* 1992;339:1245–1248.
62. Gelber RD, Goldhirsch A, Coates AS. Adjuvant therapy for breast cancer: understanding the overview. *J Clin Oncol* 1993;11:580–585.
63. Goldhirsch A, Glick JH, Gelber RD, et al. Meeting highlights: international consensus panel on the treatment of primary breast cancer. *J Natl Cancer Inst* 1998;90:1601–1608.
64. Bold RJ, Mansfield PF, Berger DH, et al. Prospective randomized double-blind study of prophylactic antibiotics in axillary lymph node dissection. *Am J Surg* 1998;176:239–243.
65. Coit DG, Peters M, Brennan MF. A prospective randomized trial of perioperative cefazolin treatment in axillary and groin dissection. *Arch Surg* 1991;126:1366–1372.
66. Rotstein C, Ferguson R, Cummings KM, et al. Determinants of clean surgical wound infections for breast procedures at an oncology center. *Infect Control Hosp Epidemiol* 1992;13:207–214.
67. Ivens D, Hoe AL, Podd TJ, et al. Assessment of morbidity from complete axillary dissection. *Br J Cancer* 1992;66:136–138.
68. McMasters KM, Giuliano AE, Ross MI, et al. Sentinel lymph node biopsy for breast cancer—not yet standard of care. *N Engl J Med* 1998;339:990–995.
69. Cabanas RM. An approach for the treatment of penile carcinoma. *Cancer* 1977;39:456–466.

70. Morton DL, Wen DR, Wong JH, et al. Technical details of intraoperative lymphatic mapping for early stage melanoma. *Arch Surg* 1992;127:392–399.
71. Giuliano AE. Sentinel lymphadenectomy in primary breast carcinoma: an alternative to routine axillary dissection. *J Surg Oncol* 1996;62:75–77.
72. Giuliano AE, Jones RC, Brennan M. Sentinel lymphadenectomy in breast cancer. *J Clin Oncol* 1997; 15:2345–2350.
73. Veronesi U, Paganelli G, Galimberti V. Sentinel node biopsy to avoid dissection in breast cancer with clinically negative lymph nodes. *Lancet* 1997;349:1864–1867.
74. Smith LF, Cross MJ, Klimberg VS. Subareolar injection is a better technique for sentinel lymph node biopsy. *Am J Surg* 2000;180:434–437.
75. Morrow M, Rademaker AW, Bethke KP, et al. Learning sentinel node biopsy: results of a prospective randomized trial of two techniques. *Surgery* 1999;126:714–720.
76. Giuliano AE, Dale PS, Turner RR, et al. Improved axillary staging of breast cancer with sentinel node lymphadenectomy. *Ann Surg* 1995;222:394–399.

14

Adjuvant Systemic Therapy for Primary Breast Cancer

William J. Gradishar

A recommendation for adjuvant systemic therapy is commonly made to women with a diagnosis of early stage breast cancer. The standard adjuvant therapies include chemotherapy and endocrine therapy, although treatment with antibody therapy (i.e., Herceptin) and vaccines is being studied in clinical trials. Data from the Surveillance, Epidemiology and End Results (SEER) registries in the United States report a reduction in breast cancer related–mortality of 7.5% since 1973, whereas during the same period, the incidence of invasive breast cancer increased by 25% (1–4). The improvement in survival for patients with early stage breast cancer coincides with the widespread use of screening mammography and the administration of adjuvant chemotherapy and tamoxifen (5–8).

The decision to offer adjuvant therapy is made after providing the patient with a thorough discussion of her prognosis based on clinical and biologic characteristics of the primary tumor. Once an estimate of the risk of recurrence and mortality secondary to breast cancer is established for a population of breast cancer patients with similar characteristics, the medical oncologist can provide the patient with an estimate of potential benefit derived from the addition of adjuvant chemotherapy or endocrine therapy. Benefit from adjuvant systemic therapy is described in terms of reducing the risk of recurrence and death from breast cancer. An equally important issue that must figure into the discussion of adjuvant systemic therapy is the associated toxicity, both acute and chronic. Only after considering both the potential benefit and toxicity related to adjuvant systemic therapy can either the medical oncologist or the patient make a rational decision regarding its use.

Hundreds of individual clinical trials involving thousands of patients have been conducted to assess the efficacy of various adjuvant chemotherapy or endocrine programs in women with early stage breast cancer. The fundamental message that is gleaned from this experience is that adjuvant systemic therapy does reduce the risk of recurrence and improve survival in women with early stage breast cancer (7, 8). This chapter provides an overview of this experience and suggests guidelines to use when evaluating patients who are potential candidates for adjuvant systemic therapy.

The three meta-analyses (overview analyses) of randomized clinical trials of chemotherapy and endocrine therapy in early stage breast cancer patients provide the largest data set showing that systemic adjuvant therapy does reduce the risk of recurrence and death related to breast cancer (7–10). Because the overview analyses include thousands of patients and events (e.g., recurrences and deaths), greater validity is assigned to estimates of benefit derived from adjuvant therapy. On the other hand, the overview analyses also have the potential weakness of obscuring important differences in the design of individual trials (i.e., drug dose, duration of therapy, and variation of schedule).

Critical to understanding the overview analyses is an appreciation of how efficacy of adjuvant therapy is reported. Two concepts are worth reviewing: proportional risk reduction and absolute risk reduction. *Proportional risk reduction* can be viewed as the percentage of negative outcomes that were avoided (recurrences or deaths) because adjuvant systemic therapy was administered. The overview analyses actually reported the proportional risk reduction for the *annual* risk of an event (e.g., recurrence or death) occurring. The annual risk *compounds* to give the risk of an adverse event at some future time. *Absolute risk reduction* of an adverse event simply states what percentage of patients, at a specific time, have avoided an adverse event (recurrence or death) by having received adjuvant therapy compared with a group of similar patients who did not receive that therapy. Absolute risk reduction is a smaller number than proportional risk reduction. Unfortunately, a misunderstanding of the terms frequently leads patients and physicians to erroneous conclusions regarding the benefits of adjuvant systemic therapy. Finally, it is important to appreciate that estimates of benefit, as reported by the overview analyses, apply to populations of patients with similar characteristics rather than an individual patient.

ROLE OF ADJUVANT POLYCHEMOTHERAPY

The 1998 overview analysis of adjuvant chemotherapy trials is based on 47 trials involving 17,723 patients (7). Many of the clinical trials included in the overview analyses now have greater than 10 years of follow-up. Collectively, thousands of recurrences and deaths have occurred in these trials. Eleven clinical trials involving 6,104 patients addressed the issue of longer versus shorter durations of chemotherapy. Eleven clinical trials involving 5,942 patients assessed the relative efficacy of anthracycline-containing (doxorubicin or epirubicin) regimens. The most recent overview analysis reported two major endpoints: reduction in recurrence and reduction in mortality (7,8). Deaths were assumed to be due to breast cancer unless otherwise defined.

The 1998 overview analysis confirmed that treatment with several months of combination chemotherapy resulted in a reduced risk of recurrence and death. Furthermore, there was no significant difference between the type of chemotherapy evaluated and the magnitude of benefit derived by the average patient participating in these clinical trials (Table 14.1). The overview analyses confirmed that the magnitude of benefit derived from adjuvant chemotherapy was greatest in younger patients, but unlike previous overview analyses, the most recent showed that adjuvant chemotherapy did benefit older patients as well (Table 14.2).

TABLE 14.1. *1998 Overview analysis: efficacy of polychemotherapy*

	Proportional risk reduction	
Regimen	Recurrence (%)	Death (%)
All polychemotherapy	25 ± 2	15 ± 2
CMF	24 ± 3	14 ± 4
CMF + additional cytotoxins	20 ± 2	15 ± 5
Other non-CMF chemotherapy	25 ± 4	17 ± 4
Longer *vs* shorter	7 ± 4	−1 ± 5

±, standard deviation; CMF, cyclophosphamide, methotrexate, 5-fluorouracil.

Effect of Age and Menopausal Status

The 1998 overview analysis also suggests that the age of the patient may be as important as menopausal status in determining the relative efficacy of adjuvant chemotherapy (7). This analysis is complicated by the difficulty of defining with precision when menopause occurs and by the small number of patients in certain subsets. If patients younger than 50 years of age are divided into premenopausal or perimenopausal and postmenopausal status, the effect of adjuvant chemotherapy is similar. This analysis cannot be made with confidence because the number of young postmenopausal patients in this age group is small ($n = 476$). Similarly, the effect of adjuvant chemotherapy would appear to be similar between premenopausal or perimenopausal and postmenopausal patients in the age group 50 to 69 years, although the number of older premenopausal patients is relatively small ($n = 1,469$) (Table 14.3).

The use of adjuvant chemotherapy in women over the age of 70 could not be adequately addressed by the overview analyses because few patients in this age group were included in randomized clinical trials ($n = 609$). In such patients, a recommendation for adjuvant chemotherapy must be individualized and must take into consideration the patient's general health status and other medical conditions.

TABLE 14.2. *1998 Overview analysis—relationship between age and efficacy of polychemotherapy*

	Proportional risk reduction	
Age (yr)	Recurrence (%)	Death (%)
<40	37 (7)	27 (5)
40–49	34 (5)	27 (5)
50–59	22 (4)	14 (4)
60–69	18 (4)	8 (4)
≥70	NS	NS
Overall	24 (2)	15 (2)

( ), standard deviation; NS, not significant.

TABLE 14.3. *1998 Overview analysis—relationship between menopausal status and efficacy of polychemotherapy*

	% Proportional risk reduction	
	Recurrence	Death
Age <50 yr		
Pre/perimenopausal	34 (4)	27 (5)
Postmenopausal	44 (13)	28 (15)
Age 50–59 yr		
Pre/perimenopausal	24 (7)	19 (8)
Postmenopausal	20 (3)	10 (3)

( ), standard deviation.

Although definitive data are lacking, one would surmise that the relative effect of adjuvant chemotherapy in women over the age of 70 would be similar to the effect observed in women 50 to 69 years of age.

Adjuvant chemotherapy reduces the relative risk of recurrence and death in both axillary node–negative and axillary node–positive patients to a similar degree, but the absolute magnitude of benefit is greater for those patients at highest risk of relapse (e.g., axillary node–positive patients). There are clinical situations, such as a patient with a very large primary tumor with negative axillary nodes, where the risk of recurrence is similar or greater compared with a patient with positive axillary nodes (i.e., microfoci of metastases in a single axillary node) (11,12). The data from the 1998 overview analysis show that the absolute risk reduction for those patients receiving adjuvant chemotherapy is greatest for patients younger than 50 years of age, regardless of axillary nodal status (Table 14.4) (7).

TABLE 14.4. *Absolute benefit derived from adjuvant polychemotherapy*

	Chemotherapy (%)	No chemotherapy (%)	Absolute benefit (%)
DFS			
<50 yr			
NN	68.3	58	10.3
NP	47.6	32.2	15.4
50–69 yr			
NN	65.6	59.9	5.7
NP	43.4	38	5.4
Overall survival			
<50 yr			
NN	77.6	71.9	5.7
NP	53.8	41.4	12.4
50–69 yr			
NN	71.2	64.8	6.4
NP	48.6	46.3	2.3

DFS, disease-free survival; NN, node negative; NP, node positive.

TABLE 14.5. *1998 Overview analysis: ER status of tumor and efficacy of polychemotherapy*

	Proportional risk reduction (%)	
ER	Recurrence	Death
<50 yr	35 (4)	27 (5)
ER-poor	40 (7)	35 (9)
ER-positive	33 (8)	20 (10)
50–69 yr	20 (3)	11 (3)
ER-poor	30 (5)	17 (6)
ER-positive	18 (4)	9 (5)

( ), standard deviation; ER, estrogen receptor.

Based on the 1998 overview analysis, adjuvant chemotherapy was similarly effective in reducing the risk of recurrence in patients with estrogen receptor (ER)-poor tumors, whether younger or older than age 50. Adjuvant chemotherapy was significantly more effective in reducing the risk of death in younger patients with ER-poor tumors compared with patients older than 50. For patients between 50 and 69 years of age, the relative risk reduction of recurrences and death from adjuvant chemotherapy was twice as great in patients with ER-poor tumors compared with those with ER-positive tumors (Table 14.5) (7).

Role of Anthracyclines

A long-standing assumption is that anthracycline-based adjuvant chemotherapy is superior to CMF (cyclophosphamide, methotrexate, 5-flourouracil)–like regimens, although little data were available to substantiate the claim. Anthracyclines (doxorubicin and epirubicin) have significant activity in metastatic disease, but the greater toxicity of anthracyclines compared with CMF (i.e., alopecia, cardiotoxicity, myelosuppression, and mucositis) raised concerns about their use in the adjuvant setting. The most recent overview analysis evaluated 11 randomized clinical trials in which anthracycline-based regimens were compared with CMF-type regimens (7). Overall, there was a 12% proportional risk reduction in the odds of recurrence and death for patients who received an anthracycline-based regimen. The relative risk reduction afforded to patients receiving an anthracycline translated into a modest absolute improvement of 3% in each endpoint. Most patients participating in these trials were premenopausal (70%); therefore, it remains unclear whether the same advantage would be observed in postmenopausal patients receiving adjuvant, anthracycline-based chemotherapy. A recent report from Canada provided additional support for anthracycline-based adjuvant therapy by demonstrating survival benefit for axillary node–positive patients receiving epirubicin-based therapy compared with CMF (13).

These data do not suggest that CMF-type regimens are outdated. When selecting an adjuvant therapy program, issues of toxicity, duration of therapy, and cost may figure into the decision. It is also important to recognize that although numerous

CMF-type regimens exist, they are not all equal in efficacy. The best results appear to be derived from "classic" CMF rather than the other permutations (14). In certain patients in whom minimizing toxicity (i.e., concerns regarding cardiotoxicity of alopecia) is of major importance, then CMF-type regimens would be appropriate.

Another area of clinical research that is evolving is the use of so-called predictive factors, such as the *HER-2* expression of the primary tumor, as a way of selecting the optimal adjuvant chemotherapy for a particular patient (15). A retrospective analysis of several clinical trials suggested that doxorubicin-based chemotherapy is more effective in patients with tumors that overexpress *HER-2* (16,17). Preliminary data support this hypothesis and also suggest that the dose of doxorubicin is important, but prospective clinical trials designed to address this issue will be required before this approach can be deemed standard. At present, there is no definitive evidence for resistance to CMF-type regimens in *HER-2*-positive breast cancers. There has also been a suggestion that *HER-2*-positive breast cancer may be relatively resistant to tamoxifen therapy (18,19). *HER-2* overexpression is inversely associated with ER positivity, but in cases where ER and *HER-2* are both expressed, it remains unclear whether tamoxifen is less effective. Several studies reported findings on this issue (18,19), but there are no definitive data or uniform conclusions at this time.

Duration of Adjuvant Chemotherapy

Many of the early adjuvant chemotherapy trials evaluated the effect of different durations of therapy. Based on this experience and the overview analysis, durations of adjuvant therapy in excess of 6 months do not appear to provide additional benefit in terms of reducing the risk of death (7). The optimal duration of chemotherapy was addressed in 11 clinical trials involving 6,104 patients in the 1998 overview analysis. Although there was a trend toward a reduced risk of recurrence with longer durations of adjuvant chemotherapy, this did not translate into an improvement in survival (Table 14.1). The optimal duration of therapy, based on currently available drugs and regimens, is between 4 and 6 months. As newer drugs are introduced into the adjuvant setting, duration of therapy will become an important question again. The antitumor activity of Herceptin (20) in patients with tumors that overexpress *HER-2* has generated a great deal of enthusiasm for evaluating the drug in the adjuvant setting. Clinical trials are now under way to assess the efficacy of Herceptin when added to adjuvant chemotherapy or tamoxifen. The optimal duration of adjuvant Herceptin therapy has not been defined.

Role of Taxanes

Much of the focus in the 1990s was directed to the development and evaluation of the taxanes (e.g., docetaxel and paclitaxel) for breast cancer treatment in both the metastatic and adjuvant setting. In the metastatic disease setting, the taxanes were shown to lack cross-resistance with doxorubicin, making them attractive agents to incorporate into adjuvant chemotherapy programs (21). The intergroup trial [Cancer and Leukemia Group B (CALGB 9344)] evaluated the effect of adding four cycles of paclitaxel following four cycles of doxorubicin and cyclophosphamide (AC) compared with four cycles of AC alone (22). In addition, all patients with ER-positive tumors received tamoxifen for 5 years. A second issue addressed by this trial focused on whether escalating the dose of doxorubicin in AC (60–90 mg/m^2) impacted on patient outcome. A total of 3,170 axillary node-positive patients were enrolled from 1994 to 1997. The first report of this trial, with 18 months of follow-up, indicated that the addition of paclitaxel to AC resulted in relative risk of recurrence and death of 22% and 26%, respectively (22). The absolute benefit accrued to patients receiving paclitaxel improved disease-free survival (DFS) from 86% to 90% and overall survival from 95% to 97%. The escalation of doxorubicin dose (60–90 mg/m^2) did not affect DFS. Based on these data, the U.S. Food and Drug Administration now approved paclitaxel for the adjuvant treatment of axillary node-positive breast cancer. An unanswered question is whether all subsets of patients benefited to the same degree from the addition of paclitaxel. The preliminary report of the data suggests that those patients with ER-positive tumors who received tamoxifen did not benefit from the addition of paclitaxel, but the trial was not designed to address this issue specifically (22).

A closed intergroup trial [Eastern Cooperative Oncology Group (ECOG 2197)] for patients with lower risk of disease recurrence (e.g., 0–3 positive lymph nodes) compared AC every 3 weeks × 4 with A/docetaxel every 3 weeks × 4. More than 2,700 patients have been enrolled in this trial, but results will not be available for a few more years. The design of this trial will examine the effect of adding docetaxel while keeping the total duration of adjuvant therapy equivalent in both treatment groups.

Role of Sequencing and Dose Density

The intergroup trial (CALGB 9344) (22) also raises the issue of using chemotherapy drugs in sequence as opposed to using them in combination. The rationale for using adjuvant combination chemotherapy include that (a) two or more drugs with potentially different mechanisms of action could be administered simultaneously, (b) combinations of drugs may have additive or synergistic antitumor activity, and (c) the total duration of adjuvant chemotherapy programs could be shortened. More recently, the use of sequential chemotherapy was evaluated in the adjuvant and metastatic disease setting. Sequential use of chemotherapy drugs is potentially more advantageous than combination chemotherapy because it allows the optimal administration of each drug individually, without compromising drug dose because of concerns with overlapping drug toxicities. Another theoretical advantage for sequential use of chemotherapy drugs is based on the premise that a breast tumor is a collection of heterogenous tumor cells with different biologic properties. As a result, optimizing the dose and exposure of the tumor to an individual drug may eradicate tumor cell clones that are particularly sensitive to that drug. An extension of this strategy is to

TABLE 14.6. *Adjuvant chemotherapy trials assessing sequential chemotherapy programs*

Study	Regimen
Intergroup	AC (60/600 mg/m^2) q21d × 4 ± paclitaxel (175 mg/m^2) q21d × 4
(CALGB 9344)	AC (75/600 mg/m^2) q21d × 4
	AC (90/600 mg/m^2) q21d × 4
NSABP B-28	AC (60/600 mg/m^2) × 4 ± paclitaxel (225 mg/m^2) q21d × 4
SWOG 9623	A (80 mg/m^2) q14d × 3 → paclitaxel (200 mg/m^2/24h) q14d × 3 →
	C (3000 mg/m^2) q14d × 3
	AC (80/600 mg/m^2) q21d × 4 → STAMP I/V → PBSCT
CALGB 9741	A (60 mg/m^2) → paclitaxel (175 mg/m^2) → C (600 mg/m^2) q21d × 4
	A (60 mg/m^2) → paclitaxel (175 mg/m^2) → C (600 mg/m^2) q14d × 4
	AC (60/600 mg/m^2) → paclitaxel (175 mg/m^2) q21d × 4
	AC (60/600 mg/m^2) → paclitaxel (175 mg/m^2) q14d × 4 + GCSF
NSABP B-27	AC (60/600 mg/m^2) q21d × 4 → surgery
	AC (60/600 mg/m^2) q21d × 4 → docetaxel (100 mg/m^2) q21d × 4 → surgery
	AC (60/600 mg/m^2) q21d × 4 → surgery → docetaxel (100 mg/m^2) q21d × 4
NSABP B-30	AC (60/600 mg/m^2) q21d × 4 → docetaxel (100 mg/m^2) q21d × 4
	A/docetaxel (60/60 mg/m^2) q21d × 4
	A/docetaxel/C (60/60/600 mg/m^2) q21d × 4

A, doxorubicin; C, cyclophosphamide; CALGB, Cancer and Leukemia Group B; GCSF, granulocyte colony-stimulating factor; NSABP, National Surgical Adjuvant Breast Project; PBSCT, peripheral blood stem cell transplant; STAMP I/V: I = cyclophosphamide, BCNU, cisplatinum; V = cyclophosphamide, carboplatin, thiotepa; SWOG, Southwestern Oncology Group.

explore reducing the interval between doses of chemotherapy, the dose-dense strategy. Pilot studies confirmed the feasibility of this strategy, and large randomized clinical trials are assessing its efficacy compared with more standard schedules (Table 14.6).

High-dose Chemotherapy

High–dose chemotherapy (HDC) and peripheral blood stem cell transplantation (PBSCT) have been evaluated extensively in the metastatic disease setting. Numerous pilot trials suggested that higher response rates could be attained with HDC/PBSCT compared with standard dose (e.g., non-bone marrow ablative) chemotherapy, but until recently, randomized studies were not available to critically evaluate the relative efficacy of these treatments in patients with metastatic breast cancer. The controversy surrounding the disclosure of research fraud in a recent South African adjuvant high-dose chemotherapy trial (23,24) raised concerns about the validity of an earlier report from the same investigator (25). A higher tumor response rate (95% versus 53%) and improved median survival (90 weeks versus 45 weeks) was reported in patients who received two courses of HDC plus PBSCT versus standard-dose chemotherapy (25).

The results of the largest randomized trial reported to date, comparing HDC/PBSCT with standard-dose CMF in patients with metastatic breast cancer, who initially responded to standard-dose CAF (cyclophosphamide, adriamycin, and fluorouracil) or CMF, were recently reported (26). After a median follow-up of 37 months, no significant difference in overall survival at 3 years or in the median time to disease progression was found (26). The French trial reported by Lotz et al. is the smallest of the randomized trials (27). Although an initial advantage was suggested for patients receiving HDC/PBSCT, the difference disappeared by 5 years of follow-up. The study reported by Peters et al. was restricted to patients who attained a clinical remission after two to four cycles of standard-dose chemotherapy (28). Eligible patients then were randomized to immediate HDC (e.g., carmustine, cyclophosphamide, cisplatin) /PBSCT or observation and HDC/PBSCT at the time of disease progression. Those patients who received immediate HDC/PBSCT had improved progression-free survival but shorter overall survival (28).

The results of these trials were disappointing and suggested that if HDC/PBSCT offered an advantage to patients with metastatic breast cancer, it was likely to be small. In recent years, the focus of attention has been redirected to evaluating the role of HDC/PBSCT in the high-risk adjuvant setting. The HDC/PBSCT strategy for patients at very high risk of relapse seemed reasonable because the potential for chemotherapy to eradicate disease is greatest when the tumor burden is low.

Five randomized trials of HDC/PBSCT for high-risk primary breast cancer have been reported (Table 14.7). The Bezwoda trial has been discounted because of research fraud (23,24). The early results of the U.S. intergroup study, reported by Peters et al., involved 783 women with primary breast cancer involving ten or more axillary lymph nodes, who were randomized to receive HDC/PBSCT or to receive an "intermediate dose" of the HDC regimen not requiring PBSCT (29). At a median follow-up of 37 months, event-free survival was equivalent in the two groups, with no detectable difference in 5-year overall survival, although fewer patients receiving HDC/PBSCT have relapsed.

TABLE 14.7. *Randomized trials of HDC/PBSCT for primary breast cancer*

Study	Regimen	Patient no.	Median F/U (mo.)	RFS (%)	Overall survival (%)
Peters et al. (29)	CAF × 4 → ID CPB	389	37	58	69
	CAF × 4 → HDC/PBSCT	394	37	60	67
Scandinavian (30)	FEC + GCSF × 9	251	24	50	70
	FEC × 3 → HDC/PBSCT	274	24	55	70
MD Anderson (31)	FAC × 8	39	78	46	52
	FAC × 8 → HDC/PBSCT × 2	39	78	52	46
Rodenhuis et al. (32)	FEC × 4	40	49	72	75
	FEC × 4 → HDC/PBSCT	41	49	76	57
Rodenhuis et al. (33)	FEC × 5	443	36	65	80
	FEC × 4 → HDC/PBSCT	442	36	72	84

CAF, cyclophosphamide, adriamycin, fluorouracil; CPB, cyclophosphamide, cisplatin, BCNU; FAC, 5-fluouracil, doxorubicin, cyclophosphamide; FEC, 5-fluouracil, epirubicin, cyclophosphamide; F/U, follow-up; GCSF, granulocyte colony-stimulating factor; HDC, high-dose chemotherapy; ID, intermediate dose; PBSCT, peripheral blood stem cell transplant; RFS, recurrence-free survival.

The Scandinavian trial (30) compared nine cycles of "tailored" (dose calculated on the basis of nadir white blood cell counts), dose-intensive 5-flourouracil, epirubicin, and cyclophosphamide (FEC) with three cycles of standard-dose FEC, followed by HDC/PBSCT in 274 patients with primary breast cancer. Eligibility criteria were heterogenous and included patients with more than eight positive axillary lymph nodes, more than five positive axillary lymph nodes, and an ER-negative tumor with a high proliferative index or a positive bone scan with negative plain films or microscopic bone marrow involvement. At a median follow-up of 23.7 months, survival rates were equivalent in the two groups (30).

The MD Anderson trial, reported by Hortobagyi et al., randomized 78 patients to 5-fluorouracil, doxorubicin, and cyclophosphamide (FAC) for eight cycles or FAC for eight cycles followed by HDC/PBSCT for two cycles (31). With a median follow-up of 78 months, there is no statistical difference in relapse-free survival (RFS) or overall survival between the two treatment arms. A Dutch study, reported by Rodenhuis et al., randomized 81 patients with infraclavicular-involved lymph nodes to treatment with FEC for four cycles or FEC for four cycles followed by HDC/PBSCT (32). With a median follow-up of 49 months, 5-year RFS favored patients receiving HDC, but overall survival was superior for patients receiving standard-dose chemotherapy (32).

A large Dutch trial was recently reported in which 885 patients with four or more positive axillary lymph nodes (570 patients with four to nine nodes and 315 patients with ten or more nodes) were randomized to receive either FEC five cycles or FEC four cycles followed by HDC/PBSCT (33). The final report is due in 2002, but the funding agency required analysis of the first 284 patients on study. Four hundred forty-three patients were randomized to the conventional arm with no crossover to the HDC/PBSCT arm, and 442 patients were randomized to the HDC/PBSCT arm (7.7% were did not have transplantation). The RFS for the entire cohort of patients at 3 years is 65% for patients receiving conventional treatment and 72% for those receiving HDC/PBSCT. The overall survival for the entire cohort of patients at 3 years was 80% for patients receiving conventional treatment and 84% for those receiving HDC/PBSCT. If the analysis is restricted to only the first 284 patients, there appears to be advantage for patients who received HDC/PBSCT. Longer follow-up of the entire cohort of patients will be required to determine whether there is a subset of patients who benefit from the HDC strategy. At present, the HDC/PBSCT cannot be viewed as standard therapy for any subset of patients with breast cancer. The results of other large randomized trials comparing adjuvant HDC/PBSCT with conventional-dose chemotherapy for the treatment of high-risk primary breast cancer are eagerly anticipated in the next few years. It is hoped that these results will define what, if any, role HDC/PBSCT has in the treatment of breast cancer.

ROLE OF ADJUVANT ENDOCRINE THERAPY

The most recent overview analysis clearly demonstrates that treatment with tamoxifen in women with ER-positive (or unknown receptor status) breast cancer substan-

TABLE 14.8. *Proportional risk reduction with adjuvant tamoxifen therapy*

Duration (yr)	% Risk reduction	
	Recurrence	Death
1	18 (3)	10 (3)
2	25 (2)	15 (2)
5[a]	42 (3)	22 (4)

( ), standard deviation.
[a] Median duration is 5 years.

tially reduces the risk of disease recurrence and death, irrespective of age, menopausal status, nodal status, and adjuvant chemotherapy administration (8). The conclusions of the overview analysis are particularly robust because significant data are now available that support the use of tamoxifen for 5 years rather than shorter durations, and many of the clinical trials included in the overview analysis have follow-up of more than 10 years.

The overview analysis compared 1, 2, and 5 years of adjuvant tamoxifen therapy. The optimal benefit to patients, in terms of reduced risk of recurrence and death, was conferred by 5 years of adjuvant tamoxifen use (Table 14.8). In addition, the risk of developing contralateral breast cancer was maximally reduced by 5 years of tamoxifen compared to shorter durations of therapy (8). The benefit derived from tamoxifen therapy was confined only to patients with ER-positive or ER-unknown tumors, whereas no benefit was conferred to patients with ER-negative tumors. Of the patients with ER-positive tumors, the magnitude of benefit from adjuvant tamoxifen therapy was also greatest for patients with tumors expressing the highest values of ER (Table 14.9). The overview analysis attempted to estimate benefit from adjuvant tamoxifen by assessing progesterone receptor (PR) expression, but relatively few patients had complete information on PR and certain subsets of patients (i.e., ER-negative/PR-positive) had little data. Nevertheless, patients with ER-positive/PR-negative disease attained benefit from tamoxifen similar to patients with ER-positive tumors (e.g., proportional risk reduction of recurrence and mortality of 46% ± 9)

TABLE 14.9. *Proportional risk reduction with adjuvant tamoxifen therapy: relationship to ER expression*

ER level	% Risk reduction	
	Recurrence	Death
Poor	6 (11)	−3 (11)
Unknown	37 (8)	21 (9)
Positive	50 (4)	28 (5)
10–99 fm/mg	43 (5)	23 (6)
≥100 fm/mg	60 (6)	36 (7)

( ), standard deviation; ER, estrogen receptor.

and 28% ± 11). Among patients with ER-negative/PR-positive tumors, adjuvant tamoxifen therapy provided benefit, mirroring the experience in patients with metastatic disease (34).

The clear relationship between the magnitude of risk reduction and the duration of tamoxifen therapy raises the question of whether longer durations of therapy beyond 5 years provide additional risk reduction. Three clinical trials have attempted to address this issue. The largest of the trials, National Surgical Adjuvant Breast Project (NSABP) B-14, rerandomized axillary node-negative patients who had received 5 years of tamoxifen with 5 additional years of tamoxifen or no additional treatment (35). The results of this trial showed a statistically significant detrimental effect from treatment with tamoxifen for 10 years compared with 5 years of treatment. There was a statistically significant higher recurrence rate and a trend toward deaths in patients receiving 10 years of tamoxifen compared with patients receiving 5 years of tamoxifen (35). Two other smaller clinical trials reported contradictory results (36,37), but at present there is no compelling evidence to support the use of tamoxifen therapy for longer than 5 years (38). An ongoing international clinical trial, Adjuvant Tamoxifen, Longer Against Shorter, randomizes patients to 5 more years of tamoxifen after treatment with at least 2 years of tamoxifen or no further therapy (39). Patients are encouraged to participate in the trial if they or their physician are uncertain about whether tamoxifen should be continued. More than 20,000 patients are expected to participate in the trial.

Tamoxifen appears to benefit women of all ages with ER-positive breast cancer. In the overview analysis, age is more reliably recorded in most trials compared with menopausal status, but the assumption can be made that most women younger than 50 years are premenopausal and most women over age 50 are postmenopausal (8). The overview analysis concludes that women younger than 50 years benefit from tamoxifen to as great a degree as women older than 50 years (Table 14.10). Interest-

TABLE 14.10. *Proportional risk reduction associated with chemoendocrine therapy*

Group	N	Proportional risk reduction %	
		Recurrence	Death
TAM *vs* Nil	3,253/3,229	46 (4)	22 (5)
<50 yr		47 (8)	30 (12)
≥50 yr		45 (4)	20 (5)
TAM + C *vs* C	485/460	52 (8)	47 (9)
<50 yr		40 (19)	39 (22)
≥50 yr		54 (8)	49 (10)
C *vs* Nil		24 (2)	15 (2)
<50 yr	1,992/1,908	37 (4)	28 (5)
≥50 yr	2,205/2,243	22 (4)	12 (4)
C + TAM *vs* TAM			
<50 yr	340/300	21 (13)	25 (14)
≥50 yr	4,582/4,610	19 (3)	11 (4)

( ), standard deviation; C, chemotherapy; Nil, no treatment; TAM, tamoxifen.

TABLE 14.11. *Proportional risk reduction (%) in odds of death due to systemic adjuvant therapy*

Age (yr)	Tamoxifen (5 yr)	Chemotherapy
<50	32 (10)	27 (5)
50–59	11 (8)	14 (4)
60–69	33 (6)	8 (4)

( ), standard deviation.

ingly, treatment with tamoxifen can increase serum levels of estrogen in some premenopausal women (40), and yet the magnitude of risk reduction from tamoxifen is similar to that in older women (8). This finding suggests that tamoxifen can inhibit breast cancer cells even in a milieu of increased estrogen and should be considered as an adjuvant treatment for premenopausal women.

The other interesting finding from the most recent overview analysis is that adjuvant tamoxifen therapy alone provided as much risk reduction for death as chemotherapy alone in premenopausal women (Table 14.11). The average relative risk reduction of death from tamoxifen therapy for all age groups was 26% and exceeded 30% for all age groups except women between the ages of 50 and 59 years. This latter inconsistent finding in the 50- to 59-year-old group is likely due to chance alone. The risk reduction derived from adjuvant chemotherapy is much more age dependent, with the greatest benefit attained by women younger than 50 years and a diminishing effect in older subsets of women (Table 14.11).

Future Directions with Adjuvant Endocrine Therapy

Other Antiestrogens

Toremifene, or chloro-tamoxifen, is another triphenylethylene drug, like tamoxifen. Toremifene has been found to have efficacy similar to tamoxifen in the metastatic disease setting and a similar side-effect profile. Holli et al. published a randomized trial comparing adjuvant toremifene and tamoxifen in axillary node-positive, postmenopausal breast cancer (41). Although the follow-up is short, the report suggests that both drugs are equally well tolerated and that toremifene does not appear to have inferior efficacy compared with tamoxifen.

Aromatase Inhibitors

In postmenopausal women, estrogens are produced through the peripheral aromatization of androgens (androstenedione) produced by the adrenal glands. Three selective aromatase inhibitors are now available to treat postmenopausal patients with ER-positive breast cancer (42–46). Exemestane is a type I, or irreversible, inhibitor of aromatase. It interacts with the substrate-binding site of the aromatase enzyme. Anastrozole and letrozole are type II aromatase inhibitors that act by reversibly binding to the aromatase enzyme. All three agents have been shown to be well tolerated and superior to traditional second-line endocrine therapy (after patients have disease progression while receiving an antiestrogen) (42–46). More recently, anastrozole has been shown to be superior to tamoxifen as first-line endocrine therapy in ER-positive, postmenopausal, metastatic breast cancer (47).

The activity of aromatase inhibitors in advanced breast cancer has generated interest for evaluating them in the adjuvant setting. A recently reported Italian trial was designed to examine the role of aromatase inhibition in the adjuvant setting (48). Postmenopausal patients were randomized to 5 years of tamoxifen therapy or 3 years of tamoxifen followed by 2 years of aminoglutethimide. Although aminoglutethimide would now be viewed as a suboptimal choice for aromatase inhibition because of the greater selectivity of third-generation aromatase inhibitors, the Italian trial does examine the concept of introducing an aromatase inhibitor into the adjuvant setting. Patients receiving aminoglutethimide after tamoxifen had similar overall survival compared with patients receiving tamoxifen alone for 5 years. This trial shows that replacing tamoxifen with an aromatase inhibitor did not seem to be detrimental to patients (48).

TABLE 14.12. *Selected clinical trials addressing sequential use of aromatase inhibitors*

Drug	Study group		Design
Anastrozole	ABCSG Study 8 GABG Study IV-C	TAM (2 yr)	┌ TAM (3 yr) └ Anastrozole (3 yr)
Exemestane	ICCG Study 96	TAM (2–3 yr)	┌ TAM (to 5 yr) └ Exemestane
	NSABP B-33	TAM (5 yr)	┌ Exemestane (2 yr) └ Placebo
Letrozole	IBCSG 18–98	R	┌ TAM (5 yr) ├ Letrozole (5 yr) ├ TAM (2 yr) → Letrozole (3 yr) └ Letrozole (2 yr) → TAM (3 yr)
	NCIC CTG MA. 17	TAM (5 yr)	┌ Letrozole (5 yr) └ Placebo (5 yr)

ABCSG, Austrian Breast Cancer Study Group; GABG, German Adjuvant Breast Cancer Group; IBCSG, International Breast Cancer Study Group; ICCG, International Collaborative Cancer Group; NCIC CTG, National Cancer Institute of Canada Clinic Trials Group; NSABP, National Surgical Adjuvant Breast Project; TAM, tamoxifen.

Several clinical trials are now under way to evaluate the role of selective aromatase inhibitors in the adjuvant setting (Table 14.12). These ongoing clinical trials examine whether an aromatase inhibitor can be substituted for tamoxifen or whether the addition of an aromatase inhibitor after tamoxifen therapy offers additional benefit.

ROLE OF ADJUVANT CHEMOENDOCRINE THERAPY

Another important issue addressed by individual clinical trials and by the overview analysis is whether chemoendocrine therapy offers additional benefit, in terms of reducing the risk of recurrence or death, over that which can be attained by either modality alone. Relatively few premenopausal women receiving tamoxifen alone versus tamoxifen plus adjuvant chemotherapy were included in the overview analysis ($n = 640$) (7,8). The largest individual trial was reported by the NSABP and showed that the combination of chemotherapy plus tamoxifen was superior to tamoxifen alone in node-negative, ER-positive breast cancer (49).

The addition of tamoxifen to chemotherapy clearly adds additional risk reduction compared with chemotherapy alone in premenopausal women with ER-positive breast cancer (7,8). Initial trials of this approach failed to show significant benefit for the addition of tamoxifen after adjuvant chemotherapy, but many of these trials administered tamoxifen for only 1 or 2 years (9,10). A recent analysis by the International Breast Cancer Study Group (IBCSG) evaluated whether chemotherapy alone was adequate for a population of very young (<35 years), premenopausal women identified in four randomized clinical trials (50). A total of 3,700 premenopausal and perimenopausal patients were treated with CMF-type regimens, with or without prednisone and oophorectomy. Of 3,700 women, 314 were younger than 35 years old. Relapse and death occurred earlier and more often in younger (<35 years) than in older (≥35 years) patients, with a 10-year DFS of 35% versus 47%, respectively, and overall survival of 49% versus 62%, respectively. Younger patients (<35 years) with ER-positive tumors had a significantly worse DFS compared with younger patients with ER-negative disease. These findings suggest that chemotherapy provides an inadequate endocrine effect in the youngest patients with ER-positive breast cancer and supports the concept of adding tamoxifen or possibly ovarian ablation to chemotherapy (50).

The ECOG recently reported the results of randomized clinical trial in which 1,537 premenopausal patients with ER-positive breast cancer were randomized to FAC six cycles or FAC plus goserelin or FAC plus goserelin and tamoxifen (51). Among women younger than 40 years, there was a substantial and statistically significant benefit from adding goserelin and tamoxifen. Among women older than 40 years, there was no advantage from adding goserelin to FAC, but the patients in the tamoxifen-containing arm had an improvement in DFS. It is also interesting to note that only 40% of the women younger than 40 years had postmenopausal estrogen levels, compared with 80% of women over the age of 40. The added benefit of tamoxifen was observed only in patients who had postmenopausal estrogen levels after chemotherapy.

Intergroup study 0102 also provides support for the use of chemoendocrine therapy in premenopausal women (52). Both premenopausal and postmenopausal women with high-risk, axillary node-negative breast cancer were randomized to receive CAF or CMF with or without 5 years of tamoxifen. The preliminary report of this trial suggests that CAF offers a marginal benefit over CMF and that tamoxifen provides additional benefit for patients who have ER-positive tumors. As a note of caution, the subset of premenopausal patients with ER-negative tumors actually had a worse outcome (DFS and overall survival) if they received tamoxifen (52). A Danish trial (DBCG 82B) of 634 premenopausal women with stage II or III primary breast cancer evaluated treatment with CMF nine cycles or CMF followed by tamoxifen (30 mg) for 1 year (53). This trial showed no benefit from the addition of 1 year of tamoxifen, but the overview analysis clearly demonstrates that longer durations of tamoxifen are optimal (8).

Many randomized clinical trials have evaluated the role of adjuvant chemoendo-crine therapy in postmenopausal patients. The most recent overview analysis reaf-firms that the addition of tamoxifen to chemotherapy in women aged over 50 years adds substantial benefit over that attained with chemotherapy alone (Table 14.10). These findings are not surprising because adjuvant chemotherapy alone provides less benefit (i.e., risk reduction) compared with tamoxifen in this age group of largely postmenopausal women.

More important is the issue of how much benefit is derived by the addition of chemotherapy to adjuvant tamoxifen in women over age 50 compared with adjuvant tamoxifen alone. Several recent trials addressed this issue. The IBCSG reported a clinical trial of node-positive, postmenopausal patients randomized to receive tamox-ifen, with or without CMF chemotherapy (54). Patients with ER-positive breast cancer benefited from chemoendocrine therapy, whereas patients with ER-negative breast cancer had a worse outcome with chemoendocrine therapy (54).

Albain et al. reported the results of an intergroup study involving ER-positive, node-positive, postmenopausal breast cancer patients who were randomized to ta-moxifen alone for 5 years versus CAF for six cycles followed by tamoxifen versus CAF concurrently with tamoxifen (55). The preliminary data showed that DFS is improved for patients who received chemoendocrine therapy versus tamoxifen alone (4-year DFS was 72% on tamoxifen and 79% on CAF plus tamoxifen). No difference in survival was detected in this analysis. Furthermore, an analysis of *HER-2* status suggested that in the subset of patients with *HER-2*-negative/ER-positive tumors, no benefit was derived from the addition of CAF (56). This latter observation will need to be validated in additional trials before it can be used to make decisions regarding the selection of adjuvant therapy.

In NSABP B-16, postmenopausal patients with ER-positive, axillary node-positive breast cancer were randomized to tamoxifen alone for 5 years or AC for four cycles plus tamoxifen or PAF (melphalan, doxorubicin, 5-flourouracil) plus tamoxifen (57). Patients who received AC plus tamoxifen had improved DFS and overall survival compared with those who received tamoxifen alone. All patients who received chemotherapy plus tamoxifen had improved outcome, although there was no difference detected between the two chemotherapy arms (57).

The overview analysis shows that the addition of chemotherapy to tamoxifen in women more than 50 years of age reduces the annual odds of recurrence and death by 19% and 11%, respectively (Table 14.10). The results of individual trials and those of the overview analysis support the use of chemoendocrine therapy in ER-positive postmenopausal patients. For an individual patient, it remains important to consider the added toxicity of chemotherapy in light of the small additional benefit over tamoxifen alone. An analysis by Gelber et al. (58) evaluated this issue by performing a meta-analysis of randomized clinical trials of adjuvant chemotherapy in postmenopausal women. It is noteworthy that the analysis took into account quality of life and confirmed that the toxicity that many women experience may outweigh the benefit gained from receiving adjuvant chemotherapy.

Table 14.13 provides a framework for current adjuvant therapy recommendations for patients with stage I or stage II primary breast cancer. These recommendations are based on the best available evidence from individual clinical trials and the most recent overview analysis (59).

TABLE 14.13. *Systemic adjuvant therapy recommendations – 2000*

	Positive axillary nodes	
	Therapy	Comment
Premenopausal		
ER negative	CMF, FEC, CEF, AC, AC → T	4–8 cycles
ER positive	Same chemo options plus TAM × 5 yr	
Postmenopausal		
ER negative	Same chemo options	
ER positive	TAM × 5 yr ± chemo options above	Overview analysis shows chemo/TAM superior to TAM

	Negative axillary nodes		
	ER status	Tumor size	Therapy
Pre-or postmenopausal	(1) Positive or negative	<10 mm	• Consider TAM for prevention • Consider chemotherapy for adverse features, such as nuclear grade, S-phase, angiolymphatic invasion, and size 6–10 mm
	(2) Negative	1–2 cm	CMF, AC, FEC, CEF
	(3) Negative	≥2 cm	CMF, AC, FEC, CEF
	(4) Positive	≥1 cm	TAM × 5 yr ± chemo (CMF, FEC, CAF, AC)

A, doxorubicin; C, cyclophosphamide; E, epirubicin; F, 5-Fluouracil; M, methotrexate; T, paclitaxel; TAM, tamoxifen.

REFERENCES

1. Landis SH, Murray T, Bolden S, et al. Cancer statistics, 1999. *CA Cancer J Clin* 1999;49:1,8–31.
2. Hankey BF, Ries LA, Edwards BK. The Surveillance, Epidemiology, and End Results Program: a national resource. *Cancer Epidemiol Biomarkers Prev* 1999;8:1117–1121.
3. Del Turco MR. Breast cancer update: encouraging trends . . . many new questions. *CA Cancer J Clin* 1999;49:135–137.
4. Mettlin C. Global breast cancer mortality statistics. *CA Cancer J Clin* 1999;49:138–144.
5. Olivotto IA, Bajdik CD, Plenderleith IH, et al. Adjuvant systemic therapy and survival after breast cancer. *N Engl J Med* 1994;330:805–810.
6. Quinn M, Allen E. Changes in incidence of and mortality from breast cancer in England and Wales since introduction of screening. United Kingdom Association of Cancer Registries. *BMJ* 1995;311: 1391–1395.
7. Early Breast Cancer Trialists' Collaborative Group (EBCTG). Polychemotherapy for early breast cancer: an overview of the randomised trials. *Lancet* 1998;352:930–942.
8. Early Breast Cancer Trialists' Collaborative Group (EBCTG). Tamoxifen for early breast cancer: an overview of the randomised trials. *Lancet* 1998;351:1451–1467.
9. Early Breast Cancer Trialists' Collaborative Group (EBCTG). Effects of adjuvant tamoxifen and of cytotoxic therapy on mortality in early breast cancer: an overview of 61 randomized trials among 28,896 women. *N Engl J Med* 1988;319:1681–1692.
10. Early Breast Cancer Trialists' Collaborative Group (EBCTG). Systemic treatment of early breast cancer by hormonal, cytotoxic, or immune therapy: 133 randomised trials involving 31,000 recurrences and 24,000 deaths among 75,000 women. *Lancet* 1992;339:71–85.
11. Carter CL, Allen C, Henson DE. Relation of tumor size, lymph node status, and survival in 24,740 breast cancer cases. *Cancer* 1989;63:181–187.
12. Rosen PR, Groshen S, Saigo PE, et al. A long-term follow-up study of survival in stage I (T1N0M0) and stage II (T1N1M0) breast carcinoma. *J Clin Oncol* 1989;7:355–366.
13. Levine MN, Bramwell VH, Pritchard KI, et al. Randomized trial of intensive cyclophosphamide, epirubicin, and fluorouracil chemotherapy compared with cyclophosphamide, methotrexate, and fluorouracil in premenopausal women with node-positive breast cancer: National Cancer Institute of Canada Clinical Trials Group. *J Clin Oncol* 1998;16:2651–2658.
14. Goldhirsch A, Colleoni M, Coates AS, et al. Adding adjuvant CMF chemotherapy to either radiotherapy or tamoxifen: are all CMFs alike? The International Breast Cancer Study Group (IBCSG). *Ann Oncol* 1998;9:489–493.
15. Pegram M, Pauletti G, Slamon D. HER-2/neu as a predictive marker of response to breast cancer therapy. *Breast Cancer Res Treat* 1998;52:65–77.
16. Thor AD, Berry DA, Budman DR, et al. erbB-2, p53, and efficacy of adjuvant therapy in lymph node-positive breast cancer. *J Natl Cancer Inst* 1998;90:1346–1360.
17. Paik S, Bryant J, Park C, et al. erbB-2 and response to doxorubicin in patients with axillary lymph node-positive, hormone receptor-negative breast cancer. *J Natl Cancer Inst* 1998;90:1361–1370.
18. Carlomagno C, Perrone F, Gallo C, et al. c-erb B2 overexpression decreases the benefit of adjuvant tamoxifen in early-stage breast cancer without axillary lymph node metastases. *J Clin Oncol* 1996; 14:2702–2708.
19. Elledge RM, Green S, Ciocca D, et al. HER-2 expression and response to tamoxifen in estrogen receptor-positive breast cancer: a Southwest Oncology Group Study. *Clin Cancer Res* 1998;4:7–12.
20. Norton L, Slamon D, Leyland-Jones B, et al. Overall survival advantage to simultaneous chemotherapy plus the humanized anti-HER-2 monoclonal antibody Herceptin in HER-2 -overexpressing metastatic breast cancer. *Proc Am Soc Clin Oncol* 1999;18:483A.
21. Munster PN, Hudis CA. Role of taxanes in adjuvant therapy. *Cancer Invest* 2000;18:32–38.
22. Henderson I, Berry D, Demetri G, et al. Improved disease-free survival and overall survival from the addition of sequential paclitaxel but not from the escalation of doxorubicin dose level in the adjuvant chemotherapy of patients with node-positive primary breast cancer. *Proc Am Soc Clin Oncol* 1998;17:390A.
23. Bezwoda W. Randomized, controlled trial of high dose chemotherapy versus standard dose chemotherapy for high risk, surgically treated primary breast cancer. *Proc Am Soc Clin Oncol* 1999;18: 4A.
24. Weiss RB, Rifkin RM, Stewart FM, et al. High-dose chemotherapy for high-risk primary breast cancer: an on-site review of the Bezwoda study. *Lancet* 2000;355:999–1003.

25. Bezwoda WR, Seymour L, Dansey RD. High-dose chemotherapy with hematopoietic rescue as primary treatment for metastatic breast cancer: a randomized trial. *J Clin Oncol* 1995;13:2483–2489.
26. Stadtmauer E, O'Neill A, Goldstein L, et al. Phase III randomized trial of high-dose chemotherapy and stem cell support shows no difference in overall survival or severe toxicity compared to maintenance chemotherapy with cyclophosphamide, methotrexate and 5-fluorouracil for women with metastatic breast cancer who are responding to conventional induction chemotherapy: the Philadelphia Intergroup Study (PBT-1). *Proc Am Soc Clin Oncol* 1999;18:1A.
27. Lotz JP, Cure H, Janvier M, et al. Intensive chemotherapy and autograft of hematopoietic stem cells in the treatment of metastatic cancer: results of the national protocol Pegase 04. *Hematol Cell Ther* 1999;41:71–74.
28. Peters W, Jones R, Vredenburgh J, et al. A large, prospective, randomized trial of high-dose combination alkylating agents (CPB) with autologous cellular support (ABMS) as consolidation for patients with metastatic breast cancer achieving complete remission after intensive doxorubicin-based induction therapy (AFM). *Proc Am Soc Clin Oncol* 1996;15:149A.
29. Peters W, Rosner G, Vredenburgh J, et al. A prospective, randomized comparison of two doses of combination alkylating afents as consolidation after CAF in high-risk primary breast cancer involving ten or more axillary lymph nodes: preliminary results of CALGB 9082/SWOG 9114/NCIC MA-13. *Proc Am Soc Clin Oncol.* 1999;18:2A.
30. 9401 TSBCSG. Results from a randomized adjuvant breast cancer study with high dose chemotherapy with CTCb supported by autologous stem cells versus dose escalated and tailored FEC therapy. *Proc Am Soc Clin Oncol* 1999;18:3A.
31. Hortobagyi GN, Buzdar AU, Theriault RL, et al. Randomized trial of high-dose chemotherapy and blood cell autografts for high-risk primary breast carcinoma. *J Natl Cancer Inst* 2000;92:225–233.
32. Rodenhuis S, Richel D, van der Wall E, et al. A randomized trial of high-dose chemotherapy and hematopoietic progenitor cell support in operable breast cancer with extensive axillary lymph node involvement. *Proc Am Soc Clin Oncol* 1998;17:470A.
33. Rodenhuis S, Bontembal M, Beex L, et al. Randomized phase III study of high-dose chemotherapy with cyclophosphamide, thiotepa and carboplatin in operable breast cancer with 4 or more axillary lymph nodes. *Proc Am Soc Clin Oncol* 2000;19:286A.
34. Osborne CK, Yochmowitz MG, Knight WAd, et al. The value of estrogen and progesterone receptors in the treatment of breast cancer. *Cancer* 1980;46:2884–2888.
35. Fisher B, Dignam J, Bryant J, et al. Five versus more than five years of tamoxifen therapy for breast cancer patients with negative lymph nodes and estrogen receptor-positive tumors. *J Natl Cancer Inst* 1996;88:1529–1542.
36. Stewart HJ, Forrest AP, Everington D, et al. Randomised comparison of 5 years of adjuvant tamoxifen with continuous therapy for operable breast cancer: the Scottish Cancer Trials Breast Group. *Br J Cancer* 1996;74:297–299.
37. Tormey DC, Gray R, Falkson HC. Postchemotherapy adjuvant tamoxifen therapy beyond five years in patients with lymph node-positive breast cancer: Eastern Cooperative Oncology Group. *J Natl Cancer Inst* 1996;88:1828–33.
38. Peto R. Five years of tamoxifen—or more? *J Natl Cancer Inst* 1996;88:1791–1793.
39. Baum M. Tamoxifen—the treatment of choice. Why look for alternatives? *Br J Cancer* 1998; 78(Suppl) 4:1–4.
40. Jordan VC, Fritz NF, Langan-Fahey S, et al. Alteration of endocrine parameters in premenopausal women with breast cancer during long-term adjuvant therapy with tamoxifen as the single agent. *J Natl Cancer Inst* 1991;83:1488–1491.
41. Holli K, Valavaara R, Blanco G, et al. Safety and efficacy results of a randomized trial comparing adjuvant toremifene and tamoxifen in postmenopausal patients with node-positive breast cancer. *J Clin Oncol* 2000;18:3487–3494.
42. Buzdar AU, Jonat W, Howell A, et al. Anastrozole versus megestrol acetate in the treatment of postmenopausal women with advanced breast carcinoma: results of a survival update based on a combined analysis of data from two mature phase III trials. Arimidex Study Group. *Cancer* 1998; 83:1142–1152.
43. Dombernowsky P, Smith I, Falkson G, et al. Letrozole, a new oral aromatase inhibitor for advanced breast cancer: double-blind randomized trial showing a dose effect and improved efficacy and tolerability compared with megestrol acetate. *J Clin Oncol* 1998;16:453–461.
44. Gershanovich M, Chaudri HA, Campos D, et al. Letrozole, a new oral aromatase inhibitor: randomised

trial comparing 2.5 mg daily, 0.5 mg daily and aminoglutethimide in postmenopausal women with advanced breast cancer: Letrozole International Trial Group (AR/BC3). *Ann Oncol* 1998;9:639–645.

45. Lonning PE, Bajetta E, Murray R, et al. Activity of exemestane in metastatic breast cancer after failure of nonsteroidal aromatase inhibitors: a phase II trial. *J Clin Oncol* 2000;18:2234–2244.

46. Kaufmann M, Bajetta E, Dirix LY, et al. Exemestane is superior to megestrol acetate after tamoxifen failure in postmenopausal women with advanced breast cancer: results of a phase III randomized double-blind trial: The Exemestane Study Group. *J Clin Oncol* 2000;18:1399–1411.

47. Buzdar A, Nabholtz J, Robertson J, et al. Anastrozole (Arimidex) versus tamoxifen as first-line therapy for advanced breast cancer in postmenopausal women. Combined analysis from two identically designed multicenter trials. *Proc Am Soc Clin Oncol* 2000;19:609A.

48. Mari E, Borrelle G, Sacco M, et al. Sitam-01: an Italian clinical trial comparing 2 versus 5 years of adjuvant tamoxifen in breast cancer patients aged >50 years: preliminary results. *Proc Am Soc Clin Oncol* 2000;19:331A.

49. Fisher B, Dignam J, Wolmark N, et al. Tamoxifen and chemotherapy for lymph node-negative, estrogen receptor-positive breast cancer. *J Natl Cancer Inst* 1997;89:1673–1682.

50. Aebi S, Gelber S, Castiglione-Gertsch M, et al. Is chemotherapy alone adequate for young women with oestrogen-receptor-positive breast cancer? *Lancet* 2000;355:1869–1874.

51. Davidson N, O'Neill A, Vukow A, et al. Effect of chemohormonal therapy in premenopausal, node(+), receptor(+) breast cancer: an Eastern Cooperative Oncology Group phase III Intergroup trial (E5188, INT-0101). *Proc Am Soc Clin Oncol* 1999;18:249A.

52. Hutchins L, Green S, Ravdin P, et al. CMF versus CAF with and without tamoxifen in high-risk, node-negative breast cancer patients and a natural history follow-up study in low-risk node-negative patients: first results of intergroup trial INT 0102. *Proc Am Soc Clin Oncol* 1998;17:1A.

53. Andersson M, Kamby C, Jensen MB, et al. Tamoxifen in high-risk premenopausal women with primary breast cancer receiving adjuvant chemotherapy: report from the Danish Breast Cancer cooperative Group DBCG 82B Trial. *Eur J Cancer* 1999;35:1659–1666.

54. International Breast Cancer Study Group. Effectiveness of adjuvant chemotherapy in combination with tamoxifen for node-positive postmenopausal breast cancer patients. *J Clin Oncol* 1997;15: 1385–1394.

55. Albain K, Green S, Osborne K, et al. Tamoxifen (T) versus cyclophosphamide, Adriamycin and 5-FU plus either concurrent or sequential T in postmenopausal, receptor (+), node(+) breast cancer: a Southwest Oncology Group phase III intergroup trial (SWOG-8814, INT-0100). *Proc Am Soc Clin Oncol* 1997;16:450A.

56. Ravdin P, Green S, Albain K, et al. Initial report of the SWOG biological correlative study of c-erbB-2 expression as a predictor of outcome in a trial comparing adjuvant CAFT with tamoxifen (T) alone. *Proc Am Soc Clin Oncol* 1998;17:374A.

57. Fisher B, Redmond C, Legault-Poisson S, et al. Postoperative chemotherapy and tamoxifen compared with tamoxifen alone in the treatment of positive-node breast cancer patients aged 50 years and older with tumors responsive to tamoxifen: results from the National Surgical Adjuvant Breast and Bowel Project B-16. *J Clin Oncol* 1990;8:1005–1018.

58. Gelber RD, Cole BF, Goldhirsch A, et al. Adjuvant chemotherapy plus tamoxifen compared with tamoxifen alone for postmenopausal breast cancer: meta-analysis of quality-adjusted survival. *Lancet* 1996;347:1066–1071.

59. National Comprehensive Cancer Network (NCCN). Update: NCCN practice guidelines for the treatment of breast cancer. *Oncology (Huntingt)* 1999;13:41–66.

15

The Role of Radiation Therapy in Breast Cancer Management

Ruth Heimann

INTRODUCTION TO RADIATION ONCOLOGY

At the end of nineteenth century (1895), Wilhelm Roentgen announced the discovery of "a new kind of ray" that allows the "photography of the invisible." The biological and therapeutic effects of the newly discovered x-rays were soon recognized, particularly because of the dermatitis and epilation they caused. In early 1896, a few weeks after the public announcement of Roentgen's discovery, Emil Grubbe in Chicago, Illinois, irradiated a patient with recurrent carcinoma of the breast. Also, Herman Gocht in Hamburg, Germany, irradiated a patient with locally advanced inoperable breast cancer and a patient with recurrent breast, cancer in the axilla (1). Despite the technical limitations of the early equipment, tumor shrinkage and, at times, complete elimination of the tumor were noticed. The full potential of radiation therapy could not be achieved in those early days, however, because of the limitations in the knowledge regarding fractionation, treatment techniques, and uncertainties about how to calculate the tissue dosage to deliver safe and effective doses of radiation.

Physics of Radiation Therapy

The x-rays and gamma rays are part of the spectrum of electromagnetic radiation that also includes radio waves, infrared, and visible and ultraviolet light. They are thought of as small packets of energy called *photons*. The x-rays reaching the tissue deposit their energy, and because their energy is quite high, they cause ejection of orbital electrons from the atoms, resulting in ionization—hence, the term *ionizing radiation*. Once the energy is deposited, many interactions occur, which generate more free electrons and free radicals. Because the human body is made mostly of water, the energy absorption leads to a chain reaction that results in the formation of multiple reactive free radical intermediates. Any of the cell constituents, such as proteins, lipids, RNA, and DNA, can be damaged. Apoptosis, signal transduction, and lipid peroxidation are altered as a result of direct or indirect effects of radiation. DNA double-strand breaks seem to the most critical damage, which, if unrepaired or incorrectly repaired, will result in cell death.

The radiation dose is measured in terms of the amount of energy absorbed per unit mass. Presently, the measurement unit is Gray (1 Gy is equal to 1 Joule/kg).

The past measurement unit was the Rad, and 100 Rads = 1 Gy. The beam energy determines its medical usefulness. The clinically useful energy ranges of the electromagnetic radiation are the following: superficial radiation, 10 to 125 keV; orthovoltage, 125 to 400 keV; and supervoltage, greater than 1,000 keV (> 1 MeV). As the beam energy increases, it penetrates deeper and more uniformly, and the skin sparing increases; this occurs because electrons that are created from the interaction between photons and the tissue travel some time before they reach the maximum intensity. In the superficial and orthovoltage ranges, most of the energy is deposited at or very close to the skin (i.e., with significant skin dose), a significant dose is absorbed in the bones, and useful beam energy cannot reach tissues at more than a couple of centimeters deep, resulting in marked dose nonhomogeneity in the tissue. The great advantage of the supervoltage/megavoltage photons is that, as the energy increases, the penetration of the x-ray increases, absorption into bone is not higher than the surrounding tissue, and skin sparing increases. Therefore, maximum dose does not occur on the skin but at depth in the tissue, and more homogeneity can be achieved in the targeted volume.

The era of modern radiation therapy started approximately 50 years ago when supervoltage machines became widely available because of advances in technology resulting from atomic energy research, the development of radar, and advances in computing. The availability of high-energy beam revolutionized the field of radiation oncology. Initially, the cobalt machine, a by-product of atomic research and subsequently the linear accelerator (LINAC)-generating beams with the energy ranging from 4 to 24 MeV became available; currently, LINACs are mostly in use. A photograph of a LINAC is shown in Fig. 15.1. In the LINAC, electrons are accelerated to very high speeds using electromagnetic waves in the frequency of the microwave range. The high-speed electrons are guided to strike a tungsten target to produce the x-rays.

For certain clinical circumstances, the electron beam is preferred. Electrons differ in the way they deposit energy in the tissue. With electrons, the maximum dose is reached close to the skin surface with minimum skin sparing; however, there is a marked fall in radiation dose at certain depth in the tissue. This depth can be carefully chosen, depending of the energy of the electron beam. Electron beams are used mostly for therapy of superficial tumors or to supplement (boost) photon therapy.

To conform to the tumor shape and anatomy, the radiotherapy beam is tailored to each individual patient by using beam modifiers placed in the path of the beam. They may include such devices as collimator, tissue compensators, individually constructed blocks, or, more recently, the multileaf collimator (MLC). An image of a MLC is shown in Fig. 15.2. From the early days of manual computing, when dose was calculated in a single point in the treated volume, recent computing advances led us to calculate dose in three dimensions (3D) in the tumor and surrounding tissue (3D treatment planning). In addition, these advances led us to account for differences in tissue density (i.e., lung, bone) as well as modify the dose inside the target area by ''dose painting'' or intensity-modulated radiation therapy (IMRT). We are now able to deliver more accurate radiation treatments and tailor treatments to individual

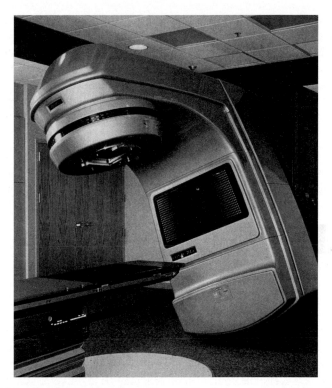

FIG. 15.1. A linear accelerator (LINAC) used for radiation therapy treatments (Courtesy of Varian Medical Systems Inc.).

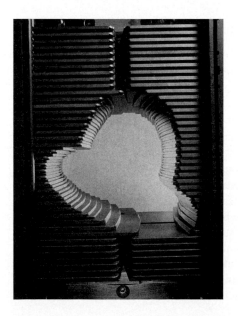

FIG. 15.2. The multileaf collimator (MLC) used to shape the treatment beam (Courtesy of Varian Medical Systems Inc.).

patients with increased efficacy and less morbidity. When dose can be delivered more accurately to the tumor and more normal surrounding tissue can be spared, dose intensification can be attempted to achieve higher cure rates without increased complications. Exclusion of as much normal tissue as possible from the path of the radiation beam is always of great importance because many patients are also receiving chemotherapy, which may result in higher probability of late complications.

Radiation, Surgery, and Chemotherapy

Radiation therapy is a locoregional curative modality that can be used either alone or in combination with surgery and chemotherapy. The rationale for combining surgery and radiation is because their patterns of failure are different. Radiation is less effective and failures occur more at the center of the tumor, where there is the largest volume of tumor cells, some necrotic, and in hypoxic conditions. Radiation is most effective at the margins where the tissue is well vascularized and the numbers of tumor cells are the lowest. Surgery, on the other hand, usually is limited by the normal structures in the proximity of the tumor. The bulk of the tumor usually can be excised, but to remove all microscopic disease may require very extensive surgery. So the failures of surgery are usually at the margins of excision, and that is where radiation is the most effective. To increase its therapeutic effectiveness, the radiation also can be sometimes combined with chemotherapeutic agents. Because these two modalities have different mechanisms of cell kill and can interfere with different phases of the cell cycle, the combined effects may be additive or synergistic or the chemotherapy may act as sensitizer to the effects of radiation.

Technical Aspects of Radiation Planning and Delivery

Radiation therapy is an integral part of the management of all stages of breast cancer. Prior to embarking on radiation treatments, careful treatment planning is necessary, including patient positioning and immobilization. Both are essential for accuracy of therapy, to ensure day-to-day reproducibility, and patient comfort. The treatment planning is done with the aid of a simulator, which is a machine with identical geometric characteristics as the treatment machine. Instead of high-energy treatment rays, it generates diagnostic x-rays to image the target (i.e., the irradiated volume). More recently, computed tomography (CT) has been incorporated into the simulator, allowing even more accurate target identification in the actual treatment position. After the target has been delineated, alternative treatment plans are generated and optimized. The plan that gives the best coverage of the target with minimal dose to the surrounding tissue and minimal inhomogeneities is chosen. The dose homogeneity is of great importance. Cold and hot spots have to be minimized because cold spots in the target will leave cancer undertreated, and, thus, a source of disease recurrence, and hot spots may increase the risk of complications. The treatment planning is a team effort between the physician, physicist, dosimetrist, and technologist. It is an interactive process that usually goes through multiple iteration until the optimal plan is reached.

In the treatment of nonmetastatic breast cancer, the radiation is aimed at the breast and chest wall and, depending on the clinical situation, also at the regional lymphatics, such as the supraclavicular, axillary, and internal mammary lymph nodes. The treatment goal is eradication of tumor with minimal side effects. The CT scanner can be used to delineate the targeted area and the critical structures to which dose should be limited. The beam arrangement that traverses the least amount of normal critical organs is chosen. In treatment of the intact breast or chest wall, medial and lateral tangential beams are used (Fig. 15.3). Tangential beams allow the encompassing of the breast tissue while including limited amounts of lung or heart. Using 3D treatment planning software the dose distribution is calculated for the entire breast volume. Beam modifiers are incorporated to minimize the volume of tissue receiving higher or lower than the prescribed dose and to minimize the dose to the skin surface while ensuring that the glandular tissue several millimeters under the skin is not undertreated. To treat the supraclavicular or axillary nodes and limit the dose to the spinal cord, a field shown in Fig. 15.4 is used. This field is usually an anterior–posterior field slightly angled to exclude the upper thoracic and

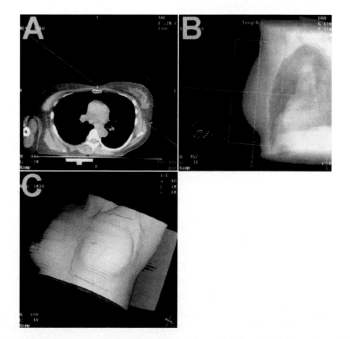

FIG. 15.3. Tangential beam arrangement for treatment of the intact breast or chest wall. **A:** Axial view showing medial and lateral tangential beams covering the breast tissue. **B:** View from the beam direction, "beam's eye view." Note the small amount of lung or heart in the treated volume. **C:** Projection of tangential beams on the patient's skin. These views were obtained from computed tomography-based simulation workstation.

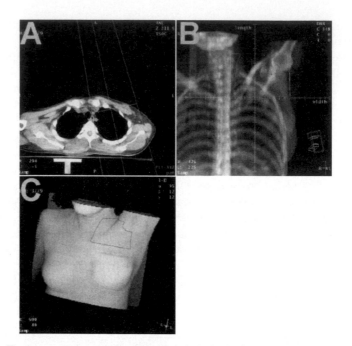

FIG. 15.4. The beam arrangement for the supraclavicular and axillary apex area. **A:** Axial view. Note how the beam is directed to avoid the spinal cord. **B:** The view from the beam angle also showing the blocking of the spinal cord and humeral head. **C:** The beam as it projects on the patient skin.

lower cervical spinal cord. Various techniques are used to match all the fields perfectly to prevent an overlap or a gap between them. Depending on the clinical situation radiation, treatments are given daily for $5\frac{1}{2}$ to $6\frac{1}{2}$ weeks. Most commonly in the United States, 1.8 Gy or 2.0 Gy fractions are used. Fractionation is necessary to keep the normal tissue complications to a minimum while still achieving maximum tumor control.

Adverse Effects of Radiation to the Breast

Treatments are usually well tolerated. Acute side effects may include fatigue, breast edema, skin erythema, hyperpigmentation, and, at times, desquamation, mostly limited to the inframammary fold and axilla. Acute skin changes should resolve 1 to 2 weeks posttreatment. Higher treatment fraction sizes may result in more moist desquamation during therapy, breast edema, and fibrosis, thus jeopardizing the cosmetic outcome. The cosmesis posttreatment is usually good to excellent in most patients. Posttherapy, the appearance of the breast gradually improves. Hyperpigmentation resolves, skin color returns to normal, and breast edema resolves. The return to normal color and texture happens in most patients but in some may take 2 or even up to 3 years.

With modern megavoltage therapy and treatment planning, the long-term side effects are limited. They depend on the radiation dose, fraction size, energy of the beam, and volume radiated. Most of the side effects can be limited with appropriate treatment planning.

Symptomatic pneumonitis is exceedingly rare, occurring in fewer than 1% of patients, particularly in those treated only with tangential fields and not receiving chemotherapy. The risk is 3% to 5% if chemotherapy is given and the supraclavicular nodes need to be treated. If chemotherapy and radiation are given sequentially instead of concomitantly, the risk is lower. In a study by Lingos at al., the risk of radiation pneumonitis was 1% if the chemotherapy and radiation were given sequentially and could be as high as 9% if the treatments were concurrent (2). The risk also depends on the type, dose, and scheduling of the chemotherapeutic agents. In patients in whom symptomatic pneumonitis develops, it is usually mild and reversible either spontaneously or after a short course of steroids. Damage to the brachial plexus may develop in less than 1% of women treated with the currently used doses and fraction sizes. Larger fraction size may result in an increased risk of brachial plexopathy. There is a very small risk of rib fractures and soft-tissue necrosis.

In more than 2,000 patients treated at the University of Chicago Center, no rib fractures or soft-tissue necrosis were noted. Radiation can cause damage to the heart. The effects are dependent on the radiation technique used. The early trials of postmastectomy radiation have shown an increase in cardiac deaths in the long-term survivors (3). In those early days, however, an anteroposterior photon beam was used to treat the internal mammary nodes (IMN) that on the left side included a large segment of the heart (4). With the currently used treatment planning techniques, excessive doses to large part of the heart can be avoided. The effects on the heart may include pericarditis (5) and acceleration of coronary artery disease. Many of the active and currently used chemotherapeutic agents (Adriamycin, Taxol, and Herceptin) can produce deleterious effects on the heart. Except in rare occasions, radiation and these chemotherapeutic agents are not given concurrently, and therefore no significantly increased risk of heart-related complications have been noted. The long-term combined effects of cardiotoxic chemotherapeutic agents and radiation are not yet completely known, however, because the newer drugs have not been used that long. Cardiac disease can become evident 10 to 20 years posttherapy. Thus, longer follow-up will be needed before firm conclusions are reached. In the interim, particular attention should be given to the treatment planning of left-sided breast cancer after cardiotoxic chemotherapy, particularly if IMNs need to be treated. New treatment planning techniques using IMRT are being studied to decrease the volume of heart and lung treated.

Lymphedema may develop following axillary dissection and can be exacerbated with radiation. Although not life-threatening, it can significantly impact the quality of life. The risk of lymphedema depends on the extent of axillary node dissection and the extent of the radiation to the axilla. With a complete axillary dissection, including all three levels of axillary nodes, and radiation therapy, the risk of lymphedema may be up to 40%. If the surgery is limited to level I and II dissection and the axilla is not radiated, however, the risk of significant lymphedema is only 3% to 5 %. This risk can be reduced by avoiding trauma and infection to the arm on the dissected side. The condition is usually chronic, and although it can be stabilized with physical therapy and manual lymphatic decompression, it can rarely be eliminated.

There is a small risk of second malignancies in long-term breast cancer survivors treated with radiation (6). In a woman with breast cancer, the risk of contralateral breast cancer is approximately 0.5% to 1% per year, of which fewer than 3% could be attributed to previous radiation (7). In the study by Boice et al. most of the risk was seen among women radiated before age 45 (7). After age 45, there was little, if any, risk of radiation-induced secondary breast cancers. This finding has been confirmed in a case–control study in a cohort of more than 56,000 mostly perimeno-pausal and postmenopausal women. The dose to the contralateral breast was calculated to be 2.51 Gy, and the overall risk of contralateral breast cancer was not increased in the patients receiving radiation therapy. The secondary tumors were evenly distributed in the various quadrants of the breast, also arguing against radiation-related contralateral breast cancer (8). In patients treated at the University of Chicago with mastectomy between 1927 to 1987, no increase was found in contralateral breast cancer in women who also received chest-wall radiation (9).

Other treatment-related malignancies include lung cancer, sarcoma, and leukemia. The risk of treatment-related lung cancer is small. Studies from the Connecticut Tumor Registry of patients treated between 1945 and 1981 show that in 10-year survivors, approximately nine cases of radiotherapy-induced lung cancer per year would be expected to occur among 10,000 treated women (10). The risk is significantly increased with smoking (11). The reported cumulative risk of sarcoma in the radiation field is 0.2% at 10 years (12), and the risk of leukemia is minimal with radiation only. In combination with alkylating agents, however, the risk may be higher (13). Many published studies tend to report the risk of second malignancies as the relative risks. It is important to realize when reading and evaluating the clinical literature that, from patients' and physicians' perspectives, the concept of relative risk is not very informative because the relative risk of an event with radiation may be very high compared with no radiation. If, however, the absolute risk is very low, it has no management or practical clinical value. Thus, absolute numbers of risk are much more relevant and enlightening.

RADIATION THERAPY IN EARLY STAGE BREAST CANCER

Ductal Carcinoma *In Situ*

Ductal carcinoma in situ (DCIS), noninvasive ductal carcinoma, and intraductal carcinoma all refer to proliferation of malignant cells confined within the basement membrane. DCIS, a premalignant condition if untreated, is likely to progress to invasive breast cancer (14,15). Management of DCIS remains one the most controversial aspects of breast cancer treatment. It is a disease of the mammographic era with a significant increase in the incidence rate in the last decade. The nonpalpable DCIS, which constitutes most currently diagnosed disease, almost unknown 25 to 30 years ago, was expected to have reached 42,600 cases in year 2000 (16). Its natural history is long, and although the incidence has been increasing in recent years, few studies have been performed to examine alternative treatment options that have sufficient power and length of follow-up to have definite answers. The treatment options include simple mastectomy or local excision, with or without radiation. Several factors are important in the management decision of a patient with DCIS. Any evidence that the disease is or could be extensive, such as diffuse, suspicious, or indeterminate microcalcifications or multicentricity, as well as a mammogram that is difficult to follow, or if there is uncertainty that the patient can comply with a program of routine mammograms for follow-up, are contraindications for breast-conserving surgery. Status of the margin following local excision and the histologic subtype are important when making treatment decisions, and, as always, patient wishes and comorbidities need to be considered. If negative margins of excision cannot be obtained, breast-conservation attempts have to be abandoned. Among histologic subtypes, high-grade nuclei and comedo necrosis appear to be more aggressive variants and seem to have a higher risk of recurrence. It is not clear, however, whether the risk of recurrence is higher with comedo DCIS or just that the recurrence appears sooner, and if the follow-up were long enough, the recurrence rate would be the same in patients with comedo or noncomedo histology.

Traditionally, mastectomy was the standard of therapy for DCIS. The recurrence rates following mastectomy were 1% or less and the cancer related mortality 2% (17). After the documented success with breast-conserving therapy in infiltrating ductal carcinoma, however, it became increasingly difficult in the daily practice to recommend mastectomy to women with DCIS. Paradoxically, women who were adhering to a strict regimen of screening and were detected as having DCIS could be "rewarded" with mastectomy, whereas if they would have waited a few years for the disease to progress to invasion, they could have had breast-sparing surgery. A decision analysis of tradeoffs shows that there is only an 1% to 2 % difference in the actuarial survival rates at 10 and 20 years if the initial therapy is breast-conserving surgery and radiation compared with mastectomy (18). The small difference is most likely because at least half of recurrences after breast conservation are DCIS; among the other half that are invasive, most are detected at an early stage. As in many other clinical dilemmas in breast cancer, the National Surgical Adjuvant Breast and Bowel Project (NSABP) investigators significantly contributed to the changes in practice and redefined the standard of care in DCIS. A large prospective, randomized trial of 818 women done by the NSABP-17, with a median follow-up of 8 years, demonstrated that radiation therapy following breast-conserving surgery reduces both invasive and noninvasive ipsilateral breast cancer recurrences, and the particular impact was on the reduction of invasive breast cancer recurrences. The incidence of noninvasive cancer was reduced from 13% to 9%, invasive breast cancer from 13% to 4% (19). Mortality from breast cancer after 8 years was 1.6%. All patients benefited from radiation, irrespective of tumor size or pathologic characteristics. No features could be identified that would allow selection of patients in whom radiation could be eliminated (20,21). A separate analysis of the effects of radiation on DCIS in the earlier NSABP-06 also showed a reduction in local failure with radiation (22). A randomized trial performed by the European Organization for Research and Treatment of Cancer breast cancer cooperative group confirmed the NSABP-17 finding (23). With radiation, local recurrences were decreased from 16% to 9%. Both noninvasive and invasive tumor recurrences were decreased. Although with longer follow-up and more information from the combined prospective and retrospective studies the data may change, the currently available information for patients who are candidates for breast conservation shows a local recurrence rate after excision alone of 20% to 30%. Radiation can reduce this rate to about 10% to 15%. To improve the outcome, NSABP performed a study in which all patients who were candidates for breast conservation were treated with local excision followed by radiation and randomized to tamoxifen or placebo. This study, NSABP-24, enrolled more than 1,800 women (24). Tamoxifen therapy resulted in 50% decrease in recurrences compared with radiation only without tamoxifen.

In several retrospective studies, attempts were made to determine in which patients radiation can be eliminated. Silverstein et al. devised a scoring system that combined the size of the DCIS, margins, grade, and necrosis (25). This system was subsequently modified to show that margins alone are the most important (26). Using the information regarding pathologic margins, these researchers attempted to develop criteria to decide when DCIS can be satisfactorily treated by local excision, when radiation therapy should be added, and when mastectomy is required. Because the number of events in relation to the number of patients was low, the differences were not statistically significant, and firm conclusions cannot be reached (27). It is important to realize that because of the pathologic characteristics of DCIS, it is frequently difficult to determine the exact size of the DCIS, and many pathologists are reluctant to do so. Thus, because many times the pathologic size is unavailable or cannot be accurately ascertained, some studies report DCIS size in millimeters, others in the number of slides with DCIS, and still others by using its mammographic size. This makes the comparison between studies and the interpretation of the literature difficult. The other criteria for breast conservation, the widths of the margins, can significantly compromise cosmesis. In breast-conservation surgery, the width of the margins is in close inverse correlation with cosmesis. When performing the surgical excision, the surgeon is carefully balancing an oncologic surgery to achieve adequate margins and cosmesis because wide margins and removal of large amount of tissue may significantly impact on cosmesis.

In general, small incidental DCIS as well as very small low-grade DCIS excised with wide margins (> 1 cm) can be followed up after local excision without radiation. In summary, DCIS size, margins, histology, mammographic presentation, age, comorbidities, life expectancy, and patient preference are all factors in determining the optimal management of each patient.

NIH Consensus Conference (1990)
Early-Stage Breast Cancer (28)

Breast conservation therapy is an appropriate method of primary therapy for the

majority of women with stage I and II breast cancer and is *preferable* because it

provides *survival equivalent* to the total mastectomy and axillary dissection while

preserving the breast.

FIG. 15.5. The National Institutes of Health Consensus Conference Statement.

Invasive Breast Cancer

Breast Conservation

In 1990, the National Institutes of Health (NIH) convened a consensus conference to address the issue of breast-conserving therapy in stage I and II breast cancers (28). The participants concluded that breast-conserving therapy is equivalent and possibly better than mastectomy. The summary statement is presented in Fig. 15.5. The conclusions were based on six randomized trials that all showed equal survival for patients treated with breast-conserving therapy compared with those who underwent mastectomies. With more follow-up and update, the results have been further confirmed and they are holding (29–34) (Table 15.1). Breast-conserving therapy means local excision of the bulk of the tumor followed by moderate doses of radiation to eradicate residual foci of tumor cells in the remaining breast. Despite the NIH

TABLE 15.1. *Overall survival (%) in six randomized trials of breast-conserving treatment compared to mastectomy*

Treatment (ref)	Stage I and II breast cancer	
	Mastectomy (%)[a]	BCT (%)[a]
NSABP B-06[a] (32)	60	62
NCI[a] (33)	75	77
Milan (29)	69	71
IGR (Paris)[a] (34)	65	73
EORTC[a] (30)	73	71
DBCCG[a] (31)	82	79

BCT, breast conservation therapy; DBCCG, Danish Breast Cancer Cooperative Group; EORTC, European Organization for Research and Treatment of Cancer; IGR, Institute Goustave Roussy; NCI, National Cancer Institute; NSABP, National Surgical Adjuvant Breast and Bowel Project.
[a] Follow-up of 6 to 15 years.

Consensus Conference conclusions, it seems the acceptance of breast-conserving therapy is far from uniform and varies greatly by geographic area (35,36). From the most recently available data, the overall breast conservation rates are still only 60% in stage I patients and less than 40% in stage II patients, indicating that there are significant barriers to the use of breast-conserving therapy (37,38). Medical contraindications and patient choice do not seem to be the major factors in the underuse of breast-conserving surgery (39). More than 80% of the women, independent of age or race, given the option, will choose breast conservation.

The role of the radiation is to decrease the risk of local failure in the breast, but it also may contribute to survival. It accomplishes what mastectomy would have done, that is, treat the entire breast. Treatments usually are delivered to the whole breast, followed with an additional radiation "boost" to the lumpectomy site. Careful pathologic studies of mastectomy specimens have shown that microscopic residual disease is present away from the primary (index) tumor; however, the highest burden is in the same quadrant less than 4 cm from the primary tumor (40). Extrapolation from early radiation therapy studies established the appropriate dose to eradicate microscopic foci of disease in the range of 45 to 50 Gy. This is the dose usually given to the entire breast. The higher burden of microscopic disease around the primary site is encompassed in the "boost" volume. Reported local control rates in the randomized trials and retrospective studies vary from 70% to 97% (19,41, 42). Many factors have been suggested as having an impact on local control rates. Some have been confirmed in multiple studies, whereas some were shown not to be of importance when longer follow-up and more data became available. Most local recurrences following mastectomy occur in the first 3 years; however, recurrences after breast-conserving therapy have been documented to occur up to 20 years. Up to 5 to 8 years from diagnosis, most recurrences are in the same quadrant as the primary. Subsequently, the proportion changes in favor of tumor "elsewhere" in the breast. These are most likely second primaries.

Determination of whether a patient is candidate for breast-conserving surgery and radiation is a multidisciplinary effort in which close communication between the surgeon, the mammographer, the pathologist, the medical oncologist, and the radiation oncologist is necessary. *Absolute contraindications* (43,44) for breast-conserving therapy are the following:

1. Multicentric disease (i.e., disease in separate quadrants of the breast, diffuse malignant appearing, or indeterminate microcalcifications)
2. Prior radiation treatments to doses that, combined with the planned dose, will exceed tissue tolerance, which may happen in women who have received radiation at younger age for lymphoma, particularly Hodgkin disease
3. Inability to obtain negative surgical margins following attempts for breast-conserving surgery. Negative excision margins appear to be the most important factor impacting on local control. If the margins are positive, the risk of local recurrence is increased (42,45). From retrospective studies, it appears that focally positive margins

can be controlled with radiation, but more extensively involved margins are indication for reexcision. If, after several attempts of reexcision negative margins cannot be obtained, the plans for breast conservation should be abandoned because both survival and cosmesis may be compromised.

4. Pregnancy is a contraindication for breast-conserving therapy because of the concerns on the effects of radiation on the fetus. Sometimes surgery can be done during the third trimester and follow with radiation after delivery. This latter is to be done only after careful consideration because chances for cure ought not be compromised for cosmetic reasons.

Relative contraindications include the following:

1. The *size of tumor* compared with the breast size may pose some challenge from the perspective of cosmetic outcome. Most randomized trials of breast-conserving therapy included women whose tumors were smaller than 4 cm, but tumor size is mainly a consideration as it relates to the cosmetic outcome. Breast conservation should be attempted only if an acceptable cosmetic outcome can be achieved. If the tissue deficit because of the size of the tumor is large in relation to the breast size, then it is preferable to perform a mastectomy followed by breast reconstruction. The ratio between tumor size and patient's breast size determines the advisability of breast-conserving therapy.

2. *Tumor location* in the vicinity of the nipple may require excision of the nipple–areola complex, which may result in less than optimal cosmesis, but it does not impact on outcome. Many women will opt for breast preservation even if the nipple is removed because it still leaves behind most of the breast tissue and native skin.

3. *Breast size.* There are some technical difficulties in the radiation treatment of women with large breasts, but if adequate immobilization can be devised and adequate dose homogeneity can be achieved, breast conservation is preferable to a mastectomy that would result in major asymmetry.

4. *Patients with history of collagen vascular disease,* particularly lupus or scleroderma, are reported to be at significantly increased risk of complications, especially soft-tissue and bone necrosis, most likely because of compromised microvasculature.

Other criteria—such as patient age, family history, positive axillary lymph nodes—are not contraindications for breast-conserving therapy. Patient age should not be considered in the decision regarding breast-conservation therapy. Although breast cancer appears to be more aggressive in very young women, there is no clear evidence that if the currently used criteria for breast-conserving therapy are followed, breast conservation should be denied to young women. Very young women (i.e., age 35 or younger) may have more aggressive disease and are at higher risk of both distant and local recurrences. Although the perception may be that cancer may be less aggressive, and that older women are not as interested in breast preservation, the studies do not support this contention. In fact, several reports have shown that survival and disease-free survival from breast cancer are lower in older women (46,

47), and there are no indications that elderly women have significantly more problems tolerating radiation compared with younger women.

A challenging question is whether mutations in the two genes that predispose to breast cancer, *BRCA-1* and *BRCA-2*, are a contraindication for radiation and thus breast conserving treatment. Hypotheses yet to be proven are whether radiation to the remaining breast tissue or scatter radiation to the contralateral breast will increase the risk of a second breast cancer or, conversely, whether radiation is more effective in patients with known mutations because the normal function of the genes is DNA repair and the mutations could prevent the escape of tumor cells from the effects of radiation. If the damaged DNA cannot be repaired, the effects of controlling the tumor with radiation may be enhanced. In a case–control study of women treated with breast-conserving surgery and radiation, it was shown that after radiation there is no increased risk of events in the ipsilateral breast in patients with known *BRCA* mutations compared with patients without mutations (48). When patients with local recurrence following radiation were matched with a group without local recurrence, mutations were found to be more common in patients with recurrences and occurred primarily in younger women, in other quadrants, and late, most likely representing new primaries (49). There is currently no evidence that women with mutations in *BRCA-1* or *BRCA-2* or with a family history of breast cancer would be at a disadvantage if offered breast-conserving therapy, including radiation (50).

Several studies attempted to define a subpopulation of patients who may not need radiation (Table 15.2). They vary in length of follow-up, inclusion criteria, and details of therapy. In studies from Sweden and Canada, investigators tried to determine whether radiation could be omitted in patients with small tumors. Thus, they limited their studies to patients with node-negative tumors smaller than 2 cm (51, 52). These trials showed a significant decrease in local failures when radiation was given but no significant difference in survival. Nevertheless, there was a trend toward overall survival benefit in the group receiving radiation (32,52). None of the trials had a sufficient number of patients and thus the power to detect 10% or lower absolute benefits in survival. In a prospective single institution study, attempts were made to select the most favorable patients with the lowest risk of recurrence and enroll them in a study of only breast-conserving surgery, that is, without radiation. The criteria for inclusion were tumor size smaller than 2 cm, negative axillary nodes, absence of lymphatic invasion, absence of extensive intraductal component, at least

TABLE 15.2. *Local recurrence (%) following local excision compared with local excision and radiation in stage I breast cancer*

	Excision	Excision and radiation	Follow-up (yr)
Liljergen et al. (51)	24	8	10
Clark et al. (52)	35	11	8
Schnitt et al. (53)	16	N/A	5

N/A, not available.

1 cm margin of normal breast tissue around the tumor, and breasts that can be easily followed mammographically. The median tumor size was 6 mm. Even in this very favorable group, the failure rate was 20% at 5 years (53), and the trial was stopped before its completion because the observed failure rate exceeded the expected rate predetermined by the trial-stopping rules. This study highlights the difficulty in selecting patients in whom radiation treatments can be eliminated.

Chemotherapy or tamoxifen may contribute to local control but, by themselves, are not sufficient. For example, in the NSABP-06 trial, the local failure rate in patients undergoing only local excision without radiation was approximately 32%. In those who underwent local excision and also received chemotherapy, it was close to 40%, demonstrating that the chemotherapy did not decrease the local failure rates. In the comparable group who, after local excision, received both chemotherapy and radiation, the cumulative risk at 12 years was only 5% (32), whereas in those receiving radiation only, the local failure rates were 12%. This finding demonstrates that radiation decreases the local recurrence rates and this is further decreased when combined with chemotherapy. Other studies confirmed better local control rates with the addition of chemotherapy to radiation (54,55). Even the very high doses of chemotherapy alone that were given as part of bone marrow transplant programs were not sufficient for local control. To increase the feasibility of breast-conserving therapy, neoadjuvant chemotherapy has been attempted, and results have been satisfactory. Some women who would not be candidates for breast conservation because of tumor size, if they first receive chemotherapy and the tumor shrinks, may become candidates for breast conservation without affecting their survival (56).

Many women who undergo breast-conserving therapy are also receiving adjuvant chemotherapy. In these women, the sequencing of chemotherapy and radiation needs to be decided. One prospective randomized trial and several retrospective studies had somewhat conflicting results. Some studies show that giving chemotherapy first, before radiation, increases the risk of local failure, whereas other studies show that the chemotherapy-first does not significantly increase local failure rates and may result in better distant disease-free survival and overall survival (57–59). If local excision with negative margins is achieved and the patient is a candidate for breast conservation, it is unlikely that the patient's survival will be affected by a delay in radiation therapy because of initial chemotherapy. Our institutional preference is that small-node-negative patients receive radiation first, whereas node-positive patients receive chemotherapy first. In some instances, concomitant chemotherapy and radiation therapy have been given, which may increase the risk of side effects and jeopardize the cosmetic outcome.

Depending on the clinical situation, radiation is delivered to the draining lymphatics, which include axilla, supraclavicular nodes, and IMNs. Axillary radiation is indicated if the axilla has not been dissected, if a limited dissection was done and includes positive nodes, or if gross disease was found, particularly in the apex of the axilla close to the axillary vein. Communication between the surgeon and the radiation oncologist regarding the findings at surgery is of great importance. The undissected axillary apex nodes and supraclavicular nodal areas are treated if the axilla has been dissected and positive nodes were found. Treatment to the IMNs is given at times if the primary lesion is medially or centrally located and the axillary lymph nodes are positive with metastatic breast cancer. CT-based 3D treatment planning is recommended, particularly for left-sided lesions where care needs to be taken to minimize the amount of treated heart. Treatment of the regional lymphatics, in addition to the tangential fields, adds technical complexity to the treatments and particular attention is paid in matching the fields so as not to undertreat or overtreat.

Good disease control in the axilla with minimum morbidity can be obtained from radiation to axilla without dissection (60). Thus, axillary dissection is indicated if the results would change the planned therapy. In patients who undergo sentinel node biopsy, if the sentinel node has no disease, radiation to the axilla is omitted. If the node is positive, complete dissection or radiation to the axilla is likely to be of equivalent efficacy.

Close follow-up after breast conservation is essential to detect local recurrences, new primaries, and contralateral disease. In general, true local recurrences occur earlier, whereas disease in other quadrants develops later (i.e., 5 years or longer after therapy). Although institutional policies for mammographic follow-up vary, a reasonable policy would be mammograms of the index breast every 6 months for the first 2 years, followed by yearly mammograms, and yearly mammograms for the contralateral breast.

Postmastectomy Radiation

Postmastectomy, the risk of local recurrence varies, depending on the number of positive nodes in the axilla, size of the tumor, length of follow-up, and how local site recurrences are being scored. As the number of nodes with metastatic disease in the axilla increases, the risk of chest wall recurrence increases. In fact, the number of positive nodes is related more to an increased risk of recurrence than to the size of the tumor. The length of follow-up and how the recurrences are being scored are also important. Frequently, if a patient develops metastatic disease, there is a tendency to overlook a local recurrence. Most locoregional recurrences occur in the first 5 years following mastectomy, but disease may recur even 10 to 15 years postmastectomy (61). Thus, long-term follow-up is important. Local recurrences have significant impact on quality of life. They may become quite large, ulcerate, and become malodorous and painful. Radiation can decrease the risk of local recurrence postmastectomy. Once recurrence is clinically manifested, the likelihood of controlling the recurrence is only 50% to 60%. Who, therefore, should be receiving radiation postmastectomy? There is reasonable consensus when it comes to patients with four or more positive nodes in the axilla or with a tumor more than 5 cm large. What, then, should we do with a patient with a 3.5- to 4-cm tumor and three positive nodes, particularly if she is young? Do we have sufficient information to counsel these younger women when the potential life expectancy is 20 to 30 years? Data on sufficient women with the various combinations of tumor size and node positivity and long enough follow-up are difficult to come by, particularly for those who also

TABLE 15.3. *Percent cumulative incidence of LRF (10 years) following mastectomy and chemotherapy*

Node positive	Size					
	≤1	1.1–2	2.1–3	3.1–4	4.1–5	>5
1	3	11	12	10	6	27
2	8	14	12	20	14	31
3	20	18	11	8	14	36
4	19	17	22	26	37	33
5–6	22	23	27	25	22	47
7–9	12	33	30	32	32	41
≥10	39	30	31	36	35	31

LRF, local regional failure.

Data from Recht A, Gray R, Davidson NE, et al. Locoreginal failure 10 years after mastectomy and adjuvant chemotherapy with or without tamoxifen without irradiation: experience of the Eastern Cooperative Oncology Group. *J Clin Oncol* 1999;17:1689, with permission.

receive chemotherapy. Recht et al. reviewed the local failure in patients treated with mastectomy and chemotherapy without radiation in the various Eastern Cooperative Oncology Group trials (62). The data are shown in Table 15.3. The cumulative rates of chest-wall failure in patients not receiving chemotherapy can be up to 30% to 35% in patients with four or more positive nodes or up to 25% to 30% if one to three nodes are positive (63).

The impact of chest-wall radiation remains controversial because the natural history of breast cancer is long; the techniques of radiation are continuously changing, allowing better coverage of the target with less morbidity; and in most women chemotherapy is also given. Meta-analyses show that radiation decreases breast cancer deaths, but in some studies an increase in the risk of cardiovascular disease was noted (3,64). Few of the studies included in the meta-analyses used the current radiation techniques or administered chemotherapy. The capability currently exists to design CT-guided treatment plans. When treatment is done with CT planning, the exact target location can be determined and the radiated volume of lung and heart in the treatment field minimized.

Two updated studies in which women were treated with chemotherapy and radiation postmastectomy show better disease-free and overall survival in patients who received radiation therapy to the chest wall and draining nodes in addition to full systemic therapy (Table 15.4) (65–67). To date, these are the most relevant trials to our current clinical practice. These studies reignited discussions regarding the benefits of postmastectomy radiation. Particularly questioned are the benefits in women with one to three positive nodes and whether the results can be extrapolated to practice in the United States because the median number of lymph nodes dissected was only seven. In United States, the axillary node dissections usually are more extensive. These investigators reanalyzed their data separately for women with one to three positive nodes and also in those with ten or more nodes dissected. They

TABLE 15.4. *Impact of postmastectomy radiation therapy on overall survival in patients also receiving systemic therapy*

	Follow-up (yr)	Overall survival (%)		*p* value
		CMF and radiation	CMF	
Overgaard et al. (65)	10	54	45	0.001
Ragaz et al. (66)	15	52	43	0.02
		TAM and radiation	TAM	
Overgaard et al. (67)	10	45	36	0.03

CMF, cytoxan, methotrexate, 5 fluorouracil; TAM, tamoxifen.

found a significant benefit in survival in women with one to three positive nodes and also in those who had the more extensive axillary dissection. Interestingly, the benefit in survival for the group receiving radiation was even larger in the women who only had one to three positive nodes compared with those with four or more positive nodes. A national trial was initiated in women with one to three positive nodes to address more fully the role of postmastectomy radiation. The benefit from radiation therapy on survival was, in fact, equivalent to the known benefit women achieve from chemotherapy (68). Because in both the Canadian and Danish trials women also were treated to their IMNs, this question also is receiving renewed interest. Radiation therapy to the IMNs benefits women with medial or central lesions in whom the axillary nodes are positive. Inclusion of the IMNs, particularly on the left side, undoubtedly will increase the volume of heart treated. Thus, treatments should be done with CT-based planning so that the IMN can be localized and the volume of lung and heart minimized.

The management of breast cancer recurrences depends on the prior therapy. Disease that recurs after breast-conserving surgery and radiation therapy is usually treated with mastectomy. Attempts have been made to perform an excision only in patients in whom a very early recurrence is found, and results have been satisfactory, but the number of patients treated in this manner is low and the follow-up too short to realize the full impact (69). A full course of radiation for the second time is difficult to deliver because of the risk of long-term complications. The breast may become fibrotic and cosmetically unappealing. If feasible, a recurrence that occurs postmastectomy should be excised. Radiation, particularly if not previously given, will decrease the risk of further recurrences. The radiation fields need to encompass the chest wall and regional lymphatics, not just the area of recurrence, because it seems that if only a small radiation field is used, recurrences may appear just outside the irradiated area (70)

Radiation and Breast Reconstruction

Many women who undergo mastectomy also opt for breast reconstruction. The techniques of reconstructive surgery have been changing. The use of silicone and saline implants has decreased significantly in favor of autologous tissue with pedicle or microanastomosis. The reconstructed, vascularized tissue is of great advantage in minimizing the risk of complications from radiation. The reported risk of complications for patients who undergo reconstruction and radiation varies anywhere from 18% to 51%. In the more recent publications, the risk of complications is at the lower end of range, probably because of improvements in techniques of both surgery and radiation. The optimal sequencing of radiation and reconstructive surgery is not well established; thus, multiple factors need to be considered. Because a general consensus is lacking, good communication between all members of the oncologic team is essential. The issue under consideration is the operation in a previously irradiated field if the reconstruction is being done following radiation. Concerns are less, however, with the techniques that are using autologous vascularized tissues. On the other hand, if the reconstruction is done immediately after mastectomy and this is followed by radiation, there are concerns regarding the cosmesis, firming, and fat necrosis after radiating the reconstruction and the possible obscuring of a recurrence. Data exist to show, however, that most recurrences are not obscured by the myocutaneous flap (71). In general, good to excellent cosmesis is being achieved in most women who have radiation to the reconstructed breast. If there are no other contraindications, breast cancer occurring in an augmented breast can be treated with breast conservation. There may be some complications, such as scarring or fat necrosis, but the risk seems to be low (72), and the cosmetic outcome very good. Thus, the augmentation does not need to be removed prior to radiation. In most patients in whom complications may later develop, the reconstruction may have to be revised or removed. This approach would leave most women with the augmentation spared.

LOCALLY ADVANCED BREAST CANCER

Locally advanced and inflammatory breast cancers, stage III disease, pose a major management challenge. Because of the very high risk of local and distant failure, no single modality satisfactorily controls the disease, and thus, all three treatment modalities (i.e., chemotherapy, radiation therapy, and surgery) need to be incorporated in a management plan. Because this disease presentation is not common and because its definition encompasses a spectrum of diseases from large primary tumors with some skin edema or small limited skin ulceration to huge necrotic masses or global inflammatory changes, large randomized trials to define the standard of care are lacking. If the patient is a candidate for mastectomy, surgery can be performed upfront, followed by adjuvant systemic therapy and radiation. Radiation alone as the local treatment modality in patients with large tumors is suboptimal. Control of the disease can be obtained in at most in 50% of the patients, and large doses are needed, which may result in long-term sequelae, including fibrosis and tissue necrosis (73). If, however, mastectomy is feasible, radiation is very effective in reducing the local failure rates. The microscopic residual disease can be well controlled with 50 to 60 Gy, and failure rates would decrease from 30% to 40% down to 10% to

15%. Because the risk of metastatic disease is very high, there is general consensus that systemic therapy is needed, despite the fact that several small randomized trials failed to demonstrate benefit for chemotherapy, probably because patient numbers were low and the disease is heterogeneous. Retrospective studies, however, show significant benefits compared with historical controls (74,75).

Despite the general consensus that there is need for aggressive control of both local and distant disease, controversies remain regarding sequencing of the various therapies and the need for both radiation and surgery for local control. In most situations, even if patients are technically operable, a few cycles of chemotherapy are given first. Response rates to chemotherapy are usually high, and complete clinical response can be achieved in up to 30% of the patients. Patients with the best response have also the best chances for survival. If a good response to chemotherapy is obtained, mastectomy is undertaken, followed by additional chemotherapy and radiation. If there is no response to initial chemotherapy, a switch to radiation or a different chemotherapy regimen is needed. Although not clearly established, retrospective reviews indicate that local control is better if both surgery and radiation are given than with either modality alone (76).

Inflammatory breast cancer has a very high risk of metastatic disease and also very high risk of local failure if surgery alone is performed. Because of the involvement of the dermal lymphatics, the disease is much more extensive than can be clinically appreciated. Therefore, even if negative margins can be obtained, the disease soon recurs. Historically, because of its systemic nature, the 5-year survival rates were at most 10%. Presently, however, with the combination of chemotherapy surgery and radiation, the 5-year survival rates are approaching 30% to 50% (75). The sequencing of treatments depends on the response to therapy. Chemotherapy is initiated as soon as possible and response assessed after each cycle. If a good response is obtained, surgery is performed, followed by additional chemotherapy and radiation to the chest wall and draining lymphatics. If, however, the response to chemotherapy is poor, radiation is added to bring the patient to operability. Because of the competing risks of both local and distant disease, several pilot research protocols are now in progress that are using concomitant aggressive chemotherapy and radiation; preliminary results are encouraging (77,78). The challenge is to give concomitantly sufficient chemotherapy to be therapeutically effective for metastatic disease and radiation therapy to control local disease, all this without severe complications.

RADIATION AS PALLIATION

Radiation treatments may contribute significantly to the palliative treatment of advanced and metastatic disease. Painful, weeping, malodorous chest-wall recurrences can be controlled with radiation, thus significantly contributing to quality of life and the ability to resume a normal lifestyle. The symptomatic effects of brain, bone, spinal cord, brachial plexus, coroidal, and liver metastases can be palliated with radiation, and the effects can be durable for the lifetime of the patient. Single brain metastases or few metastases in the same proximity can be boosted with stereotactic radiosurgery or stereotactic radiotherapy, significantly improving the outcome, particularly if the disease at the primary site is controlled or if there is no evidence of disease elsewhere. (*Stereotactic radiosurgery* refers to a single large fraction, whereas *stereotactic radiotherapy* refers to fractionated stereotactic therapy using a relocatable frame). Decisions regarding dose, fractionation, and length of therapy are determined based on the life expectancy and quality of life considerations. It is important always to keep in mind the goals of palliation. The side effects should be kept to a minimum and the treatment course kept as short as possible.

SUMMARY

Radiation therapy is an integral part of the management of breast cancer in all stages of the disease, from DCIS to metastatic disease. Treatments should be tailored to each patient's clinical situation to obtain the best disease control with minimum side effects. The new and developing technologies provide us with the tools to accomplish this goal.

REFERENCES

1. de Moulin D. *A short history of breast cancer.* Boston: Martinus Nijhoff, 1983:88–104.
2. Lingos TI, Recht A, Vicini F, et al. Radiation pneumonitis in breast cancer patients treated with conservative surgery and radiation therapy. *Int J Radiat Oncol Biol Phys* 1991;1:355–360.
3. Cuzick J, Stewart H, Rutqvist L, et al. Cause-specific mortality in long-term survivors of breast cancer who participated in trials of radiotherapy. *J Clin Oncol* 1994;12:447–453.
4. Rutqvist LE, Lax I, Fornander T, et al. Cardiovascular mortality in a randomized trial of adjuvant radiation therapy versus surgery alone in primary breast cancer. *Int J Radiat Oncol Biol Phys* 1992; 22:887–896.
5. Pierce SM, Recht A, Lingos TI, et al. Long-term radiation complications following conservative surgery (CS) and radiation therapy (RT) in patients with early stage breast cancer. *Int J Radiat Oncol Biol Phys* 1992;23:915–923.
6. Neugut AI, Weinberg MD, Ahsan H, et al. Carcinogenic effects of radiotherapy for breast cancer. *Oncology* 1999;13:1245–1256.
7. Boice JD Jr, Harvey EB, Blettner M, et al. Cancer in the contralateral breast after radiotherapy for breast cancer. *N Engl J Med* 1992;326:781–785.
8. Storm HH, Andersson M, Boice JD Jr, et al. Adjuvant radiotherapy and risk of contralateral breast cancer. *J Natl Cancer Inst* 1992;84:1245–1250.
9. Abdalla I, Thisted RA, Heimann R. The impact of contralateral breast cancer on the outcome of breast cancer patients treated by mastectomy. *Cancer J* 2000;6:266–272.
10. Inskip PD, Stovall M, Flannery JT. Lung cancer risk and radiation dose among women treated for breast cancer. *J Natl Cancer Inst* 1994;86:983–988.
11. Neugut AI, Murray T, Santos J, et al. Increased risk of lung cancer after breast cancer radiation therapy in cigarette smokers. *Cancer* 1994;73:1615–1620.
12. Taghian A, de Vathaire F, Terrier P, et al. Long-term risk of sarcoma following radiation treatment for breast cancer. *Int J Radiat Oncol Biol Phys* 1991;21:361–367.
13. Curtis RE, Boice J Jr, Stovall M, et al. Risk of leukemia after chemotherapy and radiation treatment for breast cancer. *N Engl J Med* 1992;326:1745–1751.
14. Page DL, Dupont WD, Rogers LW, et al. Continued local recurrence of carcinoma 15-25 years after a diagnosis of low grade ductal carcinoma *in situ* of the breast treated only by biopsy. *Cancer* 1995; 76:1197–1200.
15. Betsill WL Jr, Rosen PP, Lieberman PH, et al. Intraductal carcinoma. Long-term follow-up after treatment by biopsy alone. *JAMA* 1978;239:1863–1867.
16. Greenlee RT, Murray T, Bolden S, et al. Cancer statistics, 2000. *CA Cancer J Clin* 2000;50:7–33.

17. Frykberg ER, Bland KI. Overview of the biology and management of ductal carcinoma *in situ* of the breast. *Cancer* 1994;74:350–361.
18. Hillner BE, Desch CE, Carlson RW, et al. Trade-offs between survival and breast preservation for three initial treatments of ductal carcinoma-in-situ of the breast. *J Clin Oncol* 1996;4:70–77.
19. Fisher B, Dignam J, Wolmark N, et al. Lumpectomy and radiation therapy for the treatment of intraductal breast cancer: findings from National Surgical Adjuvant Breast and Bowel Project B-17. *J Clin Oncol* 1998;16:441–452.
20. Fisher ER, Costantino J, Fisher B, et al. Pathologic findings from the National Surgical Adjuvant Breast Project (NSABP) Protocol B-17. Intraductal carcinoma (ductal carcinoma *in situ*). The National Surgical Adjuvant Breast and Bowel Project Collaborating Investigators. *Cancer* 1995;75:1310–1319.
21. Fisher ER, Dignam J, Tan-Chiu E, et al. Pathologic findings from the National Surgical Adjuvant Breast Project (NSABP) eight-year update of Protocol B-17: intraductal carcinoma. *Cancer* 1999;86:429–438.
22. Fisher ER, Leeming R, Anderson S, et al. Conservative management of intraductal carcinoma (DCIS) of the breast. Collaborating NSABP investigators. *J Surg Oncol* 1991;47:139–147.
23. Julien JP, Bijker N, Fentiman IS, et al. Radiotherapy in breast-conserving treatment for ductal carcinoma *in situ*: first results of the EORTC randomised phase III trial 10853. EORTC Breast Cancer Cooperative Group and EORTC Radiotherapy Group. *Lancet* 2000;355:528–533.
24. Fisher B, Dignam J, Wolmark N, et al. Tamoxifen in treatment of intraductal breast cancer: National Surgical Adjuvant Breast and Bowel Project B-24 randomised controlled trial. *Lancet* 1999;353:1993–2000.
25. Silverstein MJ, Lagios MD, Craig PH, et al. A prognostic index for ductal carcinoma in situ of the breast. *Cancer* 1996;77:2267–2274.
26. Silverstein MJ, Lagios MD, Groshen S, et al. The influence of margin width on local control of ductal carcinoma in situ of the breast. *N Engl J Med* 1999;340:1455–1461.
27. Heimann R, Karrison T, Hellman S. Treatment of ductal carcinoma in situ [letter]. *N Engl J Med* 1999;341:999–1000.
28. NIH consensus development conference. Treatment of early stage breast cancer. *JAMA* 1991;265:391–395.
29. Veronesi U, Banfi A, Salvadori B, et al. Breast conservation is the treatment of choice in small breast cancer: long-term results of a randomized trial. *Eur J Cancer* 1990;26:668–670.
30. van Dongen JA, Bartelink H, Fentiman IS, et al. Randomized clinical trial to assess the value of breast-conserving therapy in stage I and II breast cancer, EORTC 10801 trial. *Monographs Natl Cancer Inst* 1992;11:15–18.
31. Blichert-Toft M, Rose C, Andersen JA, et al. Danish randomized trial comparing breast conservation therapy with mastectomy: six years of life-table analysis. Danish Breast Cancer Cooperative Group. *Monogr Natl Cancer Inst* 1992;11:19–25.
32. Fisher B, Stewart A, Redmond C, et al. Reanalysis and results after 12 years of follow-up in a randomized clinical trial comparing total mastectomy with lumpectomy with or without irradiation in the treatment of breast cancer. *N Engl J Med* 1995;333:1456–1461.
33. Jacobson JA, Danforth DN, Cowan KH, et al. Ten-year results of a comparison of conservation with mastectomy in the treatment of stage I and II breast cancer. *N Engl J Med* 1995;332:907–911.
34. Arriagada R, Le MG, Rochard F, et al. Conservative treatment versus mastectomy in early breast cancer: patterns of failure with 15 years of follow-up data. Institut Gustave-Roussy Breast Cancer Group. *J Clin Oncol* 1996;14:1558–1564.
35. Farrow DC, Hunt WC, Samet JM. Geographic variation in the treatment of localized breast cancer. *N Engl J Med* 1992;326:1097–1101.
36. Nattinger AB, Goodwin JS. Geographic and Hospital Variation in the Management of Older Women With Breast Cancer. *Cancer Control* 1994;1:334–338.
37. Lazovich DA, White E, Thomas DB, et al. Underutilization of breast-conserving surgery and radiation therapy among women with stage I or II breast cancer. *JAMA* 1991;266:3433–3438.
38. Lazovich D, Solomon CC, Thomas DB, et al. Breast conservation therapy in the United States following the 1990 National Institutes of Health Consensus Development Conference on the treatment of patients with early stage invasive breast carcinoma. *Cancer* 1999;86:628–637.
39. Morrow M, Bucci C, Rademaker A. Medical contraindications are not a major factor in the underutilization of breast conserving therapy. *J Am Coll Surg* 1998;186:269–274.

40. Holland R, Veling SH, Mravunac M, et al. Histologic multifocality of Tis, T1-2 breast carcinomas. Implications for clinical trials of breast-conserving surgery. *Cancer* 1985;56:979–990.
41. Kurtz JM, Amalric R, Brandone H, et al. Local recurrence after breast-conserving surgery and radiotherapy: frequency, time course, and prognosis. *Cancer* 1989;63:1912–1917.
42. Heimann R, Powers C, Halpem HJ, et al. Breast preservation in stage I and II carcinoma of the breast: the University of Chicago experience. *Cancer* 1996;78:1722–1730.
43. Winchester DP, Cox JD. Standards for breast-conservation treatment. *CA Cancer J Clin* 1992;42:134–162.
44. Winchester DP, Cox JD: Standards for diagnosis and management of invasive breast carcinoma: American College of Radiology, American College of Surgeons, College of American Pathologists, Society of Surgical Oncology. *CA Cancer J Clin* 1998;48:83–107.
45. Park CC, Mitsumori M, Nixon A, et al. Outcome at 8 years after breast-conserving surgery and radiation therapy for invasive breast cancer: influence of margin status and systemic therapy on local recurrence. *J Clin Oncol* 2000;18:1668–1675.
46. Mueller CB, Ames F, Anderson GD. Breast cancer in 3,558 women: age as a significant determinant in the rate of dying and causes of death. *Surgery* 1978;83:123–132.
47. Yancik R, Ries LG, Yates JW. Breast cancer in aging women: a population-based study of contrasts in stage, surgery, and survival. *Cancer* 1989;63:976–981.
48. Pierce LJ, Srawderman M, Narod SA, et al. Effect of radiotherapy following breast-conserving treatment in women with breast cancer and germline BRCA1/2 mutations. *J Clin Oncol* 2000;18:3360–3369.
49. Turner BC, Harrold E, Matloff E, et al. BRCA1/BRCA2 germline mutations in locally recurrent breast cancer patients after lumpectomy and radiation therapy: implications for breast-conserving management in patients with BRCA1/BRCA2 mutations. *J Clin Oncol* 1999;17:3017–3024.
50. Hellman S. The key and the lamppost. *J Clin Oncol* 1999;17:3007–3008.
51. Liljegren G, Holmberg L, Adami HO, et al. Sector resection with or without postoperative radiotherapy for stage I breast cancer: five-year results of a randomized trial. Uppsala-Orebro Breast Cancer Study Group. *J Natl Cancer Inst* 1994;86:717–722.
52. Clark RM, Whelan T, Levine M, et al. Randomized clinical trial of breast irradiation following lumpectomy and axillary dissection for node-negative breast cancer: an update. Ontario Clinical Oncology Group. *J Natl Cancer Inst* 1996;88:1659–1664.
53. Schnitt SJ, Hayman J, Gelman R, et al. A prospective study of conservative surgery alone in the treatment of selected patients with stage I breast cancer. *Cancer* 1996;77:1094–1100.
54. Fisher B, Dignam J, Bryant J, et al. Five versus more than five years of tamoxifen therapy for breast cancer patients with negative lymph nodes and estrogen receptor-positive tumors [see comments]. *J Natl Cancer Inst* 1996;88:1529–1542.
55. Fisher B, Dignam J, Mamounas EP, et al. Sequential methotrexate and fluorouracil for the treatment of node-negative breast cancer patients with estrogen receptor-negative tumors: eight-year results from National Surgical Adjuvant Breast and Bowel Project (NSABP) B-13 and first report of findings from NSABP B-19 comparing methotrexate and fluorouracil with conventional cyclophosphamide, methotrexate, and fluorouracil. *J Clin Oncol* 1996;14:1982–1992.
56. Fisher B, Bryant J, Wolmark N, et al. Effect of preoperative chemotherapy on the outcome of women with operable breast cancer. *J Clin Oncol* 1998;16:2672–2685.
57. McCormick B, Begg CB, Norton L, et al. Timing of radiotherapy in the treatment of early-stage breast cancer [letter; comment]. *J Clin Oncol* 1993;11:191–193.
58. Heimann R, Powers C, Fleming G, et al. Does the sequencing of radiotherapy and chemotherapy affect the outcome in early-stage breast cancer: a continuing question. *Int J Radiat Oncol Biol Phys* 1994;30 (S1):241.
59. Recht A, Come SE, Henderson IC, et al. The sequencing of chemotherapy and radiation therapy after conservative surgery for early-stage breast cancer. *N Engl J Med* 1996;334:1356–1361.
60. Fisher B, Redmond C, Fisher ER, et al. Ten-year results of a randomized clinical trial comparing radical mastectomy and total mastectomy with or without radiation. *N Engl J Med* 1985;312:674–681.
61. Heimann R, Hellman S. Clinical progression of breast cancer malignant behavior: what to expect and when to expect it? *J Clin Oncol* 2000;18:591–599.
62. Recht A, Gray R, Davidson NE, et al. Locoregional failure 10 years after mastectomy and adjuvant chemotherapy with or without tamoxifen without irradiation: experience of the Eastern Cooperative Oncology Group. *J Clin Oncol* 1999;17:1689–1700.

63. Arriagada R, Rutqvist LE, Mattsson A, et al. Adequate locoregional treatment for early breast cancer may prevent secondary dissemination. *J Clin Oncol* 1995;13:2869–2878.
64. Early Breast Cancer Trialists' Collaborative Group. Effects of radiotherapy and surgery in early breast cancer: an overview of the randomized trials. [Published erratum appears in *N Engl J Med* 1996;334:1003]. *N Engl J Med* 1995;333:1444–1455.
65. Overgaard M, Hansen PS, Overgaard J, et al.: Postoperative radiotherapy in high-risk premenopausal women with breast cancer who receive adjuvant chemotherapy: Danish Breast Cancer Cooperative Group 82b trial. *N Engl J Med* 1997;337:949–955.
66. Ragaz J, Jackson SM, Le N, et al. Adjuvant radiotherapy and chemotherapy in node-positive premenopausal women with breast cancer. *N Engl J Med* 1997;337:956–962.
67. Overgaard M, Jensen MB, Overgaard J, et al. Postoperative radiotherapy in high-risk postmenopausal breast-cancer patients given adjuvant tamoxifen: Danish Breast Cancer Cooperative Group DBCG 82c randomised trial. *Lancet* 1999;353:1641–1648.
68. Hellman S. Stopping metastases at their source [Editorial]. *N Engl J Med* 1997;337:996–997.
69. Salvadori B, Marubini E, Miceli R, et al. Reoperation for locally recurrent breast cancer in patients previously treated with conservative surgery. *Br J Surg* 1999;86:84–87.
70. Halverson KJ, Perez CA, Kuske RR, et al. Isolated local-regional recurrence of breast cancer following mastectomy: radiotherapeutic management. *Int J Radiat Oncol Biol Phys* 1990;19:851–858.
71. Slavin SA, Love SM, Goldwyn RM. Recurrent breast cancer following immediate reconstruction with myocutaneous flaps. *Plast Reconstr Surg* 1994;93:1191–1204.
72. Ryu J, Yahalom J, Shank B, et al. Radiation therapy after breast augmentation or reconstruction in early or recurrent breast cancer. *Cancer* 1990;66:844–847.
73. Spanos WJ Jr., Montague ED, Fletcher GH. Late complications of radiation only for advanced breast cancer. *Int J Radiat Oncol Biol Phys* 1980;6:1473–1476.
74. Touboul E, Lefranc JP, Blondon J, et al. Multidisciplinary treatment approach to locally advanced non-inflammatory breast cancer using chemotherapy and radiotherapy with or without surgery. *Radiother Oncol* 1992;25:167–175.
75. Hortobagyi GN. Multidisciplinary management of advanced primary and metastatic breast cancer. *Cancer* 1994;74:416–423.
76. Perez CA, Graham ML, Taylor ME, et al. Management of locally advanced carcinoma of the breast. I. Noninflammatory. *Cancer* 1994;74:453–465.
77. Masters G, Heimann R, Skoog L, et al. Concomitant chemoradiotherapy with vinorelbine and paclitaxel with filgrastim(G-CSF) support in patients with unresectable breast cancer. *Breast Cancer Res Treat* 1997;46:75.
78. Formenti SC, Symmans WF, Volm M, et al. Concurrent paclitaxel and radiation therapy for breast cancer. *Semin Radiat Oncol* 1999;9:34–42.

16

Unusual Presentations of Breast Cancer

R. T. Osteen

INTRACYSTIC CARCINOMA

Breast macrocysts are common, but cancers arising in cysts are rare. In a series of 2,500 women operated on at the University of Pennsylvania for breast cancer, only 0.5% had intracystic carcinomas (1). In a series of 9,000 breast cancers reported from the Mayo Clinic, for the period 1920 to 1954, the incidence of intracystic cancers was also 0.5% (2).

The lesion is a papillary tumor growing within a cystic capsule. This entity must be distinguished from a benign papilloma within a cyst, invasive papillary carcinoma within a cyst, and cystic degeneration of an adenocarcinoma. When confined within the cyst, the intracystic papillary carcinoma carries an excellent prognosis with very limited potential for axillary metastasis and systemic spread, similar to ductal carcinoma in situ (DCIS). Lefkowitz et al. consider intracystic papillary carcinoma a variant of DCIS (3). With invasion into or through the capsule, metastatic potential increases. The widely differing incidences of positive axillary nodes in (0%–30%) series reporting axillary dissection probably reflect inclusion of different degrees of invasion (4,5). Most patients with intracystic carcinoma seem to have a good prognosis (3).

Like other forms of breast cancer, intracystic papillary carcinomas tend to occur in older, postmenopausal patients. In the series from the University of Pennsylvania, 80% were over 60 years of age, and the mean age was 67 years (1). Benign cysts tend to occur in premenopausal women and are uncommon in postmenopausal women who are not taking estrogen. This age differential is an important clinical observation that makes cysts in postmenopausal patients more suspicious (6). A disproportionate number of black patients have been reported in several series of cases of intracystic carcinoma (1,2).

The evaluation of cystic masses by mammography and ultrasonography has simplified the management of these lesions. Cystic masses are often firm and difficult to distinguish from a solid mass by palpation. Ultrasonography can readily distinguish cystic from solid masses and can segregate suspicious cysts from simple cysts. Suspicious cysts have internal echoes from debris, papillary fronds, or other solid tissue. Simple cysts contain only fluid and can be safely disregarded. Cysts containing debris should be aspirated. Cysts that contain fronds of other solid contents projecting from the wall into the lumen of the cyst should be excised for histologic examination.

The routine use of aspiration cytology for the evaluation of cyst fluid has been discredited. Ciatto et al. reported the results of cytologic examination of fluid from 6,782 breast cyst fluids after excluding patients in whom a cancer was suspected on the basis of physical or mammographic findings (7). No cancers were identified. There were five cases of intracystic papillomas, all of which had bloody aspirates. Interestingly, bloody cystic fluid also was obtained from 10 of 13 cancers in intracystic lesions that had been excluded from the study because malignancy was suspected on physical examination on mammography. These findings support the recommendation to excise the cyst when bloody fluid is obtained but not to send a nonbloody fluid from aspiration for cytology if cancer is not otherwise suspected. If cancer is suspected, a negative cytology should not dissuade the surgeon from excising the lesion for histologic examination.

Before the era of high-quality mammography and ultrasonography, routine follow-up at 2 to 8 weeks was recommended to ensure that the cyst did not refill. This recommendation was derived from the concept that malignant cysts would usually refill, whereas benign cysts might collapse and the walls adhere. Pursuit of such a strategy faced several objections. Many patients with gross cystic disease have multiple cysts, and the physician cannot be sure whether a cyst in the same general area of the breast is "recurrent" or new. Follow-up is expensive, time consuming, and low yield at best. Even advocates of early follow-up, such as Hamed et al., have had difficulty presenting a convincing case (8). Of the four patients whom they reported as supporting the value of routine follow-up after aspiration, two had bloody fluid and a lump, one had a 3-cm solid mass, and the other had a 7-cm solid mass. Similarly, four patients described by Forrest et al. as having cysts that refilled after aspiration all had grossly bloody fluid (9). Refilling may be more frequent in cysts lined by an apocrine epithelium (10). Although widely advocated and clearly safe, routine short-term follow-up is neither cost effective nor necessary for patients who have nonbloody aspirates, no mass, and appropriate mammography screening.

Because intracystic papillary carcinoma is uncommon and no large series exist, treatment recommendations must be based on extrapolation from the experience with other types of breast pathology rather than from a large body of data arrived from the treatment of this specific entity. Although historically most patients have been treated by mastectomy, there is no obvious reason why intracystic carcinomas cannot be managed by local excision with or without radiation therapy. The need for axillary dissection should be dictated by the presence or absence of cyst-wall invasion. The only patient with a positive lymph node was reported by Estabrook et al.; this patient had a large ulcerated tumor (11). After analysis of 77 cases at the Armed Forces Institute of Pathology, Lefkowitz at al. believed that low-grade tumors without stromal invasion could be treated by local excision but that higher grade tumors have an increased risk for recurrence and metastasis (3). Harris et al. found no axillary metastases in seven patients undergoing axillary dissection (12). One local recurrence was seen in 13 patients undergoing local excision.

PAGET DISEASE

Paget disease is a manifestation of carcinoma *in situ* as the ducts are everted onto the nipple. It is initially an eczematoid focal change in the nipple that can spread over the entire nipple and the entire areolar. In several large series of breast cancer patients, the percentage of patients with Paget disease ranged from 1.3% to 3% (13, 14). The number of patients who present with overt Paget disease may be considerably smaller than the number of patients with microscopic pagetoid spread within the nipple. In the series of 149 patients studied by Lagios et al., using the serial subgross technique, seven patients had Paget disease, only one of which was recognized clinically (15). All the patients in that series had invasive cancers somewhere in the breast.

The association of Paget disease with an underlying invasive cancer or DCIS has been widely investigated (16,17). If Paget disease is a cutaneous manifestation of DCIS and DCIS is a segmental or lobular disease, one might predict a relatively high likelihood of DCIS or invasive cancer deeper in the breast within the affected segment. Before the availability of high-quality mammography, the likelihood of underlying disease was used as a justification for mastectomy. Indeed, finding Paget disease combined with a mass probably means the mass is malignant. High-quality mammography has opened the possibility of distinguishing between patients who have disease limited to the nipple from those patients with disease at a distance from the nipple. Theoretically, if patients who have limited disease could be identified, then those patients could be treated by limited surgery, such as resection of the nipple–areolar complex and some underlying breast tissue, followed by radiation therapy. Several small series of successfully treated patients have been reported (18–20). The frequency of underlying disease was documented by Yim et al., who found underlying invasive carcinoma or DCIS in 92% of 38 patients with Paget disease and 85% with no palpable mass (16). Mammography failed to identify the underlying pathology in 64% of cases. These researchers did not comment on the distance of the disease from the nipple or how many would have been included in a conservative nipple–areolar excision with underlying breast tissue.

Lacking other selection criteria at the present time, it would seem prudent to select breast conservation only for patients with negative mammograms and disease that appears to be confined to the nipple. Significant disease in the subareolar breast may indicate other disease in the segment more peripherally and should be considered a relative indication for mastectomy if it approaches the margin, the type of criteria that would indicate the need for mastectomy if the DCIS were presenting elsewhere in the breast.

Relatively few patients have been treated by techniques other than mastectomy. Treatment failure rates for patients treated without radiation therapy have been relatively high (19). Pierce et al. pointed out that the local recurrence rate in their series was comparable to the control group in the National Surgical Adjuvant Breast Project B-17 trial of radiation and local excision for DCIS patients who were not treated with radiation therapy (19). As they suggest, because DCIS is the predominant underlying malignancy, it is not surprising that the recurrence rates were similar.

Biopsy technique is either by wedge biopsy of the nipple or a punch biopsy under local anesthesia.

Two hypotheses have been proposed to explain Paget disease: epidermotropic migration from an underlying malignancy or an *in situ* transformation of keratinocytes in the epidermis of the nipple. The frequency of reported underlying pathology suggests the former theory. Schelfout et al. reported that Paget cells express receptors for heregulin alpha, a motility factor released by normal epidermal keratinocytes (21). That finding again supports the theory of epidermotropic growth.

INFLAMMATORY BREAST CANCER

Inflammatory breast cancer is a rare form of breast cancer characterized by presentation with a hot, red, tender breast that mimics mastitis. The diagnosis is frequently missed initially when the patient is being treated with antibiotics for a presumptive infection. The syndrome usually appears *de novo* without antecedent mass or other symptoms.

Mammography is generally unrevealing. Masses or microcalcifications are uncommon (22). Skin and trabecular thickening and general increased density are all signs of water in the tissue, which is evident on physical examination. Lymph node involvement is common, and lymphadenopathy may be seen on the mammogram. The tenderness of the breast and lack of specificity of the mammographic findings make performance of the mammogram a debatable study. An ultrasound to rule out an abscess is probably a more valuable study. A breast abscess large enough to be confused with inflammatory breast cancer is rare in the nonlactating breast and even less common in, postmenopausal women. Therefore, inflammatory carcinoma must be included in the differential diagnosis of a mastitis-like appearance in a nonlactating woman. If a trial of antibiotics is selected, then failure to achieve a prompt response should mandate a biopsy.

Cancer cells in the dermal lymphatics are the hallmark of inflammatory breast cancer. The implication is that a skin punch biopsy of the inflamed area should yield a diagnosis. Random core biopsies or image-directed core biopsies are rarely necessary and miss the opportunity to confirm the diagnosis by skin biopsy. Some patients have dermal lymphatic infiltration without an inflammatory response. The clinical behavior of those patients appears to be similar to patients who have the inflammatory response.

Inflammatory breast cancer is locally advanced and prognostically the equivalent of systemic disease. Systemic therapy is clearly the primary treatment, with radiation therapy and surgery the adjuvant for local control. Although recent improvements in survival have been reported, the prognosis remains poor. Data from the Surveillance, Epidemiology, and End Results Program shows that 3-year survival improved from 32% in 1975 through 1979 to 42% in 1988 through 1992 (23). Overall 5-year survival for patients diagnosed with locoregional inflammatory breast cancer was 45% between 1975 and 1984 as reported by Moore et al. (24). Five-year disease-free survival in that series was 37%; approximately 30% of patients have systemic metastases at presentation (25).

Improvements in survival are largely due to chemotherapy, which is generally used before any local or regional treatments (neoadjuvant chemotherapy). Dramatic improvement in the appearance of the breast is frequently seen shortly after initiation of chemotherapy. Fleming et al. recommended the use of mastectomy only for patients who have a significant response to induction chemotherapy (26). Microscopic disease frequently persists in the breast even when there is a major response to chemotherapy. Moore et al. found extensive disease in mastectomy specimens from six of seven complete responders to induction chemotherapy (24). The risk for systemic disease is sufficient that induction chemotherapy seems like a reasonable first treatment. Patients who subsequently develop overt distant metastases on induction chemotherapy have such a poor prognosis that locoregional therapy is probably unnecessary. On the other hand, patients whose breasts respond to induction chemotherapy and do not develop overt distant metastases deserve an attempt at locoregional control. Because persistent disease in the responding breast may be extensive and because of potential disease in dermal lymphatics, both mastectomy and radiation therapy should be used to try to obtain control of disease in the skin, chest wall, and axilla.

An unusual syndrome that mimics inflammatory breast cancer has been pointed out by Loprinzi et al. (27). Some patients who have recently had breast or axillary surgery develop edema and erythema of the skin of the breast similar to a mastitis or inflammatory breast cancer. The etiology is unknown but probably is related to lymphatic interruption. Antibiotics are minimally effective, and the condition slowly resolves over weeks to months.

NIPPLE DISCHARGE

Nipple discharge is yet another unusual form of presentation of breast cancer and is discussed in greater detail in Chapter 3. Although nipple discharge is common, a significant or suspicious discharge is much less common. As pointed out by Chaudary et al., for a discharge to be considered significant, it should be spontaneous, persistent, and nonlactational (28). In a series of patients from France, abnormal discharges contributed only 3% to 5% of mammary consultations at their breast clinic (29). In the absence of a mass, the type of discharge is the primary consideration in the decision to pursue the diagnosis. Serous, purulent, milky discharges generally do not require biopsy, whereas serous, sanguineous, or bloody discharges can be associated with malignancy.

Discharge from a single duct is more worrisome than discharge from multiple ducts. Intraductal papillomas, fibrocystic disease, and duct ectasia are considerably more common causes of bloody discharge than is cancer. Chaudary et al. reported that all 16 patients with carcinoma in their series of 270 patients undergoing duct resection for discharge had either gross or occult blood in the discharge (28). These researchers recommended testing all discharges for occult blood, although they did not state how many of their cancers presented with occult versus gross blood. A thin, watery discharge has been reported to be a rare type of discharge associated with cancer (30).

The age distribution of patients with benign and malignant causes of discharge is different: Younger patients tend to have benign causes and older patients, more cancers. Bloody discharge should be evaluated by duct excision in either age group. Although it may be possible using magnifying loops to identify and cannulate the duct through the nipple and then excise the duct through a circumareolar incision, it is usually easy to identify and probe the discolored and dilated lactiferous sinus by careful dissection of the ducts within the nipple through a circumareolar incision made in the quadrant of the discharge.

The role of cytology in evaluating nipple discharge is unclear. In the series of 84 patients with carcinoma presenting with nipple discharge reported by Leis, 71 patients had abnormal cytology defined as malignant or atypical cells (31). Seventy-two of 502 patients with benign disease also had malignant or atypical cytology. No abnormal cytology was seen in patients with nonsanguineous discharges. These data indicate that cytology on nonsanguineous discharges was without benefit, that the false-positive cytology rate on nonsanguineous discharges was relatively high, and that negative cytology on bloody discharges did not exclude the diagnosis of cancer. Therefore, biopsy of patients with a bloody discharge seems indicated regardless of the cytology, and cytology on nonbloody discharges appears to be unnecessary and confusing.

Patients at any age who present with a suspicious discharge should have a mammogram. Negative mammograms, however, should not be used as a reason not to perform a duct excision. Tabar et al. reported negative mammograms in approximately half of the patients who presented with nipple discharge as their first sign of cancer (32). As discussed by Jardines, ductography has been advocated as a technique for evaluating duct discharge (33). It seems unlikely that a negative ductogram in patients with a pathologic discharge will be sufficiently accurate as to exclude the need for duct excision. If there is a role for ductography, it lies in identifying lesions at the periphery of the breast or multiple lesions. If the duct excision is done under local anesthesia, tracing a duct to the periphery of the breast can be trying for the patient and surgeon. If duct excisions are done with the patient under general anesthesia, it is usually possible to identify the extent of the ductal involvement without preliminary ductography.

An important subset of patients with bloody discharge are those who are subsequently shown to have DCIS. Although most patients with DCIS are identified by screening mammography, a few patients present with a nipple discharge. In the series reported by Bauer et al., 43 of 277 patients undergoing duct exploration and biopsy for a pathologic discharge were found to have DCIS (34). Patients with DCIS and discharge have been reported to have a higher risk of breast recurrence after partial mastectomy and radiation therapy compared with patients with DCIS but no discharge (35,36). Two studies suggested that discharge is a marker for more locally extensive disease or involvement of large ducts (34,37). Either of those features would predispose toward local recurrence after breast-conserving treatment. Bauer et al. estimated that extensive, centrally located disease and intraductal spread would have precluded breast preservation in 63% of their cases with DCIS and discharge (34).

MAMMOGRAPHICALLY OCCULT CANCERS

Most breast cancers are visible by mammography. A few are missed because of errors of interpretation, malpositioning of the breast on the film, or dense breast tissue. These errors can be minimized by an alert radiologist who insists on high-quality films and possibly by review by more than one radiologist. Such steps will minimize but not eliminate false-negative readings that in retrospect showed the cancer or an examination that was technically inadequate and should have been repeated. Holland et al. estimated that 2% to 9% of symptomatic patients have negative mammograms in which a palpable cancer cannot be recognized on a mammogram even in retrospect (38). These need not be small cancers. The mean diameter of the occult invasive ductal carcinomas reported by Holland et al. was 20 mm, and the mean diameter of five invasive lobular carcinomas was 50 mm (38). The histology of mammographically occult cancers was distinctive, with a diffuse, invasive pattern and a poor desmoplastic reaction. Hollingsworth et al. also singled out diffuse histologies as contributing to false-negative mammograms (39). Although concern about the difficulty of seeing mass lesions or distortion of architecture in dense, estrogen-stimulated breasts is appropriate, the importance of histologic patterns that do not produce enough scar or desmoplastic reaction to be seen on the mammogram should not be overlooked (40).

The relatively large size of the tumors in the report by Holland et al. indicates that these tumors, especially the invasive lobular ones, are not readily palpable (38). The desmoplastic reaction that makes for a visible mass on mammogram is also the reason why cancers are hard and palpable. Not until enough cancer cells are present will a diffuse, minimally desmoplastic tumor become palpable. It is important to recognize this entity as a real limitation in the ability to detect small cancers. Such cancers are undetectable by current techniques. In a society that feels the need to compensate patients for the perception of errors in diagnosis, these undiagnosable cancers will be a prime source of lawsuits.

Another type of occult breast cancer is the one that gives off an axillary metastases without a primary being detectable in the breast (41). Obviously, this clinical situation can be defined in a number of ways. The primary may not be palpable but may be found on a mammogram; it may be mammographically occult but seen on ultrasound or magnetic resonance imaging or positron emission tomography scan; or it may be occult on all imaging modalities but found at mastectomy (42–44). Mammography is an obvious first step in the evaluation of a patient who has suspicious axillary lymph nodes (45). Mammography detects some cancers that are not palpable. Most issues arise when no lesion is seen in the breast on mammography.

The standard treatment for axillary lymph nodes from unknown primary has been to perform a modified radical mastectomy. Although a few patients have been treated by radiation therapy or observation of the breast, mastectomy has been used more commonly (46). A few patients have been treated by axillary dissection and systemic therapy with or without radiation therapy to the breast (47). Breast conservation by lumpectomy and radiation therapy generally has been reserved for the situation in which an identifiable primary is excised with negative margins. Irradiation of larger amounts of tumor has been less successful in controlling gross disease. For patients with axillary metastases and no demonstrable tumor in the breast, the obvious concern is that there may be too much occult tumor to be controlled with radiation therapy. No randomized trial comparing mastectomy with breast conserving strategies for patients with axillary metastases from an unknown primary has been performed or is likely to be performed because of the limited number of patients with this condition.

NIPPLE INVERSION

Nipple inversion is an uncommon presentation of breast cancer. In the cases reported by the Yorkshire Breast Cancer Group, nipple retraction was the presenting symptom of 43 of the 1,205 patients (4 %) (48). Nipple inversion caused by a cancer is usually associated with a palpable mass. The nipple is generally fixed and cannot be everted. Rees et al. pointed out that nipple retraction by carcinoma is more likely to be complete and accompanied by distortion of the areolar (49). The asymmetric distortion by cancer is to be distinguished from central symmetric retraction, which favors the diagnosis of duct ectasia (49). Nipple inversion is usually seen as a longstanding condition present since puberty. Retraction due to duct ectasia is usually more recent onset and may have been preceded by a subareolar infection. A recent history of developing nipple inversion should be investigated mammographically as well as by physical examination. In patients who have a palpable mass, a biopsy should be done of the mass. If an ectatic duct is suspected, excision of the infected duct system is appropriate (50). Patients who do not have a palpable mass and are mammographically negative can be divided into two groups: (a) patients who have fatty atrophic breasts need no further evaluation; and (b) patients who have dense breast tissue in the subareolar area probably should have closer follow-up and repeat mammography in 6 months.

BREAST CANCER DURING PREGNANCY

Breast cancer presenting during pregnancy is distinctly uncommon; reported incidences range from 0.07% to 0.1% (50). Breast cancer is primarily a disease of postmenopausal women and is uncommon during the main childbearing years. The modern tendency to defer pregnancy into the fourth and fifth decades may increase the frequency with which the combination is seen.

Changes in the breast during pregnancy obviously make palpation of a mass difficult and make nodular breast changes difficult to distinguish from a mass. Because of concern about radiation to the fetus, screening mammograms are suspended or delayed during pregnancy, and diagnostic mammograms for a questionable mass are avoided. The net result is that pregnant patients present with more advanced stages of breast cancer compared with nonpregnant patients. This fact probably accounts for the perception of breast cancer during pregnancy as being a particularly aggressive form of the disease. Ultrasonic evaluation of a mass poses no radiation threat to the fetus and may be able to distinguish hypertrophic breast tissue from a mass, and can be used to guide a core needle biopsy. Although a mammogram can be done with relative safety during pregnancy, there is little indication to recommend it. If a palpable mass is suspicious, a biopsy should be performed with or without a mammogram, and an ultrasound is at least as good as evaluating equivocal masses as a mammogram is. Open biopsies of the breast during pregnancy or lactation can be performed but tend to be bloody and milk tends to accumulate in the biopsy cavity. Fine-needle aspiration (FNA) is helpful if it is positive, but a negative FNA does not exclude the diagnosis of cancer (51). When possible, ultrasound-guided core biopsy is preferable. Once the diagnosis of breast cancer is established, several difficult treatment decisions must be made. Once thought by Haagenson and Stout to be incurable (52), breast cancer during pregnancy is now thought to have about the same prognosis stage for stage as breast cancer in the absence of pregnancy (53). Pregnancy does limit treatment options, however. Radiation therapy cannot be given because of potential radiation injury to the fetus. Late in the pregnancy, the lump can be removed and radiation therapy delayed until the infant is delivered. Early in the pregnancy, mastectomy or abortion and breast conservation with radiation therapy are options. At midterm, modified radical mastectomy is generally the only option strongly considered. Modified radical mastectomy can be carried out with little risk to the fetus. Concerns about fetal damage also limit the use of chemotherapy. Berry et al. reported using 5-fluorouracil (5-FU), doxorubicin, and cyclophosphamide in 22 patients during all trimesters of pregnancy, but the chemotherapy was given primarily during the second and third trimesters (54). Folic acid antagonists given during the first trimester are known to cause significant risk of abortion or teratogenesis (55). Methotrexate is avoided because of potential third-space accumulation of the drug in the amniotic fluid.

REFERENCES

1. Czernobilsky B. Intracystic carcinoma of the female breast. *Surg Gynecol Obstet* 1967;124:93–98.
2. Gatchell FG, Dokerty MD, Claggett OT. Intracystic carcinoma of the breast. *Surg Gynecol Obstet* 1958;106:555–562.
3. Lefkowitz M, Lefkowitz W, Wargotz ES. Intraductal (intracystic) papillary carcinoma of the breast and variants: a clinicopathological study of 77 cases. *Hum Pathol* 1994;25:802–809.
4. Carter D, Orr SL, Merino MJ. Intracystic papillary carcinoma of the breast: after mastectomy, radiotherapy or excisional biopsy alone. *Cancer* 1983;52:14–19.
5. Payne RA, Jackson DB. Cystic tumors of the breast. *Ann R Coll Surg Engl* 1980;62:228–229.
6. Ravichanadran D, Rubin C, Carty NJ, et al. Cystic carcinoma of the breast: a trap for the unwary. *Ann R Coll Surg Engl* 1995;77:123–126.

7. Ciatto S, Cariaggi P, Bulgaresi P. The value of routine cytologic examination of breast, cyst fluids. *Acta Cytol* 1987;31:301–304.
8. Hamed H, Coady A, Chaudary MA, et al. Follow-up of patients with aspirated breast cysts is necessary. *Arch Surg* 1989;124:253–255.
9. Forrest APM, Kirkpatrick JR, Roberts NM. Needle aspiration of breast cysts. *BMJ* 1975;3:30–31.
10. Dixon JM, Clarke PJ. Refilling of breast cysts as indication for biopsy. *Lancet* 1985;2:608–609.
11. Estabrook A, Asch T, Gump F, et al. Mammographic features of intracystic papillary lesions. *Surg Gynecol Obstet* 1990;170:113–116.
12. Harris KP, Faliakou EC, Exon DJ, et al. Treatment and outcome of intracystic papillary carcinoma of the breast. *Br J Surg* 1999;86:1274.
13. Dockerty MB, Harrington SW. Preclinical Paget's disease of the nipple. *Surg Gynecol Obstet* 1951; 93:317–320.
14. Ashikari R, Park K, Huvos AG, et al. Paget's disease of the breast. *Cancer* 1970;26:680–685.
15. Lagios MD, Gates EA, Westdahl PR, et al. A guide to the frequency of nipple involvement in breast cancer: a study of 149 consecutive mastectomies using a serial subgross and correlated radiographic technique. *Am J Surg* 1979;138:135–141.
16. Yim JH, Wick MR, Philopott GW, et al. Underlying pathology in mammary Paget's disease. *Ann Surg Oncol* 1997;4:287–292.
17. Nance FC, DeLoach DH, Welsh RA, et al. Paget's disease of the breast. *Ann Surg* 1970;171:864–874.
18. Lagios MD, Westdahl PR, Rose MR, et al. Paget's disease of the nipple: alternative management in cases without or with minimal extent of underlying breast carcinoma. *Cancer* 1984;54:545–551.
19. Pierce L, Haffty BG, Solin LJ, et al. The conservative management of Paget's disease of the breast with radiotherapy. *Cancer* 1997;80:1065–1072.
20. Stockdale AD, Brierley JD, White WF, et al. Radiotherapy for Paget's disease of the nipple: a conservative alternative. *Lancet* 1989;2:664–666.
21. Schelfout VR, Coene ED, Delaey B, et al. Pathogenecis of Paget's disease: epidermal heregulin alpha, motility factor, and the HER receptor family. *J Natl Cancer Inst* 2000;92:622–628.
22. Kushwaha AC, Whitman GJ, Stelling CB, et al. Primary inflammatory carcinoma of the breast: retrospective review of mammographic findings. *AJR Am J Roentgenol* 2000;174:535–538.
23. Chang S, Parker SL, Buzdar P, et al. Inflammatory breast carcinoma incidence and survival: the Surveillance, Epidemiology, and the End Results Program of the National Cancer Institute, 1975-1992. *Cancer* 1998;82:2366–2372.
24. Moore MP, Ihde JK, Crowe JP Jr, et al. Inflammatory breast cancer. *Arch Surg* 1991;126:304–306.
25. Sherry MM, Johnson DH, Page DL, et al. Inflammatory carcinoma of the breast. Clinical review and summary of the Vanderbilt experience with multi-modality therapy. *Am J Med* 1985;79:355–364.
26. Fleming RYD, Asmar L, Buzdar AU, et al. Effectiveness of mastectomy by response to induction chemotherapy for control in inflammatory breast carcinoma. *Ann Surg Oncol* 1997;4:452–461.
27. Loprinzi CL, Pisansky TM, Sterioff S, et al. Postsurgical changes of the breast that mimic inflammatory breast carcinoma. *Mayo Clin Proc* 1996;71:552–555.
28. Chaudary MA, Millis RR, Davies GC, et al. Nipple discharge: the diagnostic value of testing for occult blood. *Ann Surg* 1982;196:651–655.
29. Murad TM, Contesso G, Mouriesse H. Nipple discharge from the breast. *Ann Surg* 1982;195:259–264.
30. Lewison EF, Chambers RG. Clinical significance of nipple discharge. *JAMA* 1951;147:295–299.
31. Leis HP. Management of nipple discharge. *World J Surg* 1989;13:736–742.
32. Tabar L, Marton Z, Kadas I. Galactography in the examination of secretory breast. *Am J Surg* 1974; 127:282–286.
33. Jardines L. Management of nipple discharge. *Am Surg* 1996;62:119–122.
34. Bauer RL, Eckhert KH, Nemoto T. Ductal carcinoma *in situ*-associated nipple discharge: A clinical marker for locally extensive disease. *Ann Surg Oncol* 1998;5:452–455.
35. Recht A, Danoff B, Solin LJ, et al. Intraductal carcinoma of the breast: results of treatment with excisional biopsy and irradiation. *J Clin Oncol* 1985;3:1339–1343.
36. Solin LJ, Fowble BL, Schultz DJ, et al. Definitive irradiation for intraductal carcinoma of the breast. *Int J Radiat Oncol Biol Phys* 1990;19:843–850.
37. Ohuchi N, Furutu A, Mori S. Management of ductal carcinoma *in situ* with nipple discharge. *Cancer* 1994;74:1294–1302.
38. Holland R, Hendricks JHCL, Mravunac M. Mammographically occult breast cancer: a pathologic and radiologic study. *Cancer* 1983;52:1810–1819.

39. Hollingsworth AB, Taylor LDH, Rhodes DC. Establishing a histologic basis for false-negative mammograms. *Am J Surg* 1993;166:643–647.
40. Lannin DR, Harris RP, Swanson FH, et al. Difficulties in diagnosis of carcinoma of the breast in patients less than fifty years of age. *Surg Gynecol Obstet* 1993;177:457–462.
41. Knapper WH. Management of occult breast cancer presenting as an axillary metastasis. *Semin Surg Oncol* 1991;7:311–313.
42. Scoggins Cr, Vitola JV, Sandler MP, et al. Occult breast carcinoma presenting as an axillary mass. *Am Surg* 1999;65:1–5.
43. Foxcroft LM, Evans EB, Joshua HK, et al. Breast cancers invisible on mammography. *Aust NZ J Surg* 2000;70:162–167.
44. Tilanus-Linthorst MM, Obdeijn AI, Bontenbal M, et al. MRI in patients with axillary metastases of occult breast carcinoma. *Breast Cancer Res Treat* 1997;44:179–182.
45. Leibman AJ, Kossoff MB. Mammography in women with axillary lymphadenopathy and normal breasts on physical examination: value in detecting occult breast carcinoma. *AJR Am J Roentgenol* 1992;159:493–495.
46. Baron PL, Moore MP, Kinne DW, et al. Occult breast cancer presenting with axillary metastases. Updated management. *Arch Surg* 1990;125:210–214.
47. Van Ooijan B, Bontenbal M, Henzen-Logmans SC, et al. Axillary nodal metastases from an occult primary consistent with breast carcinoma. *Br J Surg* 1993;80:1299–1300.
48. Yorkshire Breast Cancer Group. Symptoms and signs of operable breast cancer. 1976–1981. *Br J Surg* 1983;70:350–351.
49. Rees BI, Gravelle IH, Hughes LE. Nipple retraction in duct ectasia. *Br J Surg* 1977;64:577–580.
50. Hartley MN, Stewart J, Benson EA. Subareolar dissection for duct ectasia and periareolar sepsis. *Br J Surg* 1991;78:1187–1188.
51. Barnavon Y, Wallack MK. Management of the pregnant patient with carcinoma of the breast. *Surg Gynecol Obstet* 1990;171: 347–352.
52. Haagenson CD, Stout AP. Carcinoma of the breast: criteria of operability. *Ann Surg* 1943;118: 859–870.
53. Petrek JA, Dukoff R, Rogatko A. Prognosis of pregnancy-associated breast cancer. *Cancer* 1991; 67:869–872.
54. Berry DL, Theriault RL, Holmes FA, et al. Management of breast cancer during pregnancy using a standardized protocol. *J Clin Oncol* 1999;17:855–861.
55. Doll DC, Ringenberg QS, Yarbro JW. Antineoplastic agents and pregnancy. *Semin Oncol* 1989;16: 337–346.

17

Metastatic Breast Cancer

Edith A. Perez and Christy A. Russell

Although fewer than 10% of patients with breast cancer initially present with metastatic disease, it will eventually develop in a substantial proportion of them (1). Therapy for metastatic breast carcinoma remains palliative. The average survival time after the diagnosis of metastatic breast cancer is 18 to 24 months, although it varies widely according to the metastatic site (1). The median survival time traditionally has been lower for patients with visceral disease (6–13 months) compared with those with bone-only disease (18–30 months) (1). Although definitive curative therapy for metastatic breast cancer is lacking, various therapies are used in an attempt to retard progression of disease, to ameliorate symptoms, and to improve the quality and duration of survival time. Therapeutic goals are directed at improving response rates and prolongation of progression-free survival and overall survival times.

Hormonal approaches have classically included antiestrogens. The newer aromatase inhibitors are increasingly being incorporated for the treatment of patients with ER-positive tumors. Although there is no rigid standard for the sequencing of therapy for the management of metastatic breast cancer, chemotherapy has a role in the treatment program for nearly all patients with this disease. Chemotherapy-based treatments have been the initial choice for patients with negative estrogen receptor (ER) status, with visceral disease, or with ER-positive disease who have progressed after endocrine therapy (1,2). Chemotherapy combinations of cyclophosphamide, doxorubicin, or methotrexate, and 5-fluorouracil [e.g., FAC (5-fluorouracil [5-FU], doxorubicin, and cyclophosphamide) or CMF (cyclophosphamide, methotrexate, and 5-FU)] result in objective responses in 40% to 60% and 50% to 70% of patients, respectively (3). At 10 years after initiation of chemotherapy, only 3% of patients treated with FAC or CMF are alive and disease free (4). Moreover, many patients with breast carcinoma will have received CMF, FAC, or similar regimens as adjuvant chemotherapy, preexposing them to the agents that are also used most commonly to treat advanced disease. This can potentially diminish their chance for a future response, and the identification of new, non–cross-resistant drugs or drug combinations is needed.

Optimism has been renewed with the emergence of novel treatment strategies. In addition to the well-defined improvements in the supportive care of patients with metastatic breast cancer, a variety of new therapeutic agents with favorable therapeutic ratios became available recently. These agents include hormonal, chemotherapeutic, and monoclonal antibody therapies. How best to incorporate these new strategies into the current management of patients is the focus of intensive preclinical and clinical research.

The single-agent activity of some of the newer agents used in metastatic breast cancer treatment rivals that of older combination chemotherapy treatments. Improved objective response rates and improved duration of response compared with older therapies have been reported in studies evaluating optimal dosing and sequencing of these newer agents, alone or in combination with other drugs. Monoclonal antibody therapy is also promising; ideally, these agents should exhibit high tumor selectivity and a favorable therapeutic ratio. A humanized version of a murine antibody directed against the extracellular domain of *HER-2* has been developed for the treatment of patients with breast cancer whose tumors overexpress *HER-2* (1).

Current research focuses on investigation of biologic targets for primary or secondary prevention along with treatment options for patients who develop metastatic disease. Standard oncology outcomes of response, survival, and time to progression remain important, along with recognition of the importance of quality of life and time without symptoms or toxicity. New agents that are cytostatic or that inhibit tumor angiogenesis, metastasis, or invasion represent a challenge in the design of clinical trials in breast cancer. Because the predominant effect of these agents may be stabilization of tumor size or prevention of metastases, radiographic response rates are a suboptimal outcome measure. Valid intermediate endpoints, including biologic correlates, will be important in dosage and scheduling of these agents and in determination of the clinical situations in which they should be evaluated. Data collected from surrogate studies involving such methodologies as positron emission tomography, biopsy with attention to blood vessel number, and morphology may be relevant in this regard.

HORMONAL THERAPY

Stimulation of growth of breast carcinomas by estrogen is well established, and the aim of hormonal therapy is to interfere with this phenomenon. Several strategies have been used to inhibit estrogen-stimulated breast cancer growth; these act by one of two mechanisms: inhibition of estrogen action or inhibition of estrogen production.

Estrogen action can be systemically blocked using antiestrogens, such as the selective ER modulators (SERMs) or downregulators (SERDs) or aromatase inhibitors (5). In premenopausal women, estrogen production can be blocked by ovarian ablation using surgery, irradiation, or more recently by the use of luteinizing hormone-releasing hormone (LHRH) agonists (1,2). In postmenopausal women, estrogen production can be blocked using inhibitors of the aromatase enzyme, which is responsible for extraovarian estrogen production after menopause (1). Because hormonal therapy is generally well tolerated, it is an attractive treatment option for patients with metastatic breast cancer (1). Approximately 40% to 50% of women with ER-positive metastatic breast cancer will respond to hormonal therapy (1,2); predictive factors that are associated with response include ER or progesterone receptor (PR) expression, long disease-free interval, and nonvisceral disease (1,2).

For both premenopausal and postmenopausal women with hormonally responsive metastatic breast cancer, one of the SERMs (tamoxifen or toremifene) is most frequently used as initial therapy (1). These agents primarily function as ER antagonists, but they also have partial agonist activity (1). A randomized trial comparing tamoxifen 20 mg per day with toremifene at 60 and 200 mg per day as first-line therapy for postmenopausal women with metastatic breast cancer reported response rates of 24%, 24%, and 26%, respectively (6). Response or stable disease occurred in 53%, 56%, and 54% of patients, with no statistical difference among the treatment arms for either of these endpoints (6). Another class of antiestrogens that are being evaluated in clinical trials (SERDs) are the "pure" antiestrogens, which compete with estrogen for the ER at both the Af-1 and Af-2 domains; unlike SERMs, however, they do not possess partial estrogen agonist activity (5). Fulvestrant, one of the first of these compounds to be studied, was tested in 19 tamoxifen-resistant patients. Responses occurred in seven patients (37%) and lasted 3 to 20 months, and stable disease occurred in six patients (32%), lasting 9 to more than 23 months (7). Although antiestrogens are considered standard first-line therapy, recent data suggest that aromatase inhibitors may prolong the time to progression and median survival in postmenopausal women compared with tamoxifen as first-line hormonal therapy for metastatic breast cancer (8,9).

After failure of antiestrogens, second-line treatment involves estrogen deprivation. This approach is based on the menopausal state of the patient, as well as disease status, at the time of progression to first-line hormonal therapy. For premenopausal women, estrogen deprivation is achieved by ovarian ablation using surgery or irradiation, which removes the major source of estrogen production, or LHRH agonists (goserelin, buserelin), which inhibit ovarian estrogen production by blocking pituitary production of the gonadotrophins luteinizing hormone and follicle-stimulating hormone (1). A multicenter randomized trial comparing goserelin and ovariectomy demonstrated similar efficacy, with response rates of 31% and 27% (nonsignificant) and median overall survival of 37 and 33 months (nonsignificant), respectively (10). LHRH agonists be may preferable because their action is reversible. The major side effects experienced with LHRH agonists are hot flashes and tumor flare (10).

For postmenopausal women who have disease progression on tamoxifen, estrogen deprivation with aromatase inhibitors is used as second-line therapy. After loss of ovarian function in postmenopausal women, extraovarian aromatase is responsible for estrogen production, catalyzing the formation of estrone and estradiol from androgen precursors in the adrenal gland (11). Historically, progestins such as megestrol acetate or medroxyprogesterone acetate have been used as second-line therapy, but clinical trials in postmenopausal women with metastatic breast cancer have demonstrated that aromatase inhibitors have an improved safety profile (12–14) and similar or improved activity (14–17) compared with progestins. Some of these agents have been under investigation and have now been approved as first-line hormonal therapies (8,9) for patients with metastatic breast cancer.

Aromatase inhibitors can be divided into two classes. Type II aromatase inhibitors, such as aminoglutethimide, anastrozole, and letrozole, are nonsteroidal agents that act by reversibly binding the cytochrome P-450 moiety of the aromatase enzyme such as exemestane. Because blockade is reversible, ongoing estrogen deprivation requires the continued presence of the drug (12,13). Type I inhibitors, such as formestane and exemestane, are highly specific steroidal agents that irreversibly inhibit aromatase by binding its substrate-binding site. Because the inhibition is irreversible, renewed estrogen production requires synthesis of new aromatase molecules. Therefore, type I aromatase inhibitors are perhaps more appropriately called *aromatase inactivators*. Development of irreversible inactivators is of particular interest because evidence suggests a partial lack of cross-resistance between these agents and type II aromatase inhibitors (18,19).

Exemestane is a type I aromatase inhibitor currently available for clinical use (20, 21). In phase 1 and 2 studies at dosages of up to 600 mg per day, exemestane was well tolerated; a maximum tolerated dose has not yet been identified (22–26). Oral exemestane at 10 to 25 mg per day suppresses plasma estrogens as much as 6% to 15% of pretreatment levels (22). In two phase 2 controlled studies, objective response rates with exemestane as second-line therapy in postmenopausal women with advanced breast cancer were 22% and 28%. Overall success rates (defined as the proportion of patients with objective response or stable disease for longer than 24 weeks, sometimes described by other authors as "clinical benefit") (11,12) were 47% and 48% (23,25). When exemestane was used as third-line hormonal therapy in postmenopausal women with advanced breast cancer who experienced failure of tamoxifen, progestins, or nonsteroidal aromatase inhibitors, the objective response rate ranged from 7% to 26% and the overall success rate from 25% to 39% (24,25, 27).

Progestins or androgens also have been used as hormonal therapy and appear to inhibit breast cancer growth by several mechanisms (1). Progestins, however, are associated with the side effects of weight gain and fluid retention; androgens are associated with virilization (1). Typically, these hormones are now considered third-line therapy after failure of estrogen deprivation (3).

Another area of investigation has been whether additional benefit can be achieved by combining different hormonal treatments. A randomized trial in premenopausal women with metastatic breast cancer demonstrated that the combination of tamoxifen with the LHRH agonist buserelin produced a higher response rate (51%) than buserelin (33%) or tamoxifen (29%) alone ($p = 0.02$) (28). A separate trial in premenopausal women demonstrated that the combination of tamoxifen and goserelin, although it produced statistically similar response rates and median overall survival compared with goserelin alone, did produce a slight, but significant, prolongation of time to progression (28 weeks versus 23 weeks, $p = 0.03$) (29). More clinical data will be necessary to determine whether hormonal treatments are more beneficial when administered sequentially or in combination.

The use of hormonal therapy plays an important role in the treatment of metastatic breast cancer. Investigation continues into new agents that block estrogen action (SERMs, pure antiestrogens) or production (LHRH agonists, aromatase inhibitors).

Questions regarding the optimal sequencing of these agents as well as possible benefits to combining them with one another, are also being addressed.

CHEMOTHERAPY

Patients with hormone-refractory metastatic breast cancer, ER-negative disease, or symptomatic progressive or visceral disease are candidates for systemic chemotherapy. Combination regimens such as FAC or CMF have been widely used and have produced response rates of 50% to 70% and 40% to 60%, respectively (3). The introduction of the taxanes paclitaxel and docetaxel into metastatic breast cancer treatment has resulted in improvements in survival (30–32). Their partial non–cross-resistance with anthracyclines has provided a substantial benefit for patients with anthracycline-resistant disease (32). Both paclitaxel and docetaxel appear to have similar efficacy with respect to response rate when administered in 3-week cycles and in phase 3 trials have yielded survival times comparable to single-agent doxorubicin (33–35). Data from randomized trials comparing taxanes to standard regimens also demonstrated improvements in patient outcome. Briefly, results of these clinical trials demonstrate a survival advantage at 2 years for single-agent paclitaxel compared with CMFP (CMF plus prednisone) (with adjustment for prognostic variables with similar quality-of-life rate scores) (30). Improvement of time to progression and 1-year survival occurred when docetaxel was compared to mitomycin-C/vinblastine (31). A multinational trial reported by Pluzanska et al. demonstrated that the combination of doxorubicin and paclitaxel was associated with significantly longer survival compared with FAC (36). Also, a multinational trial by Nabholtz et al. reported that the combination of doxorubicin and docetaxel results in improved time to progression compared with doxorubicin and cyclophosphamide (37). A recent report by Lück et al. (ASCO 2000) demonstrated an improvement of time to progression, primary failure, and 6-month survival with a combination of epirubicin/paclitaxel versus epirubicin and cyclophosphamide as first-line therapy for metastatic breast cancer (38).

Single-Agent Activity

Paclitaxel

Paclitaxel has been studied extensively in patients previously treated for metastatic disease, with complete responses observed in as many as 14% of patients and overall response rates of up to 55%. In chemotherapy-naive patients with metastatic disease, paclitaxel treatment achieved objective response rates ranging from 32% to 62%, with complete responses observed in 4% to 17% of patients (Table 17.1). A dose–response relationship exists for paclitaxel in metastatic breast cancer, and trials in previously treated and untreated patients with advanced disease determined the optimal dose range to be 175 to 210 mg/m^2 (32,39,40) administered in 3-week cycles. Although the preferred duration of administration remains uncertain, results

TABLE 17.1. *Single-agent paclitaxel in previously treated and untreated patients with metastatic breast cancer*

Regimen	No. of patients evaluated no. of trials	Response (%)		
		CR	PR	OR
Previously treated patients[a,b]				
Paclitaxel 120–250 mg/m^2 by 3-, 24-, or 96-h i.v.	1,007/13	0–14	0–48	0–55
Previously untreated patients				
Paclitaxel 135–250 mg/m^2 by 3- or 24-h i.v.	166/5	4–17	21–50	32–62

CR, complete response; i.v., intravenous infusion; PR, partial response; OR, overall response.

[a] All patients in seven trials of 248 patients were considered refractory to anthracyclines or anthracenediones.

[b] All patients in two trials of 52 patients had previously progressed on shorter taxane infusion regimens.

From Miller KD, Sledge GW, Jr. Taxanes in the treatment of breast cancer: a prodigy comes of age. *Cancer Invest* 1999;17:121–136, with permission.

of a recent randomized trial suggest that the therapeutic index may be higher with a 3-hour infusion compared with a 24-hour infusion (41). With conventional dosing schedules, the major toxicities include neutropenia, peripheral sensory neuropathy, and arthralgia/myalgia (32).

In a large randomized trial by Bishop et al., single-agent paclitaxel was compared with a CMFP regimen in 209 patients with metastatic breast cancer. Although response rates were not significantly different between the two treatments, patients in the paclitaxel arm had a 2-year survival rate of 39% compared with a 20% survival rate for patients in the CMFP arm ($p = 0.025$, after Cox proportional hazards regression) (30). Paclitaxel was associated with less severe neutropenia, thrombocytopenia, mucositis, infections, and nausea/vomiting than was CMFP but with more severe peripheral neuropathy, alopecia, and myalgia/arthralgia. Although patients in both arms were crossed over to anthracyclines after failure, very few patients in the CMFP arm were crossed over to taxanes; therefore, the contribution of paclitaxel to increased survival is less confounded than in other comparative trials, in which patients in the nontaxane arm eventually received taxanes (30).

Recent studies evaluated paclitaxel administered as a weekly 1-hour infusion schedule, which results in a higher dose density and may offer a better therapeutic index than a 3- or 24-hour infusion given every 3 weeks (Table 17.2). In phase 2 clinical trials, the weekly 1-hour infusion schedule maintained efficacy while reducing toxicity compared with every-3-week schedules. In patients with metastatic breast cancer, weekly administration resulted in complete response rates of up to 25% and overall response rates of 41% to 92% (Table 17.2) (42–48). Weekly paclitaxel administration was associated with less myelosuppression compared with every-3-week administration, with the incidence of grade 3/4 neutropenia ranging from 0% to 14% in most studies (42–47). In one trial, however, 68% of patients with locally

TABLE 17.2. *Weekly dose-dense administration of paclitaxel as first-, second-, or third-line chemotherapy in patients with metastatic breast cancer*

Study (ref)	Dose (mg/m^2 by 1-h i.v.)	n	CR (%)	OR (%)	OR in ARD (%)	Grade 3/4 neutropenia (% of patients)
Small phase 2 trials						
Lück et al., 1997 (43)	60–90	26	12	41	NR	0
Asbury et al., 1998 (44)	50–100	21	0	62	40	14
Sola et al., 1998 (45)	80	13	23	92	NR	2
Seidman et al., 1998 (42)	100	30	10	53	50	14
Alvarez et al., 1998 (46)	100	24	25	67	NA	4
Breier et al., 1998 (47)	80	27	8	50	NR	4
Sikov et al., 1999 (48)	175[a]	19	11	89	>80[b]	68[c]
Large phase 2 trials						
Perez et al., 1999 (50)	80	212	2	23	NR	11.5

ARD, anthracycline-resistant disease; CR, complete response; i.v., intravenous infusion; NA, not applicable; NR, not reported; OR, overall response.

[a] Paclitaxel was infused over 3 hours.
[b] In patients who received anthracycline-based adjuvant chemotherapy.
[c] Of 40 patients with locally advanced or metastatic disease evaluable for toxicity.

advanced or metastatic disease experienced grade 3/4 neutropenia, but only two episodes of neutropenic fever were reported (48). The dose-limiting toxicity of weekly paclitaxel in these trials was manageable neuropathy. Weekly paclitaxel achieves a 50% or greater increase in dose density over standard administration and may have a higher therapeutic index, suggesting a possible uncoupling of drug delivery from marrow suppression (42). This hypothesis will be studied in an upcoming multicenter randomized trial [Cancer and Leukemia Group B (CALGB 9840)] comparing a 3-hour infusion given every 3 weeks with a weekly 1-hour infusion (49). A recent amendment to this trial now incorporates the monoclonal antibody trastuzumab into the treatment arms. Furthermore, weekly paclitaxel may be useful as a foundation for combination chemotherapy regimens.

The first large-scale phase 2 study of a weekly 1-hour infusion schedule of paclitaxel 80 mg/m^2 was completed by Perez and colleagues (50). This prospective multicenter trial was designed to determine the response rate, toxicity, and tolerability in a large group of patients with metastatic breast cancer. This group included patients who were receiving first-, second-, or third-line chemotherapy; those who had received prior or no prior taxane therapy; and those who had undergone high-dose chemotherapy with stem cell support as well as elderly patients, patients with multiple disease sites, and those with grade 1 peripheral neuropathy. With a median follow-up of 6.7 months, this trial demonstrated tolerable toxicity and clinical benefit from weekly therapy with paclitaxel in a cohort of 212 patients, of whom 193 have been evaluated to date. Preliminary results from this study show that 55% of patients achieved clinical benefit from this therapeutic regimen: Overall response rate was 23%, and 32% of patients had disease stabilization for at least 4 months (Table

17.2). Overall, both hematologic and nonhematologic toxicities have been generally well tolerated by this patient population. This trial finished accrual in February 1999.

Docetaxel

Docetaxel has exhibited antitumor activity in previously untreated patients, producing overall response rates of 50% to 68% (51,52). In patients who had received previous chemotherapy, docetaxel achieved overall response rates of 12% to 57% (Table 17.3). Many of these responses were noted in patients who had progressed on previous anthracycline-based chemotherapy. Single-agent docetaxel compared favorably to doxorubicin, vinblastine/mitomycin, 5-FU/vinorelbine, and methotrexate/5-FU in randomized trials (31,35,53). The major toxicities of docetaxel include neutropenia, mucositis, and fluid retention syndrome (54). Docetaxel-induced adverse events occur more frequently in patients with impaired liver function, and a reduction in dosage in these patients is recommended (54).

Some trials of dose-dense docetaxel have been completed, and results of a phase 1 trial suggest that weekly docetaxel is feasible (55). Follow-up of the recently completed and ongoing phase 2 studies is necessary to determine the therapeutic ratio of docetaxel compared with that of standard administration (every-3-week) schedules.

TABLE 17.3. *Single-agent docetaxel in previously treated and untreated patients with metastatic breast cancer*

Regimen	No. of patients evaluated/ no. of trials	Response (%)			FR (% of patients)
		CR	PR	OR	
Previously treated patients					
Docetaxel 60–100 mg/m^2 ± steroids[a]	914/10	0–15[b]	8–53[b]	12–57	7–61[c]
Docetaxel 30–45 mg/m^2 weekly x6, with 2-wk rest	26/1	4	9	50	NR
Previously untreated patients					
Docetaxel 75–100 mg/m^2 ± steroids	186/5	5–16	35–62	50–68	62–89

CR, complete response; FR, clinical fluid retention; NR, not reported; OR, overall response; PR, partial response.

[a] In one study, all patients had progressed on paclitaxel, and nearly all had anthracycline-refractory disease.

[b] One study did not report the complete and partial response rates.

[c] Some studies did not report the incidence of clinical fluid retention.

From Miller KD, Sledge GW, Jr. Taxanes in the treatment of breast cancer: a prodigy comes of age. *Cancer Invest* 1999;17:121–136, with permission.

Combination Therapy

Paclitaxel-based Combinations

Paclitaxel and Doxorubicin

Paclitaxel combined with anthracyclines or anthracenediones has been assessed in at least 15 separate studies involving more than 700 patients. The combination of paclitaxel and anthracyclines is attractive because of incomplete cross-resistance. Complete responses have been reported in 4% to 41% of patients; objective responses were observed in 46% to 94% of patients (Table 17.4). The combination of paclitaxel

TABLE 17.4. *Paclitaxel combined with anthracyclines or anthracenediones in metastatic breast cancer*

Regimen	No. of patients evaluated/ no. of trials	Response (%) CR	PR	OR	Comments
Paclitaxel 130–200 mg/m^2 3-, 24-, or 72-h i.v. Doxorubicin 50–60 mg/m^2	410/6[a]	4–41	44–64	46–94	Agents given sequentially or concurrently; 0%–20% of patients developed CHF
Paclitaxel 100–225 mg/m^2 3-h i.v. Epirubicin 30–100 mg/m^2	218/6	7–18	40–74	47–93	0%–10% of patients developed CHF
Epirubicin 100 mg/m^2 Paclitaxel 135–180 mg/m^2 3-h i.v. q2wk	14/1[b]	29	57	85	Incidence of CHF was not reported
Epirubicin 25–35 mg/m^2 Paclitaxel 80 mg/m^2 1-h i.v. weekly x6, with a 2-wk rest	35/1	20	31	51	No patients developed CHF
Paclitaxel 135 mg/m^2 1-h i.v., d 1 Mitoxantrone 10 mg/m^2, d 1 5-FU 350 mg/m^2, d 1–3 Leucovorin 300 mg/m^2, d 1–3	45/1	4	47	51	4% of patients developed CHF

All regimens were repeated at 3-week intervals unless otherwise stated.
CHF, clinical congestive heart failure; CR, complete response; 5-FU, 5-fluorouracil; i.v., intravenous infusion; OR, overall response; PR, partial response.
[a] Eligible patients in one study of 73 patients had nonmetastatic locally advanced breast cancer.
[b] Eligible patients had advanced or metastatic disease.
From Miller KD, Sledge GW, Jr. Taxanes in the treatment of breast cancer: a prodigy comes of age. *Cancer Invest* 1999;17:121–136, with permission.

and anthracyclines has produced unexpected cardiac toxicity in some studies. In a study by Gianni et al. (56), 18% of patients developed significant congestive heart failure (CHF), but all responded to treatment, and 3-year follow-up found the cardiac toxicity to be reversible (57). A review of eight single-agent trials and two randomized studies including the paclitaxel/doxorubicin combination found that the incidence of clinical CHF (4%) was similar to that noted with single-agent doxorubicin (58), provided the total cumulative exposure to doxorubicin when combined with paclitaxel is limited to 360 mg/m^2 (57).

Two large randomized trials evaluated the paclitaxel and doxorubicin combination versus either agent alone or versus a FAC combination regimen. In the Eastern Cooperative Oncology Group 1193 trial, 739 patients were randomized to receive paclitaxel (T), doxorubicin (A), or paclitaxel/doxorubicin (AT) as first-line treatment. The AT combination produced a response rate of 46% compared with response rates of 34% and 33% for A and T, respectively (33). Nevertheless, median overall survival was not significantly prolonged with AT, with rates of 20.1, 22.2, and 22.4 months for A, T, and A + T, respectively. A survival benefit may not have occurred because patients who failed with single agents were crossed over to the other agent, with a response rate of 20% for those crossing from A to T and 14% for those crossing from T to A. Therefore, A and T given sequentially or in combination may have a similar impact on overall outcome. In a trial by the Eastern European and Israeli Breast Cancer Study Group, the AT combination regimen was compared with a standard FAC regimen as first-line therapy (36). Patients who received AT achieved an overall response rate of 68% and a complete response rate of 19% compared with an overall response rate of 55% and an 8% complete response rate achieved by patients who received FAC. Importantly, patients in the AT arm had a significantly longer median overall survival of 23.0 months compared with 18.3 months for patients in the FAC arm. AT was associated with higher incidences of grade 3/4 neutropenia, peripheral neuropathy, and myalgia/arthralgia than FAC but also had a lower incidence of nausea and vomiting. Similar to the results of E1193, cardiac toxicity was comparable in both arms and the incidence of CHF associated with AT treatment was 1.5%.

Paclitaxel and Platinum Agents

The combination of paclitaxel plus platinum compounds (either cisplatin or carboplatin) also has been evaluated for the treatment of patients with metastatic breast cancer. Although cisplatin and carboplatin have similar efficacy, carboplatin is generally better tolerated than cisplatin (59). Three phase 2 studies (60–62) of paclitaxel by 3-hour intravenous infusion plus carboplatin in a total of 153 patients with advanced breast cancer demonstrated considerable efficacy in both chemotherapy-naive and anthracycline-resistant patients. The North Central Cancer Treatment Group phase 2 study (NCCTG 95-32-52) of paclitaxel 200 mg/m^2 and carboplatin at a calculated area under the curve of 6, administered every 3 weeks, demonstrated similar response rates (62%; 95% CI, 48%–76%) to other first-line combination therapy with an anthracycline-taxane (paclitaxel or docetaxel) regimen (60). The NCCTG 95-32-52 trial also demonstrated a 7.3-month median time to progression, with a 72% 1-year survival rate. Two other studies of paclitaxel plus carboplatin, both conducted by Fountzilas and colleagues, produced similar results, with complete response rates of 12% and 14% and overall response rates of 43% and 53% (61, 62). Time to progression was 8 and 8.9 months, and median overall survival in one trial was 12 months and had not been reached at the time of reporting for the other trial. This demonstrated activity, along with the need for options for patients who have received anthracyclines in the adjuvant setting, make the paclitaxel/carboplatin regimen worthy of further study. Several national randomized phase 2 studies of this combination (with or without trastuzumab) have already been initiated or are planned.

Paclitaxel and Other Agents

Several trials have evaluated paclitaxel in combination with other agents that are active in metastatic breast cancer. Studies of paclitaxel combined with either high-dose or standard 5-FU have yielded overall response rates of 35% (in previously treated patients) and 60%, respectively (32). Paclitaxel combined with a regimen of 5-FU, leucovorin, and mitoxantrone resulted in an overall response rate of 51%, including a complete response rate of 4%, in previously treated and untreated patients. Paclitaxel plus cyclophosphamide resulted in a 28% overall response rate, including a 6% complete response rate, in patients previously treated for metastatic disease. Prolonged infusions of paclitaxel plus cyclophosphamide with growth factor support have yielded overall response rates of 62%, with a 3% complete response rate. Paclitaxel plus ifosfamide resulted in a 48% overall response rate in patients previously treated with anthracyclines. A phase 1 study of paclitaxel plus vinorelbine in extensively pretreated patients reported two complete responses and one partial response in ten assessable patients (32).

Docetaxel-based Combinations

Docetaxel and Doxorubicin

In previously untreated patients, docetaxel in combination with anthracyclines and anthracenediones produced complete responses in as many as 27% of patients and overall response rates of 63% to more than 80% (Table 17.5) (32). Early data showed that the combination was associated with very modest CHF and a small incidence of decreased left ventricular ejection fraction, consistent with the expected rates reported for anthracycline alone (58). In addition, docetaxel in combination with cisplatin demonstrated an overall response rate of 47%.

Docetaxel and Other Agents

Other docetaxel-based combinations include docetaxel and vinorelbine, with overall response rates of 58% to 66%, and docetaxel plus 5-FU, with an overall response

TABLE 17.5. *Docetaxel in combination with anthracyclines or anthracenediones in metastatic breast cancer*

Regimen	No. of patients evaluated/ no. of trials	Response (%) CR	PR	OR	Comments
Docetaxel 50–85 mg/m² Doxorubicin 40–60 mg/m²	42/1	NR	NR	>80[a]	No patients developed CHF
Docetaxel 75 mg/m² Doxorubicin 50 mg/m² Cyclophosphamide 500 mg/m²	48/1	6	67	73	2% of patients developed CHF
Docetaxel 75 mg/m² Epirubicin 60–110 mg/m²	62/1	13	61	69	5% of patients developed CHF
Docetaxel 100 mg/m², d1 Mitoxantrone 20 mg/m², d1	30	27	37	63	No patients developed CHF
Docetaxel 100 mg/m² Cisplatin 100 mg/m²	32/1	6	41	47	65% of patients required dose reduction for myelosuppression

CHF, clinical congestive heart failure; CR, complete response; NR, not reported; OR, overall response; PR, partial response.

[a] Response rate in the highest dose levels tested.

From Miller KD, Sledge GW, Jr. Taxanes in the treatment of breast cancer: a prodigy comes of age. *Cancer Invest* 1999;17:121–136, with permission.

rate of 33% in 15 previously treated patients. Phase 1 trials indicate that docetaxel can be safely added to cyclophosphamide or gemcitabine, producing overall response rates of 69% and 50%, respectively (32). A phase 3 trial was reported for 429 anthracycline-naive metastatic breast cancer patients who were randomly treated with AC (doxorubicin 60 mg/m² and cyclophosphamide 600 mg/m²) or AT (doxorubicin 50 mg/m² and docetaxel 75 mg/m²) every 3 weeks (37). Overall response rates were 47% (8% complete response) and 60% (11% complete response) ($p = 0.008$), respectively. Time to progression and time to treatment failure were also statistically better in the AT arm, but, at this point, no survival advantage has been reported. Cardiac dysfunction was similar in the two arms.

Other Active Agents

Epirubicin

Epirubicin is a 4′-epimer of doxorubicin that has been shown to have efficacy comparable to its parent molecule, but it is associated with lower incidences of severe toxicity than doxorubicin (63–65). Three trials administering equimolar doses of epirubicin and doxorubicin showed that epirubicin and doxorubicin produced response rates of 20% to 36% and 29% to 38%, respectively. Also, epirubicin and doxorubicin were associated with similar times to progression and median overall survival. Epirubicin demonstrated a more favorable toxicity profile than doxorubicin;

lower incidences of grade 3/4 leukopenia, nausea/vomiting, and mucositis were observed with epirubicin compared with doxorubicin. Importantly, epirubicin was associated with less cardiac toxicity than doxorubicin. Dose-escalation studies have shown that the probability of developing CHF increases substantially with a doxorubicin cumulative dose greater than 500 mg/m^2 compared with a cumulative dose of epirubicin of greater than 1,000 mg/m^2.

Based on encouraging results from single-agent trials, epirubicin has been evaluated in combination regimens. Three randomized trials compared the FAC and FEC (fluorouracil, etoposide, and cisplatin) combination regimens (66–68). Similar to single-agent trials, FEC and FAC reduced comparable response rates (45%–57% versus 44%–54%, respectively), times to progression (270–314 days versus 220–273 days, respectively), and median overall survival times (530–613 days versus 450–-591 days, respectively), but FEC exhibited a more favorable toxicity profile. Specifically, FEC was associated with less neutropenia, nausea/vomiting, and alopecia than was FAC. The incidence of CHF was also low with FEC treatment; in two of three trials, no CHF was reported (66,68), and in one trial, a CHF incidence of 0.4% was reported (67).

The combination of epirubicin with taxanes also has been investigated. The combination of epirubicin and paclitaxel is highly active, producing overall response rates of 44% to 80% with complete response rates of 0% to 17% in phase 1 and 2 studies (69–73). The most common toxicities were alopecia and neutropenia. Cardiac toxicity was reported in 0% to 13% of patients. The combination of epirubicin and docetaxel also was shown to be highly active in phase 1 and 2 trials, producing overall response rates of 52% to 79% and complete response rates of 7% to 14% (74–78). Cardiac toxicity was reported in 0% to 8% of patients. In the absence of granulocyte-colony stimulating factor (G-CSF) support, almost all patients who did not receive G-CSF support experienced grade 3/4 neutropenia (74,76,77); trials that administered docetaxel on the day following epirubicin (74) or used G-CSF support had a reduced incidence of neutropenia (78).

Capecitabine

Capecitabine is a rationally designed oral fluoropyrimidine carbamate that is enzymatically activated to 5-FU, preferentially in tumor cells. An initial phase 2 trial in 162 heavily pretreated and paclitaxel-refractory patients with metastatic breast cancer yielded an overall response rate of 20% with a median duration of response of 8.1 months (79). A recent multicenter confirmatory trial in 75 taxane-refractory patients yielded a 25% response rate with a median duration of response of 8.3 months (80). Small randomized phase 2 trials showed that capecitabine compares favorably to CMF as first-line therapy for metastatic breast cancer and also compares favorably to paclitaxel in anthracycline-resistant patients. The toxicity profile is similar to that noted for patients receiving 5-FU via continuous infusion with an ambulatory infusion pump, and it includes diarrhea, stomatitis, and hand–foot syndrome (81). Other oral 5-FU prodrugs are being actively investigated in clinical trials in an attempt to take advantage of biochemical modifications to increase 5-FU concentrations in tumor cells. These other agents include uracil/tegafur (UFT), eniluracil with oral 5-FU, and 5'-deoxy-5-fluorouridine (5'-DFUR).

Other Agents

Other agents under investigation include gemcitabine and vinorelbine. Gemcitabine has a modest toxicity profile and well demonstrated anti-tumor activity in a series of phase II studies (82); however, this agent has not yet been approved by the Food and Drug Administration (FDA) as treatment for breast cancer. Vinorelbine, a microtubule inhibitor, has clinically significant single-agent activity both in untreated (21%–44% responses) and previously treated patients (11%–64% responses) with advanced disease; it is active in combination with anthracyclines, cisplatin, mitomycin C, mitoxantrone, and ifosfamide (83). Although vinorelbine has been approved by the FDA as treatment for non–small cell lung cancer, it has not yet received approval for the treatment of breast cancer.

MONOCLONAL ANTIBODY THERAPY

The *HER-2/neu* (c-*erbB2*) protooncogene product, a transmembrane growth factor receptor involved in mitogenic signaling, is overexpressed in approximately 30% of patients with breast cancer (84,85). A thorough discussion of the biologic, prognostic, and predictive characteristics of *HER-2*, including results of completed clinical trials, was published by Perez (84). Trastuzumab, a recombinant humanized anti–HER-2/*neu* monoclonal antibody, has been developed and has been shown to inhibit the growth of breast cancer cells overexpressing HER-2. This monoclonal antibody has clinical activity and was found to be well tolerated in phase I and II clinical trials (84,86). In addition to its single activity, trastuzumab has now been demonstrated to improve the response rate, median time to progression, and median and 1-year survival when added to chemotherapy (anthracyclines, paclitaxel) compared with chemotherapy alone in patients with HER-2-overexpressing breast cancer measured by immunohistochemistry (IHC) (84). A significant increase in cardiotoxicity, however, limits the concurrent use of trastuzumab with anthracyclines. A wide variety of clinical trials are planned to optimize the use of this monoclonal antibody for the treatment of patients with metastatic (or resected) breast cancer. Some of the regimens planned for study include combinations of trastuzumab with different taxane- or nontaxane-based agents, optimization of scheduling, and potential standardization of predictive markers of response to trastuzumab.

An important factor in identifying patients who benefit from trastuzumab is the evaluation of the overexpression of the *HER-2* receptor. Overexpression of the receptor is assessed by IHC and is scored on a 4-point scale of 0, 1+, 2+, or 3+ (87). In published clinical trials, patients were eligible for enrollment if they had tumors that were rated as either 2+ or 3+. Interestingly, better outcomes were reported in patients that were 3 compared with 2 + (88). Reproducibility, however, has been a problem with IHC methods; another approach that appears to be attractive and reproducible is the fluorescence *in situ* hybridization (FISH) method in which amplification of the Her-2 gene, the mechanism of *HER-2* overexpression, can be measured (85).

Trastuzumab is administered as an outpatient loading dose of 4 mg/kg by intravenous infusion over 90 minutes, with subsequent weekly doses of 2 mg/kg over 30 minutes. Phase 1 and 2 trials of trastuzumab revealed low-grade fever at the first infusion and pain at the site of known tumor deposits as its only toxicities (85, 87). In previously treated patients with *HER-2*/neu-positive advanced breast cancer, trastuzumab therapy produced overall response rates of 12% to 15%, with median response durations of 5.1 to 8.4 months (Table 17.6) (88,89). The use of trastuzumab in combination with cisplatin in these patients resulted in objective response rates higher than those previously reported for single-agent cisplatin in a similar population, with no apparent increase in toxicity (90,91).

The ability of trastuzumab to augment first-line chemotherapy for metastatic disease was evaluated in a randomized study of 469 patients with advanced breast cancer. Patients with no prior anthracycline exposure received doxorubicin or epirubicin plus cyclophosphamide; those previously exposed to anthracyclines received paclitaxel. All patients were randomized to receive trastuzumab plus chemotherapy or chemotherapy alone. In general, patients treated with paclitaxel had received more prior adjuvant chemotherapy and had a poorer prognosis than those given an anthracycline plus cyclophosphamide. Trastuzumab plus either anthracycline-based combination chemotherapy or paclitaxel resulted in significantly higher overall response rates (62% versus 36%, respectively, $p < 0.01$), longer response durations (8.6 versus 5.5 months, respectively, $p < 0.001$), longer median survival (25.4 versus 20.9 months, respectively, $p = 0.045$), and improved 1-year survival (78% versus 67%, respectively, $p < 0.01$) than chemotherapy alone. Patients who received trastuzumab plus anthracycline-based combination chemotherapy had a 19% incidence of significant cardiac dysfunction compared with 4% in those who received trastuzumab plus paclitaxel (92,93). At a median follow-up of 25 months, chemotherapy plus trastuzumab had a superior overall survival compared with chemotherapy alone (25.4 versus 20.9 months, respectively). This survival advantage was seen despite the subsequent use of trastuzumab in patients originally randomized to chemotherapy alone who then developed progression. Studies of trastuzumab combined with other chemotherapeutic regimens (e.g., paclitaxel/carboplatin, docetaxel, and vinorelbine) are ongoing.

Trastuzumab has been approved by the FDA as a single agent for the treatment of patients with metastatic breast cancer whose tumors overexpress Her-2 protein and who have received one or more chemotherapy regimens or in combination with paclitaxel for the treatment of patients who have not received chemotherapy for their metastatic disease.

There were mild infusion-associated reactions in approximately 40% of patients, mostly with the first infusion. In the phase 3 trials, the incidence of adverse events

TABLE 17.6. *Clinical trials of trastuzumab alone or in combination for Her-2+ disease*

Study (ref)	Patients	Treatment	CR (%)	OR (%)	MDR (mo)	MS (mo)	1-yr Survival (%)
Previously treated patients							
Baselga et al., 1996 (89)	n = 43; HER-2/neu+; extensive prior therapy	Trastuzumab	2	12	5.1	NR	NR
Cobleigh et al., 1998 (88)	n = 213; HER-2/neu+; extensive prior therapy (94% had prior anthracyclines)	Trastuzumab	4	15	8.4	13	NR
Pegram, 1998 (90)	n = 37; HER-2/neu+; extensive prior therapy	Trastuzumab + cisplatin	0	24	5.3	NR	NR
Seidman, 2001 (93)	n = 88; 0–3 prior chemotherapies	Trastuzumab + paclitaxel	4	57	7.0	NR	NR
Burnstein, 2001 (94)	n = 40; 0–2 prior chemotherapies	Trastuzumab + vinorelbine	8	68	NR	NR	NR
Previously untreated patients							
Slamon et al., 2001 (92)[a]	n = 469; no prior therapy for metastatic disease; many patients had received adjuvant chemotherapy	Doxorubicin or epirubicin + cyclophosphamide (n = 145)	7	42.1	6.5	25	73
		Doxorubicin or epirubicin + cyclophosphamide + trastuzumab (n = 146)	8	64.9	9.0	33	83
		Paclitaxel (n = 89)	2	25.0	4.2	18	61
		Paclitaxel + trastuzumab (n = 89)	7	57.3	7.1	22	73
Vogel et al., 1998 (86)	n = 62[b]; no prior therapy for metastatic disease	Standard-dose trastuzumab (n = 33)	NR	21	NYR	NYR	N/A
		High-dose trastuzumab (n = 29)	NR	28	NYR	NYR	N/A

CR, complete response; MDR, median duration of response; MS, median survival; N/A, not available due to insufficient follow-up; NR, not reported; NYR, not yet reached; OR, overall response.

[a] Study had a median follow-up of 25 months.

[b] Of 114 enrolled patients, 62 were assessable for response and survival.

such as cardiotoxicity, leukopenia, anemia, and abdominal pain was higher in women receiving trastuzumab with or without chemotherapy compared with those receiving chemotherapy alone. A recent report submitted by the producer of trastuzumab, Genentech highlighted the rare occurrence of severe allergic reactions with the utilization of this monoclonal antibody in patients with preexisting pulmonary compromise due to breast cancer. Further studies to optimize the utilization of trastuzumab as a single agent or in combination with other therapies are ongoing. Recent data of trastuzumab with taxane and platinum combinations, and with trastuzumab administered once every 3 weeks (instead of weekly) are especially worthy of follow-up.

HIGH-DOSE CHEMOTHERAPY WITH STEM CELL TRANSPLANTATION FOR METASTATIC BREAST CANCER

Data from the first large randomized trial comparing high-dose chemotherapy plus stem cell transplantation with conventional-dose maintenance chemotherapy (FAC) for the treatment of metastatic breast cancer have become available (94,95). A study conducted by the Philadelphia Breast Intergroup (PBT-1) enrolled 553 patients with metastatic breast cancer who initially received either conventional-dose FAC or CMF (cyclophosphamide, methotrexate, and 5-fluorouracil) combination chemotherapy for 4 to 6 cycles. Of those patients, 296 achieved complete or partial response to this induction therapy, and 199 went on to randomization. This randomization was either to autologous stem-cell transplantation or to CMF-maintenance chemotherapy for 2 years. Patients assigned to the high-dose therapy arm underwent bone marrow or stem cell harvest, followed by high-dose carboplatin, thiotepa, and cyclophosphamide (CTCb, also called the STAMP V regimen). This trial was designed with an 85% power to detect a doubling of median survival from transplant versus CMF chemotherapy; however, the reported results did not show any significant difference in median survival between the two groups. The 3-year survival data have been reported, with a 32% survival rate for the transplant group and 38% survival for the patients receiving CMF. Time to progression was also similar, with 9.6 months reported for high-dose chemotherapy with transplant, and 9 months for CMF.

The data also were analyzed for the subgroups of patients who achieved either partial or complete responses for induction chemotherapy. Of the 45 patients who achieved complete responses to induction therapy, those who underwent transplantation had a 3-year survival rate of 42%, whereas those receiving standard-dose maintenance chemotherapy achieved a 3-year survival rate of 49%. Of the 139 patients who achieved partial responses to induction chemotherapy, patients treated with high-dose chemotherapy with stem cell transplantation achieved a 3-year survival rate of 27%, whereas those receiving standard-dose maintenance chemotherapy achieved a 3-year survival rate of 36%. These data demonstrate that CTCb with transplantation was not beneficial when used as consolidation for patients with demonstrated chemosensitivity to FAC or CMF induction therapy for metastatic breast cancer.

SUMMARY

An extensive array of basic and clinical research has been performed throughout the last decade in an attempt of improve the outcome of patients with metastatic breast cancer. Despite significant advances, cure after a diagnosis of metastatic breast cancer remains an elusive goal utilizing current therapeutic options. At this time, many therapeutic options are available, and no single method has been clearly demonstrated as being optimal. Given the novel mechanisms of action of new antitumor compounds coupled with their favorable toxicity profiles, continued improvement in survival and quality of life may be achieved in patients with advanced disease. Participation in clinical trials remains a major priority.

Phase 2 studies of the taxanes combined with other chemotherapeutic agents have begun to demonstrate higher response rates than those previously reported for single agents, but the overall impact on survival rates must be determined in competitive phase 3 trials (32). Trastuzumab plus paclitaxel has shown promising results with tumors that overexpress HER-2/*neu* (92–94). Although further research is necessary, data from recently completed large randomized trials evaluating high-dose chemotherapy with stem cell transplantation versus standard chemotherapy regimens (both in the adjuvant and metastatic settings) did not demonstrate improvements in disease-free or overall survival with the high-dose therapy approach (95,96).

Future advances in breast cancer treatment will depend on tailoring therapy to individual patients, developing new cytotoxic agents and novel combinations, and improving dose-scheduling strategies to achieve increased antitumor activity with improved tolerability. Beyond the traditional antineoplastic approach, new types of agents, such as angiogenesis inhibitors, inhibitors of tumor cell migration and invasiveness, and compounds that inhibit the signal transduction pathways involved in malignant transformation and growth may lead to significant improvements in the treatment of all patients with breast cancer.

The choice of specific agents in the management of metastatic breast cancer will be made increasingly in the context of the biology of the disease and the prior treatment received. Studies to evaluate the different alterations in the expression of genes that control the cell cycle will be of critical importance in understanding and optimizing the different treatment modalities for metastatic breast cancer.

Among the most difficult decisions physicians must make is to decide what the "optimal" duration of therapy is for patients with metastatic breast cancer. Although the available clinical literature leaves the question somewhat unsettled, data suggest that continuing chemotherapy until disease progression affords a better treatment outcome, especially in terms of time to progression and possible quality of life. The randomized studies completed have yielded improved (although not statistically significant) overall survival for patients receiving chemotherapy until progression. Data regarding optimal duration of newer treatment such as the taxanes or anti-*HER-2* monoclonal antibody are not yet available, but it appears prudent for now to recommend that women with hormone-refractory disease receive treatment until disease progression; however, it remains essential that clinicians base treatment decisions on the individual patient's circumstances and thorough informed discussions with the patient. The importance of clinical trials also should be emphasized. Participation in clinical trials is necessary for the continued investigation of novel agents and treatment approaches and is recommended for the management of metastatic breast cancer. The pace at which these new therapies are evaluated depends on patient accrual and can be enhanced by education of patients on the clinical trial process and their eligibility for open trials.

REFERENCES

1. Ellis MJ, Hayes DF, Lippman ME. Treatment of metastatic breast cancer. In: Harris J, Lippman ME, Morrow M, et al., eds. *Diseases of the breast,.* 2nd ed. Philadelphia: Lippincott Williams & Wilkins, 2000:749–797.
2. Pritchard KI. Endocrine therapy for breast cancer. *Oncology* 2000;14:483–492.
3. Hortobagyi GN. Treatment of breast cancer. *N Engl J Med* 1998;339:974–984.
4. Greenberg PA, Hortobagyi GN, Smith TL, et al. Long-term follow-up of patients with complete remission following combination chemotherapy for metastatic breast cancer. *J Clin Oncol* 1996;14: 2197–2205.
5. Olin JJ, Muss HB. New strategies for managing metastatic breast cancer. *Oncology* 2000;14:629–641.
6. Hayes DF, van Zyl JA, Hacking A, et al. Randomized comparison of tamoxifen and two separate doses of toremifene in postmenopausal patients with metastatic breast cancer. *J Clin Oncol* 1995; 13:2556–2566.
7. Howell A, DeFriend D, Robertson J, et al. Response to a specific antioestrogen (ICI 182780) in tamoxifen-resistant breast cancer. *Lancet* 1995;345:29–30.
8. Bonneterre J, Thurlimann BJD, Robertson JFR, on behalf of the Arimidex Study Group. Preliminary results of a large comparative multi-centre clinical trial comparing the efficacy and tolerability of Arimidex (Anastrozole) and tamoxifen (TAM) in postmenopausal women with advanced breast cancer (ABC). *Eur J Cancer* 1999;35(Suppl 4):S313(abst 1257).
9. Nabholtz JM, Buzdar A, Pollack M, et al. Anastrozole is superior to tamoxifen as first-line therapy for advanced breast cancer in postmenopausal women: results of a North American multicenter randomized trial. Arimidex Study Group. *J Clin Oncol* 2000;18(22):3758–3767.
10. Taylor CW, Green S, Dalton WS, et al. Multicenter randomized clinical trial of goserelin versus surgical ovariectomy in premenopausal patients with receptor-positive metastatic breast cancer: an Intergroup study. *J Clin Oncol* 1998;16:994–999.
11. Grodin JM, Siiteri PK, MacDonald PC. Source of estrogen production in postmenopausal women. *J Clin Endocrinol Metab* 1973;36:207–214.
12. Brodie AM, Njar VC. Aromatase inhibitors and breast cancer. *Semin Oncol* 1996;23:10–20.
13. Harvey HA. Aromatase inhibitors in clinical practice: current status and a look to the future. *Semin Oncol* 1996;23:33–38.
14. Thurlimann B, Castiglione M, Hsu-Schmitz SF, et al. Formestane versus megestrol acetate in postmenopausal breast cancer patients after failure of tamoxifen: a phase III prospective randomised cross over trial of second-line hormonal treatment (SAKK 20/90). Swiss Group for Clinical Cancer Research (SAKK). *Eur J Cancer* 1997;33:1017–1024.
15. Dombernowsky P, Smith I, Falkson G, et al. Letrozole, a new oral aromatase inhibitor for advanced breast cancer: double-blind randomized trial showing a dose effect and improved efficacy and tolerability compared with megestrol acetate. *J Clin Oncol* 1998;16:453–461.
16. Buzdar AU, Jonat W, Howell A, et al. Anastrozole versus megestrol acetate in the treatment of postmenopausal women with advanced breast carcinoma: results of a survival update based on a combined analysis of data from two mature phase III trials: Arimidex Study Group. *Cancer* 1998; 83:1142–1152.
17. Buzdar A, Jonat W, Howell A, et al. Anastrozole, a potent and selective aromatase inhibitor, versus megestrol acetate in postmenopausal women with advanced breast cancer: results of overview analysis of two phase III trials. Arimidex Study Group. *J Clin Oncol* 1996;14:2000–2011.
18. Geisler J, Johannessen DC, Anker G, et al. Treatment with formestane alone and in combination

with aminoglutethimide in heavily pretreated breast cancer patients: clinical and endocrine effects. *Eur J Cancer* 1996;32A:789–792.

19. Murray R, Pitt P. Aromatase inhibition with 4-OH/Androstenedione after prior aromatase inhibition with aminoglutethimide in women with advanced breast cancer. *Breast Cancer Res Treat* 1995;35: 249–253.
20. Di Salle E, Briatico G, Giudici D, et al. Novel aromatase and 5 alpha-reductase inhibitors. *J Steroid Biochem Mol Biol* 1994;49:289–294.
21. Di Salle E, Giudici D, Briatico G, et al. Novel irreversible aromatase inhibitors. *Ann NY Acad Sci.* 1990;595:357–367.
22. Johannessen DC, Engan T, Di Salle E, et al. Endocrine and clinical effects of exemestane (PNU 155971), a novel steroidal aromatase inhibitor, in postmenopausal breast cancer patients: a phase I study. *Clin Cancer Res* 1997;3:1101–1108.
23. Thurlimann B, Paridaens R, Serin D, et al. Third-line hormonal treatment with exemestane in post-menopausal patients with advanced breast cancer progressing on aminoglutethimide: a phase II multicentre multinational study. Exemestane Study Group. *Eur J Cancer* 1997;33:1767–1773.
24. Paridaens R, Thomas J, Wildiers J, et al. Safety, activity and estrogen inhibition by exemestane in postmenopausal women with advanced breast cancer: a phase I study. *Anticancer Drugs* 1998;9: 675–683.
25. Jones S, Belt R, Cooper B, et al. A phase II study of antitumor efficacy and safety of exemestane as second-line hormonal treatment of postmenopausal patients with metastatic breast cancer refractory to tamoxifen. *Breast Cancer Res Treat* 1998;50:305(abst 436).
26. Jones S, Vogel C, Arkhipov A, et al. Multicenter, phase II trial of exemestane as third-line hormonal therapy of postmenopausal women with metastatic breast cancer. Aromasin Study Group. *J Clin Oncol* 1999;17:3814–3425.
27. Jones S, Vogel C, Fehrenbacher L, et al. Antitumor efficacy of exemestane as third-line hormonal therapy in the treatment of postmenopausal women with metastatic breast cancer refractory to tamoxifen and megace. *Am Soc Clin Oncol* 1998;17(abstract 573).
28. Klijn JGM, Seynaeve C, Beex L, et al. Combined treatment with buserelin (LHRH-A) and tamoxifen (TAM) vs. single treatment with each drug alone in premenopausal metastatic breast cancer: Preliminary results of EORTC study 10881. *Proc Am Soc Clin Oncol* 1996;15:117(abst 132).
29. Jonat W, Kaufmann M, Blamey RW, et al. A randomized study to compare the effect of the luteinising hormone releasing hormone (LHRH) analogue goserelin with or without tamoxifen in pre- and perimenopausal patients with advanced breast cancer. *Eur J Cancer* 1995;31A(2):137–142.
30. Bishop JF, Dewar J, Toner GC, et al. Initial paclitaxel improves outcome compared with CMFP combination chemotherapy as front-line therapy in untreated metastatic breast cancer. *J Clin Oncol* 1999;17:2355–2364.
31. Nabholtz JM, Senn HJ, Bezwoda WR, et al. Prospective randomized trial of docetaxel versus mitomycin plus vinblastine in patients with metastatic breast cancer progressing despite previous anthracycline-containing chemotherapy. 304 Study Group. *J Clin Oncol* 1999;17(5):1413–1424.
32. Miller KD, Sledge GW Jr. Taxanes in the treatment of breast cancer: a prodigy comes of age. *Cancer Invest* 1999;17:121–136.
33. Sledge GM, Neuberg D, Ingle J, et al. Phase III trial of doxorubicin (A) vs. paclitaxel (T) vs. doxorubicin and paclitaxel (A + T) as first-line therapy for metastatic breast cancer (MBC): an Intergroup trial. *Proc Am Soc Clin Oncol* 1997;16:1a(abst 2).
34. Gamucci T, Piccart M, Brúning P, et al. Single agent taxol (T) versus doxorubicin (D) as first-line chemotherapy (CT) in advanced breast cancer (ABC): final results of an EORTC randomized study with crossover. *Proc Am Soc Clin Oncol* 1998;17:111a(abst 428).
35. Chan S, Friedrichs K, Noel D, et al. Prospective randomized trial of docetaxel versus doxorubicin in patients with metastatic breast cancer. *J Clin Oncol* 1999;17:2341–2354.
36. Jassem J, Pienkowski T, Pluzanska A, et al. Doxorubicin and paclitaxel verus fluorouracil, doxorubicin, and cyclophosphamide as first-line therapy for women with metastatic breast cancer: final results of a randomized phase III multicenter trial. *J Clin Oncol* 2001;19(6):1707–1715.
37. Nabholtz JM, Falkson G, Campos D, et al. A phase III trial comparing doxorubicin (A) and docetaxel (T) (AT) to doxorubicin and cyclophosphamide (AC) as first line chemotherapy for MBC. *Proc Am Soc Clin Oncol* 1999;18:127a(abst 485).
38. Lück HJ, Thomsenn C, Untch M, et al. Multicentric phase III study in first line treatment of advanced metastatic breast cancer (MBC): epirubicin/paclitaxel (ET) vs epirubicin/cyclophosphamide (EC). A study of the AGO Breast Cancer Group. *Proc Am Soc Clin Oncol* 2000;19:73a(abst 280).

39. Winer E, Berry D, Duggan D, et al. Failure of higher dose paclitaxel to improve outcome in patients with metastatic breast cancer—results from CALGB 9342. *Proc Am Soc Clin Oncol* 1998;17: 101a(abst 387).

40. Seidman AD, Tiersten A, Hudis C, et al. Phase II trial of paclitaxel by 3-hour infusion as initial and salvage chemotherapy for metastatic breast cancer. *J Clin Oncol* 1995;13:2575–2581.

41. Smith RE, Brown AM, Mamounas EP, et al. Randomized trial of 3-hour versus 24-hour infusion of high-dose paclitaxel in patients with metastatic or locally advanced breast cancer: National Surgical Adjuvant Breast and Bowel Project Protocol B-26. *J Clin Oncol* 1999;17:3403–3411.

42. Seidman AD, Hudis CA, Albanel J, et al. Dose-dense therapy with weekly 1-hour paclitaxel infusions in the treatment of metastatic breast cancer. *J Clin Oncol* 1998;16:3353–3361.

43. Lück H-J, Marhenke D, Petry KU, et al. Weekly paclitaxel monotherapy as salvage treatment in pretreated patients with metastatic breast cancer: experience with one hour schedule. *Br Cancer Res Treat* 1997;46:59(abst 233).

44. Asbury R, Chang A, Boros L, et al. Weekly moderate-dose paclitaxel (P) in advanced breast cancer (ABC). *Proc Am Soc Clin Oncol* 1998;17:127a(abst 486).

45. Sola C, Lluch A, Carcia-Conde J, et al. Phase II study of weekly paclitaxel (P) in recurrent breast cancer after high-dose chemotherapy (HDC). *Proc Am Soc Clin Oncol* 1998;17:174a(Abst 669).

46. Alvarez A, Mickiewicz E, Brosio C, et al. Weekly Taxol (T) in patients who had relapsed or remained stable with T in a 21 day schedule. *Proc Am Soc Clin Oncol* 1998;17:188a(abst 726).

47. Breier S, Lebedinsky C, Ayiviri C, et al. Long-term weekly paclitaxel (P) in metastatic breast cancer (MBC): a phase II trial in pretreated patients. *Proc Am Soc Clin Oncol* 1998;17:192a(abst 740).

48. Sikov W, Akerley W, Strenger R, al. High-dose weekly paclitaxel in metastatic and locally advanced breast cancer: a Brown University Oncology Group Study. *Semin Oncol* 1999;26 (Suppl 2):33(abst).

49. Seidman AD. Phase III randomized study of paclitaxel via one hour infusion every week versus three hour infusion every 3 weeks with or without trastuzumab (Herceptin) in patients with inoperable, recurrent, or metastatic breast cancer with or without overexpression of HER2-Neu. Procol CALGB 9840 *www.cancernet.nci.nih.gov.*

50. Perez EA, Vogel CL, Irwin DH, et al. A multicenter phase II trial of weekly paclitaxel in women with metastatic breast cancer. In press, *J Clin Oncol* 2001.

51. Ravdin PM, Burris HA III, Cook, G, et al. Phase II trial of docetaxel in advanced anthracycline-resistant or anthracenedione-resistant breast cancer. *J Clin Oncol* 1995;13:2879–2885.

52. Valero V, Holmes FA, Walters RS, et al. Phase II trial of docetaxel: a new, highly effective antineoplastic agent in the management of patients with anthracycline-resistant metastatic breast cancer. *J Clin Oncol* 1995;13:2886–2894.

53. Söstrom J, Blomqvist C, Mouridsen H, et al. Docetaxel compared with sequential methotrexate and 5-fluorouracil in patients with advanced breast cancer after anthracycline failure: a randomised phase III study with crossover on progression by the Scandinavian Breast Group. *Eur J Cancer* 1999;35: 1194–1201.

54. Cortes JE, Pazdur R. Docetaxel. *J Clin Oncol* 1995;13:2643–2655.

55. Loffler TM, Freund W, Droge C, et al. Activity of weekly Taxotere (TXT) in patients with metastatic breast cancer. *Proc Am Soc Clin Oncol* 1998;17:113a(abst 435).

56. Gianni L, Munzone E, Capri G, et al. Paclitaxel by 3-hour infusion in combination with bolus doxorubicin in women with untreated metastatic breast cancer: high antitumor efficacy and cardiac effects in a dose-finding and sequence-finding study. *J Clin Oncol 1995;13:2688–2699.*

57. Valagussa P, Gianni L, Capri G, et al. Three-year follow-up in women with metastatic breast cancer after bolus doxorubicin and paclitaxel infused over 3 hours. *Proc Am Soc Clin Oncol* 1998;17: 111a(abst 429).

58. Gianni L, Dombernowsky P, Sledge GW Jr, et al. Cardiac function following combination therapy with Taxol (T) and doxorubicin (A) for advanced breast cancer (ABC). *Proc Am Soc Clin Oncol* 1998;17:115a(abst 444).

59. Perez EA, Hartmann LC. Paclitaxel and carboplatin for advanced breast cancer. *Semin Oncol* 1996; 23:41–45.

60. Perez EA, Hillman DW, Stella PJ, et al. A phase II study of paclitaxel plus carboplatin as first-line chemotherapy for women with metastatic breast carcinoma. *Cancer* 2000;88:124–131.

61. Fountzilas G, Papadimitriou V, Dimopoulus MA, et al. Paclitaxel and carboplatin as first-line chemotherapy for advanced breast cancer. *Oncology* 1998;12:45–48.

62. Fountzilas G, Athanassiadis A, Kalogera-Fountzila A, et al. Paclitaxel by 3-h infusion and carboplatin

in anthracycline-resistant advanced breast cancer: a phase II study conducted by the Hellenic Cooperative Oncology Group. *Eur J Cancer* 1997;33:1893–1895.

63. Castiglione M, Schatzmann E, Goldhirsch A, et al. Adriamycin (A) versus epirubicin (E): low-dose weekly schedule in metastatic breast cancer: preliminary results of tumor response and of quality-of-life measurements. *Proc Am Soc Clin Oncol* 1990;9:48(abst 182).

64. Gasparini G, Dal Fior S, Panizzoni GA, et al. Weekly epirubicin versus doxorubicin as second line therapy in advanced breast cancer. a randomized clinical trial. *Am J Clin Oncol* 1991;14:38–44.

65. Lawton PA, Spittle MF, Ostrowski MJ, et al. A comparison of doxorubicin, epirubicin and mitoxantrone as single agents in advanced breast carcinoma. *Clin Oncol* 1993;5:80–84.

66. French Epirubicin Study Group. A prospective randomized phase III trial comparing combination chemotherapy with cyclophosphamide, fluorouracil, and either doxorubicin or epirubicin. *J Clin Oncol* 1988;6:679–688.

67. Italian Multicentre Breast Study with Epirubicin. Phase III randomized study of fluorouracil, epirubicin, and cyclophosphamide v fluorouracil, doxorubicin, and cyclophosphamide in advanced breast cancer: an Italian multicentre trial. *J Clin Oncol* 1988;6:976–982.

68. Lopez M, Papalso P, Di Lauro L, et al. 5-Fluorouracil, adriamycin, cyclophosphamide (FAC) vs. 5-fluorouracil, epirubicin, cyclophosphamide (FEC) in metastatic breast cancer. *Oncology* 1989;46: 1–5.

69. Lúck H-J, Thomssen C, duBois A, et al. Interim analysis of a phase II study of epirubicin and paclitaxel as first-line therapy in patients with metastatic breast cancer. *Semin Oncol* 1996;23(Suppl 1):33–36.

70. Carmichael J, Jones A, Hutchinson T. A phase II trial of epirubicin plus paclitaxel in metastatic breast cancer. *Semin Oncol* 1997;24(Suppl 17):S17-444–S17-447.

71. Ventriglia M, Cazap E, Esteva E, et al. Paclitaxel (P) Taxol plus epirubicin (E) as first-line therapy in patients (pts) with advanced breast cancer (ABC): a preliminary analysis. *Eur J Cancer* 1998; 33(Suppl 8):S157(abst 698).

72. Astone A, Ferro A, Fedele P, et al. Two-day epirubicin (E) plus paclitaxel (P) as first-line chemotherapy for stage IIIB-IV breast cancer (BC). *Proc Am Soc Clin Oncol* 1999;18:120a(abst 454).

73. Ries F, Duhem C, Kleiber K, et al. Phase I/II clinical trial of epirubicin and paclitaxel followed by granulocyte colony-stimulating factor in a 2-week schedule in patients with advanced or metastatic breast cancer. *Semin Oncol* 1997;24(Suppl 17):S17-48–S17-51.

74. Panagos G, Mavroudis D, Potamianou A, et al. Phase I study of docetaxel and epirubicin in advanced breast cancer. *Ann Oncol* 1998;9(Suppl 4):21(abst 97P).

75. Venturini M, Michelotti A, Papaldo P, et al. First line epirubicin (Epi) and taxotere (TXT) in advanced breast cancer: A phase I study. *Proc Am Soc Clin Oncol* 1998;17:179a(abst 690).

76. Raab G, Borquez D, Harstrick A, et al. Phase I study of docetaxel (D) in combination with epirubicin (E) as first line chemotherapy (CT) in metastatic breast cancer. *Proc Am Soc Clin Oncol* 1998;17: 168a(abst 644).

77. Kebrat P, Viens P, Roche H, et al. docetaxel (D) in combination with epirubicin (E) as 1st line chemotherapy (CT) of metastatic breast cancer (MBC): final results. *Proc Am Soc Clin Oncol* 1998; 17:151a(abst 579).

78. Pagani O. Taxoids in combination with epirubicin: the search for improved outcomes in breast cancer. *Semin Oncol* 1998;25(Suppl 12):23–26.

79. Blum JL, Jones SE, Buzdar AU, et al. Multicenter phase II study of capecitabine in paclitaxel in women with metastatic breast cancer. In press, *J Clin Oncol* 2001.

80. Blum JL, Jones SE, Buzdar AU, et al. Multicenter phase II study of capecitabine in paclitaxel-refractory metastatic breast cancer. *J Clin Oncol* 1999;17:485–493.

81. Bunnell CA, Winer EP. Oral 5-FU analogues in the treatment of breast cancer. *Oncology* 1998; 12(Suppl 7):39–43.

82. Carmichael J, Possinger K, Phillip P, et al. Advanced breast cancer: a phase II trial with gemcitabine. *J Clin Oncol* 1995;13:2731–2736.

83. Clemons M, Leahy M, Valle J, et al. Review of recent trials of chemotherapy for advanced breast cancer: studies excluding taxanes. *Eur J Cancer* 1997;33:2171–2182.

84. Perez EA. Her-2 as a prognostic, predictive, and therapeutic target in breast cancer. *Cancer Control* 1998;6:233–240.

85. Slamon DJ, Clark GM, Wong SG, et al. Human breast cancer: correlation of relapse and survival with amplification of the HER-2/neu oncogene. *Science* 1987;235:177–182.

86. Vogel CL, Cobleigh MA, Tripathy D, et al. Efficacy and safety of Herceptin (trastuzumab, humanized

anti-HER2 antibody) as a single agent in first-line treatment of HER2 overexpressing metastatic breast cancer (HER2 + /MBC). *Br J Cancer Treat* 1998;50:232(abst 23).

87. DAKO HerceptTest Product Information. DAKO HerceptTest information center. Available at: http://www.dakousa.com. Accessed March 30, 1999.

88. Cobleigh MA, Vogel CL, Tripathy D, et al. Multinational study of the efficacy and safety of humanized anti-HER2 monoclonal antibody in women who have HER2-overexpressing metastatic breast cancer that has progressed after chemotherapy for metastatic disease. *J Clin Oncol* 1999;17: 2639–2648.

89. Baselga J, Tripathy D, Mendelsohn J, et al. Phase II study of weekly intravenous recombinant humanized anti-p185HER2 monoclonal antibody in patients with HER2/neu-overexpressing metastatic breast cancer. *J Clin Oncol* 1996;14:737–744.

90. Pegram M. Phase II study of receptor-enhanced chemosensivity using recombinant humanized anti-p185-Her2/neu monoclonal antibody plus cisplatin in patients with Her2/neu-overexpressing metastatic breast cancer refractory to chemotherapy treatment. *J Clin Oncol* 1998;16:2659–2671.

91. Ostrow S, Egorin M, Aisner J, et al. High-dose cis-diamminedichloro-platinum therapy in patients with advanced breast cancer: pharmacokinetics, toxicity, and therapeutic efficacy. *Cancer Clin Trials* 1980;3:23–27.

92. Slamon DJ, Leyland-Jones B, Shak S, et al. Use of chemotherapy plus a monoclonal antibody against HER2 for metastatic breast cancer that overexpresses HER2. *N Engl Med* 2001;783–792.

93. Seidman AD, Fornier MN, Esteva FJ, et al. Weekly trastuzumab and paclitaxel therapy for metastatic breast cancer with analysis of efficacy by HER2 immunophenotype and gene amplification. *J Clin Oncol* 2001;19(10):2587–2595.

94. Burnstein HJ, Kuter I, Campos SM, et al. Clinical activity of trastuzumab and vinorelbine in women with HER2-overexpressing metastatic breast cancer. *J Clin Oncol* 2001;19(10)2722–2730.

95. American Society of Clinical Oncology. The role of high-dose chemotherapy and bone marrow transplant or peripheral stem-cell support in the treatment of breast cancer, background and preliminary results of five studies presented at ASCO's Annual Meeting May 15–18, 1999, in Atlanta, GA. Vol 1999. Available at: htt://www.asco.org/prof/me/html/m.plenabsum.htm edition, ASCO.

96. Stadtmauer EA, O'Neill A, Goldstein LJ, et al. Phase III randomized trial of high-dose chemotherapy (HDC) and stem cell support (SCT) shows no difference in overall survival or severe toxicity compared to maintenance chemotherapy with cyclophosphamide, methotrexate and 5-fluorouracil (CMF) for women with metastatic breast cancer who are responding to conventional induction chemotherapy: The 'Philadelphia' Intergroup Study (PBT-1) *Proc Am Clin Oncol* 1999;18:1a(abst 1).

18

Hormone Replacement Therapy in Patients with a Prior Breast Cancer History: A Critical Review

Joseph Ragaz

INTRODUCTION

The aim of this chapter is to establish the overall risk benefit of hormone replacement therapy (HRT) and to review the overall impact of HRT on all conditions with sufficiently reliable data on causation and mortality. Such information may permit recommendations about the applicability of HRT strategies regarding the management of menopause in breast cancer survivors.

This review accepts level I evidence for quality-of-life improvement of HRT as generated in prior studies that have confirmed a substantial improvement of most menopausal symptoms (1,2) and will focus on the HRT impact on breast cancer incidence and mortality. Discussed will be the emerging data suggesting that although the *incidence* of breast cancer may be moderately increased, the breast cancer *mortality* may not be altered substantially. Several large epidemiologic studies have shown that breast cancer mortality actually may decreased in short-term HRT users compared with nonusers and that breast cancer cases in HRT users are less advanced at diagnosis, with features of lower biological aggressiveness. If breast cancer mortality indeed is unaltered or actually reduced, then controlled trials of HRT to prove these observations are also urgently required in breast cancer survivors. This is particularly important because their numbers are rising, as seen from the new data on reduced breast cancer mortality in the Western world (3).

Reviewed also will be the HRT impact on uterine and colon cancers, as well as on nononcologic health issues, including cardiovascular mortality, thromboembolism, and osteoporosis. Published data, as well as conceptual proposals, are discussed and are required not only for a definitive conclusion of these issues but also to reassess the complexity of HRT association with breast cancer and to emphasize the need to stage more studies of HRT in breast cancer survivors.

BACKGROUND

Despite the increasing breast cancer *incidence* in developed countries, the breast cancer *mortality* is reducing sharply (3), in part because of the detection of a substantially higher proportion of low-stage invasive cancers and carcinomas *in situ* compared with decades ago and in part because of more uniform application of adjuvant therapies. The diagnostic "downstaging" is due mostly to breast cancer awareness and a greater availability of screening programs and education worldwide. The increasing implementation of adjuvant systemic and locoregional treatment policies is also of great importance because mortality reductions of 20% to 30% have been reported consistently for adjuvant cytotoxic chemotherapy (4), tamoxifen (5), and more recently also for the addition of locoregional radiotherapy (6,7).

Increased use of adjuvant chemotherapy in a large proportion of women over the age of 40 leads to premature disruption of ovarian functions and to the onset of postmenopausal symptoms. These symptoms often are exacerbated substantially by adjuvant tamoxifen, which is given with increasing frequency to most subsets of medium- and high-risk breast cancer patients of any age. As a result, large numbers of breast cancer survivors are presently alive and considered cured but suffering therapy-induced or therapy-exacerbated menopausal symptoms; yet they are not allowed palliation with HRT. Present estimates are that worldwide, their numbers may reach several millions at any given time, and their numbers are consistently on the rise.

MENOPAUSE: DEFINITION OF THE PROBLEM

Hot flashes are a reflection of the poorly understood mechanisms leading to vasomotor instability and are seen, in various degrees, in a large proportion of women in the Western world. Premature menopause after chemotherapy or oophorectomy develops more rapidly and precipitates vasomotor instability more suddenly and with more intensity. Whereas individual patient heterogeneity is seen, adjuvant chemotherapy for breast cancer induces menopause in direct relation to the age of the patient and to the selection of agents and their dose intensity. The traditional CMF [cyclophosphamide, methotrexate, and 5-fluorouracil (5-FU)] regimen, considered of medium intensity by present standards, led to amenorrhea in more than 50% women under the age of 40 years when given for 12 months as practiced originally. In women older than 40 years, however, more than 80% became postmenopausal. The anthracycline-containing regimens of AC [Adriamycin (doxorubicin) and cyclophosphamide] or FAC (5-FU, Adriamycin, and cyclophosphamide) are less commonly accompanied by menopause, with approximately 20% in the age group younger than 40 years but up to 75% in women over the age of 40 (8,9).

More recent evidence shows that intensification of adjuvant regimens with higher doses of epirubicin (10) or added taxanes (11) improves the disease-free or overall survival rates compared with the conventional CMF or AC combinations. In parallel, an increased proportion of patients becoming postmenopausal also would be expected. Their number is compounded by the tamoxifen-associated menopause symptoms because tamoxifen increases the intensity of hot flashes, vaginal dryness, mood changes, depression, insomnia, mood changes, and such symptoms in similar magnitude as the naturally occurring menopause.

HORMONE REPLACEMENT THERAPY AND BREAST CANCER

Epidemiologic Studies

The Collaborative Group on Hormonal Factors in Breast Cancer collected and reanalyzed individual data on more than 50,000 breast cancer cases and more than 100,000 healthy women as seen from 51 different epidemiologic studies (12). It, thus, represents the most comprehensive overview of HRT ever published. Of the women analyzed, 33% had used HRT at some time. The main findings of this meta-analysis were that, for current or recent HRT users compared with nonusers, the relative risk (RR) for breast cancer incidence was increased, with RR of 1.023 per year. This translates into a 2.3% increase of annual incidence of breast cancer. The overall risk increased with the duration of HRT use, so that in users of over 15 years, the RR for the incidence of 1.3 was observed. When the time of use is analyzed, the overview shows that current users of longer than 5 years of HRT had their breast cancer risk increased, with RR of 1.2 (i.e., 20% risk increase), whereas after 1 to 4 years of HRT cessation, the RR increase was much less significant, at 1.1 (i.e., 10% increase). After 5 to 9 years of HRT, the RR was the same as in women who never used HRT (RR = 1.01).

In summary, these investigators stated that the risk of having breast cancer diagnosed was increased in women using HRT, proportionate to the duration of use. This effect was reduced after cessation of HRT and largely disappeared after about 5 years.

Two points are worth emphasizing. First, although a moderate risk increase has been observed, it should be assessed in relation to other epidemiologic observations of risk increase. For instance, much higher increases of breast cancer incidence with ranges of 40% to 60% (RR = 1.4–1.6) have been reported as resulting from moderate alcohol consumption (13), the absence of exercise (14,15), nulliparity or high caloric intake (16).

Second, in human carcinogenesis, more lead time, perhaps 5 to 20 years, is required typically between the onset of carcinogenic insult and mutational DNA changes resulting in transformation and tumor formation. Such were the results from observational studies linking radiation with human leukemia (17); asbestos exposure and mesothelioma (18); smoking and lung cancer (19); hepatitis B antigenemia and hepatoma (20), and others.

The finding in this large epidemiologic overview (21) of a breast cancer incidence increase only in current HRT users shifts the emphasis to tumor *promotion* rather than carcinogenesis. This mechanism would implicate the HRT effect, primarily on the preformed malignant lesions, with resulting increased cell division of hormone sensitive clones, and subsequently formation of microcalcifications and earlier diagnosis through mammogram or physical examination. In those women, however, the carcinogenic events presumably had occurred earlier and most likely had no connection with HRT. Thus, the *promotional* effect of HRT is to be distinguished from causative role.

These data also indicate a possibility that, in the absence of HRT, the same tumor could develop later in time, but would present with a biologically more aggressive disease and at a more advanced stage clinically. The data from the old literature described in either bacteria (22) or in cancer clones (23) indicate that in time, as a result of random ongoing mutations during cellular divisions in either bacteria or malignant tumor clones, there will be an exponential increase of mutants with aggressive, therapy-resistant phenotypes. Thus, tumors diagnosed later in their history would be more aggressive and less sensitive to hormonal, chemotherapy, or radiation treatments (23). On the other hand, tumors exposed to HRT during the subclinical stage could be actually diagnosed earlier and, because of preferential stimulation of non-aggressive clones, could be less advanced biologically. Is there any evidence for these observations in breast cancer in relation to HRT?

Interaction of HRT and Breast Tumor Biology

Several recent studies confirmed lower tumor aggressiveness in HRT users (24–31), which may explain the observation in other trials of reduced breast cancer mortality in HRT users compared with nonusers (25–27,29). Magnusson et al. (32) reported in HRT users a reduced proportion of tumors larger than 2 cm (RR = 0.7) and a lower frequency of node positivity (RR = 0.7). The most significant risk reduction of aggressive tumors in HRT users was seen in patients taking estrogen–progestin combinations. HRT cases had also a lower proportion of poorly differentiated tumors and aneuploidy, characteristics all associated with adverse effects on breast cancer survival. Adjustment for lead bias or earlier detection did not alter the significance of these risk estimates (32).

In the study by Holli et al. (28), tumors in HRT users were also smaller ($p = 0.005$), had better histologic differentiation ($p = 0.04$), and had a lower proliferation fraction as measured by S-phase ($p = 0.009$). The significance of these observations persisted after adjustment, by multiple logistic regression, for age and mammography screening. The proportion of estrogen or progesterone receptor content, as well as overexpression of *erbB-2* oncogene, were not significantly different between HRT users and nonusers. Their data suggest that whereas HRT may not influence the genetic events of the primary carcinogenesis, HRT may favorably modulate the phenotype and growth characteristics of already established subclinical tumors (28).

Similar findings were documented by Gapstur et al. (31) among the 37,105 women participating in the Iowa Women's Health Study. In the 1,520 breast cancer cases, HRT use was associated with increased RR of tumors with favorable histology, permitting projection for a better outcome.

In the study of Cobleigh et al., compared to nonusers, HRT users had a significantly increased proportion of S-phase in estrogen receptor (ER)-positive tumors (RR = 5.25, $p = 0.04$) but not in ER-negative tumors (33). This is suggestive of HRT accelerating the growth fraction of subclinical ER-positive malignant clones. Typically, cancers with high S-phase not developing under the influence of HRT are associated with higher stage at diagnosis, worse differentiation, ER negativity, higher DNA index, and a more aggressive phenotype. In those tumors, the high

S-phase, measured as a high DNA or thymidine labeling index, reflects a more aggressive outcome, probably a consequence of a more aggressive genome (34). In HRT users, however, the converse is true: As seen in the study of Cobleigh et al., high S-phase was associated with higher proportion of ER-positive status reflecting better differentiation and more favorable tumor biology.

Fowble et al. (30) reported on 485 postmenopausal breast cancer patients diagnosed between 1979 and 1993, with median follow-up of 69 months. Of those, 141 had used HRT prior to the diagnosis, with a median use of 5 years. The HRT users had a significantly lower tumor stage, tumors measuring less than 2 cm seen in 77% of users versus 66% of nonusers ($p = 0.02$). There was a significant reduction of systemic metastases in users compared with nonusers, with 6% versus 17% suffering a distant relapse (p = 0.01). Of importance also is that no difference was observed in the rate of contralateral disease (6% in users versus 9% in nonusers, $p = 0.38$). This study therefore associated HRT use with smaller tumors and with a reduction of distant spread, a well-established surrogate of breast cancer mortality.

Further evidence for these concepts is provided by additional subanalyses of the collaborative reanalysis overview by the *Lancet* (12). In HRT users compared with nonusers, a substantial reduction of node-positive breast cancers tumors was reported (RR = 0.82), as were the number and proportion of tumors which were "metastatic beyond breast and lymph nodes" (i.e., stage III and IV). These advanced stages were substantially decreased in HRT users compared with nonusers (RR = 0.54).

Association of HRT with Reduced Breast Cancer Mortality

The above data provide more confirmatory data of HRT users presenting with biologically more favorable tumor subtypes, which are less advanced at diagnosis, findings that could explain the observation of HRT users having a *lower breast cancer mortality* compared with nonusers. Several studies confirm these findings. Grodstein et al. reported in the recent update of the Nurses' Health Study (26) a significant reduction of breast cancer mortality (adjusted RR = 0.76) in women taking HRT for less than 10 years, despite the moderately increased incidence rates (RR = 1.09–1.4). This is an important study because it shows that, despite the moderately increased breast cancer incidence rates in users, the actual chance of dying from breast cancer is lower than in nonusers. For users of >10 years, the survival protection of HRT disappeared. Thus, the protective effect of HRT on breast cancer mortality is restricted to the duration use of less than 10 years. In addition, the HRT users in this study had a significant reduction of all-cause mortality (adjusted RR = 0.63), with a similar survival improvement in cases with a strong family history of breast cancer (RR = 0.65) as in cases who had HRT after oophorectomy (RR = 0.71).

Jernstrom et al. analyzed 984 patients from southern Sweden who were treated between 1978 and 1997 (27). After adjustment for age at diagnosis, TNM (tumor, node, metastasis) stage, and year of diagnosis, the magnitude of HRT ever being used prior to the diagnosis was associated with a significantly improved overall survival [RR = 0.73, 95% confidence interval (CI) = 0.62–0.87, p = 0.0005). Of importance is that a similar mortality reduction in HRT users was seen in patients aged 45 to 60 years in whom breast cancer death is the main cause of mortality (27). Both mammography and HRT were independent prognostic factors, indicating that the HRT protective effect extended beyond the screening.

Other studies confirm these observations. Willis et al. reported a significant reduction of breast cancer mortality in HRT users (RR = 0.84) in a large cohort of 420,000 U.S. women (25). Schairer et al. (29) reported on 2,614 breast cancer patients participating in the Breast Cancer Detection Demonstration Project, a 5-year screening mammography program coordinated by the U.S. National Cancer Institute and the American Cancer Society between 1973 and 1981 and updated through regular interviews until 1995. The breast cancer mortality among HRT users was significantly reduced (RR = 0.5; 95% CI = 0.3–0.8). The mortality reduction was observed for 144 months among patients with node-negative disease and for 48 months for cases with node-positive disease. The mortality reduction in node-negative cases was restricted to current users only, but in the node-positive group, both the current and past users had improved survival (29).

Of great relevance is that the reduced breast cancer mortality observed over the last several years (3) is seen despite a sharp increase of HRT use in the Western world during the same period. This would suggest that HRT does not adversely affect breast cancer mortality unless evidence can be brought forward to indicate that the observed population mortality reduction due to the screening policies or adjuvant therapies would be even more substantial in the absence of HRT use. On the contrary, most HRT studies that examined breast cancer mortality in parallel with the incidence actually showed trends toward breast cancer mortality *reduction* in HRT users, providing a strong argument against this hypothetical possibility.

Impact on Mortality: Summary

Most of the preceding studies confirmed the association of favorable histology of tumors developing under HRT and reduced breast cancer mortality rates in HRT users even when controlling for age and screening mammography. These data indicate that although the screening effect in users may play a protective role, it will not provide the main explanation for the degree of mortality reduction reported. Although these observations have not yet been explained in full, and although none of the results have been obtained from randomized trials, the data as reviewed are nevertheless compatible with a modifying effect of hormones acting on early stages of promotion leading to lower aggressiveness and improved survival. These observations, although preliminary, constitute one of the most important aspects of the recent developments in breast cancer research.

ASSOCIATION OF ENDOGENOUS HORMONES AND BREAST CANCER

Most policies of *not* recommending HRT in breast cancer patients are based on the evidence linking the association of estrogens or progestins with breast cancer carcinogenesis observed *in vitro* or in animal experiments. Most of these studies have quite uniformly established the association of estrogens and progestins with higher breast cancer incidence and have determined that these hormones are, in animals, confirmed carcinogens. These conclusions have been further compounded by epidemiologic studies linking the increased breast cancer incidence with hormonal milestones such as menarche and menopause (35–37). Let us review the impact of endogenous hormones.

The 1998 hormonal meta-analysis showed a linear RR increase with the duration of menopause and a substantial reduction of RR in women with early menopause or surgical prophylactic oophorectomy (12). Thus, in age category 40 to 44 years, compared with menstruating women, those with premature menopause had a 38% risk reduction of breast cancer incidence (RR = 0.62). Compared with premenopausal women in age category 50 to 54 years, postmenopausal women of the same age had a 19% reduced breast cancer risk. Thus, the longer the duration of the menopausal state, the higher the risk of breast cancer. Similar data result for oophorectomy. Women with oophorectomy younger than 35 years of age had a 52% reduction in incidence (RR = 0.48) compared with women of the same age without oophorectomy; if oophorectomy was done later, at ages 45 to 50, then a risk reduction was still seen, but the reduction magnitude was substantially lower than in younger cohorts (RR = 0.72). The reduced risk is comparable in women with early menopause, either spontaneous or induced by early oophorectomy. The impact of early menopause provides a significantly protective effect even 10 to 15 or more than 15 years after the menopause (18) (RR = 0.59).

These data provide strong evidence that alteration of the *endogenous* hormonal milieu through earlier menopause provides a reduction of the risk and that the protective effect is *unaltered* in time and may persist for several decades. Given only a moderate short-term association of HRT with breast cancer incidence, but less with mortality (38), the data indicate that whereas a long-term reduction of endogenous hormones is highly protective, adding exogenous hormones may be less harmful.

The data linking endogenous estrogens to breast cancer are, however, more complex. The simple association of estrogen and breast cancer incidence in women may be weakened by the fact that during the life of a premenopausal woman, ovarian production of estrogens is high for several decades, and yet breast cancer incidence is significantly lower in women younger than 50 years of age. Also, pregnancy, which triples or quadruples estrogen levels is associated with a protective effect, with reduced breast cancer incidence compared with nulliparous women (16). These data provide some evidence against estrogen alone being carcinogenic. The more likely association of hormones and breast carcinogenesis could involve the interaction of multiple menopause-associated events, which actually may link carcinogenesis with a gradual reduction of physiologic estrogen levels but are followed by compensatory hormonal alterations in response to failing ovaries.

Specifically, as a result of all menopause-associated changes, a qualitatively different hormonal milieu may ensue, an environment that may become more carcinogenic than the hormonal environment of physiologically functional ovaries. Of importance in this regard is the possibility of emergence of altered hormones, the menopause-related carcinogenic estrogens (MRCEs), produced by the dysfunctional ovary at the time of menopause, during the irregular anovulatory cycles. These could not only profoundly alter the delicate balance between the physiologically produced estrogens, progestins, and their growth factors, but they could be also more directly implicated in the mechanism of breast cancer transformation. The existence of MRCEs and their proportionate increase during the perimenopausal period would support the observations linking the increased menopause duration with the higher breast cancer incidence (16). The positive correlation of late menopause with higher breast cancer incidence, however, may not be due to prolonged exposure to physiologic estrogens or progestins but probably to prolonged exposure to the more carcinogenic MRCEs in the perimenopausal state, which may be produced in higher quantity and for longer times in women with late menopause.

HORMONES AND GROWTH FACTORS: LINK WITH HRT

The interaction of estrogens with the growth of human cancer cells has been studied extensively *in vitro* and in animal experiments. In low doses, estrogen stimulates the MCF-7 human breast cancer cells, but with increasing doses, suppression was seen (39). In cell cultures and most animal models, estrogens and progestins are well-known promoters of chemical carcinogenesis (40). Although animal experiments and tissue cultures provide excellent models for hormonal actions and for hypothesis formation, the conclusions are not easily extrapolated to humans. Each clone of cultured cells, as well as most animal species, have unique properties and responses to hormones, with cells usually substantially more sensitive and responses more homogeneous than human tumors. The cellular genome of animals and most *in vitro* cultures are more prone to undergo mutational changes in response to hormones. Thus, in experimental tumors, the hormone effect is followed more uniformly with a documented transformation and the stimulation of cell division. With humans, the correlation of hormonal activity and breast epithelial cancer is certainly less straightforward. More recent evidence implicates in human carcinogenesis a complex interaction of hormones with secondary growth factors, either stimulatory or inhibitory (41–46).

These phenomena are made even more complex in humans by the metabolism and excretion of hormones and their growth factors, differing greatly not only among different species but also within humans among different individuals. The best examples of these complicating factors in human breast carcinogenesis include interaction of hormones with diet (47,48); alcohol consumption (13,49); smoking (50); or physical activity (14,15,51). Also, hormonal dose–response regarding carcinogenesis in humans is certainly more complex than in animals.

In the later stages of carcinogenesis associated with endogenous hormones, a disruption of stromal architecture is seen, with increased tumor cellular aggressiveness, invasiveness of collagen and vessel wall, increased cellular motility, and increased locoregional angiogenesis. Also, increased aggressivity of tumor cells may enhance the tumor clones' ability to survive in the distant organs and influence their response to hormonal, chemotherapy and radiation treatments. On the other hand, the modulating and differentiating effect of *exogenous* hormones may differentially affect tumor clones, endowing some with lesser aggressiveness and lower propensity to penetrate the angiogenic milieu and to undergo more easily a spontaneous or treatment-induced apoptosis. The epidemiologic observations of increased incidence (a reflection of increased growth rate) but reduced mortality (a reduction of tumor cell aggressiveness) could be explained by these mechanisms. Thus, the direct correlation between the hormonal effects seen in the animal experiments and human breast cancer cannot be made.

NONONCOLOGIC ASPECTS OF HRT

Cardiac Events

Most population-based studies examining HRT in the primary prevention of cardiac events have shown a strong risk reduction in users (RR: 0.4–0.8), representing a 20% to 60% mortality reduction (52–58). The magnitude of the HRT effect is similar among case–control or cross-sectional studies (59). Several hypotheses have been offered to explain these observations, the most plausible of which are the favorable estrogen effects on lipid metabolism (60–65) and on endothelial function (66–71), the two important factors in the pathogenesis of atherosclerogenesis. The contribution of a bias due to the selection of healthier women for HRT, who would also undergo cardiac screening more effectively (55), cannot be excluded entirely because none of these studies was randomized. Whereas these biases may exist, they do not fully account for the strong association of HRT with improved lipid profile and physiology of vessels, both surrogates for abnormal coronary artery pathology, linked in the cardiovascular literature with the improved cardiac morbidity and mortality outcomes (52,58,60,72).

Secondary prevention is more problematic. HRT may be less effective when atherosclerotic plaques have already developed. The first ever HRT randomized trial of secondary prevention [Heart and Estrogen/Progestin Replacement Study (HERS)] has been recently completed, and the results at least for the first few years of follow-up have been negative (73). The implication of those results will be discussed below.

Estrogens and Lipids

Several longitudinal studies of postmenopausal women have shown a strong effect of estrogen on lipid metabolism (74), with a reduction of the low-density lipoprotein cholesterol (LDL) and increasing the high-density lipoprotein cholesterol (HDL). Because the HDL:LDL ratio is one of the best predictors of future cardiovascular outcome (75), it is plausible that this particular effect best explains the mechanism of estrogen action in the primary prevention of cardiac events (60,76,77).

Other mechanisms indicate favorable estrogen effects. Studies have confirmed that serum LDL uptake by coronary arteries is reduced in monkeys fed atherogenic diets and randomized to estrogens (63,78). Also, estrogens are known to modulate the prostacyclin-mediated vasodilating effect (79) and also to interact with calcium channel blockers (71) and lipoprotein(a) (74,80–83). Furthermore, estrogen therapy significantly increased catabolism of LDL (84), and estrogens lowered adhesion molecules such as E-selectin, intercellular and vascular cell adhesion molecule-1 (VCAM-1), yet another mechanism known to reduce atherosclerogenesis (85).

The most convincing evidence for HRT effects on lipid metabolism comes from the recently concluded trial of Postmenopausal Estrogen/Progestin Interventions, or the PEPI trial (21). This was a multicenter randomized, double-blind, placebo-controlled trial of 875 postmenopausal women aged 45 to 64, with no known contra-indication to hormonal therapy. Women were randomly assigned to one of the following: estrogen [conjugated equine estrogen (CEE), 0.625 mg daily]; estrogen plus progesterone [medroxyprogesterone acetate (MPA)], given for 12 days of each 28 days; or estrogen plus a new progestin, the micronized progesterone (MP) 200 mg daily for 12 days. At 3 years' follow-up, CEE estrogen alone or in combination with MP was most effective in increasing HDL over placebo: HDL levels were increased by 5.6 and. 4.1 mg/dL compared with pretreatment levels. By comparison, an HDL increase of 1.2 mg/dL was seen in the CEE + MPA arm and an HDL decrease of 1.2 mg/dL with placebo.

These data confirm that CEE alone, or CEE with MP, is significantly more effective in raising HDL cholesterol levels than placebo. At the same time, LDL levels were decreased in the two HRT arms. In terms of HRT side effects, compared with the placebo or the estrogen plus progestin combination, the unopposed estrogen led to an increased risk of endometrial hyperplasia, and the rate of hysterectomy due to adenomas or hyperplasia was also increased compared to the placebo group, at 6% versus 1%, respectively.

In summary, the PEPI trial is the first placebo-controlled, randomized study to document that estrogen alone, or in combination with progestin, substantially improves the serum lipid profile, confirming after decades of reports from nonrandomized studies that HRT reduced the principal cardiovascular lipid risk factors. The study also suggests that the effect of lipids may be comparable between estrogen alone and the combination of estrogen and progestin, particularly with the newly available micronized progestin, the MP. The significance of these data for prevention of cardiac mortality is yet to be determined, and the *long-term* follow-up of the ongoing randomized trial of the 63,000 women participating in the Women's Health Initiative Trial (86) will provide the more definitive answers to this issue. In the absence of long-term follow-up data from this and other randomized trials, the PEPI trial remains an important positive study of HRT on surrogate markers of cardiac mortality. The PEPI trial is particularly important in view of other studies that have shown that even a modest incremental HDL increase of 4 to 5 mg/dL was associated with a further 20% to 25% reduction of coronary heart disease. These findings are in line with the long-term follow up of the observational HRT studies.

Estrogen Effect on Vessel Wall

The other type of evidence suggestive of a protective estrogenic effect on coronary arteries involves studies of direct effects of HRT on vessel walls. ERs are present in the muscularis of the arteries, and improved blood flow through the coronaries due to estrogen exposure is ER mediated (67,87). In support of these observations, estrogen protected vessels in ovariectomized female monkeys from vasoconstriction after exposure to acetylcholine (88). The same observations were subsequently made in postmenopausal women (57,70). Estrogen prevented coronary artery constriction induced by acetylcholine in 20 postmenopausal women, with a documentation of increased arterial blood flow and reduced coronary arterial resistance. In several animal species, estrogen exposure led to a reduction of systemic vascular resistance (59,67,88). In humans, estrogen also reduced arterial impedance and vascular tone after 6 weeks of treatment (68).

Other workers confirmed increased hyperemic response and vasodilatation as a reaction to estrogen (89). Pines et al. found improved flow velocity and improvement of the mean ejection fraction in estrogen users, as measured by aortic sonograms (90). Lastly, estrogen was found, in a placebo-controlled trial (90), to improve performance of women on a treadmill and to decrease symptoms of coronary artery disease (64), effects that may well be explained by the above-outlined estrogen mechanism on vessels.

Epidemiologic Data on Estrogen and Heart Disease: Primary Prevention

Almost all population-based and cross sectional studies show a protective association between HRT and coronary heart disease, with RR rates ranges of 0.4 to 0.8 59. Because none of these studies were prospectively, randomized placebo-controlled trials, it was proposed that the selection of patients, rather than the estrogen therapy, might have determined the outcome (91). It was suggested that hormone users live a healthier lifestyle, have a more favorable cardiovascular risk profile, have more frequent screening tests for risk factors such as cholesterol levels, and have more mammograms. It was argued that women who choose to use estrogen are from higher socioeconomic groups, are less obese, and exercise and see their physicians more regularly. It also has been shown, however, in most of those studies, that users and nonusers did not differ significantly and that patient heterogeneity could explain only a small portion of the cardiovascular benefit of HRT and the difference between users and nonusers. In many of these studies, the subjects were quite homogeneous, made eligible to participate either because of a common profession or life in a selected community. The best example of this is the Nurses' Health Study, in which lifestyle factors, occupation, cardiac risk factors, smoking, alcohol consumption, history of hypertension, body mass index, and other such factors were comparable (52,92). In this study, the age-adjusted RR for coronary heart disease in current estrogen users was 0.45 (95% CI, 0.31–0.66). Furthermore, after adjustment for cardiovascular risk factors such as cigarette smoking, age, hypertension, cholesterol levels, parental history of myocardial infarction, and past use of birth control pills, there was still a highly significant risk reduction in HRT users compared with nonusers (RR = 0.56). Similar findings were seen in the Lipid Research Clinics Follow-up Study (60) and in the Leisure World Study (93). In these studies, the age-adjusted RR of *all-cause* mortality was 0.80 (95% CI, 0.70–0.89), with the overall survival benefit derived mostly from the reduction in cardiac mortality. Little confounding impact was shown in a multivariate analysis when controlling for numerous other risk factors. This supports the hypothesis that the RR reduction in cardiovascular events, as well as in the mortality, is most likely due to the HRT.

Grodstein and Stampfer summarized available clinical trial data according to the types of studies (59). In the population-based case–control studies, the RR of cardiac events was 0.69 (95% CI, 0.54–0.89); for the cross-sectional studies, it was 0.38 (95% CI, 0.31 - 0.46); and for the internally controlled prospective studies, the RR was 0.55 (95% CI, 0.44-0.70). The pooled RR for all current HRT use combining all three types of studies was 0.50 (95% CI, 0.45–0.59), which is suggestive that in otherwise well women the HRT is associated, in long-term follow-up, with a protective role for primary prevention of cardiac events.

Epidemiological Data on Estrogen and Heart Disease: Secondary Prevention

Once the atherosclerogenic plaque and coronary occlusions develop to the degree of producing clinical symptoms, therapy is usually not curative. Indeed, most interventions for secondary prevention are expected to relieve symptoms and prevent progression of the disease but not to cure. Also, the full effects of reducing the cardiovascular risk factors may take decades, despite the data showing early clinical benefit of lipid intervention. Hence, it is possible that, compared with its effect in primary prevention, hormonal therapy will have lower impact once the process of atherosclerosis already has advanced.

The only randomized trial of secondary prevention, HERS, was published recently (73). A total of 2,763 women 65 years or older (mean age, 66.7 years) with a prior myocardial infarction were randomized in a double-blind, placebo-controlled design to be treated with either HRT (CEE, 0.635 mg, plus daily MPA, 2.5 mg daily) or placebo. At 4 years' follow-up, these researchers reported no significant differences in deaths from coronary heart disease or myocardial infarction between the two arms (RR = 0.99, 95% CI = 0.80–1.22). The lack of an overall effect was seen despite an 11% reduction of LDL levels and a 10% increase of HDL levels. More women in the HRT group had thromboembolic events (RR = 2.89, 95% CI = 1.50–5.58) and gallbladder disease (RR = 1.38, CI = 1.00–1.92). No difference was found in cancer rates or overall mortality. For the latter two parameters, however, the power of the study was greatly limited. The investigators' conclusion was that HRT does not reduce the overall rate of coronary heart disease in postmenopausal women with established coronary disease and that the risk of thromboembolism and of gallstones is increased.

Examining the interaction of RR with time, interesting trends were observed. In the first year of the study, more cardiac events were seen in the users (RR = 1.52). In the second year, however, that increase was not seen any longer, with the incidence of cardiac mortality or of the nonfatal infarctions among users versus nonusers being equal (RR = 1.0). Subsequently, in years 3 and 4, the risk of these events in HRT users was actually reduced (RR = 0.87 and 0.67, respectively), consistent with the degree of RR reduction seen in long-term follow-up observational primary prevention studies. No women treated with statins had events; all cardiac events were observed in approximately 30% of the study population not taking statins (personal communication, B. Wolfe, University of Western Ontario, Canada). Also, there was an overall survival benefit of HRT compared with controls restricted, however, to women with lipoprotein(a) above median (94).

These data indicate that in women with advanced atherosclerosis, the HRT may temporarily increase the morbidity or even mortality; however, even in this population, the long-term HRT effects show similar effects on serum lipids and mirror thus the results of the primary prevention trials. The increased event rate in the first year of the HERs study could be due to a precipitating event such as thromboembolism or minor blood pressure fluctuations, which is not uncommon in the population of patients with advanced vessel disease over the age of 65. These complications would be, however, of lesser consequence in selected younger women without advanced coronary disease, the prime population of breast cancer survivors suffering with menopausal symptoms targeted for HRT. In these women, not only substantial improvements in the quality of life but a positive effect on the lipid metabolism, and, thus, cardiac disease prevention, can be anticipated.

Thromboembolism

Estrogens are known to increase blood clotting because of their effects on several clotting factors, including fibrinogen, factor VII, factor X, and antithrombin III (95). As a result, HRT is known to increase the incidence of thromboembolism moderately with RR ranges 1.1 to 4.00 (53,73,96–99), but no increase of mortality rates has been reported (100). HERS found increased cardiac mortality in HRT cases in the first year of use, also considered to be associated with thromboembolism, an effect not detected in the second to the fourth years follow-up.

Osteoporosis

Estrogens are known to preserve bone mass and prevent bone resorption. Enhanced bone loss and resorption are known to take place with accelerated pace soon after the menopause, leading to osteoporosis and eventually to bone fractures (101–103). Prolonged immobilization and premature deaths are thus observed in large numbers of aging women.

Although the exact mechanism of estrogen action regarding bone mass protection is not known, it is evident that several mechanisms are important. These include altered osteoclast and osteoblast activity and bone protein metabolism in favor of bone mass preservation. Also, estrogens are known to enhance calcium absorption form the small intestine, with the resulting reduction of urinary calcium loss and hydroxyproline (104).

Protective effects of estrogens are evident throughout the menstrual life because very soon after menopause, a rapid loss of bone mass ensues (102,105). In untreated women, these losses could result in profound rates of osteoporosis and bone fractures, particularly affecting hip and spine. Also evident are microfractures in the pelvis, radius, distal forearm, proximal humerus, and other areas. It was estimated that a woman age 50 will have a 15% lifetime chance of sustaining a hip fracture and a 1.5% chance of dying from it unless treated aggressively from the early years of menopause (98). In absolute numbers, estimates are that about 1.5 million bone fractures occur in North America annually. In the older age group, hospitalizations for bone fracture-related complications constitute a large proportion of all hospital admissions. These will require, in thousands of women so affected, prolonged hospital or nursing care, with profound loss of quality of life. In more than 30% of cases, mortality follows fractures of the hip, often as a result of immediate postoperative complications, such as pneumonia or thromboembolism, both a consequence of prolonged immobilization. Thus, osteoporosis-related complications represent an overwhelming problem in the western world, and it has been estimated that successful therapy of osteoporosis would save tens of thousands of lives and billions of dollars annually.

Continuous use of estrogen soon after the menopause for a minimum 5 years could avoid hip fractures by half (RR = 0.5) (106). Maximum protection is seen if estrogen therapy starts within the first 5 years of menopause, with a direct correlation of protection and duration of estrogen use. Unfortunately, renewed cortical bone loss occurs soon after estrogen is discontinued, at a similar rate as before the therapy, with a fracture rate returning to the pretreatment rates several years after discontinuing estrogen therapy (98,106). Thus, continuous use of estrogen would be most effective. Nevertheless, at any age of start, even when osteoporosis is developed, estrogens do have a potential to prevent further bone loss and reverse the situation in most instances (107). Taking the benefits of hormones on hip fractures and other skeletal events (108), it is estimated that estrogen + progestin therapy in the form of HRT would reduce the bone-specific mortality by 30% to 50% (RR = 0.7) (98).

In summary, none of the therapeutic options available is as comprehensively effective as estrogen, although the full potential of HRT given in conjunction with the new generation agents such as biphosphates (109); raloxifene (110,111); or their combination is not known. As different mechanisms of action are evident, a potentiation is plausible.

UTERINE CANCER

Activation of ERs in endometrium provides a physiologic mechanism for stimulation by estrogens and tamoxifen but not by raloxifene (112). With estrogen and tamoxifen, the uterine binding to α receptors in the endometrium has been documented, leading to the endometrial stimulation. Alteration of the uterine-binding molecular domain in raloxifene results in a poorly understood alteration of the binding mechanisms, with virtually no endometrial effect (113).

Although stimulation of the uterine epithelium after estrogen exposure may increase the rate of endometrial cell division, the **carcinogenic** effect of estrogens is not necessarily equated with that stimulation. Specifically, whereas the malignant transformation of the endometrial epithelium by HRT has been documented in experimental studies, the short interval from the HRT start to the endometrial cancer diagnosis indicates that the most malignant lesions in women might have undergone carcinogenic transformation earlier. Subsequently, these preexisting malignant clones would be stimulated into activity by added estrogen or tamoxifen. Earlier diagnosis may modify the mortality rates, an effect also compounded by the evidence for enhanced differentiation of the endometrial cancers, which develop under the influence of an estrogenic milieu (98). Thus, similarly to breast cancer, HRT users' endometrial cancers may have a lower stage at diagnosis and better differentiation than in nonusers. As a result, a proportional increase of incidence over mortality is observed, with an RR of endometrial cancer incidence after estrogen alone approaching 6.0 to 8.0, whereas the mortality rates alter only a fraction of this (114–117). Thus, it was estimated that in a 50-year-old woman, the lifelong chance of getting uterine cancer is 2.6%, but the chance of dying from uterine cancer is only 0.3%. In the 1992 all-cause mortality assessment, Grady et al. estimated, as a worst case scenario, the RR of incidence was approximately 8.0, but the RR of mortality much lower, at RR $= 3.0$ (98). For the estrogen–progestin combinations, the RR for both incidences as mortality is close to 1.0 (98).

Whereas unopposed estrogen is associated with increased endometrial cancer risk, the addition of progestin modifies this risk substantially so that the RR in HRT with progestin combinations compared with nonusers is close to 1.0 (21,98,118–120).

Also, endometrial hyperplasia, a sign of estrogen stimulation, is seen in 20% to 40% of cases using estrogen alone but was not observed in women taking progestins in addition (98,118,121,122). Similarly, the incidence of endometrial adenomas, and of atypical hyperplasia, both endometrial cancer precursors, is decreased by progestins (21,122).

Taking the well-documented evidence for high cure rates of endometrial cancer if diagnosed early, it is not surprising that only a small proportion of diagnosed cases actually die from the disease.

In summary, unopposed estrogen definitely enhances the endometrial cancer risk, but the chance of dying from uterine cancer is small. Also of relevance is that most studies that provided the preceding data were conducted before the era of education and awareness of HRT association with uterine cancer, without screening and endometrial sampling as practiced nowadays. This is suggestive that, at present, the uterine cancer mortality rates in HRT users are unlikely to be increased substantially, particularly not in users of the combined estrogen–progestin combinations of less than 5 years' duration.

HORMONE REPLACEMENT THERAPY AND COLON CANCER

Several recent epidemiologic studies have shown a reduction of colorectal cancer incidence in HRT users (123–125). Most of those studies show incidence risk reduction, with RR ranges of 0.6 to 0.8.

The biochemical effects of estrogen offer an explanation for the potentially beneficial link between estrogen and colon carcinogenesis. Estrogens reduce the concentration of bile acids in the colon, with reduced synthesis and secretion into the bowel (123). There has been prior evidence from experimental studies for a correlation between colon cancer etiology and increasing concentrations of bile acids (123, 126–128).

Human studies have shown the fecal bile acid concentration to be higher in colon cancer cases than in controls (123). Other mechanisms may involve direct estrogen effects on colon mucosa. ERs have been identified both in colon cancer tissue as well as in adjacent uninvolved colon mucosal cells, with data suggesting that estrogen is acting as a negative inhibitor of promotion and possibly of carcinogenesis (129). A recent meta-analysis examining the issue of HRT and colon cancer confirmed a significant reduction of colon cancer incidence (124). Current or recent users had lower incidence rates (RR = 0.69). HRT users of 5 years or longer derived more protection than those who took the HRT for a shorter time.

Three levels of evidence suggest that estrogens may be protective. First are the biochemical observations. Second is that not only colon carcinomas but also adenomas—the precursors of invasive cancers—have been reduced. Third, although the incidence of colorectal cancer is reduced in most but not all studies, mortality reduction shows stronger trends than does incidence.

The largest of all individual studies involved women participating in the Cancer Prevention Study II, which started in 1982 by the American Cancer Society (123). More than 670,000 women were enrolled and followed up prospectively for the incidence and mortality of major cancer sites. Of all the colon cancer deaths that occurred by 1989, ever use of HRT was associated with a significant reduction of colon cancer mortality (RR = 0.71, 95% CI = 0.61–0.83). The reduction of RR was strongest among the current users (RR = 0.55, 95% CI = 0.40–0.76), and there was a significant association with increasing duration of use. Compared with nonusers, the current or ever users of HRT for more than 10 years had RR of 0.54 (95% CI = 0.39–0.76), and improved incidence rates were also found compared with users of HRT for less than 1 year (RR = 0.81, 95% CI = 0.63–1.03). None of the associations of HRT and reduction of fatal colon cancer was altered in multivariate analysis controlling for other risk factors.

The Nurses' Health Study, which was well controlled for homogeneity of profession and socioeconomic status due to restricting the study eligibility to nurses only, evaluated more than 59,000 women (125). Grodstein et al. found a significant reduction of colon cancer in current users (RR = 0.65, 95% CI 0.50–0.83), which was attenuated in past users (RR = 0.81, 95% CI 0.67–1.07). It was of great interest that, even after exclusion of patients who had regular screening sigmoidoscopy, the incidence rates still were reduced significantly in current HRT users (RR = 0.64, 95% CI 0.49–0.82), suggesting that the protective association of HRT and colon cancer is unlikely due to more intensive screening in users (125).

Strong support for a protective role of HRT and colorectal pathology comes from observational studies of adenoma polyps, the precursors to colorectal carcinomas. Peipins et al. (130) reported a reduced RR of 0.39 in HRT users. Chen et al. (131) reported a reduction of adenomas in HRT users undergoing sigmoidoscopy (RR = 0.57), with users of longer than 5 years' HRT duration benefiting most (RR = 0.49). Similarly, Potter et al. (132) reported in HRT users of more than 5 years' duration a reduced incidence of adenomas, with an RR of 0.43. Further support for a protective effect of estrogen on the incidence of adenomas is seen from the data of women with early surgical oophorectomy (130), in whom the incidence of adenomas was increased significantly (RR = 2.1).

IMPACT OF HORMONE REPLACEMENT THERAPY ON ALL-CAUSE MORTALITY

Whereas quality of life issues remain extremely important in assessing HRT impact, the mortality rates provide the more objective scale of its ultimate effect. If mortality rates are substantially affected in opposite directions for different conditions, then the quantitative expression of such effect in regard to the life gains or losses would be of great importance.

The all-cause mortality analyses are made more difficult not only by the absence of randomized trials but also by methodologic issues such as variable risk rates for a given condition, even when controlling for age or underlying risk factors. For example, women of the same age have substantially different underlying risk rates of cancers according to family or menopausal history, surface area, diet, socioeconomic status, and other cofactors (16). Also, even when controlling for risk categories, there are significantly different underlying risk rates among different age groups for most conditions impacted by hormones (133). Such issues make these analyses difficult and not easily comparable. While none of the different published methodologies for estimating overall mortality rates is ideal, they all provide some insight into the HRT overall effect.

One of the first examples of expressing all cause mortality of HRT was done by Bush et al. (134), who in 1983 estimated the HRT impact as a RR of deaths between users versus nonusers from any cause. The results obtained showed, in users, a mortality reduction of 63% (RR = 0.37). Variable rates were seen in women with hysterectomy (RR = 0.34) when compared to gynecologically intact women (RR = 0.54) or women with bilateral oophorectomy (RR = 0.12). Ettinger et al. using a similar methodology, also concluded that the HRT use was associated with a significantly reduced risk of death from any cause (RR = 0.54, CI = 0.38–0.76) (135).

Grady et al. (98) expressed the HRT impact on the basis of mortality rates in users versus nonusers, separately for endometrial and breast cancer, coronary heart disease, hip fracture, and stroke. They then used modified life table methods to estimate the effect of HRT on the probability of developing each disease and on overall life expectancy. Thus, women aged 50 at different risk for various underlying conditions typically had a benefit on overall life expectancy as a result of use of HRT, with results estimated as prolonged life ranging from several months to several years.

Ragaz and Coldman presented age-adjusted all-cause mortality impact of HRT (136) using a methodology described for all-cause mortality impact of adjuvant tamoxifen (133). In their calculations, the published HRT-associated RR rates of users were applied to the 1991 Canada population mortality rates (the nonusers) and expressed as avoided or excess deaths per 1,000 annually in users. The results were expressed for each condition; separately for age groups 50, 60, and 70 at HRT start; and estimated for follow-up duration of 10 years; and for age 90 (i.e., life-long). Results showed that for women aged 50, 60, and 70, the net avoidance of deaths per 1,000 users annually at 10-year follow up was 2.8, 11, and 36, respectively. Estimating the outcome until age 90, the numbers of avoided deaths were even more substantial.

USE OF ESTROGENS AS A TREATMENT FOR ESTABLISHED BREAST CANCER

The use of estrogen after the diagnosis of breast cancer traditionally has been discouraged, and most institutional policies disallow HRT in breast cancer patients symptomatic with menopausal symptoms. The source of these strong recommendations comes from the decades of considered links of estrogen and breast carcinogenesis observed mostly in animal studies but less clearly in humans. There are two sources of data regarding the effects of estrogen after breast cancer diagnosis. One is the poorly studied use of HRT for palliation of menopausal symptoms, the subject of this review. The other includes the old data of estrogen for therapy of established stage IV disease.

There is evidence that estrogen exerts beneficial effect on *established* breast cancer, as seen from trials of stilbestrol or other formulations of higher dose estrogen therapy for stage IV disease. Numerous studies show responses of 40% to 60% of long duration, according to the selection of patients (137–141). Although response rates in stage IV disease of tamoxifen and stilbestrol were repeatedly found to be similar, tamoxifen became the drug of choice because of its fewer side effects compared with high-dose estrogens (140,141). Of interest is the update (142) of one of the randomized trials of estrogen vs tamoxifen (139) showing improved survival in the arm of stilbestrol. The 5-year survival was 35% for the stilbestrol arm versus 16% for patients randomized in the tamoxifen arm ($p = 0.035$). Therefore, not only did estrogen fail to stimulate breast cancer progression, but it actually emerged to be more beneficial compared with tamoxifen.

These data suggest that estrogenic effect on *established* human breast cancer may be antimitogenic, an effect considered to be due to the suppressive effect of high-dose estrogen. *In vitro* cell culture studies have shown that very low estrogen doses were stimulatory in a linear fashion, but increasing the estrogen doses was accompanied by a loss the stimulating effect, with higher estrogen doses suppressing cell growth below the controls (39).

Although these studies could explain the effect of stilbestrol in stage IV disease as the doses of stilbestrol were of concentration considered suppressive, there are no data in humans to confirm these dose–response observations. The preceding *in vitro* studies have not explained the hormonal interaction with the induction of differentiation of subclinical cancers as documented in women with breast cancer developing under the milieu of HRT (24–31). Of relevance in this regard is the recent work of Yao et al. showing in MT2 breast cancer cell lines that the addition of estrogen at the time of tamoxifen resistance restored responsiveness to tamoxifen (143). These data indicate a potential of estrogen to induce cell differentiation, which is required to maintain responsiveness to tamoxifen or other hormones and thus delay hormonal autonomy and resistance. These data are also compatible with previously discussed epidemiologic results of HRT in breast and uterine cancer users, displaying in HRT users more differentiated and probably phenotypically less aggressive lesions, which are clinically less advanced at diagnosis, factors responsible for lower event mortality compared to nonusers (25–27,29).

USE OF HRT AFTER BREAST CANCER: PHASE II AND III STUDIES

As a result of these data, several phase 2 studies have been reported in breast cancer survivors (138,144–150). In follow-up ranging from 2 to 7 years, none reported an increase of breast cancer events as a result of HRT use. As a result, new phase 3 studies are slowly emerging or are in the last stage of preparation (151–153; personal communication, J. Holmberg, the HABITS trial: protocol for randomized clinical study concerning hormonal replacement therapy after previous radical breast cancer treatment, 1997; personal communication, D. Tormey, a phase 3 trial of HRT in breast cancer survivors: proposal for a multicenter trial, with all-cause mortality as a primary objective, 2000; and personal communication, J. Ragaz and K. Pritchard, proposal to the Canadian NCI, 2001.). These developments indicate, according to some investigators and patient advocates, that the time is appropriate to stage not only large HRT controlled studies in symptomatic breast cancer survivors, but also to initiate closely monitored HRT treatments in carefully selected patients (9,136). In those patients, the lowest possible dose of HRT that can be effective would be used. Particularly suited candidates for such an approach would be breast cancer patients with low-risk disease in whom a chance for long-term survival is good and who are symptomatic with severe menopause not controlled by any means. In support of such an approach, it has been indicated that although the HRT may interact with the preexisting breast cancer clones in either direction, it may **not induce new** metastases, and thus will not affect the overall survival but at worst may modify only the disease-free survival. In favor of this approach is the substantial long-term quality-of-life improvement that results from use of HRT. According to some patients, these benefits may outweigh the small hazard, as quality-life impact of HRT may permit activities such as physical conditioning, a variety of recreational activities, and more intense social and professional interaction. These are all considered of great potential not only as they alleviate the menopause symptoms, but also for their potential to increase the individual patient's intrinsic immunocompetence. The poorly researched psychosocial phenomena and physical exercise interacting with physiological neuroendocrinology and immunology mechanisms are made more complex in breast cancer survivors by immunosuppressive therapies, such as chemotherapy, radiation, or tamoxifen. Recent data indicate that increased psychosocial and professional activity actually may improve the outcome of adjuvant therapies for breast cancer (154). Also, evidence is mounting for a link between increased physical activity, considered to be enhanced in HRT users, and a reduction of breast cancer incidence (14,155,156); such information is applicable in breast cancer survivors in regard to their incidence of contralateral breast cancer.

SUMMARY

This review provides early evidence to health care providers and their patients that the HRT use in breast cancer survivors symptomatic with menopausal symptoms may not be as unsafe as considered over the last decades. On the contrary, the data reviewed indicate that in the population women taking HRT, not only the overall survival but also the breast cancer–specific survival may be improved in HRT users compared with nonusers providing the HRT use is restricted to less than 10 years. Therefore, as these data may apply also to breast cancer patients surviving their disease, the existing policies of HRT use in breast cancer survivors need serious reassessment. Some questions regarding hormonal effects in the etiology, biology, and therapy of breast cancer will need more detailed answers based on modern era genetic, epidemiologic, and clinical studies. Whereas some answers may have to come from large randomized, controlled trials of HRT in breast cancer survivors (some of which started recently or are in early stages of planning), some form of symptomatic HRT therapy may have to be considered in selected patients, even in the absence of results from those trials. In many such patients, the HRT quality life benefits may be more meaningful than the unknown risk of breast cancer, particularly because there is a distinct possibility that breast cancer mortality may be unaltered or actually improved, as evident for the population women without the breast cancer.

Overall, much larger scale of action regarding policies and studies of HRT may be required than seen at the present time. These may include steps such as allocating sufficient funding and developing expert infrastructure for controlled HRT trials, important mainly for younger patients suffering with symptoms made worse by adjuvant chemotherapy or tamoxifen or initiating regional, national, or international registries monitoring patients already taking HRT. These are particularly required because the numbers of breast cancer survivors already taking HRT are increasing without any attempts to uniformly monitor their outcome. After a careful review of the preceding data and of the risk-to-benefit assessment, the following is recommended in summary: Although it would be reasonable to offer to selected patients lowest-dose HRT, which improves symptoms, while closely monitoring all onco-logic and nononcologic events, the primary focus of institutional oncologists should be directed toward staging larger efforts than in the past to answer more definitively the position of HRT after the diagnosis of breast cancer. Ideally, the studies should be large, randomized, with implementation of early stopping rules, so that if harm resulting from HRT use or its absence is confirmed, it be halted and policies regarding the HRT use in breast cancer survivors modified swiftly. All these efforts will most likely be rewarded by a substantial improvement in quality of life of surviving breast cancer patients and very likely in saving additional lives by avoiding both oncologic and nononcologic causes of deaths.

REFERENCES

1. American College of Obstetricians and Gynecologists. *Hormone replacement therapy: statement of the American College of Obstetricians and Gynecologists.* Washington, DC: ACOG, 1992.
2. Wiklund I, Holst J, Karlberg J, et al. A new methodological approach to the evaluation of quality of life in postmenopausal women. *Maturitas* 1992;14:211–224.
3. Peto R, Boreham J, Clarke M, et al. UK and USA breast cancer deaths down 25% in year 2000 at ages 20–69 years [Letter]. *Lancet* 2000;55:1822.
4. Breast Cancer Trialists' Collaborative Group. Polychemotherapy for early breast cancer: an overview of the randomised trials: early Breast Cancer Trialists' Collaborative Group. *Lancet* 1998; 352:930–942.
5. Breast Cancer Trialists' Collaborative Group. Tamoxifen for early breast cancer: an overview of the randomised trials. Early Breast Cancer Trialists' Collaborative Group. *Lancet* 1998;351:1451–1467.
6. Overgaard M, Hansen PS, Overgaard J, et al. Postoperative radiotherapy in high-risk premenopausal women with breast cancer who receive adjuvant chemotherapy: Danish Breast Cancer Cooperative Group 82b Trial. *N Engl J Med* 1997;337:949–955.
7. Ragaz J, Jackson SM, Le N, et al. Adjuvant radiotherapy and chemotherapy in node-positive premenopausal women with breast cancer. *N Engl J Med* 1997;337:956–962.
8. Mehta RR, Beattie CW, Das Gupta TK. Endocrine profile in breast cancer patients receiving chemotherapy. *Breast Cancer Res Treat* 1992;20:125–132.
9. Cobleigh MA, Berris RF, Bush T, et al. Estrogen replacement therapy in breast cancer survivors: a time for change. Breast Cancer Committees of the Eastern Cooperative Oncology Group [published erratum appears in *JAMA* 1995;273:378]. *JAMA* 1994;272:540–545.
10. Levine MN, Bramwell VH, Pritchard KI, et al. Randomized trial of intensive cyclophosphamide, epirubicin, and fluorouracil chemotherapy compared with cyclophosphamide, methotrexate, and fluorouracil in premenopausal women with node-positive breast cancer: National Cancer Institute of Canada Clinical Trials Group. *J Clin Oncol* 1998;16:2651–2658.
11. Henderson IC, Berry D, Demetri C, et al. Improved disease free and overall survival from addition of sequential paclitaxel but not from the escalation of doxorubicin dose level in the adjuvant chemotherapy of patients with node-positive primary breast cancer. *Proc Am Soc Clin Oncol* 1999;17: 101a(abst).
12. Collaborative Group on Hormonal Factors in Breast Cancer. Breast cancer and hormone replacement therapy: collaborative reanalysis of data from 51 epidemiological studies of 52,705 women with breast cancer and 108,411 women without breast cancer [published erratum appears in *Lancet* 1997; 15;1484]. *Lancet* 1997;350:1047–1059.
13. Longnecker MP, Berlin JA, Orza MJ, et al. A meta-analysis of alcohol consumption in relation to risk of breast cancer. *JAMA* 1988;260:652–656.
14. Bernstein L, Henderson BE, Hamsch R, et al. Physical exercise and reduced risk of breast cancer in young women. *J Natl Cancer Inst* 1994;86:1403–1408.
15. Rockhill B, Willett WC, Hunter DJ, et al. A prospective study of recreational physical activity and breast cancer risk. *Arch Intern Med* 1999;159:2290–2296.

16. Henderson B, Pike M, Bernestein L, et al. *Breast Cancer* 1996:1022–1040.
17. Preston DL, Kusumi S, Tomonaga M, et al. Cancer incidence in atomic bomb survivors. Part III. Leukemia, lymphoma and multiple myeloma, 1950–1987 [published erratum appears in *Radiat Res* 1994;139:129]. *Radiat Res* 1994;137:568–597.
18. McDonald JC, McDonald AD. Epidemiology of mesothelioma from estimated incidence. *Prev Med* 1977;6:426–442.
19. Doll R, Peto R. Cigarette smoking and bronchial carcinoma: dose and time relationships among regular smokers and lifelong non-smokers. *J Epidemiol Community Health* 1978;32:303–313.
20. London WT. Primary hepatocellular carcinoma—etiology, pathogenesis, and prevention. *Hum Pathol* 1981;12:1085–1097.
21. The Writing Group for the PEPI Trial. Effects of estrogen or estrogen/progestin regimens on heart disease risk factors in postmenopausal women: the Postmenopausal Estrogen/Progestin Interventions (PEPI) Trial [published erratum appears in *JAMA* 1995;274:1676]. *JAMA* 1995;273:199–208.
22. Luria SE, Delbruck M. Mutations of bacteria from virus sensitivity to virus resistance. *Genetics* 1943; 28:491–511.
23. Goldie JH, Coldman AJ. A mathematic model for relating the drug sensitivity of tumors to their spontaneous mutation rate. *Cancer Treat Rep* 1979;63:1727–1733.
24. Magnusson C, Holmberg L, Norden T, et al. Prognostic characteristics in breast cancers after hormone replacement therapy. *Breast Cancer Res Treat* 1996;38:325–334.
25. Willis DB, Calle EE, Miracle-McMahill HL, et al. Estrogen replacement therapy and risk of fatal breast cancer in a prospective cohort of postmenopausal women in the United States. *Cancer Causes Control* 1996;7:449–457.
26. Grodstein F, Stampfer MJ, Colditz GA, et al. Postmenopausal hormone therapy and mortality. *N Engl. J Med* 1997;336:1769–1775.
27. Jernstrom H, Frenander J, Ferno M, et al. Hormone replacement therapy before breast cancer diagnosis significantly reduces the overall death rate compared with never-use among 984 breast cancer patients. *Br J Cancer* 1999;80:1453–1458.
28. Holli K, Isola J, Cuzick J. Low biologic aggressiveness in breast cancer in women using hormone replacement therapy. *J Clin Oncol* 1998;16:3115–3120.
29. Schairer C, Gail M, Byrne C, et al. Estrogen replacement therapy and breast cancer survival in a large screening study. *J Natl Cancer Inst* 1999;91:264–270.
30. Fowble B, Hanlon A, Freedman G, et al. Postmenopausal hormone replacement therapy: effect on diagnosis and outcome in early-stage invasive breast cancer treated with conservative surgery and radiation. *J Clin Oncol* 1999;17:1680–1688.
31. Gapstur SM, Morrow M, Sellers TA. Hormone replacement therapy and risk of breast cancer with a favorable histology: results of the Iowa Women's Health Study. *JAMA* 1999;281:2091–2097.
32. Magnusson C, Baron JA, Correia N, et al. Breast-cancer risk following long-term oestrogen- and oestrogen-progestin-replacement therapy. *Int J Cancer* 1999;81:339–344.
33. Cobleigh MA, Norlock FE, Oleske DM, et al. Hormone replacement therapy and high S phase in breast cancer. *JAMA* 1999;281:1528–1530.
34. Ragaz J, Ariel IM. High-risk breast cancer: definition of the risk. In: Ragaz J, Ariel IM, eds. *High-risk breast cancer.* New York: Springer-Verlag, 1989:3–25.
35. MacMahon B, Cole P, Lin TM, et al. Age at first birth and breast cancer risk. *Bull World Health Organ* 1970;43:209–221.
36. Pike MC, Spicer DV, Dahmoush L, et al. Estrogens, progestogens, normal breast cell proliferation, and breast cancer risk. *Epidemiol Rev* 1993;15:17–35.
37. Pathak DR, Osuch JR, He J. Breast carcinoma etiology: current knowledge and new insights into the effects of reproductive and hormonal risk factors in black and white populations. *Cancer* 2000; 88:1230–1238.
38. Bernstein L, Henderson B. *Exogenous hormones* 1996:462–488.
39. Lippman M BGHK. The effects of estrogens and antiestrogens on hormone-responsive human breast cancer in long-term tissue culture. *Cancer Res* 1976;36:4595–4601.
40. Welsch C, Rivera E. Differential effects of estrogen and prolactin on DNA synthesis in organ cultures of DMBA-induced rat mammary carcinoma. *Proc Soc Exp Biol Med* 1972;139:623–626.
41. Lippman M, Dickson RB, Kasid A, et al. Autocrine and paracrine growth regulation of human breast cancer. *J Steroid Biochem* 1986;24:147–154.
42. Dickson R, Lippman ME. Hormonal control of human breast cancer cell lines. *Cancer Surv* 1986; 5:617–624.

43. Lippman M. Estrogens regulate production of specific growth factors in hormone-dependent human breast cancer [Review]. *Ann NY Acad Sci* 1986;464:11–16.
44. Knabbe C, Lippman ME, Wakefield LM, et al. Evidence that transforming growth factor-beta is a hormonally regulated negative growth factor in human breast cancer cells. *Cell* 1987;48:417–428.
45. King RJ, Wang DY, Daly RJ, et al. Approaches to studying the role of growth factors in the progression of breast tumours from the steroid sensitive to insensitive state. *J Steroid Biochem* 1989;34:133–138.
46. Murphy LC, Murphy LJ, Dubik D, et al. Epidermal growth factor gene expression in human breast cancer cells: regulation of expression by progestins. *Cancer Res* 1988;48:4555–4560.
47. Goldin BR, Adlercreutz H, Gorbach SL, et al. Estrogen excretion patterns and plasma levels in vegetarian and omnivorous women. *N Engl J Med* 1982;307:1542–1547.
48. Howe GR, Hirohata T, Hislop TG, et al. Dietary factors and risk of breast cancer: combined analysis of 12 case-control studies. *J Natl Cancer Inst* 1990;82:561–569.
49. Howe G, Rohan T, Decarli A, et al. The association between alcohol and breast cancer risk: evidence from the combined analysis of six dietary case-control studies. *Int J Cancer* 1991;47:707–710.
50. Baron JA. Smoking and estrogen-related disease. *Am J Epidemiol* 1984;119:9–22.
51. Thune I, Brenn T, Lund E, et al. Physical activity and the risk of breast cancer. *N Engl J Med* 1997;336:1269–1275.
52. Stampfer MJ, Colditz GA, Willett WC, et al. Postmenopausal estrogen therapy and cardiovascular disease: ten-year follow-up from the nurses' health study. *N Engl J Med* 1991;325:756–762.
53. Barrett-Connor E, Bush TL. Estrogen and coronary heart disease in women. *JAMA* 1991;265:1861–1867.
54. Nabulsi AA, Folsom AR, White A, et al. Association of hormone-replacement therapy with various cardiovascular risk factors in postmenopausal women: the Atherosclerosis Risk in Communities Study Investigators. *N Engl J Med* 1993;328:1069–1075.
55. Grodstein F, Stampfer MJ, Manson JE, et al. Postmenopausal estrogen and progestin use and the risk of cardiovascular disease [published erratum appears in *N Engl J Med* 1996;335:1406]. *N Engl J Med* 1996;335:453–461.
56. Hu FB, Stampfer MJ, Manson JE, et al. Trends in the incidence of coronary heart disease and changes in diet and lifestyle in women. *N Engl J Med* 2000;343:530–537.
57. Reis SE, Holubkov R, Young JB, et al. Estrogen is associated with improved survival in aging women with congestive heart failure: analysis of the vesnarinone studies. *J Am Coll Cardiol* 2000;36:529–533.
58. Mosca L. The role of hormone replacement therapy in the prevention of postmenopausal heart disease. *Arch Intern Med* 2000;160:2263–2272.
59. Grodstein F, Stampfer M. The epidemiology of coronary heart disease and estrogen replacement in postmenopausal women. *Prog Cardiovasc Dis* 1995;38:199–210.
60. Bush TL, Barrett-Connor E, Cowan LD, et al. Cardiovascular mortality and noncontraceptive use of estrogen in women: results from the Lipid Research Clinics Program Follow-up Study. *Circulation* 1987;75:1102–1109.
61. Miller VT, Muesing RA, LaRosa JC, et al. Effects of conjugated equine estrogen with and without three different progestogens on lipoproteins, high-density lipoprotein subfractions, and apolipoprotein A-1. *Obstet Gynecol* 1991;77:235–240.
62. Walsh BW, Schiff I, Rosner B, et al. Effects of postmenopausal estrogen replacement on the concentrations and metabolism of plasma lipoproteins. *N Engl J Med* 1991;325:1196–1204.
63. Wagner JD, Clarkson TB, St. Clair RW, et al. Estrogen and progesterone replacement therapy reduces low density lipoprotein accumulation in the coronary arteries of surgically postmenopausal cynomolgus monkeys. *J Clin Invest* 1991;88:1995–2002.
64. Rosario GM, Panina G. Oestrogens and the heart. *Therapie* 1999;54:381–385.
65. Rosano GM, Panina G. Cardiovascular pharmacology of hormone replacement therapy. *Drugs Aging* 1999;15:219–234.
66. Harder DR, Coulson PB. Estrogen receptors and effects of estrogen on membrane electrical properties of coronary vascular smooth muscle. *J Cell Physiol* 1979;100:375–382.
67. McGill HC Jr. Sex steroid hormone receptors in the cardiovascular system. *Postgrad Med* 1989;64-8:89–90.
68. Bourne T, Hillard TC, Whitehead MI, et al. Oestrogens, arterial status, and postmenopausal women [letter] [see comments]. *Lancet* 1990; 335:1470–1471.

69. Rosario GM, Sarrel PM, Poole-Wilson PA, et al. Beneficial effect of oestrogen on exercise-induced myocardial ischaemia in women with coronary artery disease. *Lancet* 1993;342:133–136.
70. Gilligan DM, Quyyumi AA, Cannon RO III. Effects of physiological levels of estrogen on coronary vasomotor function in postmenopausal women. *Circulation* 1994;89:2545–2551.
71. Collins P, Rosano GM, Jiang C, et al. Cardiovascular protection by oestrogen—a calcium antagonist effect? *Lancet* 1993;341:1264–1265.
72. Stampfer MJ, Colditz GA, Willett WC. Menopause and heart disease: a review. *Ann NY Acad Sci* 1990;592:193–203; discussion 257–262.
73. Hulley S, Grady D, Bush T, et al. Randomized trial of estrogen plus progestin for secondary prevention of coronary heart disease in postmenopausal women. Heart and Estrogen/Progestin Replacement Study (HERS) Research Group. *JAMA* 1998;280:605–613.
74. Mosca L, Jahnige K, Giacherio D, et al. Beneficial effects of hormone replacement on lipoprotein(a) levels in postmenopausal women. *Prev Cardiol* 1999;2:51–58.
75. Crouse JR III, Furberg CD. Treatment of dyslipidemia: room for improvement? *Arterioscler Thromb Vasc Biol* 2000;20:2333–2335.
76. Clarkson TB, Williams TB, Adams MR, et al. Experimental effects of estrogens and progestins on the coronary artery wall. 1993:169–174.
77. Wagner JD. Rationale for hormone replacement therapy in atherosclerosis prevention. *J Reprod Med* 2000;45:245–258.
78. Adams J, Carder PJ, Downey S, et al. Vascular endothelial growth factor (VEGF) in breast cancer: comparison of plasma, serum, and tissue VEGF and microvessel density and effects of tamoxifen. *Cancer Res* 2000;60:2898–2905.
79. Steinleitner A, Stanczyk FZ, Levin JH, et al. Decreased in vitro production of 6-keto-prostaglandin F1 alpha by uterine arteries from postmenopausal women. *Am J Obstet Gynecol* 1989;161: 1677–1681.
80. Mijatovic VKP, Netelenbos JC, et al. Oral 17b-estradiol continuously combined with dydrogesterone lowers serum lipoprotein(a) concentrations in healthy postmenopausal women. *J Clin Endocrinol Metab* 1997;82:3543–3547.
81. Mijatovic V, van der Mooren MJ, Stehouwer CD, et al. Postmenopausal hormone replacement, risk estimators for coronary artery disease and cardiovascular protection. *Gynecol Endocrinol* 1999; 13:130–144.
82. Mosca L, Grundy SM, Judelson D, et al. Guide to preventive cardiology for women: AHA/ACC Scientific Statement Consensus panel statement. *Circulation* 1999;99:2480–2484.
83. Shlipak MG, Simon JA, Vittinghoff E, et al. Estrogen and progestin, lipoprotein(a), and the risk of recurrent coronary heart disease events after menopause. *JAMA* 2000;283:1845–1852.
84. Tikkanen MJ, Nikkila EA, Kuusi T. High-density lipoprotein-2 and hepatic lipase:reciprocal changes produced by estrogens and norgestrel. *J Clin Endocrinol Metab* 1982; 4:1113–1117.
85. Gaulin-Glasser T, Farrel WJ, Pfau SE. Modulation of circulating cellular adhesion molecules in postmenopausal women with coronary artery disease. *J Am Coll Cardiol* 1998;31:1555–1560.
86. McGowan JA, Pottern L. Commentary on the Women's Health Initiative. *Maturitas* 2000;34: 109–112.
87. Losordo DW, Kearney M, Kim EA. Variable expression of the estrogen receptor in normal and atherosclerotic coronary arteries of premenopausal women. *Circulation* 1996;89:1501–1510.
88. Williams JK, Adams MR, Klopfenstein HS. Estrogen modulates responses of atherosclerotic coronary arteries. *Circulation* 1990;81:1680–1687.
89. Sarrel PM, Lindsay D, Rosano GM, et al. Angina and normal coronary arteries in women: gynecologic findings. *Am J Obstet Gynecol* 1992;167:467–471.
90. Pines A, Fisman EZ, Levo Y, et al. The effects of hormone replacement therapy in normal postmenopausal women: measurements of Doppler-derived parameters of aortic flow. *Am J Obstet Gynecol* 1991;164:806–812.
91. Posthuma WF, Westendorp RG, Vandenbroucke JP. Cardioprotective effect of hormone replacement therapy in postmenopausal women: is the evidence biased? *BMJ* 1994;308:1268–1269.
92. Grodstein F, Stampfer MJ. Estrogen for women at varying risk of coronary disease. *Maturitas* 1998; 30:19–26.
93. Henderson BE, Paganini-Hill A, Ross RK. Decreased mortality in users of estrogen replacement therapy. *Arch Intern Med* 1991;151:75–78.
94. Grundy SM, Pasternak R, Greenland P, et al. Assessment of cardiovascular risk by use of multiple-

risk-factor assessment equations: a statement for healthcare professionals from the American Heart Association and the American College of Cardiology. *Circulation* 1999;100:1481–1492.

95. Meade TW. Haemostatic function and ischaemic heart disease. *Adv Exp Med Biol* 1984;164:3–9.
96. Petitti DB, Wingerd J, Pellegrin F, et al. Oral contraceptives, smoking, and other factors in relation to risk of venous thromboembolic disease. *Am J Epidemiol* 1978;108:480–485.
97. Barrett-Connor E. Hormone replacement and cancer. *Br Med Bull* 1992;48:345–355.
98. Grady D, Rubin SM, Petitti DB, et al. Hormone therapy to prevent disease and prolong life in postmenopausal women. *Ann Intern Med* 1992;117:1016–1037.
99. Grady D, Wenger NK, Herrington D, et al. Postmenopausal hormone therapy increases risk for venous thromboembolic disease: the Heart and Estrogen/Progestin Replacement Study. *Ann Intern Med* 2000;132:689–696.
100. Devor M, Barrett-Connor E, Renvall M, et al. Estrogen replacement therapy and the risk of venous thrombosis [see comments]. *Am J Med* 1992;92:275–282.
101. Melton LJ, Eddy DM, Johnston CC Jr. Screening for osteoporosis. *Ann Intern Med* 1990;112:516–528.
102. Bilezekian JP, Silverberg SJ. Osteoporosis: a practical approach to the perimenopausal woman. *J Women's Health* 1992;1:21–27.
103. Ettinger B, Genant HK, Steiger P, et al. Low-dosage micronized 17 beta-estradiol prevents bone loss in postmenopausal women. *Am J Obstet Gynecol* 1992;166:479–488.
104. Crilly R, Marshall DH, Nordin BEC. The effects of oestradiol valerate and cyclic oestradiol valerate/DL-norgestrel on calcium metabolism. *Postgrad Med J* 1978;2(Suppl):47–49.
105. Melton LJ, Eddy DM, Johnston CC Jr. Screening for osteoporosis. *Ann Intern Med* 1990;112:516—528.
106. Cummings SR, Kelsey JL, Nevitt MC, et al. Epidemiology of osteoporosis and osteoporotic fractures. *Epidemiol Rev* 1985;7:178–208.
107. Schneider DL, Barrett-Connor EL, Morton DJ. Timing of postmenopausal estrogen for optimal bone mineral density: the Rancho Bernardo Study. *JAMA* 1997;277:543–547.
108. Cauley JA, Seeley DG, Ensrud K, et al. Estrogen replacement therapy and fractures in older women: Study of Osteoporotic Fractures Research Group. *Ann Intern Med* 1995;122:9–16.
109. Cummings SR, Black DM, Thomson DE, et al. Effect of alendronate on bone mineral density and the incidence of fractures in postmenopausal osteoporosis. *JAMA* 1998;280:2077–2082.
110. Ettinger B, Black DM, Mitlak BH, et al. Reduction of vertebral fracture risk in postmenopausal women with osteoporosis treated with raloxifene. *JAMA* 1999;282:637–645.
111. Scott JA, Da Camara CC, Early JE. Raloxifene: a selective estrogen receptor modulator [see comments]. *Am Fam Physician* 1999;60:1131–1139.
112. Jordan VC, Morrow M. Tamoxifen, raloxifene, and the prevention of breast cancer. *Endocr Rev* 1999; 20:253–278.
113. Jordan VC. Designer estrogens. *Sci Am* 1998;279:60–67.
114. Collins J, Donner A, Allen LH, Adams O. Oestrogen use and survival in endometrial cancer. *Lancet* 1980;2:961–964.
115. Hulka BS, Kaufman DG, Fowler WC Jr, et al. Predominance of early endometrial cancers after long-term estrogen use. *JAMA* 1980;244:2419–2422.
116. Kelsey JL, LiVolsi VA, Holford TR, et al. A case-control study of cancer of the endometrium. *Am J Epidemiol* 1982;116:333–342.
117. Kennedy DL, Baum C, Forbes MB. Noncontraceptive estrogens and progestins: use patterns over time. *Obstet Gynecol* 1985; 65:441–446.
118. Gambrell RD Jr., Massey FM, Castaneda TA, et al. Use of the progestogen challenge test to reduce the risk of endometrial cancer. *Obstet Gynecol* 1980;55:732–738.
119. Persson I, Adami HO, Bergkvist L, et al. Risk of endometrial cancer after treatment with oestrogens alone or in conjunction with progestogens: results of a prospective study. *BMJ* 1989;298:147–151.
120. Pike MC, Peters RK, Cozen W, et al. Estrogen-progestin replacement therapy and endometrial cancer. *J Natl Cancer Inst* 1997;89:1110–1116.
121. Thom MH, White PJ, Williams RM, et al. Prevention and treatment of endometrial disease in climacteric women receiving oestrogen therapy. *Lancet* 1979;2:455–457.
122. Paterson ME, Wade-Evans T, Sturdee DW, et al. Endometrial disease after treatment with oestrogens and progestogens in the climacteric. *BMJ* 1980;280:822–824.
123. Calle EE, Miracle-McMahill HL, Thun MJ, et al. Estrogen replacement therapy and risk of fatal

colon cancer in a prospective cohort of postmenopausal women. *J Natl Cancer Inst* 1995;87: 517–523.

124. Hebert-Croteau N. A meta-analysis of hormone replacement therapy and colon cancer in women. *Cancer Epidemiol Biomarkers Prev* 1998;7:653–659.

125. Grodstein F, Martinez ME, Platz EA, et al. Postmenopausal hormone use and risk for colorectal cancer and adenoma [see comments]. *Ann Intern Med* 1998;128:705–712.

126. Narisawa T, Magadia NE, Weisburger JH, et al. Promoting effect of bile acids on colon carcinogenesis after intrarectal instillation of N-methyl-N'-nitro-N-nitrosoguanidine in rats. *J Natl Cancer Inst* 1974;53:1093–1097.

127. Reddy BS, Watanabe K, Weisburger JH. Effect of high-fat diet on colon carcinogenesis in F344 rats treated with 1,2-dimethylhydrazine, methylazoxymethanol acetate, or methylnitrosourea. *Cancer Res* 1977;37:4156–4159.

128. Reddy BS, Watanabe K, Weisburger JH, et al. Promoting effect of bile acids in colon carcinogenesis in germ-free and conventional F344 rats. *Cancer Res* 1977;37:3238–3242.

129. Meggouh F, Lointier P, Pezet D, et al. Status of sex steroid hormone receptors in large bowel cancer. *Cancer* 1991;67:1964–1970.

130. Peipins LA, Newman B, Sandler RS. Reproductive history, use of exogenous hormones, and risk of colorectal adenomas. *Cancer Epidemiol Biomarkers Prev* 1997;6:671–675.

131. Chen MJ, Longnecker MP, Morgenstern H, et al. Recent use of hormone replacement therapy and the prevalence of colorectal adenomas. *Cancer Epidemiol Biomarkers Prev* 1998;7:227–230.

132. Potter JD, Bigler J, Fosdick L, et al. Colorectal adenomatous and hyperplastic polyps: smoking and N-acetyltransferase 2 polymorphisms. *Cancer Epidemiol Biomarkers Prev* 1999;8:69–75.

133. Ragaz J, Coldman A. Survival impact of adjuvant tamoxifen on competing causes of mortality in breast cancer survivors, with analysis of mortality from contralateral breast cancer, cardiovascular events, endometrial cancer, and thromboembolic episodes. *J Clin Oncol* 1998;16:2018–2024.

134. Bush TL, Cowan LD, Barrett-Connor E, et al. Estrogen use and all-cause mortality: preliminary results from the Lipid Research Clinics Program Follow-Up Study. *JAMA* 1983; 249:903–906.

135. Ettinger B, Friedman GD, Bush T, et al. Reduced mortality associated with long-term postmenopausal estrogen therapy. *Obstet Gynecol* 1996;87:6–12.

136. Ragaz J, Coldman AJ. Age-matched all-cause mortality impact of hormone replacement therapy: applicability to breast cancer survivors. *Breast Cancer Res Treat* 1999;57:30.

137. Carter AC, Sedransk N, Kelley RM, et al. Diethylstilbestrol: recommended dosages for different categories of breast cancer patients: report of the Cooperative Breast Cancer Group. *JAMA* 1977; 237:2079–2080.

138. Stoll BA. Hormone replacement therapy in women treated for breast cancer. *Eur J Cancer Clin Oncol* 1989;25:1909–1913.

139. Ingle JN, Ahmann DL, Green SJ, et al. Randomized clinical trial of diethylstilbestrol versus tamoxifen in postmenopausal women with advanced breast cancer. *N Engl J Med* 1981;304:16–21.

140. Henderson IC, Canellos GP. Cancer of the breast: the past decade (first of two parts). *N Engl J Med* 1980;302:17–30.

141. Henderson IC, Canellos GP. Cancer of the breast: the past decade (second of two parts). *N Engl J Med* 1980;302:78–90.

142. Peethambaram PP, Ingle JN, Suman VJ, et al. Randomized trial of diethylstilbestrol vs. tamoxifen in postmenopausal women with metastatic breast cancer: an updated analysis. *Breast Cancer Res Treat* 1999;54:117–122.

143. Yao K, Lee ES, Bentrem DJ, et al. Antitumor action of physiological estradiol on tamoxifen-stimulated breast tumors grown in athymic mice. *Clin Cancer Res* 2000;6:2028–2036.

144. DiSaia PJ, Grown EA, Odicino F, et al. Replacement therapy for breast cancer survivors. A pilot study. *Cancer* 1995;76:2075–2078.

145. Powles TJ, Hickish T, Casey S, et al. Hormone replacement after breast cancer [letter; comment]. *Lancet* 1993;342:60–61.

146. Wile AG, Opfell RW, Margileth DA. Hormone replacement therapy in previously treated breast cancer patients. *Am J Surg* 1993;165:372–375.

147. Eden JA, Bush T, Nand S, et al. A case-controlled study of combined continuous hormone replacement therapy amongst women with personal history of breast cancer. *Menopause* 1995;2:67–72.

148. Eden JA. Estrogen replacement therapy in survivors of breast cancer: a risk-benefit assessment. *Drugs Aging* 1996; 8:127–133.

149. Ursic-Vrscaj M, Behar S. A case-control study of hormone replacement therapy after primary surgical breast cancer treatment. *Eur J Surg Oncol* 1999;25:146–151.
150. Decker DA, Pettinga JE, Cox TC, et al. Hormone replacement therapy in breast cancer survivors. *Breast J* 1997;3:63–68.
151. Vassilopoulou-Sellin R. Randomized trial of HRT in patients surviving breast cancer. 1997.
152. Vassilopoulou-Sellin R, Asmar L, Hortobagyi GN, et al. Estrogen replacement therapy after localized breast cancer: clinical outcome of 319 women followed prospectively. *J Clin Oncol* 1999;17: 1482–1487.
153. Cobleigh M. The ECOG randomized trial of HRT in breast cancer survivors. 1999.
154. Hislop TG, Waxler NE, Coldman AJ, Elwood JM, Kan L. The prognostic significance of psychosocial factors in women with breast cancer. *J Chronic Dis* 1987;40:729–735.
155. Kushi LH, Fee RM, Folsom AR, et al. Physical activity and mortality in postmenopausal women. *JAMA* 1997;277:1287–1292.
156. Rockhill B, Colditz GA, Rosner B. Bias in breast cancer analyses due to error in age at menopause. *Am J Epidemiol* 2000;151:404–408.

19

Breast Diseases in Males

John T. Vetto

THE MALE BREAST

The male breast is normally a rudimentary structure composed of small ducts and fibrous tissue with variable amounts of periductal fat, identical histologically to the breast of prepubertal females (1). In the absence of estrogenic stimulation, lobules are not seen. The incidences in males of absent breasts or nipples and of supernumerary nipples are identical to the incidences in females (2). In the absence of enlargement, breast tissue in the male is confined to the area directly behind the areola; therefore, clinical breast examination (CBE) is very easy in males and usually can be performed with just one or two examining fingers.

GYNECOMASTIA

Gynecomastia, the most common clinical and pathologic benign condition of the male breast (3), is defined as an enlargement of the ductal and fibrous stromal components and is clinically and histologically distinct from pseudogynecomastia, in which clinical breast enlargement is due to swelling of the surrounding subcutaneous fat (2). True gynecomastia may range in size from a small retroareolar disc to enlargement that approximates that of an adult female breast (4). Primary (idiopathic) gynecomastia occurs in 30% to 70% of male children and is thought to occur during developmental periods of relative estrogen excess or androgen deficiency (1). Typically, it resolves spontaneously, and, in the presence of an otherwise normal history and physical examination (PE), requires no specific workup or treatment unless it persists or is severe.

Secondary gynecomastia can be due to a myriad of underlying conditions and medications (1–3,5–7) listed in Table 19.1. Careful history and PE often disclose the underlying cause without the need for additional testing or sex-steroid chemistry panels, and treatment consists of correction of the underlying condition or discontinuation of the causative medication. Treatment of secondary gynecomastia, however, may not be necessary or even possible in situations in which the underlying condition is not correctable or the patient is asymptomatic, and the causative medication should not be discontinued. In symptomatic patients, a variety of hormonal options are available (testosterone, clomiphene, tamoxifen, danazol), none of which have been studied in a systematic manner and some of which can be associated with significant side effects (2). In our hands, surgical excision (by subcutaneous mastectomy, spar-

TABLE 19.1. *Benign conditions of the male breast*

Benign breast masses

Fibroadenomas	Hemangiopericytomas	Lipomas
Myofibroblastomas	Mesenchymomas	Phylloides tumors

Conditions associated with gynecomastia

Adrenal insufficiency	Chronic renal failure	Chronic liver diseases
Kleinfelter syndrome	Malnutrition	Testicular failure
Thyrotoxicosis	Transverse myelitis	Trauma

Pulmonary diseases (bronchiectasis, bronchitis, tuberculosis)
Tumors (CNS, especially hypothalmus, pituitary; lung; testicular, especially seminomas, teratomas)

Drugs associated with gynecomastia

Androgens	Amphetamines	Cyclophosphamide	Cyproterone
Diazepam	Digitalis	Exogenous estrogens	Griseofulvin
Heroin	H_2-blockers	Isoniazid	LSD
Marijuana	Methadone	Metaclopramide	Methlydopa
Phenothiazides	Penicillamine	Reserpine	Spironolactone
Thiazides	Tricyclic antidepressants		

Other benign conditions

Abscess	Adenoma of the nipple	Duct ectasia
Epithelial hyperplasia	Fibrocystic changes	Florid papillomatosis[a]
Mondor disease	Nipple discharge[a]	Paget disease
Papilloma		

CNS, central nervous system; LSD, lysergic acid diethylamide.
[a] Associated with malignancy in many cases; see text.
From references 3,10,11,13,97.

ing the nipple) is the treatment of choice because it is definitive (provided care is taken to remove all the enlarged tissue) and, in many cases, can be accomplished with the patient under local anesthesia.

Because secondary gynecomastia may be unilateral and painless in many cases, the major clinical concern regarding this lesion is distinguishing it from breast cancer (6–9). This topic is discussed in detail subsequently (see "Differential Diagnosis of Breast Masses in Males" and "FNA-Based Evaluation of Breast Masses in Males").

OTHER BENIGN BREAST CONDITIONS

A variety of benign conditions common to the female breast are also seen in males and, with the exception of gynecomastia, are similar in both genders in terms of presentation, histology diagnosis, and treatment (3). These are listed in Table 19.1.

Another occasional exception is nipple discharge; benign milky discharge can occur in males (especially the colostrum-like "witch's milk" of male neonates (1), and benign nonmilky discharge is occasionally seen in males, but bloody discharge in a male is more commonly associated with malignancy than it is in females (10–12). For example, in a review by Treves et al. of 42 cases of nipple discharge in males, more than half (57%) were associated with a clinical breast cancer. Of the discharges associated with benign conditions, all nonbloody discharges were due to gynecomastia (and had often been present for years), whereas bloody but benign discharges were due to papilloma (13). Accordingly, males presenting with bloody nipple discharge have carcinoma until proven otherwise; those in whom a cancer is not found can be evaluated and treated in a fashion similar to females (i.e., ductography and papilloma excision) (12). Nipple discharge in males is also discussed throughout the sections that follow.

BREAST CANCER IN MALES

Breast cancer in males (BCM) is one of the oldest diseases in recorded history. First reported in the Smith Papyrus, European reports date back to a 1307 case report by an English surgeon, John of Aderne. Subsequent case reports by Ambroise Pare and Fabrius Hildanus in the sixteenth and seventeenth century, respectively, followed (5). Periodic reporting continued in the latter half of the twentieth century, when large series began to appear (5,14–24), leading to our current understanding of the disease.

Although fewer than 1% of breast cancer occurs in men, this disease accounts for 0.15% of all cancer deaths in males (approximately 400 cancer deaths in the United States per year) (25–27). The widely held notion of BCM as a late-presenting disease with a dismal prognosis is largely a result of earlier (14–19,28–31) and even some more recent (23,32,33) series consisting mostly of patients presenting with advanced stage disease. Much of the previous data are flawed by single-institution experience, repeated reports from the same institutional series, small sample size, and failure to control for stage and patient age. The well-known tendency for this disease to present late in older males (who already may possess comorbid conditions leading to subsequent death from noncancer causes) may explain in part the previously reported low crude survival for BCM.

As discussed later, newer series (20,21,24), including our own (8), refute this notion and indicate that breast cancer in men carries the same prognostic factors as the disease in women and that the stage-for-stage outcomes are also the same. This newer information leads to the question of whether breast cancer is the same or a different disease in men and women. This issue is also discussed in this chapter, including a detailing of how breast cancer in men is similar to and how it differs from, breast cancer in females (BCF).

A grammatical note: Tumors do not possess gender, and therefore, the *term male breast cancer* is not as correct as *breast cancer in males* or even *cancer of the male breast* (5) Thus, throughout this chapter, the disease is referred to as BCM, as opposed to BCF.

Global Distribution

In a meta-analysis, Sasco and colleagues determined that BCM accounts for about 1% of all breast cancer worldwide (34). The global distribution of BCM is similar to that of BCF (i.e., BCM is very rare in areas with a low incidence of breast cancer in general), with a few exceptions. For example, BCM is common in Egypt, an area of relatively low BCF incidence, probably because of high rates of schistosomiasis-related liver failure (35). In contrast, BCM rates are low and fairly even in European countries (1.5–3 per million) and reflect variances in the rates for BCF, with higher rates found in France, Hungary, Austria, and Scotland (36).

U.S. Incidence

Fewer than 1% of U.S. cases of breast cancer occur in men; for example, in 1999, there were 175,000 new cases in women and 1,300 cases in men (i.e., 0.74% of new breast cancer patients were males). During that same period, there were 43,700 deaths from BCF and approximately 400 deaths from BCM. Thus, the current likelihood of dying from BCF and from BCM are similar (25% and 31%, respectively) (27).

Associated Factors and Conditions

Factors associated with the development of BCM (Table 19.2) include the following:

1. **Advanced age**. The annual incidence of BCM increases steadily (lacking the premenopausal peak seen in females) (27) between 35 years of age (0.1 case per 100,000 men) and 85 years of age (11.1 cases per 100,000) (35). The mean age of diagnosis was 64.5 years in our series (8) and 61.8 years in the series by Borgen et al., compared with 55.5 years for matched female breast cancer controls in that same study (20). The greatest incidence occurs 5 to 10 years later in males than in females.

TABLE 19.2. *Factors associated with the development[a] of breast cancer in males (BCM) age[b]*

Prolonged heat exposure
Previous chest wall radiation
Positive family history for breast cancer (in male or female relatives)
BRCA2 mutations
Conditions of relative hyperestrogeny
Testicular abnormalities
Exogenous estrogens
Obesity
Liver disease
Kleinfelter syndrome[c]

[a] Direct causation has not been established for some factors.
[b] Incidence of BCM is directly related to age.
[c] Increases BCM risk by 50-fold.

It is rarely found before the age of 26, although it was reported in a 5-year old boy (37).

2. **Prolonged heat exposure**, which may have a suppressive effect on testicular function. (28,38,39). The role of electromagnetic field exposure remains controversial (5,38,40).

3. **Previous chest wall radiation**, especially radiation given for the treatment of childhood malignancies (41,42). The risk for breast cancer after radiation appears to be similar for men and women, as is the indirect relationship between age of exposure and risk and the lag time between exposure and disease (12–36 years) (40, 43–46). Accordingly, it is generally recommended that males with such exposure history should be carefully observed (34).

4. **Conditions of relative hyperestrogeny**. These conditions include testicular abnormalities, such as the sequelae of mumps infections and infectious orchitis (5), undescended testes (34), orchiectomy, late puberty, and infertility (28,47), disorders that cause gynecomastia (gynecomastia itself is associated with up to 43% of BCM cases, but there are no data for direct causation) (3,14), exogenous estrogen, obesity, liver disease (due to cirrhosis, bilharziasis, schistosomiasis, and chronic malnutrition) (34,41,42), and Klinefelter syndrome, which (despite its rarity) accounts for 3% of BCM cases (48) and is associated with a 50-fold increased risk of BCM (49). In fact, the risk of breast cancer in men with Klinefelter syndrome approaches that of females, probably due in part to the fact that these men actually develop hypertrophied breasts that contain both acini and lobules (the normal male breast does not contain lobules) (48). This histologic event explains the fact that lobular carcinoma in men is rare and usually only associated with Klinefelter-related cases (see ''Histologies'' section to follow).

The preceding associations would lead one to the conclusion that BCM is caused by relative estrogen excess. Although breast cancer can be easily promoted in a number of animal species by hormone administration, clear data indicating causation in humans are lacking, probably because of the relative rarity of BCM and the corresponding small sample sizes in most studies. For example, breast cancer is rarely reported among men receiving estrogens for prostate cancer, and breast masses in these patients are more often metastatic deposits than BCM (50). Similarly, reports of BCM and fibroadenomas among males taking estrogen for transsexual male-to-female surgery have been anecdotal only (51–53). Data from blood chemistry studies attempting to demonstrate hormonal differences among BCM patients compared with control subjects have been sparse and conflicting. Taken together, most studies show no difference in testosterone, estradiol, and luteinizing hormone levels (54, 55), whereas one study showed increased prolactin and follicle stimulating hormone levels in patients compared with matched controls (56).

Isolated reports also suggest links between BCM and occupational exposure to gasoline and combustion products (57) and employment in blast furnaces, steel works, and rolling mills (58). To date, no link between BCM and any specific dietary factors has been found (59).

Family History and Genetics

A family history of BCM or females is present in about 30% of cases of BCM (34), with 14% reporting breast cancer in a first-degree relative in one series (60). Whereas multiple cases of BCM within families has been reported (30,61), it is rare; more typically (as one would expect from the rarity of BCM), the risk for BCM is associated with a history of BCF. Similarly, a family history of BCM imparts increased breast cancer risk to the female relatives (62,63).

Taken together, this information suggests that (a) similar to the situation in BCF, most cases of BCM are "sporadic" (i.e., a specific gene mutation is not identified), and (b) a familial form of breast cancer exists in which both males and females show an increased risk for developing breast cancer (35). Recent work has focused on identifying the mutated gene for this latter situation. Similar to BCF, studies reveal the association of BCM with a multitude of chromosomal and gene abnormalities (25, 49,64), especially on the 13q chromosome (64). The best characterized of these mutations are in the *BRCA2* gene, which, although these mutations may be associated with up to 20% of BCM cases, have a low penetrance: Only one in seven *BRCA2* carriers have a family history of breast cancer (65). The usefulness of *BRCA2* testing for relatives of BCM patients is discussed later (see "Testing of Family Members").

There appears to be little if any association between BCM and *BRCA1* mutations (66). A hereditary nonpolyposis colon cancer (HNPCC) kindred has been identified in which a male member had both an *MLH1* mutation and breast cancer, suggesting that BCM may be part of the HNPCC syndrome (67). Loss of the Y chromosome and another 13q chromosomal abnormality, del(16)(q13), have been recurrent findings in BCM patients (68). An androgen receptor (AR) gene mutation has been found in BCM associated with Reifenstein syndrome (inherited androgen resistance) (69), but at least one report suggests no correlation between AR expression and either the clinicopathologic features or outcome for BCM (70). Although *p53* mutation rates are similar for BCM (43%) and BCF (71), BCM is rarely seen in Li-Fraumeni syndrome (72), probably because of the relative rarity of both BCM and this syndrome.

Histologies

Because the male breast contains only ductal tissue, most cases if BCM are ductal type, predominantly ductal invasive [85%–90% of most series (5), 79% in our series (8)], with the remainder usually "pure" ductal carcinoma *in situ* (DCIS) or ductal variants (10,41,73). All histologies of breast cancer have been encountered in males, however, including Paget disease (both alone and associated with either DCIS or invasive tumors) and phylloides tumors (41,74,75). "Pure" DCIS accounts for 5% to 15% of BCM (5) and is less common among BCM compared with BCF cases, probably because of greater detection of ductal neoplasms at the DCIS stage in females by screening mammography (15). As expected, lobular cancers are extremely rare in men (who lack lobular tissue) and usually are not found at all in many series (20,33), including our own (8), but have been described in case reports (41) and in large data sets (21). As mentioned previously, this event probably occurs in diseases associated with the formation of lobules in the male breast, notably Klinefelter syndrome (48). BCM is bilateral at diagnosis in about 2% of cases, similar to the incidence for BCF.

Secretory carcinoma, a rare variant of breast cancer that is the most common type seen in children, has been reported in boys (76–78) and in a 51-year-old man (79). Because of its rarity, neither the natural history of this tumor nor the optimal management is well established, although the tumor generally behaves in an indolent fashion and the prognosis appears to be good (77).

Tumor Biology

Most cases of BCM are estrogen receptor (ER) positive [65%–94% in recent studies (20,33,41,80) and 85% in our series (8)]; therefore, a greater percentage of male patients will be treated with tamoxifen or will respond to hormonal manipulation than will female patients (80,81). Similarly, BCM is more commonly progesterone receptor positive (PR) [93% of cases in one series (82)]. Unlike the situation for BCF, hormone receptor expression in BCM does not seem to correlate with patient age or with histologic grade of the lesion, tumor stage, or lymph node status (35), a finding that further suggests that BCM in general is associated with relative estrogen excess. AR expression has been reported in 39% of BCMs and seems more common on tumors from older patients (83), but a clinical importance for AR expression in BCM has not been clearly demonstrated (69,70). The incidence of high-grade histology among BCM varies widely among series (20%–73%) (8,33) but is probably overall similar to the incidence in BCF (20). One study, however, reported proportionately more high-grade histology among a cohort of lower-stage BCM patients compared with a BCF cohort of similar low stage (84). Whereas breast cancer tends to present at later stages in males than in females (due, in part to the low index of suspicion and lack of screening in males), the discrepancy in stage distribution, and thus the difference in overall prognosis between BCM and BCF is shrinking as more and more recent series are examined (discussed in more detail in the section on ''Prognosis'').

Staging

BCM is staged using the same TNM (tumor, nodes, metastases) staging system of the American Joint Committee on Cancer (AJCC) as for BCF (85).

Physical Findings

Because BCM is not a screened-for disease, it presents primarily (up to 79%–85% of cases) as a unilateral firm, painless or minimally tender, subareolar mass (21,81) found on either self-examination or CBE. Seventy percent of the men in our own series presented in this fashion (8). The mass is often eccentric (i.e., not directly behind the nipple, especially when there is coexisting gynecomastia or other condition of ductal hypertrophy), slightly irregular, and firm. (35). Whereas nipple discharge in females is usually nonbloody and associated with benign conditions, discharge in men is more often bloody and a sign of malignancy, including DCIS, and discharge cytology may be diagnostic (10,11,13). Between 18% and 30% of the cases present with pain or nipple discharge (8,13), and a bloody discharge in a male has an 80% likelihood of indicating an underlying tumor (13).

Imaging

Mammography has a limited role in the diagnosis of BCM for a variety of reasons. First, it is a rare disease for which general population screening is unlikely to be cost-effective. Second, the breast is not significantly enlarged in most cases and is therefore difficult to image (5). Finally, the utility of mammography for detecting BCM is questionable; although there are indeed characteristic mammographic features of BCM, these features are not always present, or there is substantial overlap between these features and the mammographic appearance of benign lesions (86). For example, suspicious microcalcifications were found in only four of 50 cases of BCM evaluated by mammography by Borgen and colleagues (60), and Cooper et al. found no malignant findings among 263 mammograms in males obtained for abnormal findings on CBE, even among those cases found to be cancer on biopsy (87). In our diagnostic test study of breast masses in males (see section on ''Fine-needle Aspiration–Based Evaluation''), mammography was found to add no additional diagnostic information to the combination of PE and fine needle aspiration (FNA) (88).

Similarly, although ultrasound and ductography are helpful in evaluating masses and discharge in females, respectively, they have a limited role in men (5). The role of technetium-99 sestamibi scanning for the detection of BCM is limited by false-positive results caused by gynecomastia, lymphoma, and other benign and malignant conditions; compounds other than methoxyisobutyl (MIBI) may provide more accurate results (89–91).

DIFFERENTIAL DIAGNOSIS OF BREAST MASSES IN MALES

Besides BCM, masses in the male breast may represent primary lymphomas (92), metastases from other primaries (50), and a variety of benign conditions (Table 19.1) (1–3), including hemangiopericytomas (93), myofibroblastomas (94,95), and mesenchymomas (also known as *hamartomas* or *angiolipomas*) (96). Juvenile papillomatosis (''Swiss cheese disease''), which presents as a localized palpable mass, was recently reported in the breasts of male infants. This lesion often is associated with a family history of breast cancer and coexists with malignancy in almost half of cases (97).

The major point on the differential for BCM is gynecomastia, which (unlike BCM) has a bimodal age distribution. At presentation, however, older patients with gynecomastia have a similar mean age as BCM patients, and as many as 80% (63% in our study) (8) do not have pain or tenderness (6). Although gynecomastia is typically rubbery and less firm than BCM, this distinction is not always clear on PE, and (as noted earlier), mammograms that are negative or show gynecomastia do not necessarily rule out malignancy. Thus, in the older male patient who presents to a surgeon or breast clinic with a unilateral palpable breast mass, the main diagnostic task is to rule out BCM (rare, but often treatable for cure) while avoiding open biopsy if possible (unnecessary in asymptomatic benign lesions, which will constitute the majority of masses seen) (7,9).

Patient history does not reliably distinguish between gynecomastia and BCM, for two important reasons. First, the incidence of use of medications known to be associated with gynecomastia (Table 19.1) has been found to be similar between patients with benign breast conditions and BCM (7). Second, whereas some of the conditions known to be associated with gynecomastia (Table 19.1) are not directly associated with BCM risk, other such conditions (especially chronic liver diseases and Klinefelter syndrome) have also been linked to the development of BCM (5).

In experienced hands, FNA (Fig. 19.1) can distinguish between gynecomastia

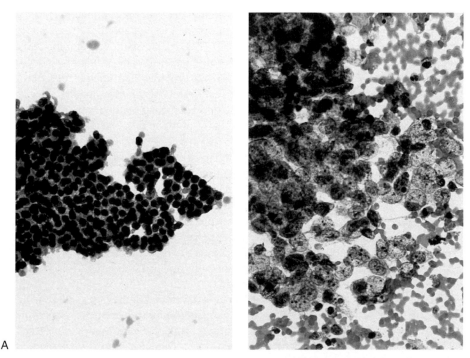

A

B

FIG. 19.1. Fine-needle aspiration can distinguish between gynecomastia (**A**) and breast cancer in males (BCM) (**B**). Hematoxylin and eosin, 400×.

and BCM with good reliability (98–101). For example, sensitivity, specificity, and accuracy rates were 100% in a recent study by Joshi and colleagues (102), although there is a small tendency in many reported series toward false-positive results, likely secondary to the high cellularity and epithelial hyperplasia commonly found in aspirates of gynecomastia (101). Whereas some researchers believe that this "diagnostic dilemma" can be addressed only by routine open biopsy (7,103), in our breast clinics we favor a multidisciplinary nonsurgical approach that combines PE with needle biopsy.

FINE-NEEDLE ASPIRATION–BASED EVALUATION OF BREAST MASSES IN MALES

Because of our experience and success with FNA-based "triple testing" of palpable breast masses in female patients (104–106), we studied the accuracy and cost-effectiveness of the elements of the triple test (PE, FNA, and mammography) for the evaluation of breast masses in males. As noted previously, although some investigators advocate mammography for the evaluation of these lesions (6), experience is limited (7), sensitivity is at best 88% (i.e., no better than PE alone in ours and other studies) (88,107), no benefit has been demonstrated for patients younger than 50 years of age (87) false-positive results are the rule with certain benign lesions, such as gynecomastia (18) and epidermal cysts (9), and published information on the relationship between calcifications and malignancy is conflicting (6,41,108). Accordingly, we chose to study a diagnostic approach to palpable breast masses in males that used the combination of PE and FNA (PE + FNA) without mammography since we believed mammography would add only increased patient charges. Indeed, in the 13 cases in our study where the referring provider had already ordered a mammogram, the test added no additional diagnostic information to that already provided by PE + FNA, nor did it change the clinical management of any case (88). We do recommend bilateral mammography as a preoperative test in cases where PE + FNA indicate the presence of a malignancy.

We performed a diagnostic test study and cost-effectiveness analysis in three participating multidisciplinary breast clinics, involving a consecutive sample of 51 males with unilateral breast masses. Each lesion was tested with both PE and FNA. Fine-needle aspirates were performed in triplicate using Diff-Quik (Fisher HealthCare, Swedesboro, NJ) staining to ensure specimen adequacy prior to the patient leaving the clinic; therefore, no patients had to be excluded for inadequate aspirates. Each test was scored as either benign or suspicious. Lesions for which both tests were benign were followed up clinically (mean 19 months). Lesions for which any test was suspicious were excised.

Both tests were benign in 38 cases. No cancers developed at the index sites during follow-up of these lesions, including eight excisional biopsies done for symptoms [negative predictive value (NPV) and specificity 100%]. Open biopsy confirmed malignancy in all six cases for which both tests were suspicious [positive predictive value (PPV) and sensitivity 100%]. In all seven cases where the tests were not in agreement, open biopsy was benign. In these cases, FNA (two false-positives) proved

TABLE 19.3. Analysis of PE, FNA, and PE+FNA for the detection of malignant breast lesions in males

Measure[a]	PE	FNA	PE+FNA	PE+FNA (females)[b]
Positive PV	55	75	46	78
Negative PV	100	100	100	100
Sensitivity	100	100	100	100
Specificity	89	96	84	67
Accuracy	90	96	86	85

FNA, fine-needle aspiration; PE, physical examination; PV, predictive value.
[a] See text. All values percentages.
[b] Results of a previous study (104) on this test combination for palpable breast masses in females, for comparison.
Reprinted from Vetto J, Schmidt W, Pommier R, et al. Accurate and cost-effective evaluation of breast masses in males. *Am J Surg* 1998;175:383–387, with permission.

more accurate than PE (five false-positives). Accordingly, Table 19.3 displays the PPVs, NPVs, sensitivities, specificities, and accuracy rates for the detection of malignant lesions by the combination of PE + FNA, in addition to those values for either test alone. For comparison, these same parameters from our previous study of this diagnostic doublet applied to palpable breast lesions in women (104) are also shown. Compared with routine open biopsy, the combination of PE and FNA avoided surgical biopsy in 30 of the 51 lesions and therefore was associated with an average decrease in patient charges of up to $510 per case. We concluded that the combination of PE and FNA for the evaluation of breast masses in males is diagnostically accurate and results in a reduction in patient charges compared with routine open biopsy (88).

The nonoperative evaluation of breast masses can employ either cytology (FNA) or core biopsy, depending on with which modality a given institution has more experience. Whereas core needle biopsy is advocated by many, we (104,105), like others (109–111), favor FNA-based diagnostic schemes for the evaluation of breast masses in females and therefore have applied this same approach to such masses in males. The use of this approach to evaluate breast masses in males is associated with two caveats. First, lesions with concordant negative evaluations are followed clinically, resulting in a "true-negative" rate that is not based on pathology results. Although this method introduces potential error compared with routine open biopsy, in our study, no cancers were detected after up to 60 months of follow-up (which included eight subsequent open biopsies, all benign) (88), consistent with the findings of a study by Somers et al., which showed no tumors developing in female patients with concordant negative triple tests (TTs) after up to 74 months of follow-up (112).

Second, concern may be expressed over the fate of lesions left unbiopsied and the potential effect this could have on patient care and potential charge reductions. The calculated reductions in our study took into account the above-mentioned "failure" rate for observation of benign concordant lesions (21%, or 8 of 38 masses) during the mean follow-up period of 19 months (88). This number is similar to the percentage of older male patients with benign breast conditions who present with pain (20%–34%) as reported in ours and other series (6,8); in fact, we have not had any more "failures" with additional follow-up. Further, given the potential charge reduction of $510 per case with the use of PE + FNA, it would have taken an additional 31 requests for open biopsy in our study (i.e., all remaining observed patients, plus one) to negate the observed cost-effectiveness of this diagnostic approach (88).

Interestingly, the only other report on combined modality evaluation of breast masses in males, a retrospective review from Italy of various combinations of PE, FNA, ultrasonography, and mammography recorded a sensitivity rate (100%) only for the combination of PE and mammography (107). We found the same sensitivity for PE + FNA (Table 19.3) and favor cytologic over mammographic information for the purposes of confidently reassuring patients that they do not need open biopsy and for avoiding disaster in centers where patients diagnosed clinically as having gynecomastia are treated by liposuction (113). Further, the information provided by FNA can be used to distinguish benign from malignant breast masses (114), primary breast cancers from metastases to the breast (115,116), and to determine accurately grade and other tumor features prior to neoadjuvant therapy (especially by adding DNA image cytometry to cytologic evaluation of the material) (117). The combination of history, PE, and mammography has also recently been advocated as being highly accurate for the evaluation of unilateral breast masses in males, but this conclusion was reached retrospectively, and without considering FNA in the analysis (118).

In summary, although open biopsy remains the gold standard for the evaluation of male breast cancer (3,119), it is the most expensive choice and often unnecessary, and use of FNA-based diagnosis can safely avoid it in most cases.

TREATMENT AND OUTCOMES

Surgery

Surgical excision is the mainstay for resectable BCM. For example, most (50 of 54, or 93%) of patients in our review had some type of primary surgical therapy (all three patients who presented with stage IV and one patient with stage IIIB disease did not) (8). Although radical mastectomy (RM) was traditionally the treatment of choice because of the paucity of male breast tissue and the resultant proximity of these lesions to the chest wall, surgical therapy has evolved in both the United States and Europe toward more limited procedures. For example, a 30-year review of 170 cases treated at the National Cancer Institute of Italy in Milan noted a trend from RM to modified radical mastectomy (MRM) and, finally, total mastectomy (TM; for smaller and DCIS lesions) in the later period of the study (14). A similar surgical trend was noted during approximately the same time period in the United States (60,120), and more recent series report that RM is now used infrequently, (8,10,20) probably because of the reported equivalent survival after MRM compared with RM (121) and the fact that most of these tumors do not invade beyond the pectoralis fascia and can be resected with limited in-continuity muscle excision when they do.

The National Cancer Data Base (NCDB) recently reported on a large BCM treatment study in which the treatments received by 3,627 matched pairs of BCM and BCF patients were compared. In this study, men were more likely to be treated with mastectomy than women (MRM, 65% of men versus 55.15% of women; RM, 2.5% of men versus 0.9% of women; TM, 7.6% of men vs. 3.4% of women; $p < 0.001$) (122).

Although two-level axillary dissection remains the gold standard for pathologic staging of the clinically negative axilla in BCM (as it does for BCF as of this writing), a recent case report describes the use of sentinel lymph node biopsy (SLNB) in a BCM case (the sentinel node was negative for tumor, and axillary dissection was not performed) (123). Thus, if SLNB replaces two-level axillary dissection as the standard of care for BCF in the future, it is likely that it will also be applied in males as well, leading in turn to further "downsizing" of the magnitude and morbidity of breast operations in males.

Recommendations already exist for the treatment of DCIS in males with TM rather than MRM (124), and theoretically, one could extend current surgical recommendations for DCIS in females, such as the Van Nuys Prognostic Index (VNPI), (125) to males. Indeed, in our series of recently treated BCMs, five patients with stage T0 or small T1 disease ("minimal breast cancer") were treated with lumpectomy alone, with no local recurrences during the 4.5-year follow-up period (8).

Similar to the management of BCF, potentially curative operative therapy for BCM must be postponed or modified in the event of a concurrent immediately life-threatening condition. This judgment consideration is of particular importance in older men with frequent comorbid conditions. For example, a recent case report from Japan documents a "two-stage" approach to BCM in an 61-year-old man suffering acutely from an aortic dissection. After successfully addressing the dissection, the surgeons removed the tumor with the patient under local anesthetic, completing a definitive breast procedure 1 month later (126)

Radiation

Radiation therapy (RT) has two potential (and opposite) applications for the treatment of BCM. It can and has been used to reduce the reported 4% to 26% postoperative local recurrence rate (5,66), especially when the pectoralis muscle and chest wall are found to be involved at operation. As one would expect, adjuvant use of RT in this setting improves local control, but not disease-related survival (66,127). Conversely, radiation theoretically could be used for breast preservation, especially in cases of DCIS with intermediate VNPI scores (125). In practice, breast preservation requiring RT has not been widely applied to BCM, probably because lumpectomy in men usually requires excision of the nipple; therefore, RT given to avoid mastectomy would not offer significant cosmetic benefit compared with its risks. In our review, RT was used in a minority of patients (13%) and usually only postresection for pectoralis muscle involvement (8). Similarly, men in the previously mentioned NCDB study were more likely to receive RT postmastectomy than their matched female controls (men, 29%; women, 11%; $p < 0.041$) but were less likely to receive RT after lumpectomy (men, 54%; women 68%; $p < 0.001$) (122).

Adjuvant Tamoxifen

Tamoxifen is currently accepted as first-line adjuvant therapy for receptor-positive (i.e., most cases) BCM (81,82) and is often used alone, in part because of the older mean age of patients (i.e., similar to tamoxifen alone in postmenopausal BCF patients), the attendant higher incidences of comorbidity (precluding more aggressive therapy), and the relative lack of data for adjuvant chemotherapy in BCM (see next section). Thirty-nine percent of patients in our series were treated with tamoxifen; not surprisingly, most of these patients were treated in the latter half of the time frame of the database and had receptor-positive tumors (8). An early report by Ribiero and Swindell indicated a 15% improvement in the overall 5-year survival (from 44% to 61%) and a 28% (from 28% to 56%) improvement in the 5-year disease-free survival of tamoxifen-treated patients compared with historical controls. These patients received a relatively short course of treatment (1–2 years) (128). Whereas the current trend is to treat with a more conventional 5-year course, noncompliance with this regimen for BCM is higher than in BCF (25% versus 4%) because tamoxifen is associated with a greater frequency and severity of its well-known dose-limiting side effects in men compared with women. These include (in descending order) decreased libido, weight gain, hot flashes, altered mood, and depression (26).

Adjuvant Chemotherapy

Because of the rarity of BCM, the perceived role of tamoxifen as the cornerstone of adjuvant therapy, and the higher mean age of BCM patients (with attendant lower overall performance status), information on the use of adjuvant cytotoxic chemotherapy for BCM is sparse and retrospective. In a combined experience from Memorial Sloan-Kettering Cancer Center in New York, New York and the Ochsner Clinic in New Orleans, Louisiana, Borgen et al. found a reduction in distant relapse from adjuvant chemotherapy of 11% (from 57% to 46%) for node-positive patients (60). Similarly, an improved 5-year survival rate (80%) compared with stage-matched historical controls has been reported for a cohort of 24 node-positive patients treated with Cytoxan-methotrexate-fluorouracil (129). Similar to the situation in BCF, some data in BCM also suggest a benefit of adjuvant chemotherapy for node-negative disease (130). In our own series, 20% of patients received adjuvant chemotherapy, and one additional patient received it for palliation (8). In the NCDB study, men were less likely to receive chemotherapy than their matched female controls (men, 26.7%; women, 40.6%; $p < 0.001$) after any form of surgical therapy (122).

Autotransplantation

Although the data are limited, one recent study from Roswell Park Cancer Institute in Buffalo, New York, regarding the use of high-dose chemotherapy and autotransplantation for BCM suggested that results are similar to those in BCF patients. These researchers treated 13 BCM patients; six had stage II disease, four were stage III, and three had metastatic disease. Of the 12 tumors tested for hormone receptors, all were positive. The median age at transplantation was 50 years. Five patients received cyclophosphamide, thiotepa, and carboplatin; the other eight patients received other alkylator-based regimens. There were no cases of nonengraftment and no treatment-related deaths. Three of the 10 patients receiving autotransplantation for adjuvant therapy relapsed 3, 5, and 50 months posttransplant and died of disease; the remaining patients were alive with no evidence of disease at the median follow-up time of 23 months (range, 6–50 months). Of the three men treated for metastatic disease, one progressed and the other two relapsed at 7 and 16 months posttransplant (131).

Palliative Therapy

''Downsizing'' tumors with chemotherapy and subsequent salvage mastectomy or palliative chest wall radiation are strategies that have been described for the treatment of advanced local disease (5,60). As one would expect from the high rate of ER and PR expression in BCM, hormonal manipulation has been the cornerstone of the treatment of distant disease since its first description in 1942 by Farrow and Adair, who noted disease regression after orchiectomy (132). Tamoxifen is the current mainstay of palliative hormonal therapy, with overall response rates of 70% for receptor positive tumors (81). Although exact data are lacking, patients with metastatic disease tumors who relapse on tamoxifen probably should be treated with second-line hormonal therapy (similar to the situation for postmenopausal BCF patients), with palliative chemotherapy reserved for nonresponders and receptor-negative tumors.

Prognostic Factors

Similar to BCF, the most significant prognostic factors for BCM are AJCC stage and its elements, tumor size and lymph node status (8,10,20,41,133,134). Lymph node status seems to be particularly important (133,134). This major similarity between BCF and BCM was first established in 1987, when Hultborn and colleagues demonstrated that age, tumor size, and lymph node status were the most important prognosticators by multivariate analysis among a group of 166 BCM patients (133). In 1993, Guinee et al. reported that tumor size greater than 3 cm significantly impaired prognosis and that 5-year survival was directly related to the number of nodes involved: 55% when four or more nodes were positive, 73% for one to three positive nodes, and 90% for node-negative patients (84% at 10 years). Skin involvement, chest wall fixation, and tumor ulceration (all of which are more common in BCM than BCF) were not independently prognostic in their study (134).

More recently, our group reported on a multivariate analysis relating a number of factors to disease-tree survival. We examined the impact of several patient and tumor factors, including the elements of TNM stage, tumor grade (low to intermediate versus high), receptor status (positive versus negative), personal or family history of breast cancer (positive versus negative), age (younger or older than 60), and presentation (asymptomatic versus pain and nipple discharge versus painless mass) for prognostic impact in multivariate analysis using the Cox proportional hazards model (135). Only AJCC stage and its components (tumor size, nodal status, and presence of metastases) correlated with survival (8). We hypothesized that by controlling for the effect of age (by relating to disease-free rather than crude survival), age "dropped out" as significant, unlike earlier studies that used crude survival (see next section) (133). Other recent multivariate analyses have come to similar conclusions (20,41,136,137).

One recent study from South Africa found no major impact of race on median age at presentation, the spectrum of histopathological type, or stage-for-stage 5-year survival in BCM, although blacks tended to present at later stages than did whites (similar to many reports for BCF) (24).

In terms of cellular factors, the importance of hormone receptor positivity has been difficult to ascertain, probably because it is so prevalent in BCM (5). Data regarding the prognostic importance of DNA index and S-phase also has been conflicting (136,138). As of this writing, the importance of *HER2/neu* overexpression (and the role of anti-*HER2/neu* agents) in BCM is unclear. Some reports suggest that the level of tumor expression (by immunohistochemistry) of apolipoprotein D or pepsinogen C may inversely correlate with tumor grade and directly correlate with both relapse-free and overall survival in BCM (139,140).

Prognosis: Are BCM and BCF "Different" Diseases? A Critical Appraisal of the Literature

In terms of prognosis, the essential question in BCM is whether or not the disease is biologically distinct from BCF. As mentioned previously, in part because BCM is a disease of older men (with, by definition, frequent comorbid conditions) who tend to present late [at a mean of 10.2 months in one series (21)], older series, which examined only crude survival (which does not control for age, stage, or comorbidity), reached the inevitable conclusion that it carries a worse prognosis than BCF (14–18, 28–30). This concept also has been fostered by the occasional case report emphasizing widespread and unusual metastases in BCM patients (32,141–143). By the early 1990s, however, some studies were reporting a worse prognosis only for men with positive nodes (19,60) These investigators hypothesized that because most cases of BCM were centrally located, node positivity was a worse sign than in cancers in women.

Subsequent series found similar survival between males and females afflicted with breast cancer when the cases in men were controlled for age and stage (20,21, 144). For example, Borgen et al., reviewing a 16-year, two-institution database, found similar AJCC stage-related survivals between 58 cases of BCM and matched BCF controls (20). Donnegan et al., in an 18-institution review of 217 patients with

BCM, also showed similar stage-related survival to cases of BCF, but they also found late presentation and advanced stage to be a common theme, resulting in a low 10-year survival as a result of censored events (25% of the patients in his series died during follow-up due to noncancer causes) (21).

Accordingly, at our institution, we chose to study a more "recent" cohort of patients who presented mostly to multidisciplinary breast clinics for evaluation of their masses (8). These factors may explain why the mean tumor size in our series (2.7 cm) was smaller than that in even fairly recent reports (15–19,73), that more than half (57%) of our cases were early stage (AJCC stage groupings 0–IIA; half of tumors were stages T0 or T1 at presentation), and 62% were node negative (118 of 604 total lymph nodes removed [19.5%] were pathologically positive for tumor). Whereas these figures are still higher than those for BCF, taken together with the literature as a whole, especially studies of BCM seen at different time frames (19), they do suggest a much called-for trend of increased awareness and earlier diagnosis (81,144). Some of the lower stages seen in our series may be attributable to our previously published standardized approach to breast masses in males, which involves a high index of suspicion combined with rapid and accurate evaluation of the mass in question by aspiration cytology (see "FNA-Based Diagnosis," above). (47,88). This approach has been used for the past nine years at the institutions that contribute data to our studies.

We calculated survival by the method of Kaplan and Meier, counting deaths from other causes as censored events (145). Any significant differences between survival curves were determined by log-rank analysis (146). The overall 5-year disease-free survival for our entire patient group was 87%. As demonstrated in Fig. 19.2, 5- and 10-year disease-related survival rates were AJCC stage-related; 100% and 71%, respectively. for early stage (stage groupings 0–IIA) disease, and 71% and 20% respectively for advanced stage (stage groupings IIB–IV) disease. This difference in survival was highly statistically significant by log-rank test ($p = 0.0051$). Further, Table 19.4 lists the 5-year survivals of the patients in our study by the Surveillance, Epidemiology, and End Results (SEER) database staging system (localized, regionally metastatic, and distant disease), compared with published survival numbers by SEER stages for BCF during approximately the same time as our study (147). As can be seen in Table 19.5, the stage-related 5-year survivals for BCM and BCF were similar.

To reach this finding in our study, we needed only to control only for stage, not age. As alluded to above under "Prognostic Factors," however, it should be noted that the Kaplan-Meier method does control for age in a BCM series somewhat by censoring deaths from other causes, which probably accounts for the low 10-year survivals seen in ours and Donnegan's series (21,145).

All existing data on BCM are marred by its retrospective, historical, and "patchy" nature. We applaud the Commission on Cancer for their efforts in performing a Patient Care Evaluation Study in BCM (81,122) and also Memorial Sloan-Kettering Cancer Center's (New York) ongoing Male Breast Cancer Registry (see section entitled "Tumor Registries" to follow). Based on the trend (Fig. 19.3) we have

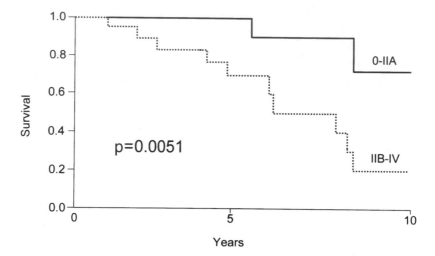

FIG. 19.2. Disease-free survival of males with breast cancer, by American Joint Committee (AJCC) on Cancer stages for early (stage groupings 0–IIA) and late (stage groupings IIB–IV) disease, by the method of Kaplan and Meier. The significance of difference between curves was calculated by the log-rank test. (From Vetto J, Jun S-Y, Paduch D, et al. Stages at presentation, prognostic factors, and outcomes of breast cancer in males. *Am J Surg* 1999;177:379–383, with permission.)

seen in the literature, including our own study (8), one wonders whether future data will show a further decrease in the presenting size and stage of BCM, with survival rates approaching those of BCF, without the necessity for even a stage correction.

At present, this seems doubtful. Although the mean size of tumors in BCF cases is expected to decrease from 1.5 to 1.0 cm in the next 10 years, such a trend for

TABLE 19.4. *Five-year disease-free survival for breast cancer by surveillance, epidemiology, and end results (SEER) stages*

SEER stage	Males[a]	Females[b]
Localized	100%	97%
Regional	81%	78%
Metastatic	33%	22%

[a] Data from the method of Kaplan and Meier.
[b] SEER data for 1989–1994, by the method of Kaplan and Meier, from Fritz A. *SEER cancer statistics review 1973–1995.* Bethesda, MD: NCI Cancer Statistics Branch, 1998, with permission.
  Reprinted from Vetto J, Jun S-Y, Paduch D, et al. Stages at presentation, prognostic factors, and outcomes of breast cancer in males. *Am J Surg* 1999;177:379–383, with permission.

TABLE 19.5. *Comparison of breast cancer in males and females*

Similarities	Differences
Associated factors	Incidence
Age	Association with BRCA1, other syndromes
Exposure to estrogens	Incidence of lobular histology
Chest-wall radiation	Incidence of pure DCIS
Association with BRCA2 mutations	Incidence of hormone receptor expression
Mostly ductal histologies	Ability for early detection
Staging system	Role of mammography
Usefulness of FNA-based diagnosis	Most common location within the breast
Stage-for-stage treatment	Differential diagnosis
Main prognostic factors	Secondary prognostic factors
Stage-for-stage prognosis[a]	
Usefulness of tamoxifen (for receptor positive tumors)	

DCIS, ductal carcinoma *in situ*; FNA, fine-needle aspiration.
[a] When controlled for stage and comorbidity; see text, Table 19.4, and Fig. 19.2.

BCM is unlikely because this is an uncommon disease that is not screened for and therefore will continue to present in most cases as a palpable mass. Nonetheless, a high index of suspicion (81,144) combined with a uniform approach to diagnosis (88) and education of the high-risk population, (41) may bring about continued decreases in stage at presentation and attendant mortality.

For the present, one of the most important implications of the recent information that BCM is not a biologically more aggressive disease than the same condition in

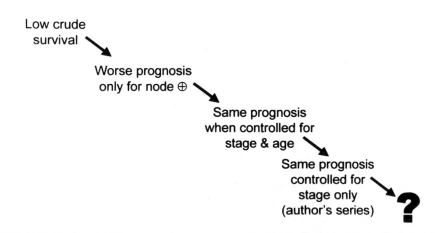

FIG. 19.3. Trends in the outcomes for breast cancer in males, as reported in the literature. See text for discussion.

females is to emphasize to providers that BCM should be treated for cure in most cases. Similar to the situation in females, such treatment should include optimal (but not overly aggressive) local control (19), adjuvant tamoxifen for receptor-positive tumors (most breast tumors in men) (22,81), and consideration of adjuvant chemotherapy for high-risk patients (41,148).

Similarities and Differences between BCM and BCF: A Summary (Table 19.5)

Like BCF, usually BCM is of ductal histology (5,8,10,41,73), is associated with relative estrogen excess (5,14,17,28,34,42,47), is staged by the TNM system (85), and is best treated by multimodality therapy (most often surgery followed by adjuvant therapy). Cases not resectable for cure can be treated by a combination of palliative therapies (surgery, chemotherapy, RT, or hormonal therapy). BCM and BCF appear to have similar prognostic factors (8,10,20,41,133,134) and similar stage-for-stage survival (8,20,21,144), especially if one controls for age and comorbid conditions.

There are also several clear clinical differences between BCM and BCF. Besides the previously noted older mean age for BCM patients, this disease is by definition usually centrally located and often involves the nipple (41). Accordingly, whereas nipple discharge in BCF is usually nonbloody and associated with benign conditions, discharge in BCM is more often bloody and a sign of malignancy, including DCIS, and discharge cytology may be diagnostic (10,11). The vast majority of cases of BCM are hormone-receptor positive [65%–93% in recent studies (20,33,41) and 85% in our series (8)]. Thus, tamoxifen has become the mainstay of therapy for most patients (81,82), although it may be associated with a greater frequency and severity of dose-limiting side effects in men than in women (26).

ISSUES AFTER BREAST CANCER IN MALES

Follow-Up

There are no recommendations for follow-up that are specific to BCM; rather, the same follow-up schedule used for BCF is generally recommended for BCM. For patients with invasive tumors, such schedules usually involve a history and PE (especially clinical breast examination) every 3 months for the first 2 years, then every 6 months for the next 2 years, and then yearly. This follow-up is based on the theory that 75% of recurrences of breast cancer occur in the first 2 years and 10% in the next 2-year period, and the recurrence rate is approximately 1% per year thereafter (149).

Although follow-up for women includes at least yearly mammography, the value of this test for male patients has not been studied and would be expected to be lower than for BCF (see preceding discussion in section entitled "Diagnosis"). Alternatively, CBE would be expected to be particularly important in male patients. An American Society of Clinical Oncology consensus panel on breast cancer follow-up has not found clear follow-up efficacy of other tests, such as liver function tests, alkaline phosphatase levels, and chest radiographs (150), although such tests are commonly ordered (149). Both randomized and nonrandomized studies have demonstrated that more intensive tests for detecting recurrence, such as bone scans, computed tomography scans, and tumor markers, do not confer survival benefit and are best reserved for the detection of metastases in symptomatic patients (149,151).

Testing of Family Members

As noted previously, although there is a known association between BCM development and mutations in the *BRCA2* gene, most cases of BCM are "sporadic" (i.e., not associated with known gene mutations) (152) and *BRCA2* gene mutations appear to have low penetrance in terms of actually causing the disease (65). Accordingly, the questions of whether BCM patients and their relatives should be tested for *BRCA2* mutations and what should be recommended to individuals found to be mutation positive remain open.

For men, the overall risk of BCM among *BRCA2* mutation carriers is 6%. There is no confirmed increased risk among these persons for colon or prostate cancer, two tumors of much higher prevalence (153,154). Thus, the finding that a male individual in a BCM family is a mutation carrier gives little useful preventative information beyond emphasizing that CBE and a low threshold for biopsy of any masses or areas of discharge should be a routine part of that person's regular medical care. Such increased awareness and measures are likely to be instituted for these individuals even without genetic testing.

For female patients, however, the implications of discovering a *BRCA2* mutation are much greater because such mutations confer on these persons a 56% to 87% BCF risk by age 70 (155), a 2% to 12% risk of contralateral BCF within 5 years of a diagnosis of BCF (156), and a 27% ovarian cancer risk by age 70 (157). In a study in Denmark, Storm and Olsen found female, but not male, offspring of BCM patients to have an increased relative risk (16.4) of breast cancer compared with the general population (158).

Accordingly, we would agree with Diez and colleagues that "all new male cases of breast cancer should be regarded as being possibly inherited and should be fully investigated," especially if potential transmissions of *BRCA2* mutations to female offspring are involved (159). In our hands, that investigation involves referral of the BCM patient or offspring to a genetic counselor for complete family history, risk calculation, risk benefit discussion of genetic testing, and *possible BRCA2* gene testing of female offspring. Research on *BRCA2* mutations linked to BCM [such as 3374delA in codon 1049 (exon 11), 6857delAA in codon 2010 (exon 11), 9254delATCAT in codon 3009 (exon 23) (159) and 3414delTCAG (160)], their relative importance in terms of risk, and other gene linkages to BCM, is ongoing.

Tumor Registry

As mentioned previously, Memorial Sloan-Kettering Cancer Center maintains a registry of BCM cases. For further information, contact the National

Male Breast Cancer Registry at *http://mskcc.org/patient_n_public/male_ breast_cancer_cmf.*

Patient Information

Because BCM is similar to BCF in terms of histology, prognostic factors, stage-for-stage prognosis, and treatment recommendations, information regarding breast cancer in general is useful to male patients. The educational Web pages of national breast cancer awareness and support organizations such as the American Cancer Society *(http://acs.org)* and the Susan G. Komen Foundation *(http://www.breast cancer info.com)* also contain sections on BCM. Internet information resources specific to BCM include the Male Breast Cancer Information Page *(http://www.withus. com/interact/mbc) and the Association of Cancer Online Resources' Male Breast Cancer News Group (http://www.empower.acor.org).*

Support Groups

The Bridging the Gap Male Breast Cancer Awareness Group, a group formed in the Portland, Oregon, area by BCM patients and their families, seeks to raise awareness of BCM to promote earlier diagnosis and treatment. The author has had the privilege of serving as a medical advisor for this group. In general, male patients wish to avoid the term *support*; hence, the members have chosen the term *awareness* instead. Initial meetings of the group identified issues for BCM survivors, including several that are common to those of BCF survivors. These include treatment-related fatigue, fear of recurrence, depression (particularly in patients receiving tamoxifen), lymphedema, issues of genetic counseling and testing, concerns about sexual attractiveness, and concerns over long-term side effects of treatment. Issues somewhat unique or of particular importance to male patients include embarrassment related to diagnosis disclosure and discrimination from breast cancer support and information groups (men often feel alone, uncomfortable, or unwanted in such groups because breast cancer is statistically a "female" disease). This group can be reached through Paula Beaulieu, Public Relations Coordinator, at *ironjaw@teleport.com* and through their Web page at *(http://www.geocities.com/bridge_gap_mbcg).*

The John W. Nick Foundation, a not-for-profit private foundation headquartered in Vero Beach, Florida, and named after a BCM patient who died in 1991, is dedicated to breast cancer education for both male and female patients. The group has designed an awareness ribbon that is pink throughout (like the well-known ribbon) except for the left tip, which is blue, symbolizing the fact that breast cancer on occasion affects males as well. The foundation can be reached through its Web page at *http://www.johnwnickfoundation.com.*

RECOMMENDED READING FOR PATIENTS AND THEIR PROVIDERS

Allen T. This man survived breast cancer. *Esquire* 2000;133:103–109.
This is a BCM awareness article that focuses on the various awareness and

support efforts, especially on the part of a particular survivor, Dave Lyons, who is known to me (see Acknowledgments).

Cope JR. *A warrior's way: insights for cancer patients, cancer survivors, and those who love them.* Lake Oswego: Hearts That Care Publishing, 2000.

This book relates the personal story and insights of a BCM survivor who was diagnosed with metastatic disease 14 years ago and has overcome three relapses. Mr. Cope candidly discusses what it is like to have a disease that usually strikes women and emphasizes that all cancer survivors, regardless of their gender or exact diagnosis, must have a "warrior's attitude" rather than allow themselves to become victims.

Landay DS. The complete financial, legal, and practical guide to living with a life-challenging condition. New York: St. Martin's Press, 1998.

A valuable resource for all cancer survivors, regardless of diagnosis, gender, or age.

ACKNOWLEDGMENTS

I gratefully acknowledge the assistance of Si-Youl Jun, M.D., Darius Paduch, M.D., Heidi Eppich, and Richard Shih for their assistance in collection of the Oregon data on breast cancer in males; Waldemar Schmidt, M.D., Ph.D., Rodney Pommier, M.D., John DiTomasso, M.D., Heidi Eppich, William Wood, M.D., and Dane Moseson, M.D., for their contribution to the diagnostic test data for the evaluation of breast masses in males; and Excerpta Medica for granting permission to reprint parts of the resulting publications (8,88). I also thank George Hughes, M.D.; Paula Beaulieu; James Lowery; Dave and Theresa Lyons; Lowell Gere; Bob Miller; Richard Gilbert; and Dr. Duffy Hughes for their assistance and input on the "Issues after Breast Cancer" section of this chapter. The assistance of Irene Perez Vetto R.N., M.N., O.C.N., in reviewing and editing the manuscript is also gratefully acknowledged.

REFERENCES

1. Ellis H. Anatomy of the breast. In: Isaacs JH, ed. *Textbook of breast disease.* St. Louis: Mosby Year Book, 1992:2.
2. Hughes LE, Mansel RE, Webster DJT. *Benign disorders and diseases of the breast: Concepts and clinical management.* London: Bailliere Tindall, 1989:167.
3. Rosen PP, Oberman HS. *Tumors of the mammary gland (atlas of tumor pathology, series 3, fascicle 7).* Washington, DC: Armed Forces Institute of Pathology, 1993:282.
4. Hall R, Anderson J, Smart GA, et al. *Fundamentals of clinical endocrinology.* London: Pitman Medical, 1980:198.
5. Wilhelm MC, Langenburg SE, Wanebo HJ. Cancer of the male breast. In: Bland KI, Copeland EM, eds. *The breast: comprehensive management of benign and malignant disease.* Philadelphia: WB Saunders, 1998:1416–1420.
6. Chantra PK, So JS, Wollman JS, et al. Mammography of the male breast. *AJR Am J Roentgenol* 1995;164:853–858.
7. O'Hanlon DM, Kent P, Kerri MJ, et al. Unilateral breast masses in men over 40: a diagnostic dilemma. *Am J Surg* 1995;170:24–26.

8. Vetto J, Jun S-Y, Paduch D, et al. Stages at presentation, prognostic factors, and outcomes of breast cancer in males. *Am J Surg* 1999;177:379–383.
9. Braunstein GD. Gynecomastia. *N Engl J Med* 1993;328:490–495.
10. Cutuli B, Dilhuydy JM, DeLafontan B, et al. Ductal carcinoma *in situ* of the male breast: analysis of 31 cases. *Eur J Cancer* 1997;33:35–38.
11. Lopez-Rios F, Vargas-Castrillon J, Gonzalez-Palacios F, et al. Breast carcinoma *in situ* in a male: report of a case diagnosed by nipple discharge cytology. *Acta Cytol* 1998;42:742–744.
12. Detraux P, Benmussa M, Tristant H, et al. Breast disease in the male: galactographic evaluation. *Radiology* 1985;154:605–606.
13. Treves N, Robbins GF, Amoroso WL. Serous and serosanguinous discharge from the male nipple. *Arch Surg* 1956;90:319–329.
14. Heller KS, Rosen PP, Shattenfeld DD, et al. Male breast cancer: a clinicopathologic study of 97 cases. *Ann Surg* 1978;188;60–65.
15. Adami HO, Holmberg L, Malker B, et al. Long-term survival in 406 males with breast cancer. *Br J Cancer* 1985;52:99–103.
16. Salvadori B, Saccozzi R, Manzari A, et al. Prognosis of breast cancer in males: an analysis of 170 cases. *Eur J Cancer* 1994:30A:930–935.
17. Cutuli B, Lacroze M, Dilhuydy JM, et al. Male breast cancer: results of the treatment and prognostic factors in 397 cases. *Eur J Cancer* 1995;31A:160–164.
18. Stierer M, Rosen H, Weitensfelder W, et al. Male breast cancer: Australian experience. *World J Surg* 1995;19;687–693.
19. Gough DB, Donohue JH, Evans MM. A 50-year experience of male breast cancer: is outcome changing? *Surg Oncol* 1993;2:325–333.
20. Borgen PI, Senie RT, McKinnon WMP, et al. Carcinoma of the male breast: analysis of prognosis compared to matched female patients. *Ann Surg Oncol* 1997;4:385–388.
21. Donegan WL, Redlich PN, Lang PJ, et al. Carcinoma of the breast in males: a multiinstitutional survey. *Cancer* 1998;83:498–509.
22. Ribeiro G. Male breast carcinoma—a review of 301 cases from the Christie Hospital and Holt Radium Institution, Manchester. *Br J Cancer* 1985;51:115–119.
23. Goss PE, Reid C, Pintilie M, et al. Male breast carcinoma: review of 229 patients who presented to the Princess Margaret Hospital during 40 years: 1955–1996. *Cancer* 1999;85:629–639.
24. Vaizey C, Burke M, Lange M. Carcinoma of the male breast—a review of 91 patients from Johannesburg Hospital breast clinics. *S Afr J Surg* 1999;37:6–8
25. Teixeira MR, Pandis N, Dietrich CU, et al. Chromosome banding analysis of gynecomastia and breast carcinomas in men. *Genes Chromosomes Cancer* 1998;23:16–20.
26. Anelli TF, Anelli A, Tran KN, et al. Tamoxifen administration is associated with a high rate of treatment-limiting symptoms in male breast cancer patients. *Cancer* 1994;74:74–77.
27. Greenlee RT, Murray T, Bolden S, et al. Cancer statistics, 2000. *CA J Clin* 200;50:7–33.
28. Thomas DB, Jimenez LM, McTiernan A, et al. Breast cancer in men: risk factors with hormonal implications. *Am J Epidemiol* 1992;135:734–738.
29. Anderson DE, Badzioch MD. Breast cancer risks in relatives of male breast cancer patients. *J Natl Cancer Inst* 1992;74:1114–1117.
30. Rosenblatt KA, Thomas DB, McTieman A, et al. Breast cancer in men: aspects of familial aggregation. *J Natl Cancer Inst* 1991;83:849–854.
31. Demers PA, Thomas BD, Rosenblatt KA, et al. Occupational exposure to electromagnetic fields and breast cancer in men. *Am J Epidemiol* 1991;134:340–347.
32. DiBenedetto G, Perangeli M, Bertani A. Carcinoma of the male breast: an underestimated killer. *Plast Reconstruct Surg* 1998;102:696–700.
33. Willsher PC, Leach IH, Ellis IO, et al. Male breast cancer: pathological and immunohistochemical features. *Anticancer Res* 1997;17:2335–2338.
34. Sasco AJ, Lowenfels AB, Pasker-deJong P. Epidemiology of male breast cancer. A meta-analysis of published case-control studies and discussion of selected aetiologic factors. *Int J Cancer* 1993; 53:538–549.
35. Moore MP. Male breast cancer. In: Harris JR, Lippman ME, Morrow M, et al., eds. *Diseases of the breast*. Philadelphia: Lippincott–Raven, 1996:859–863.
36. LaVecchia C, Levi F, Luccini F. Descriptive epidemiology of male breast cancer in Europe. *Int J Cancer* 1992;51:62–66.

37. Saltzstein EC, Tanof M, Latomoca R. Breast carcinoma of a young male. *Arch Surg* 1978;113: 880–881.
38. Rosenbaum FF, Vena JE, Zielezny MA, et al. Occupational exposures associated with male breast cancer. *Am J Epidemiol* 1994;139:30–36.
39. Mabuchi A, Bross D, Kessler I. Risk factors in male breast cancer. *J Natl Cancer Inst* 1985;74: 371–375.
40. Tynes T. Electromagnetic fields and male breast cancer. *Biomed Pharmacother* 1993;47:425–427.
41. Memon MA, Donohue JH. Male breast cancer. *Br J Surg* 1997;84:433–435.
42. Hsing AW. McLaughlin JK, Cocco P, et al. Risk factors for male breast cancer. *Cancer Cause Control* 1998;9:269–275.
43. Greene M, Goedert J, Bech-Hansen N, et al. Radiogenic male breast cancer with in vitro sensitivity to ionizing radiation and bleomycin. *Cancer Invest* 1983;1:379–386.
44. Edlar S, Nash E, Abrahamson J. Radiation carcinogenesis in the male breast. *Eur J Surg Oncol* 1989;15:274.
45. Hauser A, Lerner I, King R. Familial male breast cancer. *Am J Med Genet* 1992;44:839–840.
46. Yahalom J, Petrek JA, Biddinger PW, et al. Breast cancer in patients irradiated for Hodgkin's disease: a clinical and pathologic analysis of 45 events in 37 patients. *J Clin Oncol* 1992;10: 1674–1681.
47. Casagrande J, Hanische R, Pike M, et al. A case–control study of male breast cancer. *Cancer Res* 1988;48:1326–1330.
48. Evans DB, Critchlow RW. Carcinoma of male breast and Kleinfelter's syndrome-Is there an association? *CA Cancer J Clin* 1987;37:246–250.
49. Hultborn R, Hanson C, Kopf I, et al. Prevalence of Kleinfelter's syndrome in male breast cancer patients. *Anticancer Res* 1997;17:4293–4297.
50. Schlappack OK, Braun O, Maier U. Report of two cases of male breast cancer after prolonged estrogen treatment for prostatic carcinoma. *Cancer Detect Prev* 1986;9:319–322.
51. Pritchard TJ, Pankowsky DA, Crowe JP, et al. Breast cancer in a male to female transsexual. *JAMA* 1988;259:2278–2280.
52. Symmers W. Carcinoma of the breast in transsexual individuals after surgery and hormonal interference with primary and secondary sex characteristics. *BMJ* 1968;2:82–85.
53. Kanhai RC, Hage JJ, Biomena E, et al. Mammary fibroadenoma in a male-to-female transexual. *Histopathology* 1999;35:183–185.
54. Ballerini P, Recchione C, Cavalleri A, et al. Hormones in male breast cancer, *Tumori* 1990;76: 26–28.
55. Scheike O, Svenstump B, Frandson B. Metabolism of estradiol 17-beta in men with breast cancer. *J Steroid Biochem* 1973;4:489–501.
56. Olsson H, Alm P, Aspergren K, et al. Increased prolactin levels in a group of men with breast cancer: a preliminary study. *Anticancer Res* 1990;10:59–62.
57. Hansen J. Elevated risk for male breast cancer after occupational exposure to gasoline and vehicular combustion products. *Am J Ind Med* 2000;37:349–352.
58. Cocco P, Figgs L, Dosemeci M, et al. Case–control study of occupational exposures and male breast cancer. *Occup Environ Med* 1998;55:599–604.
59. Rosenblatt KA, Thomas DB, Jimenez LM, et al. The relationship between diet and breast cancer in men. *Cancer Causes Control* 1999;10:107–113.
60. Borgen PI, Wong GY, Vlamis V, et al. Current management of male breast cancer. *Ann Surg* 1992; 215:451–457.
61. LaRaja RD, Pagnozzi JA, Rothenberg RE, et al. Cancer of the breast in three siblings. *Cancer* 1985;55:2709–2711.
62. lsson H, Anderson H, Johansson O, et al. Population-based cohort investigations of the risk for malignant tumors in first degree relatives and wives of men with breast cancer. *Cancer* 1993;71: 1273–1278.
63. Kozak FK, Hall JG, Baird PA. Familial breast cancer in males: a case report and review of the literature. *Cancer* 1986;58:2736–2739.
64. Wingren S, vanden Heuvel A, Gentile M, et al. Frequent allelic losses on chromosome 13q in human male breast cancer. *Eur J Cancer* 1997;33:2393–2396.
65. Haraldsson K, Loman N, Zhang QX, et al. BrCa2 germ-line mutations are frequent in male breast cancer patients without a family history of the disease. *Cancer Res* 1998;58:1367–1371.

66. Stratton MR, Ford D, Neuhasen S. Familial male breast cancer is not linked to the BrCa1 locus on chromosome 17q. *Nat Genet* 1994;7:103–107
67. Boyd J, Rhei E, Federici MG, et al. Male breast cancer in the hereditary nonpolyposis syndrome. *Breast Cancer Res Treatment* 1999;53:87–91.
68. Adeyinka A, Mertens F, Bonderson L, et al. Cancer heterogeneity and clonal evolution in synchronous bilateral breast carcinomas and their lymph node metastases from a male patient without ant detectable BRCA2 mutation. *Cancer Genet Cytogenet* 2000;118:42–47.
69. LoBaccaro JM, Lumbroso S, Belon C, et al. Androgen receptor gene mutations in male breast cancer. *Hum Mol Genet* 1993;2:1799–1802.
70. Pich A, Margaria E, Chiusa L, et al. Androgen receptor expression in male breast cancer: lack of clinicopathological association. *Br J Cancer* 1999;79:959–964.
71. Anelli A, Anelli TF, Youngson B. Mutations in the p53 gene in male breast cancer. *Cancer* 1995; 75:2233–2238.
72. Malkin D. p53 and the Li-Fraumeni syndrome. *Biochem Biophys Acta* 1994;1198:197–213.
73. Kollmorgen DR, Varanasi JS, Edge SB, et al. Paget's disease of the breast: a 33 year experience. *J Am Coll Surg* 1998;187:171–177.
74. Takeucki T, Komatsuzaki M, Minesaki Y, et al. Paget's disease arising near a male areola without an underlying carcinoma. *J Dermatol* 1999;26:248–252.
75. Bodnar M, Miller OF III, Tyler W. Paget's disease of the male breast associated with intraductal carcinoma. *J Am Acad Dermatol* 1999;40:829–831.
76. Yildirim E, Turhan N, Pak I, et al. Secretory breast carcinoma in a boy. *Eur J Surg Oncol* 1999; 25:98–99.
77. Bhagwandeen BS, Fenton L. Secretory carcinoma of the breast in a nine year old boy. *Pathology* 1999;31:166–168.
78. Titus J, Sillar RW, Fenton LE. Secretory breast carcinoma in a 9-year-old boy. *Aust N Z J Surg* 2000;70:144–146.
79. Kameyama K, Mukai M, Iri H, et al. Secretory carcinoma of the breast in a 51-year-old male. *Pathol Int* 1998;48:994–997.
80. Winchester DJ. Male breast carcinoma: a multiinstitutional challenge. *Cancer* 1998;83:399–400.
81. Sandler B, Carman C, Perry RR. Cancer of the male breast. *Am Surg* 1994;60:816–820.
82. Mercer RJ, Bryan RM, Bennett RC. Hormone receptors in male breast cancer. *Aust NZ Surg* 1984; 54:215–218.
83. Munoz de Toro MM, Maffini MV, Kass L, et al. Proliferative activity and steroid hormone receptor status in male breast carcinoma. *J Steroid Biochem Mol Biol* 1998;67:333–339.
84. Wick MR, Sayadi H, Ritter JH, et al. Low-stage carcinoma of the male breast: a histologic, immunohistochemical, and flow cytometric comparison with localized female breast carcinoma. *Am J Clin Pathol* 1999;111:59–69.
85. American Joint Committee on Cancer. *AJCC cancer staging manual,* 5th ed. Philadelphia: Lippincott–Raven, 1997:171–180.
86. Appelbaum AH, Evans GF, Levy KR, et al. Mammographic appearances of male breast disease. *Radiographics* 1999;19:559–568.
87. Cooper RA, Gunter BA, Ramamurthy L. Mammography in men. *Radiology* 1994;191:651–656.
88. Vetto J, Schmidt W, Pommier R, et al. Accurate and cost-effective evaluation of breast masses in males. *Am J Surg* 1998;175:383–387.
89. Gellett LR, Farmer KD, Vivian GC. Tc-99m sestimibi uptake in a patient with gynecomastia: a potential pitfall in the diagnosis of breast cancer. *Clin Nucl Med* 1999;24:466.
90. Du Y, Long Y, Ma R. Tc-99m MIBI uptake by a male breast lymphoma accompanied by diffuse bone marrow metastases. *Clin Nucl Med* 1999;24:454–455.
91. Liu M, Hussain SS, Hameer HR, et al. Detection of male breast cancer with Tc-99m methoxyisobutyl isonitrile. *Clin Nucl Med* 1999;24:882–883.
92. Kim SH, Ezekial MP, Kim RY. Primary lymphoma of the breast: breast mass as an initial symptom. *Am J Clin Oncol* 1999;22:381–383.
93. Talwar S, Prasad N, Gandhi S, et al. Hemangiopericytoma of the adult male breast. *Int J Clin Pract* 1999;53:485–486.
94. Vourtsi A, Kehangias D, Antoniou A, et al. Male breast myofibroblastoma and MR findings. *J Comp Assist Tomogr* 1999;23:414–416.
95. Eyden BP, Shanks JH, Ioachim E, et al. Myofibroblastoma of the breast: evidence favoring smooth-muscle rather than myofibroblastic differentiation. *Ultrastruct Pathol* 1999;23:249–257.

96. Chalkiadakis G, Petrakis I, Chrysos E, et al. A rare case of benign mesenchymoma of the breast in a man. *Eur J Surg Oncol* 1999;25:96–97.
97. Rice HE, Acosta A, Brown RL, et al. Juvenile papillomatosis of the breast in male infants: two case reports. *Pediatr Surg Int* 2000;16:104–106.
98. Gupta RK, Saran S, Dowel CS, et al. The diagnostic impact of needle aspiration cytology of the breast on clinical decision making with an emphasis on the aspiration cytodiagnosis of male breast masses. *Diagn Cytopathol* 1991;7:637–639.
99. Das DK, Junaid TA, Mathews SB, et al. Fine needle aspiration cytology diagnosis of male breast lesions: a study of 185 cases. *Acta Cytol* 1995;39:870–876.
100. Slavin JL, Baird LI. Fine-needle aspiration cytology in male breast carcinoma. *Pathology* 1996; 28:122–124.
101. Sneige N, Holder PD, Katz RL, et al. Fine-needle aspiration cytology of the male breast in a cancer center. *Diagn Cytopathol* 1993;9:691–697.
102. Joshi A, Kapila K, Verma K. Fine needle aspiration cytology in the management of male breast masses: nineteen years of experience. *Acta Cytol* 1999:43:334–338.
103. Cooper RA, Ramamurthy L. Epidermal inclusion cysts in the male breast. *Can Assoc Radiol* 1996; 47:92–93 .
104. Vetto JT, Pommier RP, Schmidt W, et al. Use of the "triple test" for palpable breast lesions yields high diagnostic accuracy and cost savings. *Am J Surg* 1995;169:519–522.
105. Vetto JT, Pommier RF, Schmidt WA, et al. Diagnosis of palpable breast lesions in younger women by the modified triple test is accurate and cost effective. *Arch Surg* 1996;131:967–974.
106. Morris A, Pommier RF, Schmidt WA, et al. Accurate evaluation of palpable breast lesions by the "triple test score." *Arch Surg* 1998;133:930–934.
107. Ambrogetti D, Ciatto S, Catarzi S, et al. The combined diagnosis of male breast lesions: a review of a series of 748 cases. *Radiol Med* 1996;91:356–359.
108. Tukel S, Ozcan H. Mammography in men with breast cancer: review of the mammographic findings in five cases. *Aust Radiol* 1996;40:387–390.
109. Layfield LJ. Can fine-needle aspiration replace open biopsy in the diagnosis of palpable breast lesions? *Am J Clin Pathol* 1992;98:145–147.
110. Costa MJ, Tadras T, Hilton G, et al. Breast fine needle aspiration cytology: utility as a screening tool for clinically palpable lesions. *Acta Cytol* 1993;37:461–471.
111. Sneige N. Fine needle aspiration of the breast: a review of 1,995 cases with emphasis on diagnostic pitfalls. *Diagn Cytopathol* 1994;9:106–112.
112. Somers RG, Sandler GL, Kaplan MJ, et al. Palpable abnormalities of the breast not requiring excisional biopsy. *Surg Gynecol Obstet* 1992;174:325–328.
113. Samdal F, Kleppe G, Amland PF, et al. Surgical treatment of gynecomastia: five years experience with liposuction. *Scan J Plastic Reconstruct Surg Hand Surg* 1994;28:123–130.
114. McCluggage WG, Sloan S, Kenny BD, et al. Fine needle aspiration cytology (FNAC) of mammary granular cell tumor: a report of three cases. *Cytopathology* 1999;10:383–389.
115. Deshpande AH, Munshi MM, Lele VP, et al. Aspiration cytology of extramammary tumors metastatic to the breast. *Diagn Cytopathol* 1999;21:319–323.
116. Gupta RK. Immunoreactivity of prostate-specific antigen in male breast carcinomas: two examples of a diagnostic pitfall in discriminating a primary breast cancer from metastatic prostate carcinoma. *Diagn Cytopathol* 1999;21:167–169.
117. Dey P, Luthra UK, Prasad A, et al. Cytologic grading and DNA image cytometry of breast carcinoma on fine needle aspiration cytology smears. *Anal Quant Cytol Histol* 1999;21:17–20.
118. Volpe CM, Rafetto JD, Collure DW, et al. Unilateral male breast masses: cancer risk and their evaluation and management. *Am Surg* 1999;65:250–253.
119. Dershaw DD, Borgen PI, Deutch BM, et al. Mammographic findings in men with breast cancer. *AJR Am J Roentgenol* 1993;160:267–270.
120. Kinne D, Hakes T. Male breast cancer. In: Harris J, Hellman S, Henderson IC, eds. *Breast diseases*. Philadelphia: JB Lippincott, 1991:782–789.
121. Hodson GR, Urdaneta LF, Al-Jurf AS, et al. Male breast carcinoma. *Am Surg* 1985;51:47–49.
122. Scott-Conner CE, Jochimsen PR, Menck HR, et al. An analysis of male and female breast cancer treatment and survival among demographically identical pairs of patients. *Surgery* 1999;126: 775–780.
123. Hill AD, Borgen PI, Cody HS III. Sentinel node biopsy in male breast cancer. *Eur J Surg Oncol* 1999;25:442–443 .

124. Camus MG, Joshi MG, Mackarem G, et al. Ductal carcinoma in situ in the male breast. *Cancer* 1994;74:1289–1293
125. Silverstein MJ, Lagios MD, Craig PH, et al. Developing a prognostic index for ductal carcinoma in situ. *Cancer* 1996;78:1138–1140.
126. Uematsu M, Okada M, Ataka K. Two-step approach for the operation of male breast cancer: report of a case at high risk for surgery. *Kobe J Med Sci* 1998;44:163–168.
127. Stranzl H, Mayer R, Quehenberger F, et al. Adjuvant radiotherapy in male breast cancer. *Radiother Oncol* 1999;53:29–35.
128. Ribiero G, Swindell R. Adjuvant tamoxifen for male breast cancer. *Br J Cancer* 1992;65:252–254.
129. Bagley C, Wesley M, Young R, et al. Adjuvant chemotherapy in males with cancer of the breast. *Am J Clin Oncol* 1987;10:55–60.
130. Jaiyesimi IA, Buzdar A, Sahin A, et al. Carcinoma of the male breast. *Ann Intern Med* 1992;117: 771–777.
131. McCarthy P, Hurd D, Rowlings P, et al. Autotransplantation in men with breast cancer. ABMRT Breast Cancer Working Committee. Autologous Blood and Marrow Transplant Registry. *Bone Marrow Transplant* 1999;24:365–368.
132. Farrow J, Adair F. Effects of orchiectomy on skeletal metastases from cancer of the male breast. *Science* 1942;95:654–657.
133. Hultborn R, Friberg S, Hultborn KA, et al. Male breast carcinoma. II. A study of the total material reported to the Swedish Cancer Registry 1958–1967 with respect to treatment, prognostic factors, and survival. *Acta Oncol* 1987;26:327–341.
134. Guinee VF, Olsson H, Moller T, et al. The prognosis of breast cancer in males. *Cancer* 1993;71: 154–161.
135. Cox DR. Regression models and life-tables. *J R Stat Soc* 1972;4:187–220.
136. Hatschek T, Wingren S, Carstensen J, et al. DNA content and S-phase fraction in male breast carcinomas. *Acta Oncol* 1994;33:609–613.
137. Hill A, Yagmur Y, Tran KN, et al. Localized male breast carcinoma and family history. *Cancer* 1999;86:821–825.
138. Hecht RJ, Winchester DJ. Male breast cancer: review. *Am J Clin Pathol* 1994;102(Suppl):S25–S30.
139. Serra Diaz C, Vizoso F, Lamelas ML, et al. Expression and clinical significance of apolipoprotein D in male breast cancer and gynecomastia. *Br J Surg* 1999;86:1190–1197.
140. Serra Diaz C, Vizoso F, Rodriguez JC, et al. Expression of pepsinogen C in gynecomastias and male breast carcinomas. *World J Surg* 1999;23:439–445.
141. Garcia GH, Weinberg DA, Glasgow BJ, et al. Carcinoma of the male breast metastatic to both orbits. *Opthal Plast Reconstruct Surg* 1998;14:130–133.
142. Kim JH, Benson PM, Beard JS, et al. Male breast carcinoma with extensive metastases to the skin. *J Am Acad Dermatol* 1998;38:995–996.
143. Kreusel KM, Heimann H, Bornfeld N, et al. Choroidal metastasis in men with metastatic breast cancer. *Am J Opthalmol* 1999;128:253–255.
144. Fullerton JT, Lantz J, Sadler GR. Breast cancer among men; raising awareness for primary prevention. *J Am Acad Nurse Pract* 1997;9:211–216.
145. Kaplan EL, Meier P. Nonparametric estimation from incomplete observations. *J Am Statist Soc* 1958;53:457–481.
146. Peto R, Peto J. Asymptotically efficient rank invariant test procedures. *J R Statist Soc* 1972;35: 185–206.
147. Fritz A. *SEER cancer statistics review, 1973–1995.* Bethesda: NCI Cancer Statistics Branch, 1998.
148. Wagner JL, Thomas CR Jr, Koh W-J, et al. Carcinoma of the male breast: update. *Med Pediatr Oncol* 1995;24:123–132.
149. Joseph E, Hyacinthe M, Lyman GH, et al. Evaluation of an intensive strategy for follow-up and surveillance of primary breast cancer. *Ann Surg Oncol* 1998;5:522–529.
150. American Society of Clinical Oncology. Recommended breast cancer surveillance guidelines. *J Clin Oncol* 1997;15:2149–2156.
151. The Givio Investigators. Impact of follow up testing on survival and health-related quality of life in breast cancer patients: a multicenter randomised controlled trial. *JAMA* 1995;271:1587–1592.
152. Tirkkonen M, Kainu T, Loman N, et al. Somatic genetic alterations in BRCA2-associated and sporadic male breast cancer. *Gene Chromosomes Cancer* 1999;24:56–61.
153. Easton DF, Steele L, Fields P, et al. Cancer risks in two large breast cancer families linked to BRCA2 on chromosome 13q12-13. *Am J Hum Genet* 1997;61:120–128.

154. Couch FJ, Farid LM, DeShano ML, et al. BRCA2 germline mutations in male breast cancer patients and breast cancer families. *Nat Genet* 1996;13:123–125.
155. Struewing JP, Hartge P, Wachholder S, et al. The risk of cancer associated with specific mutations of BRCA1 and BRCA2 among Ashkenazi Jews. *N Engl J Med* 1997;336:1401–1408.
156. Verhoog LC, Brekelmans CTM, Seynaeve C, et al. Survival in hereditary breast cancer associated with germline mutations of BRCA2. *J Clin Oncol* 1999;17:3396–3402.
157. Ford D, Easton DF, Stratton M, et al. Genetic heterogeneity and penetrance analysis of the BRCA1 and BRCA2 genes in breast cancer families. *Am J Hum Genet* 1998;62:676–689.
158. Storm HH, Olsen J. Risk of breast cancer in offspring of male breast-cancer patients (letter). *Lancet* 1999;353:209.
159. Diez O, Cortes J, Domenech M, et al. BRCA2 germ-line mutations in Spanish male breast cancer patients. *Ann Oncol* 2000;11:81–84.
160. Balchi A, Huusko P, Pakkonen K, et al. Mutation analysis of BRCA1 and BRCA2 in Turkish cancer families: a novel mutation BRCA2 3414del4 found in male breast cancer. *Eur J Cancer* 1999;35:707–710.

20

Psychosocial Support for the Breast Cancer Patient

Patricia A. Ganz

Breast cancer is the most common cancer in women, accounting for about one third of all incident cancers each year (1). With advances in the early detection of breast cancer, as well as highly successful adjuvant therapies, many women can expect long-term survival from this disease. The price of such success, however, is increasingly complex therapy. Gone are the days of surgery alone, with recovery from primary treatment in about a month's time. Because of intense media attention, breast cancer screening campaigns, and greater openness in discussing a diagnosis, women have heightened awareness and anxiety about the risk of breast cancer. Thus, although somewhat more informed about breast cancer, women still are not prepared psychologically when a screening mammogram detects cancer.

Breast cancer treatment is usually multidisciplinary and necessitates careful coordination of treatment among several types of specialists (e.g., surgery, radiation therapy, chemotherapy). The increased number of doctors and the disparate opinions they sometimes provide to the patient can lead to increased psychological distress. Often the primary care provider will not have the expertise to make specific treatment recommendations for the cancer patient; however, it is his or her role to make sure the patient's situation is adequately reviewed by cancer treatment specialists and that certain standards of care are maintained. Understanding that the processes set in motion by an abnormal mammogram can "snowball" into a long, protracted diagnostic process (with attendant psychological distress) can help health professionals support their patients at this time. The increased complexity of primary breast cancer treatment is a major contributor to the psychosocial distress most women experience. Nevertheless, the extensive literature on the psychosocial aspects of breast cancer does not demonstrate major excess in psychiatric morbidity or psychological distress in women with breast cancer (2–5). This chapter focuses on the most frequent psychosocial issues facing women with breast cancer, including their informational needs at the time of diagnosis and thereafter as well as psychological distress associated with primary treatment, survivorship, and recurrence. As each topic is reviewed, strategies to provide support for the patient are addressed.

INFORMATIONAL NEEDS OF THE WOMAN WITH BREAST CANCER

In a 1980 review of the psychosocial correlates of breast cancer (6), Meyerowitz described the critical role of the doctor–patient relationship as a source of support for the patient. Meyerowitz noted that multiple "authors have pointed out that the attitudes of physicians are carefully scrutinized and can have a tremendous impact on the attitudes and emotional states of patients" (6). The physician is in a pivotal position to provide guidance and emotional support. Ervin (7) suggests that the surgeon is in the best position to apply preventive counseling by presenting an honest but hopeful presentation of the physical and psychological aspects of the disease and its treatment. Other researchers suggest that physicians must be aware of individual patient differences in the response to cancer and to avoid common misconceptions and biases (6).

Since the early 1980s, the treatment of breast cancer has become more complex, with most women receiving some form of postoperative adjuvant therapy (8). As a result, the breast cancer patient interacts with several different physicians who may vary in their ability to provide information and counseling. In addition, different physicians may provide conflicting information or opinions. Concurrent social trends—the consumer movement, increasing patient autonomy, greater openness about breast cancer—have influenced the content of physician–patient interactions at the time of breast cancer diagnosis (5). The early diagnostic and treatment phase of breast cancer management is the point of highest psychological distress and uncertainty for most women today (5,9,10).

Rowland and Holland (5) reviewed the informational needs and decision-making patterns for women with early breast cancer and noted the following: "The current climate which dictates a single approach to all women fails to take into account the fact that reactions of women to the decision-making process vary widely. Ideally, information should be conveyed in different ways for each patient" (5). Although shared decision making is the goal in current doctor–patient encounters, it is often not feasible. For one reason, the patient has the disadvantage of having less information and experience than the physician and is often in a "crisis mode" after being told that the diagnosis is breast cancer. For the woman who has an information-seeking style of interaction, assuring her that the decision-making process need not be rushed and allowing her time to gather information, including second opinions, is often an important strategy. Other women may feel more comfortable deferring to the physician's recommendation without questioning; nevertheless, it is important that these women are given adequate information about their diagnosis and prognosis, along with including a significant family member if she wishes.

Numerous strategies are useful in communicating complex information that can facilitate shared decision making. These strategies include providing written information or tape recording the consultation, so it can be replayed at home, the use of multidisciplinary breast clinics to coordinate medical consultation and consolidate recommendations, and the use of nurse specialists in breast cancer to provide continuity of care and support. Further research on the decision-making process and the methods by which information about treatment options are conveyed is warranted (11).

Dramatic changes have occurred in the extent to which cancer patients are informed of their diagnosis; however, the amount and type of information disclosed beyond the diagnosis vary widely (12,13). Simonoff (13) suggests that there are four essential components of satisfactory communication between doctor and patient: (a) discussing the rationale for the procedure, (b) making sure that the patient underand stands the risks involved, (c) communicating the potential benefits of the procedure, and (d) explaining any treatment alternatives available. The benefits of effective communication include improved recall and understanding of what was said, increased patient and physician satisfaction and reduction of patient anxiety, increased adherence to medication and treatment plans, and improved patient survival and quality of life (12,13).

The communication process between patients and physicians is complicated, and cancer patients often present a special set of problems because of the seriousness of the illness and the complexity of the treatment. Miller (14) showed that patients differ in their informational style (monitors versus blunters) and decision-making preferences, without expected concordance between styles and preferences. The key to effective physician–patient communication seems to be the match between the patient's needs and style and the physician's response. Physicians vary in the amount of information they provide to patients (15), but it is clear that most patients desire information, with several studies documenting improved patient outcomes from more accurate information (16,17). In a study that examined communication between breast cancer surgeons and their patients, it was found that these physicians communicated in the same way to all patients rather than tailoring their communications to the individual patient (18).

Several studies documented poor patient understanding of information as an important barrier in this process (13). Multiple studies demonstrate poor patient recall of chemotherapy side effects or expected outcomes from therapy, even when the information communication has been documented by audiotape (12). Others also observed that numeric rather than verbal descriptors are most effective (13). Several studies point to the need for additional patient education materials (written, audio, and videotape) to enhance patient understanding of her particular situation. Attention to these communication issues is critical in reducing the anxiety and distress that accompany the diagnosis of breast cancer and the attendant treatment decisions that follow.

MANAGING PSYCHOSOCIAL CONCERNS DURING PRIMARY TREATMENT OF BREAST CANCER

Once the treatment plan is decided for the woman with breast cancer, she will experience some relief of anxiety and distress, but she now has to face the hurdle of receiving the planned treatment. Surgery, particularly lumpectomy and axillary dissection, is often done as an outpatient or short stay procedure. Even the length of hospital stay for mastectomy has been shortened from what it was just a few years ago. This means that someone must be available to assist the woman at home, particularly with household tasks and some nursing care (e.g., drains). Women undergoing mastectomy and immediate reconstruction, especially with flaps, will have longer hospitalizations and a more protracted recovery from surgery. Women need to be prepared for what to expect with each of these procedures, and such preparation is important for her psychological well-being and recovery.

Similarly, women benefit from being prepared for the experience of radiation therapy. Many women feel anxiety associated with being in the treatment room "all alone" while the therapy is being delivered. They must become comfortable with the loss of modesty associated with baring their breast and disrobing among technical staff. In addition, the variation in skin reactions and local symptoms associated with 6 weeks of daily radiation therapy need to be explained to women, so that they understand what to expect as treatment proceeds. It is important for the medical staff to attend to these symptoms when they arise and to provide reassurance about their normalcy and the expected eventual recovery and successful result. Some women electing breast conservation will experience lingering doubts about the comparable efficacy of this treatment approach to mastectomy, and they may need continued support and reassurance about their treatment choice. Finally, the waiting room of the radiation therapy department can sometimes be distressing to breast cancer patients, especially when they share their visits with patients who are much sicker and who are receiving palliative therapy for advanced cancer. Nursing and physician staff should acknowledge these issues and address them directly when breast cancer patients report their concerns about their own health and mortality.

Adjuvant therapies for breast cancer vary considerably, depending on the unique characteristics of each woman's tumor. In support groups and waiting rooms, many breast cancer patients compare notes with other patients and often learn that their treatments differ from that of the other women in their support group or in the office waiting room. It is important to reassure women about the varied prognoses of women with breast cancer and that many different treatment strategies can be used for the same stage of disease. It is best for a woman to receive as much information and consultation as necessary before embarking on a course of adjuvant treatment. This can ensure that she understands what is the most appropriate treatment for her (given medical, personal, and social factors). The process of gathering information will be stressful but usually leads to better understanding and acceptance of the treatment plan.

Most adjuvant chemotherapy is well tolerated and women often continue to do many of their usual activities (child care, household activities, paid employment) albeit on a reduced schedule, especially modified by treatment administration. Hair loss, nausea, and vomiting are among the most distressing side effects, followed by fatigue and changes in body image. The difficulty here is that this treatment takes someone who is healthy and who is trying to recover physically and psychologically from surgery and a diagnosis of cancer, and adds additional physical symptoms for a period of 4 to 6 months. While perceived by most women as a reasonable "insurance policy" against subsequent breast cancer recurrence, adjuvant treatment decreases quality of life while it is being given. Many women have a love–hate relationship with adjuvant treatment, feeling protected by it and even wanting more intensive therapies, but nevertheless feeling distressed and overwhelmed by some of the physical symptoms they experience while receiving treatment. The medical and nursing staff can help the patient by vigorously addressing side effects and symptoms, referring her to a support group during this time and reassuring her about the medical rationale for the treatment and its likely benefit.

Tamoxifen therapy may be the sole adjuvant therapy or can be combined with chemotherapy in some women. Whereas the medical evidence for its benefits in improving survival and reducing the risk for breast cancer recurrence is overwhelming, in the eyes of many women it is still seen as a controversial and potentially toxic therapy. Women may be especially concerned about the risk of endometrial cancer, and physicians must directly address the risks and benefits of tamoxifen therapy with each patient. Other frequent concerns about tamoxifen expressed by women relate to possible depression, weight gain, hot flashes, and decreased sexual functioning. Many of these problems are common in breast cancer survivors and are not specifically related to the drug tamoxifen. The recently reported Breast Cancer Prevention Trial is the only randomized, placebo-controlled trial to study the effects of tamoxifen on symptoms and quality of life (19). In this study of more than 13,000 healthy women at high risk for breast cancer, only hot flashes and vaginal dryness were significantly increased in women taking tamoxifen (19). There was no increase in depression or weight gain as a result of taking this medication and no serious changes in sexual functioning. Thus, we can now use this information to reassure women who are recommended to take tamoxifen as adjuvant therapy.

SPECIAL NEEDS OF PATIENTS WITH DUCTAL CARCINOMA *IN SITU*

With the increasing use of screening mammography, the rate of diagnosis of noninvasive ductal carcinoma *in situ* (DCIS) has increased tremendously. In some communities, DCIS cases account for as many as 20% of the incident cases of breast cancer. Although the potential benefits of diagnosing an early noninvasive cancer are clear, for many women the anxiety associated with this condition is tremendous. Many women feel placed in limbo, where they are told that their condition is not serious, and yet they receive local treatments that are analogous to the woman with invasive breast cancer. Despite the efficacy of local treatment with breast conservation, they face a continuous risk of recurrent disease in the involved breast. For many younger women, this situation can be very distressing, with the uncertainty and risk labeling effect of this diagnosis. As women with DCIS face menopause, they often struggle with whether hormone replacement therapy is safe given their medical history. The combination of the breast cancer risk status and uncontrolled menopausal symptoms can severely affect quality of life for this unique group of breast cancer patients. Specialized support groups are often very helpful under these circumstances and can allow these women to share their concerns and apprehensions with women who have a similar diagnosis.

PREPARING FOR SURVIVORSHIP: GOING OFF PRIMARY TREATMENT

At the end of primary breast cancer treatment–whether it is at the conclusion of 6 weeks of radiation therapy or after 4 to 6 months of adjuvant chemotherapy–most women experience a mixture of elation, fear, and trepidation. Although they have mastered the many aspects of their treatment regimen, they have little preparation and information to guide them in their recovery from treatment. This is coupled with their planned discharge from intensive interaction with the health care system. No longer do they have daily visits or visits every 3 weeks to the treatment center, and they may not have a scheduled return visit for several months after the completion of therapy. In some managed care settings, the woman may have no further contact with the oncology treatment team and will be referred back to her primary care physician. With whom will she talk about the nonspecific joint pains bothering her or the fatigue and difficulty sleeping she is still experiencing? Could these be signs of recurrence? Why is she still experiencing so much fatigue when her treatments ended several weeks ago? Why is her family not paying as much attention to her, and why do they expect life to go back to normal when for her it has been forever changed?

During the past decade, the oncology care system has developed many structured ways to educate newly diagnosed patients about the rationale for primary breast cancer treatments. In addition, a variety of supporting staff (nurses, social workers, support groups) and written materials are available to inform and guide patients through this stressful and physically challenging period. At this time, little systematic information is available about the time when women go off treatment and make the transition from patient to survivor. So little is known about this time that this is one focus of my current research program. Clinically experienced physicians are well aware of the stressful features of this transition time, and they attempt to prepare women by telling them that it may take several months to a year to recover fully from the effects of treatment. For women initiating therapy with adjuvant tamoxifen, additional new symptoms may be a problem. Information and reassurance are often very helpful by providing the patient with realistic expectations about the trajectory of recovery. A program of research at the University of California Los Angeles sponsored by the National Cancer Institute is currently investigating an intervention strategy to prepare women for this transitional period.

LONGER-TERM SURVIVORSHIP

There has been growing interest in the late effects of breast cancer treatment and the quality of life of long-term survivors beyond the acute phase of treatment. Several published studies have compared breast cancer survivors to healthy, age-matched populations of women and have found few differences in their physical or emotional well-being (3,4,10,20). There is some evidence that women who receive adjuvant therapy may have more physical disruption than those who receive no further therapy

(21) and that women who receive chemotherapy may have more sexual dysfunction than survivors who did not receive similar therapy (4). Other ongoing concerns for these survivors relate to their menopausal status and the relative prohibition of hormone replacement therapy. In addition to vasomotor symptoms and vaginal dryness, which can be clinically troubling, a more serious medical consequence for some women is premature osteoporosis and fractures. Ongoing systematic research with survivors, especially those who become menopausal prematurely as a result of chemotherapy, may help to delineate preventive interventions that can modify this risk. Cognitive dysfunction is another identified late effect of adjuvant therapy (22). The etiology and specific mechanisms and drugs that are responsible are other areas of active investigation. Trials to address the efficacy and safety of hormone replacement in breast cancer survivors are also under way, and these studies may provide better guidance about how to treat the symptoms of estrogen deficiency in this patient population.

BREAST CANCER RECURRENCE

Recurrence of breast cancer is undoubtedly the most stressful time for patients and their doctors. For both, it is perceived as a failure of primary therapy, and most sophisticated patients know that recurrent disease is seldom curable. Whereas shock and disbelief are common emotions at diagnosis, hopefulness and a treatment plan that is touted to forestall recurrence often counter these emotions. In contrast, recurrent breast cancer is usually insidious in its onset, occurs despite careful follow-up and past treatment, and often is associated with clinical symptoms such as pain, cough, or the development of soft tissue metastases. The clinical symptoms of recurrence provide tangible evidence of the seriousness of the situation, and all the emotions that were associated with the time of diagnosis are likely to recur and be intensified.

This time is often challenging for the patient, her family, and the treatment team. Women who faced their initial treatment with aggressive treatments are often unwilling to accept less intensive treatments at recurrence. In recent years, many of them sought high-dose therapy programs despite insufficient evidence for their treatment efficacy. Often this occurred because these women were reluctant to face long-term and unending therapies. They perceived intensive but time-limited, ''potentially curative'' therapies as an alternative to protracted course of chemotherapy. To some extent, this approach is probably fulfilling a psychological need to gain some control over an uncontrolled situation. For many of these women, taking an action, obtaining second opinions, and seeking experimental therapies becomes the focus of their efforts. Other women will be more accepting of their situation and will see breast cancer as chronic condition that can be controlled long-term, even if it is not cured.

It is important for the treatment team to gauge the psychological needs of the patient with recurrence. She should be supported in her efforts to obtain as much information about the types of treatments available for her situation. Control of pain and symptoms should be attended to while restaging and information gathering are occurring. Support groups and individual counseling can be particularly useful at this time in the breast cancer experience. Some studies have demonstrated improved survival for women with metastatic breast cancer participating in support groups (23). Similar to the transition from patient to survivor, the time of breast cancer recurrence has had limited systematic study. A trial currently under way in the Southwest Oncology Group is testing a psychoeducational telephone counseling intervention in this population to determine whether it will have an impact on quality of life.

PALLIATIVE CARE

Attention to the symptomatic and pain relief needs of the woman with advanced breast cancer is central to her emotional well-being. With uncontrolled pain, she will function at a lower level and will be more withdrawn for those around her. Many women try to maintain their usual social roles as mother, spouse, or caretaker and will continue working until they have major functional impairments. Spiritual and existential matters often mark this phase of the illness, as women focus on their legacy to their families and children. Support groups can be useful in this phase of the illness; however, individual counseling from mental health professionals or clergymen may be more appropriate as women look for ways to specify their wishes for those they leave behind. Active preparation for the end of life can give many women a sense of personal and emotional control at a time when they have little control over their symptoms or the disease course. The medical team is crucial for its role in addressing physical symptoms and ensuring that the woman is able to find emotional closure for difficult relationships or ongoing worries. Listening to the woman and supporting her in the resolution of her psychosocial concerns are critical. Hospice services can assist the medical team in carrying out these responsibilities, and they should be called in as early as possible when curative intent therapy is no longer appropriate.

CROSS-CUTTING PSYCHOSOCIAL ISSUES

Sexuality and Intimacy

Establishing or continuing intimate relationships is sometimes difficult for the woman with breast cancer. The lack of a secure and healthy future, as well as the feeling of increased vulnerability, can interfere with the establishment of new relationships. For women with a supportive partner, the cancer experience often enhances the relationship and the quality of the sexual relationship (24,25). If tensions were present in the relationship prior to the cancer diagnosis, however, breast cancer often exacerbates the situation. It is rare that the cancer itself is the cause of divorce or separation. Rather, the breast cancer survivor is likely to reevaluate the good and bad aspects of the relationship and make a decision about its continuation based on long-standing issues as well as the cancer crisis.

Sexual functioning is a topic of considerable concern to most breast cancer patients (26,27). Nonetheless, physicians rarely address sexual matters with patients, assuming that all is going well if the patient is disease free and not on treatment. In our research with breast cancer survivors (26), issues related to sexual functioning were the most persistent and severe problems reported, and these difficulties often worsen in the years after breast cancer treatment (10). Only the most vocal or severely distressed patients will discuss these problems with their physician; yet, when asked about how their sex life is, most women will provide specific information about the difficulties they are having. Sexual dysfunction is common in the general population, and the treatments for breast cancer often make normal situations worse (e.g., increased fatigue, premature menopause, withdrawal of hormone replacement therapy). Many sexual problems can be addressed with counseling or with medications. In a recently completed randomized trial, we found that providing information, counseling, and pharmacologic management of menopausal symptoms (including vaginal dryness) in breast cancer survivors significantly improved sexual functioning (28). Most often, the physician can address these problems directly or refer the patient to an appropriate resource. Provision of information and reassurance are important starting points for most patients.

Parenting Issues

Cancer is a family disease in that everyone is affected when a member of the family has cancer. The woman's role in the family and the severity of her disease and treatment will affect the family's functioning. To a certain extent, the age of the children, their life stage, and the role of the other parent during the cancer experience can modify the effects on children. Early on, the physician should inquire about the welfare of the children of the patient. In many communities, there are resources for younger and older children whose parents have cancer. In general, women should be encouraged to be open with their children about their medical history, with a level of information that is age appropriate. Sometimes patients face difficult situations, such as during custody disputes or adoption proceedings. It is not unheard of for the health of the patient to be challenged and their ability to parent questioned. The physician can be supportive by providing accurate information about the patient's status and capabilities.

Fertility and Childbearing

The future ability to have children is a critical issue for some women with breast cancer. Some women become infertile as a result of adjuvant chemotherapy; this can be the complete cessation of menses or menstrual irregularity with anovulatory cycles. Even if menstrual cycles are maintained, many women receive conflicting information about the risk of breast cancer recurrence with pregnancy (29,30). Limited scientific data are available on this subject, and often patients are presented with anecdotal information from a variety of sources. Nevertheless, the desire to bear a child is very strong for many women, and the choice is a personal one. Women must be supported in whatever decision they make regarding this matter.

Fear of Recurrence

This is one of the most persistent psychological consequences of a cancer diagnosis. The intensity of this fear tends to diminish with time; however, many seasoned breast cancer survivors will recount their anxiety and fear during an annual checkup decades after the initial cancer diagnosis. It is common for minor aches and pains to generate considerable anxiety early on in the survivorship experience. A reassuring relationship with the physician, with open discussion of how to manage and assess these aches and pains, can assure the patient that transient and fleeting complaints are common in everyone. Patients have different levels of anxiety; often reaching certain landmarks (e.g., 5-year survivorship) leads to diminishment of these fears.

CONCLUSIONS

The overwhelming majority of women face a breast cancer diagnosis with courage and dignity. They learn how to cope with the threat of death as well as the toxicities of various treatments. Through much of their experience with breast cancer, they "put on a brave front" and try not to burden others with their physical and emotional problems. Nevertheless, when asked to share their experiences with researchers, they often reveal the physical and emotional scars of their illness. Most of them tell us that life is never the same after a breast cancer diagnosis and that, despite some difficulties, they have found new meaning in life and a changed outlook as a result of facing death. For those women who have recurrent disease and die of breast cancer, their fighting spirit is often an inspiration to others. To the extent possible, the health care team needs to allow women to share their feelings and unburden themselves with respect to the emotional challenges of breast cancer. Because we face this illness with them, we are often better able than family and friends to understand what they are experiencing. When appropriate, we need to facilitate their obtaining appropriate counseling and support for emotional distress. Ideally, this should be a central and integrated component of the medical treatment program.

REFERENCES

1. American Cancer Society. *Cancer facts and figures 2000.* Atlanta: American Cancer Society.
2. Lansky SB, List MA, Herrmann CA, et al. Absence of major depressive disorder in female cancer patients. *J Clin Oncol* 1985;3:1553–1560.
3. Wolberg WH, Romsaas EP, Tanner MA, et al. Psychosexual adaptation to breast cancer surgery. *Cancer* 1989;63:1645–1655.
4. Ganz PA, Rowland JH, Desmond K, et al. Life after breast cancer: understanding women's health-related quality of life and sexual functioning. *J Clin Oncol* 1998;16:501–514.

5. Rowland JH, Holland JC. Psychological reactions to breast cancer and its treatment. In: Harris JR, Hellman S, Henderson IC, et al. *Breast diseases,* 2nd ed. Philadelphia: JB Lippincott, 1991:849–866.
6. Meyerowitz BE. Psychosocial correlates of breast cancer and its treatment. *Psychol Bull* 1980;8: 108–131.
7. Ervin CV. Psychologic adjustment to mastectomy. *Med Aspects of Human Sexuality* 1973;7:42–65.
8. Harris JR, Lippman ME, Veronesi U, et al. Breast cancer (medical progress). *N Engl J Med* 1992; 327:319–328,390–398,437–480.
9. Northouse LL. Psychological impact of the diagnosis of breast cancer on the patient and her family. *JAMA* 1992;47:161–164.
10. Ganz PA, Coscarelli A, Fred C, et al. Breast cancer survivors: psychosocial concerns and quality of life. *Breast Cancer Res Treat* 1996;38:183–199.
11. Sepucha KR, Belkora JK, Tripathy D, et al. Building bridges between physicians and patients: results of a pilot study examining new tools for collaborative decision making in breast cancer. *J Clin Oncol* 2000;18:1230–1238.
12. Siminoff LA, Fetting JH, Abeloff MD. Doctor-patient communication about breast cancer adjuvant therapy. *J Clin Oncol* 1989;7:1192–1200.
13. Simonoff LA. Improving communication with cancer patients. *Oncology* 1992;6:83–87.
14. Miller SM. Monitoring and blunting: validation of a questionnaire to assess styles of information seeking under threat. *J Pers Soc Psychol* 1987;52:345–353.
15. GIVIO Italy. What doctors tell patients with breast cancer about diagnosis and treatment: findings from a study in general hospitals. *Br J Cancer* 1986;54:319–326.
16. Cassileth BR, Zupkis RV, Sutton-Smith K, et al. Information and participation preferences among cancer patients. *Ann Intern Med* 1980;92:832–836.
17. Kaplan SH, Greenfield S, Ware JE Jr. Assessing the effects of physician-patient interactions on the outcomes of chronic disease. *Med Care* 1989;27:5110–5127.
18. Taylor KM. Telling bad news: physicians and the disclosure of undesirable information. *Sociol Health Illn* 1988;10:109–132.
19. Day R, Ganz PA, Costantino JP, et al. Health-related quality of life and tamoxifen in breast cancer prevention: a report from the National Surgical Adjuvant Breast and Bowel Project P-1 Study. *J Clin Oncol* 1999;17:2659–2669.
20. Dorval M, Maunsell E, Deschênes L, et al. Long-term quality of life after breast cancer: comparison of 8-year survivors with Population Controls. *J Clin Oncol* 1998;16:487–494.
21. Ganz PA, Rowland JH, Meyerowitz BE, et al. Impact of different adjuvant therapy strategies on quality of life in breast cancer survivors. *Recent Results Cancer Res* 1998;152:396–411.
22. van Dam FS, Schagen SB, Muller MJ, et al. Impairment of cognitive function in women receiving adjuvant treatment for high-risk breast cancer: high-dose versus standard-dose chemotherapy. *J Natl Cancer Inst* 1998;90:210–218.
23. Kogon MM, Biswas A, Pearl D, et al. Effects of medical and psychotherapeutic treatment on the survival of women with metastatic breast carcinoma. *Cancer* 1997;80:225–230.
24. Ganz PA, Desmond KA, Belin TR, et al. Predictors of sexual health in women after a breast cancer diagnosis. *J Clin Oncol* 1999;17:2371–2380.
25. Meyerowitz BE, Desmond KA, Rowland JH, et al. Sexuality following breast cancer. *J Sex Marital Ther* 1999;25:237–250.
26. Schag CAC, Ganz PA, Polinsky ML, et al. Characteristics of women at risk for psychosocial distress in the year after breast cancer. *J Clin Oncol* 1993;11:783–793.
27. Schover LR. The impact of breast cancer on sexuality, body image, and intimate relationships. *CA Cancer J Clin* 1991;41:112–120.
28. Ganz PA, Greendale GA, Petersen L, et al. Managing menopausal symptoms in breast cancer survivors: results of a randomized controlled trial. *J Natl Cancer Inst* 2000;92:1054–1064.
29. Petrek JA. Pregnancy safety after breast cancer. *Cancer* 1994;74:528–531.
30. Petrek JA. Pregnancy after breast cancer. In: Perry MC, ed. *ASCO educational book.* Alexandria: American Society of Clinical Oncology, 2000:408–412.

21

Genetic Testing for Breast Cancer Predisposition

Vickie L. Venne and Saundra S. Buys

Women who have close relatives with breast cancer are at an increased risk of developing breast cancer themselves. Familial clustering of breast cancer may be coincidental, with several members in the family all developing the same relatively common disease by chance. Shared environmental or lifestyle factors may result in multiple cases of breast cancer within a family, particularly among siblings. Genetic factors that indirectly influence the incidence of breast cancer, such as those regulating estrogen metabolism, may play a role in many familial clusters of breast cancer. Finally, major breast cancer predisposition genes that are inherited in an autosomal dominant fashion may be responsible for an increased risk of breast cancer in some families. Of all women with breast cancer, about 25% to 30% have a close family member with cancer (1), but only about 5% to 10% of breast cancer is due to a major genetic predisposition (2).

SOMATIC AND GERM-LINE GENETICS

All cancer is genetic; that is, all cancer is caused by the accumulation of genetic mutations in a specific cell. Only rarely, however, is cancer the result of an inherited mutation. Cancer can occur in any cell, either somatic or germ line, that contains a nucleus, but heritability requires a mutation in the germ line. Mutations in the germ line may be passed on to the next generation at the time of conception, resulting in an individual having the mutation in each somatic cell in the body. Persons with an inherited predisposition to cancer therefore have a germline mutation in each of their somatic cells and require one less *acquired* mutation before a given cell will become malignant. Families in which there is an inherited predisposition to cancer therefore usually have more cases of cancer than would be expected by chance, cancer in several generations, and cancer at early ages of onset.

BREAST CANCER SYNDROMES

There are more than 60 diseases with a mendelian inheritance pattern that are associated with a predisposition to cancer. A smaller number have been clearly defined and are amenable to genetic testing. The best known of these is breast/ovarian cancer syndrome. Other syndromes involve breast cancer in addition to cancer or benign disease in other organ sites. Therefore, an evaluation of the complete

TABLE 21.1. *Breast cancer syndromes*[a]

Syndrome	Gene (chromosome) involved	Inheritance pattern	Organ sites involved
Hereditary breast/ovarian cancer syndrome	BRCA1 (17q21) BRCA2 (13q12–13)	Autosomal dominant	Breast, ovary, colon, prostate, pancreas
Cowden syndrome	PTEN (10q22–23)	Autosomal dominant	Hamartomas of skin, throat, breast, thyroid; cancers of breast, thyroid; intestinal polyps
Ataxia telangiectasias	ATM (11q22–23)	Autosomal recessive	Cerebellar ataxia, telangiectasias, immunodeficiency, breast cancer in heterozygotes
Peutz-Jeghers syndrome	LKB-1/STK1 1 (19p)	Autosomal dominant	GI polyps and cancers; breast, uterus, ovary, testes cancer; also abnormal melanin deposits
Li-Fraumeni syndrome brain,	TP53 (17p13.1)	Autosomal dominant	Cancers of breast, adrenal cortex, sarcomas, leukemia
Muir-Torre syndrome	MSH2/MLH1	Autosomal dominant	Breast, skin, GI/GU tracts

GI, gastrointestinal; GU, genitourinary.
[a] This table identifies several of the syndromes that include breast cancer, the causative genes, the pattern of inheritance, and other organ sites at risk for those who have mutations.
From Greene MH. Genetics of breast cancer. *Mayo Clin Proc* 1997;72:51–65, with permission.

family cancer history is necessary to determine the chance that a particular family has a predisposition gene mutation.

Table 21.1 identifies several of the syndromes that include breast cancer, the causative genes, the pattern of inheritance, and other organ sites at risk for those who have mutations (3).

BRCA1 and *BRCA2*

Mutations in *BRCA1* and *BRCA2* may be responsible for as much as 75% to 80% of inherited breast cancer (4). Both are tumor-suppressor genes. *BRCA1* was cloned in 1994 (5) and *BRCA2* in 1995 (6), and more than 1,600 *BRCA1* and *BRCA2* mutations and polymorphic variations have been identified to date (http://www.nhgri.nih.gov/Intramural__research/Lab__transfer/Bic/). The risk of breast and ovarian cancer associated with *BRCA1* and *BRCA2* mutations have been estimated in both high-risk families (4,7) and in women identified from a general population (8,9). Studies are continuing to refine risk estimates, but currently, it is estimated that the cumulative risk of developing breast cancer among women with *BRCA1* mutations is 50% at age 50 and 87% at age 70; for women with *BRCA2* mutations, it ranges between 40% and 80% at age 70. In addition, men with *BRCA2* mutations have a 2% to 3% risk of developing breast cancer. The lifetime risk of ovarian cancer in female *BRCA1* mutation carriers is around 30% to 40%, and in *BRCA2* carriers, it is approximately 20%. Because ovarian cancer is much less common in the general population than breast cancer, the presence of ovarian cancer in breast cancer families is strong evidence supporting the possibility of a gene mutation. Colon cancer and prostate cancer in *BRCA1* mutation carriers may be increased about twofold over the general population. In addition, *BRCA2* families appear to have an excess of pancreatic and stomach cancer as well as melanomas (10). *BRCA1* and *BRCA2* are currently the breast cancer predisposition genes for which clinical testing is most readily available.

GATHERING DATA

One of the key questions asked by many women who are members of families in which there seems to be an excess of cancer is, "What is the chance I will get cancer?" An accurate response will require collecting information about the family history and the patient's own medical history. Estimates of risk can then be made and communicated in a manner that is clear to the patient. The level of detail will be based on the interest level of the patient, her ability to provide accurate family and personal health history information, and her desire to receive quantitative risk information.

Eliciting a Comprehensive Medical Family History

When women present with concerns about their risk of developing cancer because of a family history of cancer, obtaining a complete, three-generation history of both her maternal and paternal family is essential (11). Information should be collected about the health status of all first-degree relatives (children, siblings, parents) and second-degree relatives (uncles and aunts, grandparents or grandchildren, nieces and nephews) as well as information about extended family members who have cancer. Health status includes the vital status and cause of death, the presence of cancer, the cancer site and age of onset, the existence of multiple primaries or bilaterality and rare cancers, and documentation of other major health conditions.

A woman's risk of developing breast cancer is strongly related to the number of affected relatives, their genetic proximity, and the ages at which they were diagnosed. Small family size and misidentified paternity complicate the analysis of a family history, as does accuracy of reporting about the health status of family members. A common cancer genetic myth is that "You don't have to worry about breast cancer because it came from your father's side of the family." Even though breast cancer is more common in women, it is essential that information is collected about the paternal side of the family as well because the vast majority of inherited cancers are autosomal dominant. For families in whom a mutation already has been identified, genetic counseling and testing are possible without an extensive pedigree analysis.

A graphic representation of the family history allows for assessment of inheritance patterns (12) and is an easier way to capture family history information than writing the relationship of the family members who have cancer, for example ''my mother's youngest sister's second daughter.'' Review of the pedigree also can help the clinician make a diagnosis and identify other family members at risk. The process of collecting a family history will alert the clinician about the social dynamics of a family: who knows what about whom and how the family interprets the cancers in the family. By using recognized pedigree nomenclature, outlined in Fig. 21.1, family history information can be communicated to other clinicians and to patients in a clear and consistent manner.

Most individuals can accurately report breast cancers of second-degree relatives (13) and disclose when they are uncertain, which occurs with increasing frequency with the distance of the relative. For more distant family relationships and other organ sites, such as ovarian cancer, it may be necessary to obtain medical records to verify the diagnoses (14). Pathology reports are the most valid method for documenting cancers, although other medical records, death certificates, and tumor registry data are other options to confirm the reported cancers.

Family medical histories are dynamic (15), and it is important to remind the patient that if additional cases of cancer are diagnosed or discovered, the patient should recontact the provider because that information may alter the risk calculation.

Family history can be collected in several ways either prior to the visit or during the initial consultation. Obtaining the information prior to the clinic visit allows time to confirm suspicious diagnoses and analyze the data with the available risk models. The disadvantage of this method is that the complexity and amount of information required may present a barrier to patients actually completing and returning forms. If family history information is to be collected during the initial consultation, it is important to inform the patient that this information will be requested so she can gather it. A benefit of collecting a family history during a consultation is that it allows a better sense of family knowledge and dynamics. A disadvantage is that, based on the initial reporting, it may be necessary to confirm the uncertain diagnoses and schedule a second visit to provide the risk assessment.

Personal Health History

In addition to information about the extended family, a cancer risk assessment includes a personal health history. The presence of cancer, the cancer site and age of onset, the existence of multiple primaries or bilaterality are important as is the history of previous biopsies and the presence of proliferative breast disease. Hormone-related factors such as age of menarche, nulliparity or age at first birth, number of pregnancies, duration of breast-feeding, age of menopause, and exogenous hor-

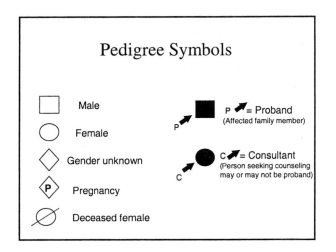

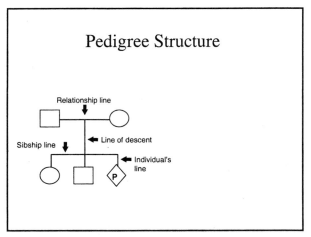

FIG. 21.1. By using recognized pedigree nomenclature, family history information can be communicated to other clinicians and to patients in a clear and consistent manner.

mone use (oral contraception, hormone replacement therapy) also have an impact on the risk of developing cancer.

RISKS

Communication of risk requires an understanding of ways to present risk, the various models used to assess risk, the manner in which numbers can be interpreted, and the factors that are necessary to put them into context of the patient's perception of her risk. Early in a breast cancer risk assessment and counseling session, it is valuable to learn the patient's sense of her own risk of developing breast cancer, which may be correlated with her level of concern. Some women believe that developing breast cancer is inevitable, whereas others focus on a specific risk figure or age at which they expect to develop cancer. Most women who have a family history of breast or ovarian cancer significantly overestimate the genetic component of their risk (16). Understanding how much of the personal risk assessment is intellectual as opposed to emotional will frame the manner in which the scientific information is presented.

Absolute Risks

An *absolute risk* is the probability of an event, such as that of developing breast cancer, occurring during a specific interval. A well-known risk figure associated with breast cancer is 11%, a cumulative incidence statistic (American Cancer Society, *Cancer Facts & Figures 2000*). It should be interpreted to mean that about one in nine women in the general population will develop breast cancer at some point during her lifetime, from birth to death.

Relative Risks

Most population-based studies of familial cancer evaluate risks by comparing the frequency of cancers within affected families to the frequencies expected in the general population. An observed-to-expected ratio (odds ratio) is used to demonstrate the risk based on a particular environmental factor (parity, oral contraceptive use, diet, pesticide exposure) or the distance of an affected relative (sister, mother, aunt, grandmother), typically described as twofold to threefold up to 14-fold over that of the general population (17). This is shown in Table 21.2.

Risk Models

Several mathematical models have been developed to estimate both the risk of developing cancer and the risk of having a *BRCA1* or *BRCA2* mutation. Early models

TABLE 21.2. *Selected lifetime risk ratios for breast cancer*

Relationship of affected relative	Risk ratio
Mother	1.7–4
Sister, premenopausal	3.6–5
Sister, postmenopausal	2
Sister and mother	2.5–14
Second degree	1.4–2
Third degree	1.35

From Slattery ML, Kerber RA. A comprehensive evaluation of family history and breast cancer risk: the Utah Population Database. *JAMA* 1993;270:1563–1568, with permission.

were based primarily on immediate family history or selected personal health factors. As more genetic information has become available, the models have become more sophisticated.

Gail

The Gail model was one of the first to compute individualized absolute risk (18). It uses five specific risk factors (age at evaluation, age at menarche, age at first live birth, number of prior breast biopsies, and number of first-degree relatives with breast cancer). A modification of the model also includes the presence of proliferative breast disease on biopsy. This model provides a risk figure that a specific woman will develop breast cancer during a specified future period. Tables as well as several computer programs are available to estimate individualized age-specific risks based on this model (19,20). Although the model is a useful tool for defining risk estimates in the general population, it has several limitations in the context of a high risk setting (21). It does not address the risk for younger women who are not undergoing regular mammogram examinations and, most relevant to a high risk population, does not accurately assess risk for families in whom there is a known or suspected inherited predisposition gene mutation.

Claus

A second model, based solely on family relationships, was subsequently developed that is more appropriate for estimating risk in women with a family history of breast cancer (22). This model includes first- and second-degree relatives and can be used to estimate risk over 10-year intervals. It can only be used for relatives in the same lineage (either maternal or paternal) but not mixed. The model uses a single locus, dominant genetic assumption, but those cases are limited to only about 5% to 10% of breast cancers. Also, the model does not include the impact of modifier genes. With those caveats, it is valuable in that it provides cumulative risks.

BRCAPro

A recently developed computer model (BRCAPro) includes age-specific cancers as well as positive and negative family history information of both first- and second-degree relatives from both sides of the family. This information is then evaluated using a Bayesian approach to calculate carrier probabilities (23). The model incorporates current knowledge of the prevalence and penetrance of the *BRCA1* and *BRCA2* genes.

Figure 21.2 demonstrates the variability of risk estimates for the same individual using the three different models.

Communicating Risk Figures

An assessment of the family and personal history will result in an estimate of cancer risk. Sharing probability figures may be challenging if patients do not under-

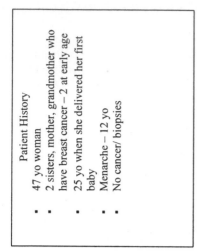

Patient History

- 47 yo woman
- 2 sisters, mother, grandmother who have breast cancer – 2 at early age
- 25 yo when she delivered her first baby
- Menarche – 12 yo
- No cancer/ biopsies

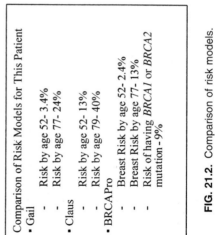

Comparison of Risk Models for This Patient

- Gail
  - Risk by age 52- 3.4%
  - Risk by age 77- 24%
- Claus
  - Risk by age 52- 13%
  - Risk by age 79- 40%
- BRCAPro
  - Breast Risk by age 52- 2.4%
  - Breast Risk by age 77- 13%
  - Risk of having *BRCA1* or *BRCA2* mutation - 9%

FIG. 21.2. Comparison of risk models.

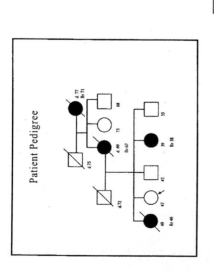

Patient Pedigree

466

stand statistics and related concepts such as independent segregation (24). For some individuals, percentages (20%, 50%) are most useful, whereas others better understand odds (1 in 5, 1 in 2). It is often helpful to use both or ascertain early in the visit which type is best understood by the patient (25). Placing the risks in context with other life events (other health risks, being in an accident, winning the lottery) also may be useful for some patients (26). Lifetime risk (e.g., 40%) is often a more frightening number than risk in a given period (e.g., 1% in the next year). During the counseling session, it is essential to obtain patient feedback to ensure that patients discriminate the numbers and interpret them correctly. Relative risks are often impressive but anxiety provoking, especially for persons with inherited mutations, so absolute numbers may provide a more accurate understanding. Using specific percentages (24.6%) may be academically correct based on the most recent literature, but it can provide a false sense of scientific accuracy in an evolving field. Using a range of risks may provide a more accurate sense of the current literature. It is useful to know what a patient initially perceives her risk to be, especially if the assessed risk is significantly different (27). This will also help the patient interpret the risk number–for some, 20% will be considered a low risk, whereas it is unacceptably high for others. Previous life experience, either personal or with other family members, may have significant influence on the manner in which the number is interpreted.

How to Better Define Risk: Genetic Testing

Who Should Be Tested

The identification of a gene mutation in a family allows much more precise risk estimation than simply knowing a family history or individual risk factors. Relatively few families, however, are appropriate candidates for genetic testing (28). In general, genetic testing is most informative for families in whom there appears to be an excess of cancer (sometimes defined as three or more closely related persons in two generations who have breast or ovarian cancer), particularly if some of the cancers occurred at an early age or were bilateral (29). Small families or families in whom most members are males may not meet these criteria but still may be appropriate for genetic testing.

The first person to receive genetic testing in a family should be someone affected with cancer because these persons are more likely than unaffected individuals to have a mutation. Almost always, this person will be a woman, but if a mutation is identified, testing is then available to all appropriate relatives, male and female, based on the inheritance pattern of the gene. Because some members of mutation-carrying families do *not* have the mutation but develop cancer anyway, it may be appropriate to offer testing to a second affected person in a family if the first person tested does not have a mutation but the family history is strongly suggestive of an inherited predisposition gene (11).

Most families with a suspected genetic predisposition to cancer will *not* have an identifiable mutation (11). A negative test result in an unaffected patient from a family that has not been previously tested provides little information to the individual or the family. Is it negative because no mutation exists in the family, is it negative because there is a mutation in a gene for which testing was not performed, or is it negative because a mutation exists in the family but the patient did not inherit it from a carrier parent? Unaffected individuals become testing candidates once a mutation is identified in a family.

Under some circumstances, it may be appropriate to test an unaffected individual in a family not known to carry a mutation, for example, if the family history is extremely suggestive of a mutation and there are no living affected members available for testing. Also, if an unaffected patient is a member of a particular ethnic group, such as Dutch or Ashkenazi Jewish, in which specific mutations have been identified, she may be a testing candidate. The individual being tested should understand, however, that a negative result does not guarantee that their risk of cancer is lowered.

From a genetic perspective, it is also ideal for the first testing candidate in a family, or a branch of a family, to represent the oldest generation. This information then provides data for all the descendants. If the parent has a mutation, all children become testing candidates, but if there is no mutation, none would have inherited a mutated gene. From a psychosocial perspective, there are also advantages to testing a member of the oldest generation first because it is often easier to share information from a parent to a child than from a child to a parent. If the person in the older generation is not particularly interested in testing, it may be reasonable to test a member of a younger generation whose diagnosis occurred at an early age.

Clinical testing is currently available primarily for *BRCA1* and *BRCA2*. Each of these genes is large, and hundreds of specific mutations have been identified. Mutation testing involves sequencing the entire gene and is complicated and expensive. Once a mutation is identified in a family, techniques to analyze specific mutations, which are usually less expensive, can be offered to other family members. Recognized high-frequency mutations in specific ethnic populations, such as those of Ashkenazi Jewish, Dutch, or Icelandic ancestry, can be evaluated initially. If a mutation is not identified, it may then be necessary to request a full-sequence analysis.

When to Test

Some women and their physicians wish to obtain genetic testing at the time a cancer is diagnosed. The reasons for this should be explored in detail before performing testing. Immediate medical management only rarely will be affected by the result of a genetic test (30); some women may consider bilateral mastectomy at the time one cancer is diagnosed, but this is generally based more on family history than on a genetic test result. The impact of a mutation on prognosis is not well understood, and the presence of a mutation does not clearly affect the choice of local therapy (lumpectomy or mastectomy) or systemic therapy (type of adjuvant chemotherapy or use of tamoxifen) (31). In addition, the logistics of obtaining genetic testing often delays definitive therapy by several weeks, and the psychosocial implications of obtaining genetic tests results are often overwhelming at a time a women is having to face a new cancer diagnosis. In general, a woman is likely to be more ready for genetic testing when she is not dealing simultaneously with the diagnosis and treatment of cancer. The readiness of the woman with cancer to receive her test results is key to offering genetic testing.

How to Obtain Testing

The vast majority of genetic testing can be accomplished with a blood specimen or, under some circumstances, a buccal smear obtained from a cheek swab. DNA also can be extracted from stored tissues blocks and used for specific tests if necessary. Testing should be performed only after appropriate genetic education and pretest counseling has been provided and informed consent has been obtained. The number of laboratories providing genetic testing is geographically dispersed and limited. One resource to help identify available laboratories is Gene Tests (www.genetests.org). This web site, developed with National Library of Medicine and Maternal & Child Health Bureau funding by the University of Washington, Seattle, is a genetic testing resource that includes a directory of clinical and research laboratories that offer specific medical genetic tests. The resource is available free of charge to registered users. Because genetic testing is still relatively new, identifying and contacting the laboratory directly are essential prior to sending specimens to ensure that the biospecimen is collected and sent appropriately. Many of the specialized genetic testing laboratories also have technical and genetic counselor support provided by the laboratory.

GENETIC EDUCATION AND COUNSELING

Genetic Education

The purpose of genetic education is to provide factual information about cancer etiology, including environmental and genetic factors. Verbal discussion, written information, and video or computer programs may be used to explain potential reasons the family may have an excess of cancer; basic genetics, including carcinogenesis and heritability; and the existence of breast cancer predisposition genes.

Pretest Counseling

Genetic counseling, as opposed to genetic education, is interactive and addresses psychosocial as well as factual issues. Components of genetic counseling include obtaining an individual and family social and health history; assessing the risk; educating the patient and family; ensuring that they understand the laboratory and clinical procedures and options for testing and screening as well as the risks, benefits, and limitations of the options; assessing psychosocial needs and intervening when appropriate; counseling to facilitate medical decision making; providing anticipatory grief or crisis counseling; and facilitating medical screening, testing, or management options as desired (32). A core genetic counseling tenet is that of nondirectiveness, a paradigm that highlights the physician–patient partnership as a model of shared decision making with the beliefs and values of the patient being the major factor in the decision to have genetic testing. The session will be impacted by the patient's previous experiences with cancer and emotions such as unresolved grief, fear, anxiety, or anger. It is valuable to assess these potential barriers early in the session.

It is also important in the genetic counseling session to clarify the reasons for the counseling and testing. Reasons for testing are numerous and probably will be different for women with and without cancer. A new personal or family cancer diagnosis may be the reason for the referral. Some patients who have cancer do not perceive any personal benefits from testing but assume that the genetic information is valuable only for extended family members. Discussions about the increased risk of cancers in other organ sites will be medically important for those patients. Often, however, patients realize that genetic testing will provide significant information for others in the family and a discussion of the importance of the various factors will improve the psychosocial outcome of the testing (33).

In addition to reviewing the purpose of the test, the consent process should include a discussion of the risks and benefits, accuracy and limitations of testing (34). Benefits can include enhanced cancer risk management, reproductive decision making, relief from uncertainty, and information for other family members. Risks include psychological distress, discrimination by employers and insurers, and social and family issues. Accuracy and limitations are often related to laboratory methodology and include the discovery of mutations of uncertain significance.

Other issues to consider in the pretest counseling include the following:

- Potential outcomes of genetic testing and the patient's response to the result
- Predictive value of a negative test
- Impact of a positive test on the risk of developing cancer
- Results of risk assessment without testing
- Medical management options based on the results
- Costs of testing

Test results can demonstrate a deleterious mutation, the absence of a mutation, or a mutation for which the clinical significance is unknown. Individuals differ about whether they consider identification of a mutation as good or bad news. For a woman with breast cancer, having a mutation will explain the etiology of her cancer, which may be good news for her. On the other hand, a woman who is the only one of her four sisters who does not have a mutation may experience survivor guilt. For many, the most frustrating result can be the one of uncertain significance, especially if there is a clear autosomal dominant pattern of cancer based on the family history. Testing for *BRCA1* and *BRCA2* is relatively new, and there are many alterations in the genes that are of uncertain significance. Some may cause a significant structural or functional change in the protein and therefore increase the risk for cancer, whereas others are probably minor variations in the DNA (polymorphisms) of no clinical consequence. Exploring the potential response to all these results, as well as how ready the patient is to hear any of these results, is an important part of the pretest session. Individuals who have the most significant distress are those who do not receive the result they expect, regardless of whether the test demonstrated the presence or absence of a mutation (35).

The predictive value of a negative test will differ based on whether or not a mutation already has been identified in the family. If the mutation in the family is known, a negative test result usually means (with > 99% accuracy) that the patient did not inherit that mutation and therefore would have a risk of developing cancer similar to the risk of a woman in the general population. Exceptions would be if the patient had a significant cancer history on the parental side different from that in which the mutation was identified or if she has first-degree family members with cancer who also did not have the mutation seen in the family. The predictive value of a negative test is lower if the patient is the first one in the family being offered testing, as discussed previously in the section on who should be tested. There are a number of other possible explanations for a negative test result, including the possibility that the cancers in the family are not due to an inherited gene mutation but rather to chance occurrences, that limitations of the technology do not allow a mutation to be identified, that the mutation is in a gene different from the one analyzed, or that the susceptibility gene that is predisposing to cancer in that family has not yet been discovered.

Prior to testing, it is important to discuss the impact of a positive test on the risk of developing cancer (33). For many women who have several family members with cancer, developing cancer seems inevitable; so assuring that they have a good understanding of penetrance is important. Because most cancers are age dependent, it is often valuable not only to provide a lifetime risk but also the risk of developing cancer in the next 5 to 10 years. In addition, interventions such as surgery or chemoprevention may reduce this risk, although specific numbers are still being estimated.

For some women, pretest counseling should include consideration of the risk assessment and management options available without testing. Concerns about genetic or employment discrimination keep some patients from considering genetic testing (36); for others, the management options that they would consider would not change in the face of having a mutation. Surveillance for early detection, as well as surgical or chemoprevention strategies and the efficacy of the various options, may impact the decision for some women. In addition, if a woman presents because of a strong history of breast cancer, but the mutation that is being analyzed includes risks for cancer in other organs, that information should be reviewed as well. Given no management changes, testing for some women may not be useful.

Major principles of genetic testing include autonomy, privacy, and confidentiality, which may be challenging aspects of genetic testing within a family construct. *Privacy* is that information that a person knows; the perceived degree of sensitivity of the information can vary (weight, genetic test results, sexual habits). *Confidentiality* is the expectation that disclosed information will not be shared with a third party, be it an insurance company or another family member, without permission. With the "right" of confidentiality comes the responsibility, that is, the health impact on other family members as a consequence of having access to the information. Because genetic testing often is performed for the express purpose of providing information for other family members, a discussion about the manner in which the test result will be shared–when, with and by whom–prior to the testing is a critical part of the pretest counseling. Autonomy takes a unique twist in the context of a family dynamic, especially if the values within a family differ. Attention to the issue of coercion is important when balancing the benefits to both the individual and the family. Genetic testing, especially for individuals who are not symptomatic, should be voluntary, and, in some families, the communication and relationship dynamic are such that independent decision making is something for which the health care provider needs to advocate.

One reason genetic testing should be especially voluntary in presymptomatic persons is the potential for employer or insurance carrier discrimination. Although the chance of this event is low, the consequences are significant, and this is often a key reason that individuals elect not to have genetic testing (37). A number of laws have been drafted to provide some protection, both nationally and in many states, but they differ significantly and many have not been tested in the court system (38). The status of these laws changes frequently, and the Ethical, Legal and Social Issues web site of the National Human Genome Research Institute (http://www.nhgri.nih.gov/ELSI/) or the National Partnership for Women & Families (www.nationalpartnership.org) can provide current information. Because of potential insurance discrimination, some individuals elect to pay for these services out of pocket instead of submitting them to their payers; costs for clinical services range from $75 to $300 and the cost of testing ranges from $150 to $3,000.

Offering genetic testing to minors is complicated, especially if the clinical manifestations for the genetic disorder do not occur until later in life. Usually, the testing decision is made by the parents, and there is controversy surrounding whether such tests are appropriate. Some argue that, in the absence of a medical benefit, offering genetic testing to minors would compromise the autonomy of the child or future access to insurance or educational opportunities (39). The psychological consequences could include stigmatization within a family or anxiety to treat as a fragile child (40). Many studies have presented hypothetical situations to assess testing in minors in health care professionals and parents, and the one study of parents who knew their mutation status indicated that about one fourth of the parents would support testing minors (41). Testing for *BRCA1* and *BRCA2* should not be performed in minors because there is virtually no risk of cancer in minors and medical management would not be affected.

Posttest Counseling

Once results are available, scheduling a posttest counseling session as a face-to-face discussion with sufficient time to address scientific, medical, and psychosocial issues is important. Some centers schedule an initial result session with a more extensive follow-up a few weeks later; others schedule one result session to address many of the issues with an invitation to the patient to return if she feels the need (35,42). When the results are provided, responding to the initial reaction of the patient is important, recognizing that there may be several psychological responses, such as anxiety and fear, stigmatization, guilt (both survivor and transmitter), regret, and personal identity issues (43,44). In addition to addressing the emotional reactions, the medical management and genetic implications should be reviewed.

Medical management aspects for all the potentially involved organs is detailed in the following section, but it usually can be separated into surveillance, surgery, and chemoprevention, taking into account the age of the patient and previous cancer or surgery. With respect to the genetic issues, other at-risk persons (children, siblings, extended family members) should be identified and a strategy defined for the manner in which they might be informed.

When counseling with families in which there is an identifiable mutation, it is important to clarify the concept that each pregnancy is a separate and unique event. Because many of the known breast cancer susceptibility mutations are inherited in a dominant manner, if a parent has an identifiable mutation, *each* child, regardless of gender, has a 50% chance of inheriting the mutation. The risk that a child who has inherited a mutation will develop cancer may vary and is based on gender and age as well as other environmental factors.

The familial nature of genetics carries an additional professional burden when counseling about the extended family. When a significant clinical finding impacts other family members, it is important to identify a mechanism to communicate this information to them. This is usually not the responsibility of the physician, but issues of confidentiality may be challenging if the physician provides care to extended family members. Part of the posttest counseling session should include information about the importance and methods of sharing genetic information with extended family members. Try to ensure that the patient has resources (such as a sample letter containing the information), especially if the extended family members do not live locally.

MEDICAL MANAGEMENT OF MUTATION CARRIERS

Medical management options for mutation carriers usually fall into one of three categories: enhanced surveillance, prophylactic surgery, or chemoprevention. The efficacy of these options in reducing mortality is not well defined, and enrollment of high-risk subjects into clinical trials should be encouraged.

Screening for Breast Cancer: Mammography

The utility of screening for disease depends on the combination of the effectiveness of the screening test and the incidence of the disease in the population to be screened. In the general population, mammographic screening for breast cancer in women over age 50 has been proven to be effective in reducing breast cancer mortality (45).

Screening between ages 40 and 49 is controversial but generally recommended. There is no debate that women with gene mutations should be screened at least as intensively as women in the general population, with mammograms starting at least by age 40.

The utility of mammograms for screening younger women with breast cancer gene mutations is entirely unknown. The increased density of breast tissue in young women and the higher likelihood of lobular carcinoma (which is frequently mammographically occult) in women with gene mutations may contribute to a higher false-negative rate in young, genetically at-risk women. Furthermore, the incidence of cancer at a given age in these women is not well defined. There is, therefore, no good way to estimate the effectiveness of screening for breast cancer using mammograms in mutation-carrying women under age 40. Several groups have published suggested guidelines (46,47) which, until more definitive data are available, should be followed. Current recommendations include, for women with mutations in *BRCA1* or *BRCA2* or women who are at 50% risk of having a mutation (i.e., women who have a first-degree relative with a gene mutation), annual mammograms starting at age 25. Members of families in whom breast cancer has been diagnosed earlier than age 25 often inquire about obtaining mammograms at a younger age. Because the incidence of breast cancer at very young ages (under 25) is low and the carcinogenic risk of breast radiation increases with younger ages, mammograms are generally not recommended before this age.

Most families with an apparent excess of breast and ovarian cancer will not have a known genetic predisposition to cancer. Some families will not have an appropriate testing candidate available or willing to undergo testing, and other families in whom testing is performed will not have an identifiable mutation. Women from these families should initiate mammograms 5 to 10 years younger than the earliest onset of breast cancer, starting at least by age 40, but not before age 25. For example, women who have family members with breast cancer in the mid-40s should start screening in their mid-30s.

Several methods of breast cancer imaging are currently being evaluated, including breast magnetic resonance imaging, ultrasound, and electrical impedance. These still are considered research tools and are not recommended for screening outside of research studies.

Screening for Breast Cancer: Clinical Breast Examination and Breast Self-Examination

Although there is no proof that breast self-examination (BSE) or clinical breast examination (CBE) reduces mortality from breast cancer in women either with or without a genetic predisposition to breast cancer, they are recommended components of screening for breast cancer. The current recommendation is that BSE be performed monthly from age 18 and CBE twice yearly starting at age 25.

Screening for Ovarian Cancer: CA125 and Transvaginal Ultrasound

The efficacy of screening for ovarian cancer is even more uncertain. In addition to a physical examination, the currently used screening tools are serum CA125 analysis and transvaginal ultrasound (TVU). Multiple studies in women at standard or slightly elevated risk have shown no significant reduction in mortality in women screened with CA125, TVU, or both. Because of the higher incidence of ovarian cancer in mutation carriers, however, these women constitute a group for whom screening may provide some benefit. Despite the absence of data, the National Comprehensive Cancer Network recommends screening for ovarian cancer with CA125 and TVU every 6 to 12 months starting at age 30 to 40 (47). A yearly pelvic examination is also recommended.

Prophylactic Surgery: Mastectomy

The most effective means of preventing breast cancer is with prophylactic mastectomy. A retrospective study of 639 women with a family history of breast cancer found a 90% reduction in breast cancer incidence compared with the incidence in sisters of women who did not have such surgery (48). Mutation status in these women was not known, but the reduction of risk was seen both in those with a moderate family history as well as those with a strong family history suggestive of genetic predisposition. Most women in this series underwent subcutaneous mastectomy, a procedure that preserves the nipple–areolar complex and therefore leaves more breast tissue than a total mastectomy. If a woman is going to the fairly aggressive step of prophylactic mastectomy, most surgeons believe a total mastectomy should be done. It is likely that this procedure will reduce the risk of breast cancer by at least 90% and lead to substantial gains in life expectancy in young women (49). Women considering this procedure should understand the options for reconstruction (including no reconstruction, implants, or tissue flaps; any of which are appropriate), the small risk of developing breast cancer in residual breast tissue, and the possibility of finding unsuspected cancer. A preoperative mammogram may be considered since identifying an unsuspected cancer may alter the type of surgery that is performed.

Prophylactic mastectomy is appropriate for some women and not for others (50). Principles that may assist in making a recommendation about this procedure include the following:

- Prognosis of the original breast cancer. Many women consider prophylactic mastectomy after being diagnosed with breast cancer, either at the time of diagnosis or some time after treatment. The prognosis of the diagnosed cancer should be considered in making this decision. The risk of cancer recurrence in women with inflammatory cancer or with involvement of numerous lymph nodes is high and may vastly outweigh the risk of developing a second primary cancer. Women with highly aggressive tumors, however, are more likely to request bilateral mastectomy than women with low-risk cancers, and this needs to be approached sensitively.

- Risk of developing breast cancer. In families in whom mutation status is known, testing is strongly recommended before considering prophylactic mastectomy. Prophylactic mastectomy almost never is warranted in a mutation-negative woman who is a member of a family in whom a mutation has been identified. Assuring that the woman understands her age-specific risks, as well as her lifetime risks, is also important.
- Ease of cancer detection. Breast cancer may be more or less difficult to detect, depending on the density of breast tissue on physical examination and mammogram. Detection is much easier in women with fatty-replaced breasts than in women with extremely dense breasts. Density of breast tissue has a genetic component (51), and difficulty in detecting cancer may therefore be a familial trait. Women may choose mastectomy over screening if screening tools are less likely to detect cancer at an early stage. Other women fear *developing* cancer, and the probability of early detection is not reassuring.
- Chemoprevention options. Risk reduction with tamoxifen or other as yet undefined agents is a good option for many women and may be considered instead of mastectomy.
- Psychological factors. Women consider prophylactic mastectomy for many reasons. For some, the family culture is to have prophylactic surgery, and the pressure to have it performed may be significant. Other women have cared for family members with terminal cancer and may wish to spare their own families. All these issues should be explored in depth. Counseling or grief therapy may be appropriate in some cases. There is never an absolute medical indication for this procedure, and the final decision about prophylactic mastectomy is always, therefore, a psychological one.

Prophylactic Surgery: Oophorectomy

Ovarian cancer is generally less common in families with *BRCA1* or *BRCA2* mutations than breast cancer, although in some families the predominant cancer is ovarian cancer. The lifetime incidence ranges from 30% to 40% in *BRCA1* mutation carriers and is about 20% in *BRCA2* mutation carriers. Although there are few reliable data, oophorectomy is estimated to reduce the risk of ovarian cancer by as much as 90%, although there is still a risk of peritoneal carcinomatosis (52). Although the psychological issues in women contemplating prophylactic oophorectomy are generally less significant than for women considering mastectomy, several important questions must be addressed, including the appropriate surgical approach and the use of postprocedure hormone replacement therapy.

The age-specific risk of ovarian cancer in mutation carriers increases sharply around age 40, and if prophylactic oophorectomy is to be performed, it is reasonable to have this done by this age. Some investigators suggest age 35 because of the added advantage that the risk of breast cancer is reduced in women who have the ovaries removed at this age, an observation seen even in women who take hormone replacement therapy after oophorectomy.

The best surgical approach is debated, but in general laparoscopy is adequate and much less morbid than an open procedure. The fallopian tubes should be resected with the ovaries, but there is, in general, no need to perform a hysterectomy.

Following removal of the ovaries, hormone replacement should be strongly considered. The risk of breast cancer is reduced after oophorectomy performed before age 40, even if estrogen replacement therapy is used, and the risk of osteoporosis is extremely high in women who undergo menopause between ages 35 and 40. One reasonable approach is to use estrogen (with cyclic progesterone in women with a uterus) from the time of oophorectomy until around age 40 and then to initiate tamoxifen for 5 years.

Breast Cancer Chemoprevention: Tamoxifen

Tamoxifen is a selective estrogen receptor modulator that has been used for more than 30 years for treatment of breast cancer, both as adjuvant therapy and for treatment of advanced disease. Women treated with tamoxifen were unexpectedly found to have a reduction in the incidence of contralateral breast cancer. This observation led to studies of tamoxifen as a breast cancer chemopreventive agent in women who were at high risk but who did not have breast cancer. The largest such study, conducted by the National Surgical Adjuvant Breast and Bowel Project, demonstrated approximately a 50% reduction in incidence of breast cancer in women who, because of age or other personal risk factors, had an *a priori* 5-year risk of 1.7% or greater as calculated by the Gail model (53). This study led to approval by the U.S. Food and Drug Administration in October 1998 for tamoxifen to reduce risk of breast cancer.

The utility of tamoxifen in women with gene mutations has been debated. Tamoxifen reduces only the risk of developing hormone receptor positive breast cancer; estrogen receptor–negative breast cancers develop as frequently in women on tamoxifen as in women not taking tamoxifen. Because a disproportionate number of cancers in mutation carriers may be estrogen receptor negative, some groups have suggested that tamoxifen would not reduce risk. A recent case–control study showed that women with *BRCA1* or *BRCA2* gene mutations who took tamoxifen for breast cancer had a reduction in the risk of contralateral breast cancer similar to women without such mutations (54). It is not known whether this will apply to unaffected women with mutations, but until more information is known, it is appropriate to recommend tamoxifen for mutation carriers starting around age 35 to 40.

Preliminary data on raloxifene, another selective estrogen receptor modulator, have shown a reduction in the risk of breast cancer in women with a low *a priori* risk (55). It is currently being compared with tamoxifen as a means of reducing risk, but it is not known to be effective in high-risk women. It is not approved as a means of risk reduction and should not be used for this purpose outside of a clinical trial.

Ovarian Cancer Chemoprevention: Oral Contraceptives

Women who take oral contraceptives, particularly for more than 5 years, have a significant reduction in risk of ovarian cancer (56). There has been some concern that prolonged use of oral contraceptives may increase the risk of breast cancer. It appears, however, that modern low-dose estrogen pills have minimal impact on the risk of breast cancer, probably reduce the risk of ovarian cancer even in women with mutations, and are an excellent means of contraception in women with mutations.

SUMMARY

As the public becomes more aware of and informed about the genetics of breast cancer, there will be an increasing demand for genetic counseling and clinical testing. Whether as part of a comprehensive clinical breast care clinic or as a component of a primary practitioner's service, high-risk families will be identified and should be offered appropriate services. A variety of resources from both the oncology and genetic communities are available to provide specialized care to women who need genetic counseling, result interpretation, or psychological support related to testing decisions (Table 21.3). The future of genetic testing will be in the primary care physician's office, whether it is obtaining a family and personal health history to determine the magnitude of risk, referring patients to specialized services for genetic counseling and testing, or providing long-term medical management of the patient or her extended family members.

TABLE 21.3. *Other resources: web sites*

Gene clinics: *www.geneclinics.org.* This web site is a companion to Gene Tests, funded by the National Institutes of Health and developed at the University of Washington, Seattle. Gene Clinics is a clinical information resource relating genetic testing to the diagnosis, management, and genetic counseling of individuals and families with specific inherited disorders. It contains information related to molecular testing, genetic counseling, and management options for specific diseases.

National Society of Genetic Counselors: *www.nsgc.org.* This site contains a resource link to assist consumers and professionals locate genetic counseling services.

National Institutes of Health: *http://cancernet.nci.nih.gov/pdq.html.* Cancer Net PDQ contains selected information about cancer, clinical trials, and providers of cancer genetic services.

The National Comprehensive Cancer Network: *www.nccn.org.* NCCN is an alliance of cancer centers, which was established in 1995 to provide state-of-the-art cancer care to the greatest number of patients in need and to advance the state-of-the-art in cancer prevention, screening, diagnosis and treatment through excellence in basic and clinical research. This site contains practice guidelines for the management of high risk patients.

American Society of Clinical Oncologists: *www.asco.org.* This interactive resource for oncology professionals and cancer patients provides a range of professionally edited information about a variety of cancers.

REFERENCES

1. Lynch HT, Lynch JF. Breast cancer genetics in an oncology clinic: 328 consecutive patients. *Cancer Genet Cytogenet* 1986;22:369–371.
2. Madigan MP, Ziegler RG, Benichou J, et al. Proportion of breast cancer cases in the United States explained by well-established risk factors. *J Natl Cancer Inst* 1995;87:1681–1685.
3. Greene MH. Genetics of breast cancer. *Mayo Clin Proc* 1997;72:54–65.
4. Ford D, Easton DF, Stratton M, et al. Genetic heterogeneity and penetrance analysis of the BRCA1 and BRCA2 genes in breast cancer families: the Breast Cancer Linkage Consortium. *Am J Hum Genet* 1998;62:676–89.
5. Miki Y, Swensen J, Shattuck-Eidens D, et al. A strong candidate for the breast and ovarian cancer susceptibility gene BRCA1. *Science* 1994;266:66–71.
6. Wooster R, Bignell G, Lancaster J, et al. Identification of the breast cancer susceptibility gene BRCA2. *Nature* 1995;378:789–792.
7. Ford D, Easton DF, Bishop DT, et al. Risks of cancer in BRCA1-mutation carriers: Breast Cancer Linkage Consortium. *Lancet* 1994;343:692–695.
8. Struewing JP, Hartge P, Wacholder S, et al., The risk of cancer associated with specific mutations of BRCA1 and BRCA2 among Ashkenazi Jews. *N Engl J Med* 1997;336:1401–1408.
9. Hopper JL, Southey MC, Dite GS, et al. Population-based estimate of the average age-specific cumulative risk of breast cancer for a defined set of protein-truncating mutations in BRCA1 and BRCA2. Australian Breast Cancer Family Study. *Cancer Epidemiol Biomarkers Prev* 1999;8:741–747.
10. The Breast Cancer Linkage Consortium. Cancer risks in BRCA2 mutation carriers. *J Natl Cancer Inst* 1999;91:1310–1316.
11. Hoskins KF, Stopfer JE, Calzone KA, et al. Assessment and counseling for women with a family history of breast cancer: a guide for clinicians. *JAMA* 1995;273:577–585.
12. Bennett RL, et al. Recommendations for standardized human pedigree nomenclature. *Journal of Genetic Counseling* 1995;4:267–278.
13. Parent ME, Ghadirian P, Lacroix A, et al. The reliability of recollections of family history: implications for the medical provider. *J Cancer Educ* 1997;12:114–120.
14. Theis B, Boyd N, Lockwood G, et al. Accuracy of family cancer history in breast cancer patients. *Eur J Cancer Prev* 1994;3:321–327.
15. Acheson LS, Wiesner GL, Zyzanski SJ, et al. Family history-taking in community family practice: implications for genetic screening. *Genet Med* 2000;2:180–185.
16. Iglehart JD, Miron A, Rimer BK, et al. Overestimation of hereditary breast cancer risk. *Ann Surg* 1998;228:375–384.
17. Slattery ML, Kerber RA. A comprehensive evaluation of family history and breast cancer risk: the Utah Population Database. *JAMA* 1993;270:1563–1568.
18. Gail MH, Benichou J. Validation studies on a model for breast cancer risk. *J Natl Cancer Inst* 1994;86:573–575.
19. Benichou J, Gail MH, Mulvihill JJ. Graphs to estimate an individualized risk of breast cancer. *J Clin Oncol* 1996;14:103–110.
20. Benichou J. A computer program for estimating individualized probabilities of breast cancer [published erratum appears in *Comput Biomed Res* 1994;27:81]. *Comput Biomed Res* 1993;26:373–382.
21. Rockhill B, Spiegelman D, Byrne C, et al. Validation of the Gail et al. model of breast cancer risk prediction and implications for chemoprevention. *J Natl Cancer Inst* 2001;93:358–366.
22. Claus EB, Risch N, Thompson WD. Autosomal dominant inheritance of early-onset breast cancer. Implications for risk prediction. *Cancer* 1994;73:643–651.
23. Parmigiani G, Berry D, Aguilar O. Determining carrier probabilities for breast cancer-susceptibility genes BRCA1 and BRCA2. *Am J Hum Genet* 1998;62:145–158.
24. Rockhill B. The privatization of risk. *Am J Public Health* 2001;91:365–368.
25. Lloyd S, Watson M, Waites B, et al., Familial breast cancer: a controlled study of risk perception, psychological morbidity and health beliefs in women attending for genetic counseling. *Br J Cancer* 1996;74:482–487.
26. Phillips KA, Glendon G, Knight JA. Putting the risk of breast cancer in perspective. *N Engl J Med* 1999;340:141–144.
27. Ritvo P, Robinson G, Irvine J, et al. Psychological adjustment to familial genetic risk assessment: differences in two longitudinal samples. *Patient Educ Couns* 2000;40:163–172.
28. Couch FJ, DeShano ML, Blackwood MA, et al. BRCA1 mutations in women attending clinics that evaluate the risk of breast cancer. *N Engl J Med* 1997;336:1409–1415.
29. Statement of the American Society of Clinical Oncology: genetic testing for cancer susceptibility, Adopted on February 20, 1996. *J Clin Oncol* 1996;14:1730–1740.

30. Breast Cancer Linkage Consortium. Pathology of familial breast cancer: differences between breast cancers in carriers of BRCA1 or BRCA2 mutations and sporadic cases. *Lancet* 1997;349:1505–1510.
31. Matloff ET. The breast surgeon's role in BRCA1 and BRCA2 testing. *Am J Surg* 2000;180:294–298.
32. Peters J. Inherited susceptibility to cancer: clinical, predictive and ethical perspectives. In: Foulkes WD, Hodgson SV, eds. *Genetic Counselling*. Cambridge: Cambridge University Press, 1998:60–95.
33. Lerman C, Narod S, Schulman K, et al. BRCA1 testing in families with hereditary breast-ovarian cancer: a prospective study of patient decision making and outcomes. *JAMA* 1996;275:1885–1892.
34. Biesecker BB, Boehnke M, Calzone K, et al. Genetic counseling for families with inherited suscepti-bility to breast and ovarian cancer [published erratum appears in *JAMA* 1993;18;270:832]. *JAMA* 1993;269:1970–1974.
35. Dorval M, Patenaude AF, Schneider KA, et al. Anticipated versus actual emotional reactions to disclosure of results of genetic tests for cancer susceptibility: findings from p53 and BRCA1 testing programs. *J Clin Oncol* 2000;18:2135–2142.
36. Lapham EV, Kozma C, Weiss JO. Genetic discrimination: perspectives of consumers. *Science* 1996; 274:621–624.
37. The Ad Hoc Committee on Genetic Testing/Insurance Issues. Genetic testing and insurance. *Am J Hum Genet* 1995;56:327–331.
38. Rothenberg K, Fuller B, Rothstein M, et al. Genetic information and the workplace: legislative approaches and policy changes. *Science* 1997;275:1755–1757.
39. Wertz DC, Fanos JH, Reilly PR. Genetic testing for children and adolescents. Who decides? *JAMA* 1994;272:875–881.
40. Michie S, McDonald V, Bobrow M, et al. Parents' responses to predictive genetic testing in their children: report of a single case study. *J Med Genet* 1996;33:313–318.
41. Hamann HA, Croyle RT, Venne VL, et al. Attitudes toward the genetic testing of children among adults in a Utah-based kindred tested for a BRCA1 mutation. *Am J Med Genet* 2000;92:25–32.
42. Baty B, et al. BRCA1 testing: genetic counseling protocol development and counseling issues. *J Genetic Counseling* 1997;6:223–244.
43. Croyle RT, Smith KR, Botkin JR, et al. Psychological responses to BRCA1 mutation testing: prelimi-nary findings. *Health Psychol* 1997;16:63–72.
44. Lerman C, Croyle RT. Emotional and behavioral responses to genetic testing for susceptibility to cancer. *Oncology (Huntingt)* 1996;10:191–195,199;–202.
45. Kelsey JL, Bernstein L. Epidemiology and prevention of breast cancer. *Annu Rev Public Health* 1996;17:47–67.
46. Burke W, Daly M, Garber J, et al. Recommendations for follow-up care of individuals with an inherited predisposition to cancer. II. BRCA1 and BRCA2. Cancer Genetics Studies Consortium. *JAMA* 1997;277:997–1003.
47. Daly M. NCCN practice guidelines: genetics/familial high-risk cancer screening. *Oncology* 1999; 13:161–171.
48. Hartmann LC, Schaid DJ, Woods JE, et al. Efficacy of bilateral prophylactic mastectomy in women with a family history of breast cancer. *N Engl J Med* 1999;340:77–84.
49. Schrag D, Kuntz KM, Garber JE, et al. Decision analysis—effects of prophylactic mastectomy and oophorectomy on life expectancy among women with BRCA1 or BRCA2 mutations [published erratum appears in *N Engl J Med* 1997;7:434]. *N Engl J Med* 1997;336:1465–1471.
50. Meiser B, Butow P, Friedlander M, et al. Intention to undergo prophylactic bilateral mastectomy in women at increased risk of developing hereditary breast cancer. *J Clin Oncol* 2000;18:2250–2257.
51. Boyd NF, Lockwood GA, Martin LJ, et al. Mammographic densities and risk of breast cancer among subjects with a family history of this disease. *J Natl Cancer Inst* 1999;91:1404–1408.
52. Rebbeck TR, Levin AM, Eisen A, et al. Breast cancer risk after bilateral prophylactic oophorectomy in BRCA1 mutation carriers. *J Natl Cancer Inst* 1999;91:1475–1479.
53. Fisher B, Costantino JP, Wickerham DL, et al. Tamoxifen for prevention of breast cancer: report of the National Surgical Adjuvant Breast and Bowel Project P-1 Study. *J Natl Cancer Inst* 1998; 90:1371–1388.
54. Narod SA, Brunet JS, et al. Tamoxifen and risk of contralateral breast cancer in BRCA1 and BRCA2 mutation carriers: a case-control study. Hereditary Breast Cancer Clinical Study Group. *Lancet* 2000; 356(9245):1876–1881.
55. Cummings SR, Eckert S, et al. The effect of raloxifene on risk of breast cancer in postmenopausal women: results from the MORE randomized trial. Multiple Outcomes of Raloxifene Evaluation [see comments]. *JAMA* 1999;281(23):2189–2197.
56. Narod SA, Risch H, et al. Oral contraceptives and the risk of hereditary ovarian cancer. Hereditary Ovarian Cancer Clinical Study Group. 1998;339(7):424–428.

22

Chemoprevention of Breast Cancer

Paul E. Goss and Kathrin Strasser

Breast cancer is one of the most common cancers of women in the Western world. Approximately 170,000 new cases are reported annually in the United States, and there are about 1 million incident cases (1). Although important gains have been made both in early detection and treatment of breast cancer, the impact of these measures to date on reduction in mortality has been modest (2). Furthermore, despite data implicating diet and other environmental risk factors discussed in this and other chapters, no lifestyle changes have yet been shown to reduce the risk of breast cancer significantly. Chemoprevention of breast cancer is therefore a logical goal that may address more significantly this urgent public health issue.

In time, a detailed understanding of the initiation, promotion, and growth of breast cancer will likely provide the rationale on which to base prevention strategies. In the interim, chemoprevention has focused on applying the antiestrogen tamoxifen, an established treatment in breast cancer patients. Cohorts of women at high risk for the disease have been studied. In this chapter, we review known breast cancer risk factors, in particular the critical role of estrogen in the pathogenesis of the disease, and preclinical models of chemoprevention. The data related to breast cancer prevention from the clinical trials with tamoxifen and raloxifene are presented. Finally, the potential for new agents and strategies in chemoprevention is discussed and possible future clinical trial designs outlined.

ESTROGEN AND BREAST CANCER RISK

Estrogen in the Pathogenesis of Breast Cancer

The exact mechanisms involved in estrogen-induced carcinogenesis are not yet fully elucidated. Exogenous estrogens cause breast cancer in rat mammary tumor models (see next section), increasing both the number of breast tumors and the rapidity of their growth (3). Endogenous or exogenous estrogens may enhance cell proliferation, which increases the number of cell divisions and thereby the number of mutations (4). With an enhanced rate of proliferation, the time available for DNA repair is reduced. The single-stranded DNA present during cell division is particularly susceptible to damage (5). The metabolism of estrogens to genotoxic products has also been suggested as a mechanism of estrogen-induced carcinogenesis (6).

Epidemiologic Factors

Epidemiologic evidence strongly favors a role for estrogens in the development and growth of breast cancers. The almost 150-fold incidence of breast cancer in women compared with men reflects the relationship between female sex steroids and breast cancer. The model proposed is that total exposure to estrogens during a lifetime is related to breast cancer risk. Thus, known risk factors that positively correlate with breast cancer risk, such as earlier age at menarche and late age at menopause, high bone mass, obesity in menopause, long-term use of hormone replacement therapy, high free levels of estradiol in postmenopausal women, and possibly breast density, all may be considered as measures of total estrogen exposure (Table 22.1) (7–19). Taken together, these data suggest that antagonizing the effects of estrogen is a logical target for breast cancer chemoprevention.

Cohort Selection

As an attempt to translate these risk factors into a useful clinical selection tool for chemoprevention trials, a model of relative risks for various combinations of

TABLE 22.1. *Risk factors for breast cancer*

Factor	Variable	Approximate relative risk estimate
Family history	One first-degree relative	1.5–2.0
	Two first-degree relatives	5.0
Diet	High-fat Western-style	~1.2
	Premenopausal obesity	1.2
	Postmenopausal obesity	1.2
Alcohol	Consumption	1.3
Oral contraceptives	General use	1.0
Hormone replacement therapy	Use	1.1–1.4
Oophorectomy	Prior to age 40	0.5
Age at menarche	Younger	Risk ↑ 4%–5%/yr
Age at menopause	Older	Risk ↑ 4%–5%/yr
Age at first birth	<20 yr	1.0
	>20 yr and multiparous	1.6
	Nulliparous ≥35 yr	1.9
Breastfeeding	Yes	0.8
Benign breast disease	Hyperplasia	1.5–2.0
	Atypia	3–5
Previous breast cancer	Yes	0.7% risk/yr
Irradiation of breast	Age 10–20 yr	>20
	Age 20–30 yr	15
	≥50 yr	1.0
Bone mass	Highest *vs* lowest quartile	2–3.5
Breast density	Highest *vs* lowest quartile	~5
Postmenopausal levels of estradiol	Highest *vs* lowest quartile	~3
Gene mutation (BRCA1)		70% risk by age 70

- Age
- Age at menarche
- Number of first-degree relatives with breast cancer.
- Nulliparity or age at first live birth
- Number of breast biopsies
- Pathologic diagnosis of atypical hyperplasia

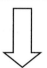

Five-Year Risk of Breast Cancer

FIG. 22.1. Variables included in the original Gail model.

these and other factors was developed by Gail et al. (20). The risk factors used in this model include age at menarche, age at first live birth, number of previous breast biopsies, and number of first-degree relatives with breast cancer. With the Gail model, the chance of a woman of a given age and with specific risk factors of developing breast cancer over a specified period can be determined (Fig. 22.1). The Gail model of risk assessment was used in the most definitive breast cancer prevention trial (National Surgical Adjuvant Breast Project, or NSABP P-1) and now is also being used in the ongoing Study of Tamoxifen and Raloxifene (STAR) trial as described in a later section (20,21).

PRECLINICAL MODELS OF POTENTIAL CHEMOPREVENTATIVES

Breast Cancer Xenografts

In breast cancer research, the most widely used hormone-dependent human tumor cell line is MCF-7. These cells can be inoculated in the mammary fat pad of cycling *athymic nude mice*. Being immunodeficient, these animals are not able to reject the human xenograft. MCF-7 breast cancer xenografts are hormone dependent and similar to human breast tumors with respect to many histologic and phenotypic features. Therefore, the ability of novel endocrine agents to shrink established tumors or to prevent tumor formation by newly inoculated cells can be usefully studied in this model (22).

Recently, a model for postmenopausal, hormone-dependent breast cancer in nude mice was established. In this model, MCF-7 cells transfected with the aromatase gene (MCF-7AROM) are inoculated in ovariectomized nude mice. The cells then serve as a source of estrogen in the "postmenopausal" mouse and produce sufficient estrogen to form tumors. This model is particularly useful to determine the effects of both antiestrogens and estrogen synthetase (aromatase) inhibitors on tumor growth (23).

An important limitation of human xenograft models is that cells might have adapted to growth *in vitro* before being inoculated and might not fully reflect human disease (6).

Carcinogen-induced Rat Mammary Tumors

The two most widely used chemical carcinogens for tumor induction in the rat mammary gland are 12-dimethylbenz(a)anthracene (DMBA) and *N*-methylnitrosurea (MNU). The tumors induced by these agents occur with latencies between 8 and 21 weeks and final tumor incidences are close to 100%. Tumor latency is in general inversely related to carcinogen dose, whereas tumor incidence is directly related if an earlier endpoint is used. As is the case with MCF-7 xenografts, these tumors have also been shown to be strongly hormone dependent for both induction and growth. Investigational antiendocrine chemopreventives can be given to animals prior to carcinogen administration (prevention of tumor initiation) or following it (inhibition of tumor promotion) (24).

SERMS IN THE CHEMOPREVENTION OF BREAST CANCER

The term *SERM* is an abbreviation for selective estrogen receptor (ER) modulator. These agents, for example, tamoxifen or raloxifene, bind to the ER and exert either estrogenic or antiestrogenic effects, depending on the specific end-organ. The most widely studied SERM is tamoxifen, a nonsteroidal antiestrogen, which has been shown in a large randomized trial to be effective in the chemoprevention of breast cancer. Raloxifene, currently under evaluation for this purpose, and other SERMs discussed later in this section, show estrogenic and antiestrogenic effects on end-organs that differ in part from those caused by tamoxifen. The efficacy and multiorgan effects of tamoxifen and raloxifene are presented and compared in detail later. It is hoped that ongoing and future clinical trials will demonstrate whether one of the newer drugs will have a superior therapeutic index compared with tamoxifen.

Tamoxifen

Tamoxifen and Breast Cancer Risk Reduction

Tamoxifen citrate was first approved by the U.S. Food and Drug Administration (FDA) for use in advanced breast cancer in 1978. In 1982, the NSABP initiated a randomized, double-blind, placebo-controlled trial, NSABP B-14, to determine the effectiveness of tamoxifen in women with operable primary breast cancer with negative nodes and positive ER status. Within 6 years, 2,818 patients were assigned to treatment with either tamoxifen 20 mg daily for 5 years or placebo. Comparable to a similar trial reported from Scotland in 1987, B-14 showed a significant difference ($p < 0.00001$) between the treatment groups in disease-free survival in favor of the patients receiving tamoxifen (a 26% reduction in treatment failure at 4 years). In addition to a reduction in local and distant treatment failures, the incidence of tumors in the contralateral breast was decreased. These findings, together with the results of the Stockholm trial of 1991, strongly support the hypothesis that tamoxifen might serve as a tumor-preventive agent (25–28).

In 1992, the NSABP initiated the P-1 trial, which randomly assigned women at increased risk for breast cancer to receive either tamoxifen 20 mg daily or placebo for 5 years (Fig. 22.2). Women were deemed at increased risk either because they were 60 years of age or older or 35 to 59 years of age with a predicted 5-year-risk for breast cancer of at least 1.66% or if they had a history of lobular carcinoma *in situ* (LCIS) (21). The algorithm for estimating 5-year risk was based on the work of Gail et al., with the average risk of breast cancer in P-1, as measured in the Gail model, being 3.2% over 5 years (20). The duration of 5 years of tamoxifen was selected because previous trials showed that there was a significant trend toward increased benefit (fewer contralateral cancers) with longer tamoxifen duration (up to 5 years) in the adjuvant setting (29,30). Through the duration of P-1, 78% of the 13,388 participants continued on therapy. When the trial was terminated in 1997, tamoxifen had reduced the overall risk of invasive breast cancer by 49% ($p < 0.00001$), with cumulative incidence rates through 69 months of follow-up of 43.4 versus 22.0 per 1,000 women in the placebo and tamoxifen groups, respectively. When age, history of LCIS, history of atypical hyperplasia, and levels of predicted risk of breast cancer were taken into consideration, tamoxifen was found to be effective in all subgroups. The reduction in breast cancer incidence was confined

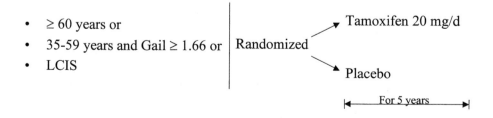

FIG. 22.2. Design of the National Surgical Adjuvant Breast Project (NSABP) P-1 study.

Type of Event	Placebo	Tamoxifen	Risk Ratio
Invasive breast cancer	175	89	0.51
Noninvasive breast cancer	69	35	0.50
Invasive endometrial cancer	15	36	2.53
Fractures[1]	137	111	0.81
Stroke	24	38	1.59
Transient ischemic attack	25	19	0.76
Pulmonary embolism	6	18	3.01
Deep vein thrombosis	22	35	1.60

FIG. 22.3. Numbers of events in National Surgical Adjuvant Breast Project (NSABP) P-1. [1]Hip, spine, radius Colles, and other lower radius.

to ER-positive tumors (69% less in the tamoxifen group) with no demonstrable difference in ER-negative disease. The greatest differences were seen in small tumors (<2 cm) and breast cancers without axillary involvement, with only small benefits from tamoxifen in larger tumors or higher nodal status. A reduction of 50% ($p <$ 0.002) in noninvasive breast cancer [ductal carcinoma *in situ* (DCIS) and LCIS] was also noted. The results of the P-1 trial are shown in Fig. 22.3 (21).

Two additional European trials evaluated tamoxifen in breast cancer chemoprevention (31,32). Overall, both failed to show any effect on breast cancer incidence. In the Italian trial, 5,408 women who had had a total hysterectomy for reasons other than neoplasm were randomized to receive tamoxifen 20 mg daily or a placebo, both orally for 5 years. Eligibility criteria in this study did not include any risk factors, and hormone-replacement therapy (HRT) was allowed. The lack of effect of tamoxifen on the incidence of breast cancer in this trial can be explained by the relatively small size of this study compared with P-1, the low-risk population (48.3% had had a bilateral oophorectomy and no specific risk factors were required), and the limited compliance (only 149 participants completed 5 years of treatment). In this study, a subset analysis showed a definite trend toward chemoprevention of breast cancer by tamoxifen in women taking concurrent HRT (21,31).

In the UK trial, 2,494 women with a strong family history of breast cancer were randomized to receive tamoxifen 20 mg per day orally or a placebo for up to 8 years. Postmenopausal women taking HRT were eligible without having to stop such therapy and also were allowed to initiate concurrent HRT for relief of symptoms while on study. No reduction in breast cancer incidence was noted in this trial. Several possible explanations have been offered for the apparently contradictory results of the UK trial compared with P-1. One reason could relate to the study populations, with the risk assessment of the UK trial predominantly based on a strong family history of breast cancer, whereas in NSABP P-1, the entry criteria were based mostly on nongenetic risk factors. In addition, there was a considerable difference in the duration of follow-up between the two trials. The average follow-up for P-1 was only 3.5 years compared with the UK median of nearly 6 years. One other reason for failure of the European studies to show a positive result could be the fact that 41% of the participants in the UK trial and 14% in the Italian trial received HRT (21,31,32).

Additional evidence of the chemopreventive effects of tamoxifen has been obtained from trials in women with DCIS, in particular in the NSABP B-24 study (33). Women with DCIS were not eligible for any of the three prevention trials, but their 5-year risk of contralateral breast cancer of 3.3% is comparable to the risk of invasive cancer in the placebo group of P-1 (3.2%). Among 1,804 patients with DCIS treated with lumpectomy and radiation in B-24, tamoxifen significantly reduced subsequent invasive breast cancers by 47% (3.4% and 2.1% incidence for placebo and tamoxifen given for 5 years, respectively), which is very consistent with the results obtained in P1 (49%) (21,33). Therefore, despite the discrepancies between the trials, the results of the P-1 trial are consistent with preclinical observations and with the reduction of contralateral breast cancer seen with 5 years of adjuvant tamoxifen therapy (30)

Tamoxifen Effects Other Than on the Breast

Endometrial Cancer Risk

In P-1, participants who received tamoxifen had a 2.53 times greater risk of developing invasive endometrial cancer [95% confidence interval (CI), 1.35–4.97). This was more common in women over 50 years of age compared with younger women [relative risk (RR), 4.01 versus 1.21). All invasive endometrial cancers that occurred in the group receiving tamoxifen were International Federation of Obstetrics and Gynecology (FIGO) stage I, none of which resulted in a death (21). The overview of adjuvant breast cancer trials by the Early Breast Cancer Trialists' Collaborative Group (EBCTCG) (30) confirmed this tamoxifen-related endometrial cancer risk. An annual excess of death from endometrial cancer of about 0.2 per 1,000 postmenopausal women treated with tamoxifen who had not been hysterectomized was observed. In general, the absolute increase in endometrial cancer was about half the decrease in contralateral breast cancer in these adjuvant trials (30).

Lipid Metabolism and Cardiovascular Risk

Although for over a decade tamoxifen has been thought to influence lipid levels, a benefit on cardiovascular mortality has not been demonstrated consistently. Although in retrospective analyses of three randomized breast cancer trials a reduction in coronary heart disease (CHD) was observed, no benefit was demonstrated in P-1 (21,34–37). In the EBCTCG overview of 1998, it was reported that mortality rates for causes "not attributed to breast or endometrial cancer" were nearly identical in patients receiving tamoxifen or placebo in the adjuvant setting (30). Therefore, it remains to be established whether the favorable influence of tamoxifen on lipid metabolism translates into a reduction in CHD.

Bone Metabolism and Fracture Risk

Tamoxifen has been shown to preserve bone mineral density (BMD) in postmenopausal breast cancer patients (38–40). P-1 is the only prospective trial that evaluated the effect of tamoxifen on bone fractures, and it showed a reduction in the risk of long bone and symptomatic vertebral fractures of borderline statistical significance (RR = 0.81, 95% CI, 0.63–1.05) (21). To date, tamoxifen has not been evaluated in a prospective trial in women with osteoporosis.

Coagulation and Thromboembolic Risk

In the tamoxifen group of P-1, pulmonary embolism (PE) was three times as frequent (RR = 3.01, 95% CI, 1.15–9.27) and strokes nearly twice as common among women older than 50 years (RR = 1.75; 95% CI, 0.98–3.20). In addition, more women receiving tamoxifen developed deep venous thrombosis (DVT) (RR = 1.6; 95% CI, 0.91–2.86). Overall, the increase in vascular events on tamoxifen was comparable to that seen with HRT (21,41).

Cataract Incidence

An additional risk of tamoxifen that was identified during P-1 was a small excess risk of cataracts (RR-1.14; 95% CI, 1.01–1.29) (21).

Quality of Life

Day et al. analyzed health-related quality of life in the P-1 study. The most important findings are listed in Table 22. 2. Tamoxifen significantly increased bothersome

TABLE 22.2. *Tamoxifen and health-related quality of life*

Symptoms reported	Placebo (%)	Tamoxifen (%)
Vaginal discharge	34.13	54.77
Cold sweats	14.77	21.40
Genital itching	38.29	47.13
Night sweats	54.92	66.80
Hot flashes	65.04	77.66
Pain in intercourse	24.13	28.19
Problems in bladder control (laugh)	46.65	52.51
Problems in bladder control (other)	47.79	52.83
Weight loss	41.97	44.94
Vaginal bleeding	21.26	21.96

hot flashes and vaginal discharge, but this did not effect overall physical and emotional well-being as reported by study participants. Weight gain and depression, two side effects commonly believed to be tamoxifen related, were not confirmed (42).

On October 29, 1998, the FDA approved tamoxifen "for reducing the incidence of breast cancer in women at high risk for the disease." It should be noted, however, that the effect of tamoxifen on overall or breast cancer specific survival has not been ascertained from these studies. Although experience with tamoxifen in the adjuvant breast cancer setting suggests a favorable impact on survival, these results cannot yet be projected to the chemoprevention setting. An ongoing trial, the International Breast Cancer Intervention Study, should provide more information in this regard.

Raloxifene

Raloxifene and Breast Cancer Risk Reduction

Raloxifene hydrochloride is a SERM that is chemically distinct from tamoxifen. It appears to act as an estrogen antagonist in breast tissue but as an estrogen agonist with respect to its effects on circulating lipids and bone and minimal agonist effects on the uterus. Based on initial laboratory studies and subsequent clinical evaluation, raloxifene received FDA approval for the prevention of osteoporosis in postmenopausal women in 1997.

In the Multiple Outcomes of Raloxifene Evaluation (MORE) study, 7,705 postmenopausal women with existing osteoporosis and no history of breast or endometrial cancer were randomized to receive either raloxifene (60 or 120 mg) or placebo daily (Fig. 22.4). The MORE trial was designed to test whether raloxifene would lower the risk of fractures in this patient population. Participants were also monitored for the occurrence of breast cancer, a secondary endpoint of the trial. After a median

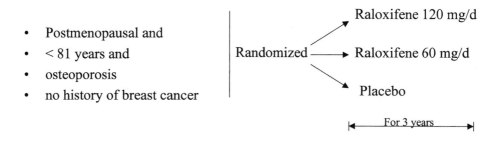

N=7,705   Primary Endpoint: Risk of Vertebral Fractures

FIG. 22.4. Design of the Multiple Outcomes of Raloxifene Evaluation (MORE) randomized trial.

Type of Event	Placebo N=2576	Raloxifene N=5129	Risk Ratio
Invasive breast cancer	27	13	0.24
Invasive endometrial cancer	4	6	0.8
New vertebral fracture	10.1%	5.4/6.6%[1]	0.7/0.5[1]
Deep vein thrombosis and pulmonary embolism	8	55	3.1

FIG. 22.5. Results of the Multiple Outcomes of Raloxifene Evaluation (MORE) randomized trial. [1]For groups receiving raloxifene 60 mg per day and 120 mg per day, respectively.

follow-up of 40 months, there were 12 DCIS and 40 invasive tumors reported. There were substantially fewer invasive cancers in women receiving raloxifene (RR = 0.24; 95% CI, 0.13–0.44; $p < 0.001$). This difference was entirely attributable to a 90% reduction in ER-positive invasive breast cancers (RR = 0.1; 95% CI, 0.04–0.24) with no difference in the occurrence of ER-negative tumors (Fig. 22.5) (43). At the 1998 American Society of Clinical Oncology meeting, a partially over-lapping analysis reviewing data from nine raloxifene trials (including MORE) was presented. Taken together, these studies demonstrate a significant reduction in newly diagnosed breast cancers in women on raloxifene (44).

Raloxifene Effects Other Than on the Breast

Endometrial Cancer Risk

Preclinical studies suggest that raloxifene may have limited effects on endometrial proliferation. In the initial clinical reports, endometrial thickening was unchanged during raloxifene therapy compared with placebo (45,46). Raloxifene did not in-crease the risk of endometrial cancer (RR = 0.8; 95% CI, 0.2–2.7) during the first 3 years of the MORE trial, but the total number of cases was small. In the women who underwent transvaginal ultrasound, endometrial thickness was increased by 0.01 mm in the raloxifene arm and decreased by 0.27 mm in the placebo group ($p < 0.01$) (43). It has not yet been established whether animal models and clinical endometrial proliferation are reliable predictors of endometrial cancer, especially in view of limited follow-up.

Bone Metabolism and Fracture Risk

Raloxifene is approved for the prevention of osteoporosis in postmenopausal women because the MORE trial showed a significant increase in BMD of the lumbar spine in women on raloxifene (47).

Lipid Metabolism and Cardiovascular Risk

Like tamoxifen, raloxifene influences serum lipid levels in a favorable way (45, 48,49), although whether this change in secondary markers can be translated into a reduction in CHD remains to be established. In the prospective, placebo-controlled RUTH (Raloxifene Use for the Heart) trial, raloxifene is being tested for its effects on CHD in high-risk postmenopausal women.

Coagulation and Thromboembolic Risk

The STAR trial (see later) will provide a direct comparison between tamoxifen and raloxifene on vascular events such as PE and deep vein thrombosis. The available data indicate a similar increase in these serious side effects from the two drugs. Among postmenopausal women on tamoxifen in the P-1 trial, the RR of PE was 3.19, and for DVT, it was 1.71 (21). For raloxifene, the RR of a thromboembolic event (including PE and DVT) was 3.1 (43).

Quality of Life

A pooled analysis from several clinical trials demonstrated a tamoxifen-like effect for raloxifene on symptoms of menopause in postmenopausal women (50). The greatest increase in hot flashes in the tamoxifen group of P-1 was seen in premeno-pausal women (21); therefore, a similar effect of raloxifene can be expected in this setting.

Comparison of Tamoxifen and Raloxifene

The reduction in breast cancer incidence was greater in the MORE trial than in P-1, but these two studies cannot be directly compared. Women in the P-1 trial were, on average, at higher risk for developing breast cancer and were generally younger. In addition, MORE was not designed to test the effect of raloxifene on breast cancer incidence, and the number of breast cancer events in the MORE study was low compared with that in P-1 (21,43). In the recently initiated STAR trial, which is comparing these two drugs as breast cancer preventatives, breast cancer incidence is the primary endpoint of the study (Fig. 22.6). Secondary endpoints and entry criteria are similar to the P-1 study, but only postmenopausal women are eligible. The safety of raloxifene use in premenopausal women is being evaluated in an ongoing study, which may allow entry of younger women into the STAR trial.

In summary, the available data suggest comparable effects of tamoxifen and raloxi-fene on organs other than the uterus, where raloxifene clearly appears less uterotropic and carcinogenic. In hysterectomized women, raloxifene has to date no demonstrable advantages over tamoxifen.

Alternative SERMS

Besides tamoxifen and raloxifene, several other SERMs have been, or are being, evaluated. Toremifene, an analog of tamoxifen, has been shown to have equivalent

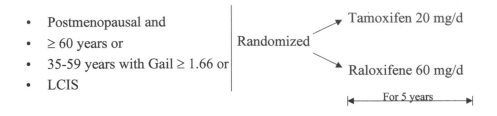

- Postmenopausal and
- ≥ 60 years or
- 35-59 years with Gail ≥ 1.66 or
- LCIS

Randomized

Tamoxifen 20 mg/d

Raloxifene 60 mg/d

|◄—————— For 5 years ——————►|

N=22,000   Primary Endpoint: Breast Cancer Incidence

FIG. 22.6. Design of the National Surgical Adjuvant Breast Project (NSABP) P-2 study.

efficacy in metastatic breast cancer compared with tamoxifen and is approved at a 20-mg dose for this indication (51,52). Currently, several adjuvant trials with toremifene are in progress. Interim analyses have shown no difference between tamoxifen and toremifene in terms of efficacy and side effects (53,54). In two other trials, toremifene appeared to have a more favorable effect on lipid metabolism than tamoxifen but was less bone preserving (55,56). Attempts to find improved SERMs as chemopreventive agents led to clinical testing of droloxifene, levormeloxifene, and idoxifene, but development has been discontinued for all three of these agents. Droloxifene did not show beneficial effects compared with tamoxifen in breast cancer patients, and both levormeloxifene and idoxifene caused somewhat unexpected gynecologic effects (57,58). EM-800 (SCH 57050) and its derivative SCH 57068, originally thought to be pure antiestrogens, have now been shown to have SERM properties. They have potent anti–breast cancer effects in preclinical models, cause uterine atrophy, and have a positive effect on bone metabolism. This profile gives these compounds the potential to be better chemopreventive agents than tamoxifen. SCH 57068 is likely to be the agent tested because it does not cause a reduction in serum free-carnitine levels, known to be a problem with the parent SCH 57050 (59–63). Likewise lasofoxifene (CP 336156) and the raloxifene analog LY 117018 have profiles in preliminary preclinical and clinical studies to make them promising chemopreventives with improved end-organ profiles (64–67).

OTHER POSSIBLE AGENTS FOR FUTURE CHEMOPREVENTION TRIALS

Pure Antiestrogens

ICI 182 780 (Faslodex), the most potent known steroidal antiestrogen, is an analog of estradiol without agonist activity. In athymic nude mice, inhibitory effects of ICI 182 780 on the growth of MCF-7 human breast cancer xenografts have been demonstrated (68) and ICI 182 780 has shown efficacy as a second-line agent after tamoxifen failure in advanced breast cancer. Unexpectedly, ICI 182 780 produced no significant changes in bone density and gonadotropin levels (69–71). Further evaluation of this potent antiestrogen is warranted. It may have a role in chemoprevention if its therapeutic index is favorable, but one definite disadvantage is the need to administer it parenterally.

Aromatase Inhibitors

Antagonizing the effects of estrogen on the breast is a principle of chemoprevention that has been established by tamoxifen and other SERMs. In addition, catecholestrogens, metabolites of estrogen, are thought to be genotoxic and tumorigenic (6). Therefore targeting estrogen synthesis is a way of preventing estradiol from stimulating the receptor and reducing the formation of these cancer-causing metabolites. To this end, estrogen synthetase (aromatase) inhibitors have been developed. Aromatase is the enzyme complex responsible for the final step in estrogen biosynthesis: the conversion of androgens to estrogens. Preclinical experiments have been conducted to determine the chemopreventive efficacy of new potent and selective aromatase inhibitors. For example, vorozole decreased tumor incidence from 100% to 10% and tumor multiplicity from 5 tumors to 0.1 tumors per animal in the MNU-induced rat mammary tumor model (72) and showed similar effects in the DMBA-induced tumor model (73). Similarly, letrozole inhibited new mammary tumor development in the DMBA rat model (74,75). To date, clinical development of aromatase inhibitors has focused on their use in postmenopausal women with hormone receptor positive breast cancer (76). The third-generation aromatase inhibitors letrozole, anastrozole, and exemestane are approved for use as second-line therapy in metastatic disease after tamoxifen (77–79). Large randomized phase 3 trials are now examining the role of aromatase inhibitors in the adjuvant treatment of breast cancer. Reduction of contralateral breast cancer in these trials will provide the first clinical data on the potential chemopreventive effects of this class of compounds. Preclinical experiments have demonstrated ''estrogen hypersensitivity'' and ''tamoxifen dependence'' in prolonged tamoxifen-exposed breast cancer cells (80). Therefore, several adjuvant trials are also exploring the role of aromatase inhibitors after tamoxifen. If this sequential strategy proves to be the optimal approach, it may translate into the chemopreventive setting.

In all the adjuvant studies, rigorous companion studies are being conducted to determine other end-organ effects of aromatase inhibitor therapy. For example, bone density, bone biomarkers, lipid metabolism, and quality of life are being carefully evaluated and will help to define the therapeutic index of this class of antiestrogen therapy.

Retinoids

Retinoids are a class of compounds that includes vitamin A and its analogs. Although their mechanisms of action at the molecular level are largely unknown, it is evident that retinoids influence cell differentiation, apoptosis and cell proliferation (81).

Exogenous retinoids have been shown to inhibit the proliferation of human breast cancer cells *in vitro* and in animal models (81). Furthermore, in preclinical breast cancer prevention studies, the addition of retinoids to both tamoxifen and raloxifene resulted in a decrease in mammary tumor incidence as compared to the use of SERMS alone (82,83). Their chronic toxicity and poor pharmacodynamic profile, however, limit the administration of pharmacologically active doses of exogenous retinoids in humans. Despite the synthesis of thousands of new retinoids in the past 20 years, these obstacles have not been overcome. In a clinical trial, the efficacy of adjuvant fenretinide, a new retinoid, in preventing a second breast malignancy in women with breast cancer was evaluated. After a median follow-up of 97 months, no statistically significant reduction in the occurrence of contralateral breast cancer could be shown compared with the no-treatment arm (81,84).

Recently, retinoic acid metabolism blocking agents (RAMBAs) have been developed. They act by inhibiting the catabolism of retinoic acid and, unlike retinoids, they do not induce their own metabolism. Consequently, they increase both tissue and plasma levels of endogenous retinoids (85,86). The first member of this class of compounds, liarozole fumarate, is not only a RAMBA but also a powerful third-generation aromatase inhibitor (86–88). Liarozole has been shown to have antitumor activity against ER-positive and ER-negative breast cancer in the preclinical and clinical setting (89,90). RAMBAs, therefore, may be the preferable approach to investigate the chemopreventive effects of retinoic acid.

Dietary Prevention

Dietary modification as a possible approach to breast cancer prevention is obviously attractive. To date, numerous compounds in food have been shown to have anticancer effects in animal studies, yet only few of them have been investigated in humans as potential chemopreventives.

Flaxseed

Flaxseed is a source of plant lignans, which are estrogenic compounds in plants called phytoestrogens. Epidemiologic evidence suggests that breast cancer incidence is low among populations with high flaxseed consumption and urinary lignan levels (91). Flaxseed has been shown to have chemopreventive effects on mammary tumor development in the preclinical setting (92). It has been suggested that some of its effects may be mediated by influence on endogenous hormone metabolism. The lignans enterolactone and enterodiol bind the ER and weakly inhibit aromatase (93). Flaxseed also increases total urinary estrogen excretion and lengthens the luteal phase of the menstrual cycle in humans (94,95). Given the strong association between estrogen levels and breast cancer risk (see also section 2), this influence on sex-steroid metabolism, together with its other antiestrogen effects, makes dietary flaxseed ingestion a chemoprevention strategy worth exploring. Currently, there are several ongoing studies examining the effects of dietary flaxseed intake on surrogate markers for breast cancer chemoprevention, such as breast density.

Soya

Soy beans contain isoflavones, which are converted to antiestrogenic and antioxidative compounds in the bowel. They have cytostatic activity in mammary cancer cell lines and inhibit growth and progression of mammary tumors in rodents (96–98). In addition, soy milk supplements have been reported to reduce serum estradiol levels in premenopausal women (99). Therefore, like flaxseed, soy protein appears to be a dietary component suitable for clinical trials to investigate a potential breast cancer chemopreventive effect (100).

Vitamin E

Vitamin E is a lipid-soluble antioxidant with the potential to protect breast tissue from oxidant damage, which has been proposed as a possible cause of breast cancer (101). In preclinical studies, vitamin E has been shown to reduce proliferation of breast cancer cell lines and to decrease mammary carcinogenesis in the DMBA-induced mammary tumor model (102,103). The influence of vitamin E on breast cancer risk has been explored in several clinical studies, some of which found an inverse association of dietary intake of vitamin E and breast cancer incidence (104).

Reduction of Fat Intake

Breast cancer incidence is associated with dietary fat intake, as shown in Table 22.1 (105). To explore whether this relationship can be exploited for chemopreventive purposes, a study is being conducted in women with higher than average mammographic density (Table 22.1). Women in this trial were randomly assigned to a low-fat, high carbohydrate diet or a control group. After 2 years, a significant reduction in breast density and serum estradiol levels was observed in the intervention group as compared to control (106,107). Whether these findings are associated with a reduction in breast cancer incidence remains to be determined by further follow-up.

Oophorectomy

The estrogen-antagonizing strategies discussed under SERMs and aromatase inhibitors may be of advantage in premenopausal women as well but probably are most effectively employed in conjunction with ovarian function ablation. The most likely cohort of premenopausal women in whom preventative strategies would be used are those at genetic risk for breast cancer.

Oophorectomy has been known for a long time to prevent recurrence of breast cancer after primary diagnosis and to reduce the risk of second, new primaries (29). Chemical oophorectomy with luteinizing hormone-releasing hormone (LHRH) analogs, such as goserelin and buserelin, that inhibit the production of LH and follicle-stimulating hormone in the pituitary gland is a reversible alternative to oophorectomy. Thus, an LHRH analog with a SERM or an aromatase inhibitor might prove to be a chemoprevention strategy for high-risk young women. Because premature loss of ovarian function is of particular concern in young women, the use of a bone-preserving and lipid-lowering SERM in combination with an LHRH analog is most attractive (see also Chapter 23).

CONSIDERATIONS FOR FUTURE CHEMOPREVENTION TRIALS

The positive results of the P-1 tamoxifen prevention trial are of major significance. Not only is it a "proof of concept" that antiendocrine agents can substantially reduce the risk of breast cancer, but it also raises important issues with respect to future chemoprevention studies. Improved agents, alternative cohort selection, and different trial designs merit consideration. Figure 22.7 illustrates parameters affecting the clinical development of future chemopreventives, and some key questions pertaining to them are discussed in more detail as follows:

What is optimal risk assessment for breast cancer? The prevention trials conducted to date have been based on identification of women at higher than average risk for breast cancer. The term *high risk*, however, has not yet been unanimously agreed on, and many risk factors that might be included into an estimation of an individual patient's risk have been proposed. In the P-1 trial, for example, *high risk* was defined as a Gail score greater than 1.66, although the Gail model has been criticized for omitting or incompletely accounting for additional factors, such as *BRCA1* or *2* status, ethnicity, and family history of male breast and ovarian cancer (20,21). Differences in risk assessment might explain the discrepant North American and European tamoxifen prevention trial results. In future clinical studies, it will be necessary to decide whether women with different risk factors should be included in the same trials as in P-1 and STAR or whether the target populations should be confined to specific risk factors. This decision is based in part on whether the selected agent is believed to act similarly in women with diverse risks. Furthermore, the addition of newly identified clinical markers of risk, such as breast density, bone density, and elevated plasma estrogen levels, may be used as entry criteria for future chemoprevention trials. Finally a study subject's perception of risk also influences the conduct of the trial in terms of compliance and the final evaluation of the therapeutic index of a study drug.

What are the features of an ideal chemopreventive drug? Originally, the term *chemoprevention* was defined as the use of specific natural or synthetic chemical agents to reverse, suppress, or prevent carcinogenic progression to invasive cancer

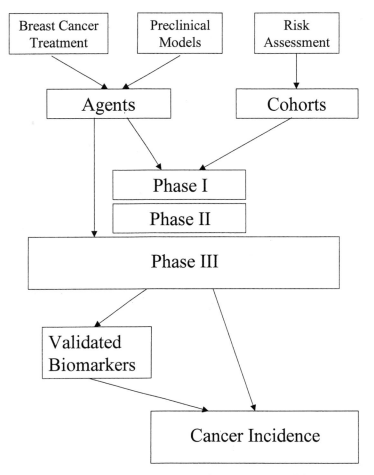

FIG. 22.7. Key parameters in chemoprevention trials.

(108). It has been debated as to whether the P-1 study has shown tamoxifen to be "chemopreventive" rather than treating incident cases of cancer. From a clinical standpoint, however, it may not be relevant whether an agent prevents the initiation of a cancer or inhibits its promotion or both because reduction in the incidence of cancer is clearly of importance. The pharmacologic profile of an ideal breast cancer chemopreventive agent should include oral availability, an excellent therapeutic index, and absence of long-term toxicities, the two last points being difficult to evaluate without costly long-term exposure and follow-up in clinical trials. Ideally, unlike tamoxifen, and apparently raloxifene, it should also reduce the incidence of both ER-positive and ER-negative tumors.

How can potential chemopreventive agents be identified? Two major tools have been used to assess potential breast cancer chemopreventives: preclinical models (see also preceding section entitled Estrogen and Breast Cancer Risk) and efficacy in the treatment of breast cancer patients. Results obtained with the currently used preclinical models have not always been predictive of efficacy in humans. Thus, improving these models is an important future challenge because it could help to select successful agents and shorten the interval between discovery of a new agent and its ultimate clinical application.

A positive effect of an agent in breast cancer treatment is obviously a powerful piece of evidence to support its potential as a chemopreventive. This was exemplified by the activity of tamoxifen in advanced disease in the adjuvant setting and most importantly in the prevention of contralateral new primary breast cancer. For the selection of future agents, however, this lengthy and costly model may not be necessary. Efficacy against advanced breast cancer may not be realistic for some agents, in which case this should not be inappropriately used as a selection tool. Where it is, a simple phase 2 response trial may be adequate to select a promising agent. In any case, outstanding questions will always remain from breast cancer studies, and additional clinical trials will be necessary. This subsequent clinical trial path, helpful in selecting an agent, is discussed next.

What studies are necessary and feasible to move forward to a large breast cancer prevention trial? In the case of tamoxifen, phase 1 and 2 trials in healthy women were not performed prior to the definitive prevention study. That left several issues unanswered at the end of the trial. Is 20 mg the minimal effective dose for chemoprevention? Is the duration of 5 years and the continuous once-daily administration the optimal chemoprevention strategy? For future agents, phase 1 and 2 dose finding studies for safety and efficacy on other end-organs should be conducted in healthy women. These could be stand-alone trials or assessed in a vanguard cohort within the context of phase 3 trials (109). Ultimately, long and costly phase 3 trials with breast cancer occurrence as an endpoint will always be required unless truly validated surrogate markers can be identified and relied on for the registration of a new chemopreventive agent (110,111). Should this happen, then the clinical trial strategy could focus on dose finding, schedule optimizing studies in healthy women, and the definitive trials could be much shorter.

What are possible secondary endpoints in breast cancer chemoprevention? Most agents evaluated in breast cancer chemoprevention to date have been endocrine agents with secondary effects on other organs, like bone, lipid metabolism, the cardiovascular system, and the uterus. Chemoprevention trials should evaluate these endpoints and cohorts should be selected with regard to risk factors in organs such as osteoporosis, high plasma lipid levels, history of myocardial infarction, or history of endometrial malignancy. Matching designer drugs with specific end-organ effects to cohorts with specific profiles of risk such as osteoporosis or cardiovascular disease may be feasible in the future.

Other future considerations: It will remain difficult but desirable to define the duration of cancer risk reduction (prevention) with future agents in novel cohorts. The risk of ER-negative breast cancer has not been reduced by either tamoxifen or raloxifene and, in addition, this form of breast cancer carries a greater risk of death.

Thus, finding ways to prevent these tumors is imperative, and ultimately, reduction in breast cancer mortality not just incidence must be achieved. This might require combinations or sequences of endocrine agents with or without other novel classes of drugs. Of course, in addition to achieving these important goals, the benefit of chemopreventives must be shown clearly both to outweigh the risks and to be affordable within the context of a health care budget. These critical questions will continue to challenge researchers attempting to prevent breast cancer in the foreseeable future.

REFERENCES

1. Ries LAG, Kosary CL, Hankey BF, et al. *SEER cancer statistics review, 1973–1996: tables and graphs.* Bethesda, MD.: National Cancer Institute, 1999.
2. Chu KC, Tarone RE, Kessler LG, et al. Recent trends in U.S. breast cancer incidence, survival and mortality rates. *J Natl Cancer Inst* 1996;88:1571–1579.
3. Hulka BS, Liu ET, Lininger RA. Steroid hormones and risk of breast cancer. *Cancer* 1994;74(3 Suppl):1111–1124.
4. Brzozowski AM, Pike AC, Dauter Z, et al. Molecular basis of agonism and antagonism in the oestrogen receptor. *Nature* 1997;389:753–758.
5. Santen RJ, Yue W, Naftolin F. The potential of aromatase inhibitors in breast cancer prevention. *Endocrine-Related Cancer* 1999;6:235–243.
6. Yager JD, Liehr JG. Molecular mechanism of estrogen carcinogenesis. *Annu Rev Pharmacol Toxicol* 1996;36:203–232.
7. Adami HO, Signorello LB, Trichopoulos D. Towards an understanding of breast cancer etiology *Semin Cancer Biol* 1998;8:255–262.
8. Boyd NF, Byng JW, Jong RA, et al. Quantitative classification of mammographic densities and breast cancer risk: results from the Canadian National Breast Screening Study. *J Natl Cancer Inst* 1995;87:670–675.
9. Cauley JA, Lucas FL, Kuller LH, et al. Bone mineral density and risk of breast cancer in older women: the study of osteoporotic fractures. Study of Osteoporotic Fractures Research Group. *JAMA* 1996;276:1404–1408.
10. Zhang Y, Kiel DP, Kreger BE, et al. Bone mass and the risk of breast cancer among postmenopausal women. *N Engl J Med* 1997;336:611–617.
11. Toniolo PG, Levitz M, Zeleniuch-Jacquotte A, et al. A prospective study of endogenous estrogens and breast cancer in postmenopausal women. *J Natl Cancer Inst* 1995;87:190–197.
12. Cauley JA, Lucas FL, Kuller LH, et al. Elevated serum estradiol and testosterone concentrations are associated with a high risk for breast cancer. *Ann Intern Med* 1999;130(4 part 1):270–277.
13. Hsieh C-C, Trichopoulos D, Katsouyanni K, et al. Age at menarche, age at menopause, height and obesity as risk factors for breast cancer: associations and interactions in an international case-control study. *Int J Cancer* 1990;46:796–800.
14. Byrne C, Schairer C, Wolfe J, et al. Mammographic features and breast cancer risk: effects with time, age, and menopause status. *J Natl Cancer Inst* 1995;87:1622–1629.
15. Easton D, Ford D, Peto J. Inherited susceptibility to breast cancer. *Cancer Surv* 1993;18:95–113.
16. Goss PE, Sierra S. Current perspectives on radiation-induced breast cancer. *J Clin Oncol* 1998;16: 338–347.
17. Collaborative Group on Hormonal Factors in Breast Cancer. Breast cancer and hormone replacement therapy: collaborative reanalysis of data from 51 epidemiological studies of 52,705 women with breast cancer and 108,411 women without breast cancer. *Lancet* 1997;350:1047–1059.
18. Colditz G, Hankinson S, Hunter D. The use of estrogens and progestins and the risk of breast cancer in postmenopausal women. *N Engl J Med* 1995;332:1589–1593.
19. Schairer C, Lubin J, Troisi R, et al. Menopausal estrogen and estrogen-progestin replacement therapy and breast cancer risk. *JAMA* 2000;283:485–491.
20. Gail MH, Brinton LA, Byar DP, et al. Projecting individualized probabilities of developing breast cancer for white females who are being examined annually *J Natl Cancer Inst* 1989;81:1879–1886.
21. Fisher B, Costantino J, Wickerham L, et al. Tamoxifen for prevention of breast cancer: report

of the National Surgical Adjuvant Breast and Bowel Project P-1. *J Natl Cancer Inst* 1998;90: 1371–1388.

22. Clarke R. Human breast cancer cell line xenografts as models of breast cancer: the immunobiologies of recipient mice and the characteristics of several tumorigenic cell lines. *Breast Cancer Res Treat* 1996;39:69–86.

23. Lu Q, Liu Y, Long BJ, et al. The effect of combining aromatase inhibitors with antiestrogens on tumor growth in a nude mouse model for breast cancer. *Breast Cancer Res Treat* 1999;57:183–192.

24. Russo J, Russo IH. Experimentally induced mammary tumors in rats. *Breast Cancer Res Treat* 1996;39:7–20.

25. Fisher B, Costantino J, Redmond C, et al. A randomized clinical trial evaluating tamoxifen in the treatment of patients with node-negative breast cancer who have estrogen-receptor-positive tumors. *N Engl J Med* 1989;320:479–484.

26. Rutqvist LE, Cedermark B, Glas U, et al. Contralateral primary tumors in breast cancer patients in a randomized trial of adjuvant tamoxifen therapy. *J Natl Cancer Inst* 1991;83:1299–1306.

27. Breast Cancer Trials Committee, Scottish Cancer Trials Office (MRC), Edinburgh. Adjuvant tamoxifen in the management of operable breast cancer: The Scottish Trial. *Lancet* 1987;2:171–175.

28. Fisher B, Redmond C. New perspective on cancer of the contralateral breast: a marker for assessing tamoxifen as a preventive agent. *J Natl Cancer Inst* 1991;83:1278–1280.

29. Early Breast Cancer Trialists' Collaborative Group. Systemic treatment of early breast cancer by hormonal, cytotoxic, or immune therapy: 133 randomised trials involving 31000 recurrences and 24000 deaths among 75000 women. *Lancet* 1992;339: 1–15,71–78.

30. Early Breast Cancer Trialists' Collaborative Group. Tamoxifen for early breast cancer: an overview of the randomised trials. *Lancet* 1998;351:1451–1467.

31. Veronesi U, Maisonneuve P, Costa A, et al. Prevention of breast cancer with tamoxifen: preliminary findings from the Italian randomised trial among hysterectomised women. Italian Tamoxifen Prevention Study. *Lancet* 1998;352:93–97.

32. Powles T, Eeles R, Ashley S, et al. Interim analysis of the incidence of breast cancer in the Royal Marsden Hospital tamoxifen randomised chemoprevention trial. *Lancet* 1998;352:98–101.

33. Wolmark N, Dgnam J, Fisher B. The addition of tamoxifen to lumpectomy and radiotherapy in the treatment of ductal carcinoma in situ (DCIS): preliminary results of NSABP Protocol B-24. San Antonio Symposium Proceedings. *Breast Cancer Res* 1998;21:227(abst).

34. McDonald CC, Alexander FE, Whyte BW et al. Cardiac and vascular morbidity in women receiving adjuvant tamoxifen for breast cancer in a randomized trial: the Scottish Cancer Trials Breast Group. *BMJ* 1994;311:977–537.

35. McDonald CC, Stewart HJ: Fatal myocardial infarction in the Scottish adjuvant tamoxifen trial: The Scottish Breast Cancer Committee. *BMJ* 1991;303:435–437.

36. Costantino JP, Kuller LH, Ives DG, et al. Coronary heart disease mortality and adjuvant tamoxifen therapy. *J Natl Cancer Inst* 1997;89:776–782.

37. Ruqvist LE, Matteson A. Cardiac and thromboembolic morbidity among postmenopausal women with early-stage breast cancer in a randomized trial of adjuvant tamoxifen: The Stockholm Breast Cancer Study Group. *J Natl Cancer Inst* 1993;85:1398–1406.

38. Love RR, Barden HS, Mazess RB, et al. Effect of tamoxifen on lumbar spine bone mineral density in postmenopausal women after 5 years. *Arch Intern Med* 1994;54:2585–2588.

39. Love RR, Mazess RB, Barden HS, et al. Effects of tamoxifen on bone mineral density in postmenopausal women with breast cancer. *M Engl J Med* 1992;326:852–856.

40. Love RR, Mazess RB, Torney DC, et al. Bone mineral density in women with breast cancer treated with adjuvant tamoxifen for at least two years. *Breast Cancer Res Treat* 1998;2:297–302.

41. Chlebowski RT, Collyar DE, Somerfield MR, et al. American Society of Clinical Oncology Technology Assessment on Breast Cancer Risk Reduction Strategies: Tamoxifen and Raloxifene. *J Clin Oncol* 1999;17:1939–1955.

42. Day R, Ganz PA, Costatino JP, et al. Health-related quality of life and tamoxifen in breast cancer prevention: a report from the National Surgical Adjuvant Breast and Bowel Project P-1 Study. *J Clin Oncol* 1999;17:2659–2669.

43. Cummings R, Eckert S, Krueger K, et al. The effect of raloxifene on risk of breast cancer in postmenopausal women: results form the MORE randomized trial. *JAMA* 1999;281:2189–2197.

44. Jordan VC, Glusman, JE, Eckert S, et al. Raloxifene reduces incident primary breast cancer: Integrated data from multicenter, double-blind, placebo-controlled, randomized trials in postmenopausal

women. San Antonio Breast Cancer Symposium Proceedings. *Breast Cancer Res Treat* 1998;21: 227(abst).

45. Delmas PD, Bjamasan NG, Mitlak BH, et al. Effects of raloxifene on bone mineral density, serum cholesterol concentrations, and uterine endometrium in postmenopausal women. *N Engl J Med* 1997;337:1641–1647.
46. Boss SM, Huster WJ, Neild JA, et al. Effects of raloxifene hydrochloride on the endometrium of postmenopausal women. *Am J Obstet Gynecol* 1997;177:1458–1464.
47. Ettinger B, Black DM, Mitlak BH, et al. Reduction of vertebral fracture risk in postmenopausal women with osteoporosis treated with raloxifene: results from a 3-year randomized clinical trial: Multiple Outcomes of Raloxifene Evaluation (MORE) Investigators. *JAMA* 1999;282:637–645.
48. Draper MW, Flowers DE, Huster WJ, et al. A controlled trial of raloxifene (LY139481) HCl: impact on bone turnover and serum lipid profile in healthy postmenopausal women. *J Bone Miner Res* 1996;11:835–842.
49. Walsh BW, Kuller LH, Wild RA et al. Effects of raloxifene on serum lipids and coagulation factors in healthy postmenopausal women. *JAMA* 1998;279:1445–1485.
50. Glusman J, Lu Y, Huster W, et al. Raloxifene effects on climacterial symptoms compared with hormone or estrogen replacement therapy (HRT or ERT) *Proceedings of the North American Menopause Society,* 8th Annual Meeting Program, 1997:65. (abst).
51. Buzdar AU, Hortobagyi G. Update on endocrine therapy for breast cancer. *Clin Cancer Res* 1998; 4:527–534.
52. Hayes DF, Vvan Zyl JA, Hacking A, et al. Randomized comparison of tamoxifen and two separate doses of toremifene in postmenopausal patients with metastatic breast cancer. *J Clin Oncol* 1995; 13:2556–2566.
53. Holli K. Evolving role of toremifene in the adjuvant setting. *Oncology* 1997;11(5 Suppl 4):48–51.
54. Holli K. Adjuvant trials of toremifene vs. tamoxifen: the European experience. *Oncology* 1998; 12(3 Suppl 5):23–27.
55. Saarto T, Blomqvist C, Ehnholm C, et al. Antiatherogenic effects of adjuvant antiestrogens: A randomized trial comparing the effects of tamoxifen and toremifene on plasma lipid levels in postmenopausal women with node-positive breast cancer. *J Clin Oncol* 1996;14:429–433.
56. Marttunen M, Hietanen P, Tiitinen A, et al. Comparison of effects of tamoxifen and toremifene on bone biochemistry and bone mineral density in postmenopausal breast cancer patients. *J Clin Endocrinol Metab* 1998;83:1158–1162.
57. Bruning PF. Droloxifene, a new anti-oestrogen in postmenopausal advanced breast cancer: preliminary results of a double-blind dose-finding phase II trial. *Eur J Cancer* 1992;28A:1404–1407.
58. Haarstad H, Lonning PE, Gundersen S, et al. Influence of droloxifene on metastatic breast cancer as first-line endocrine treatment. *Acta Oncol* 1998;37:365–368.
59. Simard J, Labrie C, Belanger A, et al. Characterization of the effects of the novel non-steroidal antiestrogen EM-800 on basal and estrogen-induced proliferation of T-47D, ZR-75-1 and MCF-7 human breast cancer cells in vitro. *Int J Cancer* 1997;73:104–112.
60. Simard J, Sanchez R, Poirier D, et al. Blockade of the stimulatory effect of estrogens, OH-tamoxifen, OH-toremifene, droloxifene and raloxifene an alkaline phosphatase activity by the antiestrogen EM-800 in human endometrial adenocarcinoma Ishikawa cells. *Cancer Res* 1997;57:3494–3497.
61. Tremblay A, Tremblay GB, Labrie C, et al. EM-800, a novel antiestrogen, acts as a pure antagonist of the transcriptional functions of estrogen receptors a and b. *Endocrinology* 1998;139:111–118.
62. Labrie F, Labrie C, Belanger A, et al. EM-652 (SCH 57068), a third generation SERM acting as a pure antiestrogen in the mammary gland and endometrium. *J Steroid Biochem Mol Biol* 1999; 69:51–84.
63. Luo S, Sourla A, Labrie C, et al. Effect of twenty-four-week treatment with antiestrogen EM-800 on estrogen-sensitive parameters in intact and ovariectomized mice. *Endocrinology* 1998;139: 2645–2656.
64. Rosati RL, Da Silva Jardine P, et al. Discovery and preclinical pharmacology of a novel, potent, nonsteroidal estrogen receptor agonist/antagonist, CP-336156, a diaryltetrahydronaphthalene. *J Med Chem* 1998;41:2928–2931.
65. Ke HZ, Paralkar VM, Grasser WA, et al. Effects of CP-336156, a new, nonsteroidal estrogen agonist/antagonist, on bone, serum cholesterol, uterus and body composition in rat models. *Endocrinology* 1998;139:2068–2076.
66. Curiel MD, Calero JA, Guerrero R, et al. Effects of LY-117018 HCl on bone remodeling and mineral density in the oophorectomized rat. *Am J Obstet Gynecol* 1998;178:320–325.

67. Hodsman AB, Drost D, Fraher LJ, et al. The addition of a raloxifene analog (LY117018) allows for reduced PTH(1-34) dosing during reversal of osteopenia in ovariectomized rats. *J Bone Miner Res* 1999;14:675–679.
68. Osborne CK, Coronado-Heinsohn EB, Hilsenbeck SG, et al. Comparison of the effects of a pure steroidal antiestrogen with those of tamoxifen in a model of human breast cancer. *J Natl Cancer Inst* 1995;87:746–750.
69. Howell A, De Friend DJ, Robertson JF, et al. Pharmacokinetics, pharmacological and anti-tumour effects of the specific anti-oestrogen ICI 182780 in women with advanced breast cancer. *Br J Cancer* 1996;74:300–308.
70. Howell A, De Friend D, Robertson J, et al. Response to a specific antioestrogen (ICI 182780) in tamoxifen-resistant breast cancer. *Lancet* 1995;345:29–30.
71. Nicholson RI, Gee JM, Manning DL, et al. Responses to pure antiestrogens (ICI 164384, ICI 182780) in estrogen-sensitive and resistant experimental and clinical breast cancer. *Ann NY Acad Sci* 1995;761:148–163.
72. Lubet RA, Steele VE, Casebolt TL, et al. Chemopreventive effects of the aromatase inhibitors vorozole (R-83842) and 4-hydroxyandrostenedione in the methylnitrosourea (MNU)-induced mammary tumor model in Sprague-Dawley rats. *Carcinogenesis* 1994;15:2775–2780.
73. De Coster R, Van Ginckerl RF, Callens MJ, et al. Antitumoral and endocrine effects of (+)-vorozole in rats bearing dimethylbenzanthracene-induced mammary tumors. *Cancer Res* 1992;52: 1240–1244.
74. Bhatnagar AS, Hausler A, Schieweck K, et al. Highly selective inhibition of estrogen biosynthesis by CGS 20267, a new non-steroidal aromatase inhibitor. *J Steroid Biochem Mol Biol* 1990;37: 1021–1027.
75. Schieweck K, Bhatnagar AS, Batzl C, et al. Anti-tumor and endocrine effects of non-steroidal aromatase inhibitors on estrogen-dependent rat mammary tumors. *J Steroid Biochem Mol Biol* 1993; 44:633–636.
76. Goss PE, Winer EP, Tannock IF, et al. on behalf of the North American Vorozole Study Group. A randomized phase III trial comparing the new potent and selective third-generation aromatase inhibitor vorozole with megestrol acetate in postmenopausal advanced breast cancer patients. *J Clin Oncol* 1999;17:52–63.
77. Buzdar A, Jonat W, Howell A, et al. for the Arimidex Study Group. Anastrozole, a potent and selective aromatase inhibitor, versus megestrol acetate in postmenopausal women with advanced breast cancer: results of overview and analysis of two phase III clinical trials. *J Clin Oncol* 1996; 14:2000–2011.
78. Dombernowsky P, Smith I, Falkson G, et al. Letrozole, a new oral aromatase inhibitor for advanced breast cancer: double-blind randomized trial showing a dose effect and improved efficacy and tolerability compared with megestrol acetate. *J Clin Oncol* 1998;16:453–461.
79. Scott LJ, Wiseman LR. Exemestane. *Drugs* 1999;58:675–680.
80. Yue W, Santen R. Aromatase inhibitors: rationale for use following anti-oestrogen therapy. *Semin Oncol* 1996;23(4 Suppl 9):21–27.
81. Miller WH Jr. The emerging role of retinoids and retinoic acid metabolism blocking agents in the treatment of cancer. *Cancer* 1998;83:1471–1482.
82. Anzano MA, Byers SW, Smith JM, et al. Prevention of breast cancer in rats with 9-cis-retonoic acid as a single acid and in combination with tamoxifen. *Cancer Res* 1994;54:4614–4617.
83. Anzano MA, Peer CW, Smith JM, et al. Chemoprevention of mammary carcinogenesis in the rat: combined use of raloxifene and 9-cis-retinoic acid. *J Natl Cancer Inst* 1996;17;88:123–125.
84. Veronesi U, De Palo G, Marubini E, et al. Randomized trial of fenretinide to prevent second breast malignancy in women with early breast cancer. *J Natl Cancer Inst* 1999;91:1847–1856.
85. Van Wauwe JP, Coene MC, Goossens J, et al. Effects of cytochrome P-450 inhibitors on the *in vivo* metabolism of all-*trans*-retinoic acid in rats. *J Pharmacol Exp Ther* 1990;252:365–369.
86. Van Wauwe J, Van Nyen G, Coene MC, et al. Liarozole, an inhibitor of retinoic acid metabolism, exerts retinoid-mimetic effects *in vivo J Pharmacol Ther* 1992;261:773–779.
87. Bruynseels J, De Coster R, Van Rooy P, et al. G: R75251, a new inhibitor of steroid biosynthesis. *Prostate* 1990;16:345–357.
88. Van Wauwe J, Coene MC, Cools W, et al. Liarozole fumarate inhibits the metabolism of 4-keto-all-trans-retinoic acid. *Biochem Pharmacol* 1994;47:737–741.
89. Goss PE, Oza A, Goel R, et al. Liarozole fumarate (R85246): a novel imidazole in the treatment

of receptor positive postmenopausal metastatic breast cancer. *Breast Cancer Res Treat* 2000;59: 55–68.

90. Goss PE, Strasser K, Marques R, et al. Liarozole fumarate (R85246): in the treatment of ER negative, tamoxifen refractory or chemotherapy resistant postmenopausal metastatic breast cancer. *Breast Cancer Res Treat* 2001;64:177–188.

91. Ingram D, Sanders K, Kolybaba M, et al. Case-control study of phyto-oestrogens and breast cancer. *Lancet* 1997;350:990–994.

92. Serraino M, Thompson LU. The effect of flaxseed supplementation on the initiation and promotional stages of mammary tumorigenesis. *Nutr Cancer* 1992;17,153–159.

93. Wang C, Makela T, Hase T, et al. Lignans and flavonoids inhibit aromatase enzyme in human preadipocytes. *J Steroid Biochem Mol Biol* 1994;50:205–212.

94. Haggans CJ, Hutchins AM, Olson BA, et al. Effect of flaxseed consumption on urinary estrogen metabolites in postmenopausal women. *Nutr Cancer* 1999;33:188–195.

95. Serraino M, Thompson LU. The effect of flaxseed supplementation on early risk markers for mammary carcinogenesis. *Cancer Lett* 1991;60:135–142.

96. Lamartiniere CA, Moore JB, Brown NM, et al. Genistein suppresses mammary cancer in rats. *Carcinogenesis* 1995;16:2833–2840

97. Hawrylewicz EJ, Zapata JJ, Blair WH. Soy and experimental cancer: animal studies. *J Nutr* 1995; 125(Suppl 3):698–708

98. Barnes S. Effect of genistein on *in vitro* and *in vivo* models of cancer. *J Nutr* 1995;125 (Suppl 3): 777–783.

99. Lu LJW, Anderson KE, Grady JJ, et al. Effects of soya consumption for one month on steroid hormones in premenopausal women: implications for breast cancer risk reduction. *Cancer Epidimiol Biomarkers Prev* 1996;5:63–70.

100. Stoll BA. Eating to beat breast cancer: Potential role for soy supplements. *Ann Oncol* 1997;8: 223–225.

101. Baum M, Ziv Y, Colletta A. Prospects for the chemoprevention of breast cancer. *Br Med Bull* 1991; 47:493–503.

102. Knekt P. Role of vitamin E in the prophylaxis of cancer. *Ann Med* 1991;23:3–12.

103. Charpentier A, Groves S, Simmons-Menchaca M, et al. RRRα-Tocopheryl succinate inhibits proliferation and enhances secretion of transforming growth factor-β (TGF-β) by human breast cancer cells. *Nutr Cancer* 1993;19:225–239.

104. Kimmick GG, Bell RA, Bostick RM. Vitamin E and breast cancer: a review. *Nutr Cancer* 1997; 27:109–117.

105. Prentice RL, Kakar F, Hursting S, et al. Aspects of the rationale for the women's health trial. *J Natl Cancer Inst* 1988;80:802–814.

106. Boyd NF, Greenberg C, Lockwood GA, et al. Effects at two years of a low-fat, high carbohydrate diet on radiologic features of the breast: results from a randomized trial. *J Natl Cancer Inst* 1997; 89:488–496.

107. Boyd NF, Lockwood GA, Greenbert CV, et al. Effects of a low-fat high carbohydrate diet on plasma sex hormones in premenopausal women: results from a randomized controlled trial. *Br J Cancer* 1997;76:127–135.

108. Lippman SM, Benner SE, Hong WK. Cancer chemoprevention. *J Clin Oncol* 1994;12:851–873.

109. Goodman GE. The clinical evaluation of cancer chemoprevention agents: defining and contrasting phase I, II, and III objectives. *Cancer Res* 1992;52(9 Suppl):2752s–2757s.

110. Lippman SM, Lee JS, Lotan R, et al. Biomarkers as intermediate and points in chemoprevention trials. *J Natl Cancer Inst* 1990;82:555–560.

111. Schatzkin A, Freedman LS, Schiffman MH, et al. Validation of intermediate endpoints in cancer research. *J Natl Cancer Inst* 1990;82:1746–1752.

23

Management of Women at Increased Risk for Breast Cancer

Carol E. H. Scott-Conner

From observations of familial clusters of breast and ovarian cancer, the deduction was made that an autosomal dominant mutation might explain some of these events. *BRCA1* and subsequently *BRCA2* were identified (1–4). Although specific tests are available for *BRCA1* and *BRCA2*, most women present for evaluation of breast problems without a detailed genetic analysis. Because most cases of breast cancer occur in women who lack these genes, an overall assessment of risk is in order. From this will follow naturally a decision as to whether or not to discuss and offer the option of genetic counseling or referral to a high-risk familial cancer clinic. The first part of this chapter briefly summarizes the known risk factors, tools for assessing risk, and the decision to refer for genetic counseling. The second part deals with options in the management of the woman who has been identified to be at increased risk.

The two strongest risk factors are family and personal history of breast cancer. Most women with a family history of breast cancer generally do not have the genetically transmitted form of the disease because of a currently identifiable mutation (4). Thus, a strategy for identifying women at sufficiently high risk to justify genetic testing has evolved. Familial clusters of cancer due to an identifiable gene share these characteristics: young age of onset, multicentricity or bilaterality, multiple cases of cancer on the same side of the family, and a cluster of tumors at sites considered rare (5). Applying this logic, the likelihood of *BRCA1* or *2* mutation increases with more breast cancer on one side of the family, early onset or bilateral disease, and a personal or family history of ovarian cancer. It is now thought that approximately 50% of such families carry a disease-associated allele. Special populations have significantly higher rates of carriage of known specific mutations, for example, Ashkenazi Jewish women (3). In one study, even in families with four or more breast cancer cases, a *BRCA1* or *2* mutation was identified in only 44% (6). From these data, general guidelines have evolved using algorithms involving the age of onset of affected family members, the number of affected first-degree relatives, or the presence of ovarian or male breast cancer (7). Reactions to genetic counseling vary; women found to be carriers do not appear to develop more depression or anxiety, and the reaction in women found not to be carriers spans a spectrum from relief through survivor guilt (8,9).

It appears likely that not all mutations of *BRCA1* and *2* are equally severe (10).

Variable penetrance of even known mutations implies that not all women who carry these mutations are at equal risk. In some affected families, breast cancer predominates, whereas in others, ovarian cancer is the dominant problem. Some affected families have a low incidence of breast cancer, and it has been hypothesized that mutation carriers from such families are likely to be at decreased risk (11). How much of this is due to other genetic factors, phenotype, environment, or differing mutation severity is unknown.

Two other autosomal-dominant syndromes that may increase the risk of breast cancer are Li Fraumeni (*p53*) and Cowden (*PTEN*). Ataxia–telangiectasia, an autosomal recessive gene that is present in high frequency in the population, may increase risk to both heterozygotes and homozygotes (12–14). Because several of these mutations involve repair genes and, hence, increase radiation sensitivity, the presence of these mutations has implications for early mammographic screening and possibly for therapy of breast cancer with radiation in affected persons (discussed later).

The incidence of any particular gene is low in the general population, and the large size and variety of mutations of several of these genes create a potential for a high false-negative rate in the absence of a known mutation. It has been estimated that genetic screening may miss 5% to 15% of significant *BRCA* mutations (15). Therefore, genetic screening is not advocated in the absence of a known mutation within a particular family or high-risk subgroup. The general strategy has been to identify the mutation in a known affected carrier before screening other members of the family. Exceptions may be made for high-risk populations such as Ashkenazi Jewish women, in whom the frequency of a known mutation is high (12).

Other, as yet unidentified genes that slightly increase the risk of breast cancer actually may be responsible for most cases of familial breast cancer. Finally, the absence of a strong family history may be misleading if small family sizes or adoption preclude accurate assessment of risk (16).

Cancer of one breast puts a woman at increased risk of cancer of the opposite breast, particularly if there is a family history of breast cancer. Until genetic testing was available, this was often stated to be the strongest predictor of increased risk. Some subsets of women, for example, women who undergo mantle radiation for Hodgkin disease at a young age, are at high risk for breast cancer, which is frequently bilateral.

Other risk factors include age (half of a woman's lifetime risk of breast cancer occurs after age 65) (4) and prolonged uninterrupted menses. Fewer than 25% of women with breast cancer will have a prior history of contralateral breast cancer, a family history, or the other risk factors previously mentioned (17). For most cases of breast cancer, an interaction between environmental and genetic factors is likely (14). Minor, but controllable, factors that increase risk include cigarette smoking, high dietary fat intake, obesity, and exogenous hormone administration. Exercise and prolonged lactation slightly decrease risk (14,17).

Tumor markers have been sought for risk assessment, screening, prognostic and therapeutic information (17). One such marker is overexpression of *HER-neu* protooncogene. There is a complex relationship between overexpression of *HER-neu* and response to hormonal or chemotherapy. Tumors with this trait are less likely to be estrogen or progesterone receptor positive; however, expression of the gene itself is modulated by estrogen. Better response to various chemotherapeutic agents and a potential target for gene-directed therapy make this an active area of investigation (18).

To put the problem into perspective, it has been estimated that a family practitioner with a panel of 1,000 women will diagnose one case of breast cancer every 1 to 2 years and one case of breast cancer due to an inherited susceptibility gene every 20 years (7). Risk may not be equivalent for all mutations, and family history should be considered (10). The decision to undergo genetic testing must be made with readiness to accept and work through the implications of a positive result (19); thus, a considerable amount of counseling should occur before actual testing. All this underscores the importance of a readily available tool that the individual practitioner can use to estimate risk in an individual woman.

Two commonly used risk-assessment tools, the Gail and Claus models, are available on the Internet (6,20). The Gail model was derived from breast cancer detection data from the 1970s and includes age, previous biopsies, and hormonal factors. The Clause model incorporates more data from family history, such as age of onset of affected family members. Neither model is perfect. American Society of Clinical Oncology guidelines suggest that genetic counseling be offered to patients with a strong family history, particularly with a young age of onset (21). As previously mentioned, population-based screening is not justified (22).

Biopsy evidence of particular kinds of benign breast disease correlates with increased risk. Proliferative lesions such as moderate or florid hyperplasia or a papilloma with a fibrovascular core are associated with a slight increase in risk (4). Proliferative lesions with atypia significantly increase risk (4). The multistep model of carcinogenesis has been more difficult to prove in breast cancer than in colon cancer because of the heterogeneous nature of the tissue (23). A plausible sequence would be normal → hyperplasia of the usual types → atypical ductal hyperplasia (ADH), which shares many of the genetic alterations of ductal carcinoma *in situ* (DCIS) → low nuclear grade DCIS → high nuclear grade DCIS → invasive carcinoma (17). Risk of invasive carcinoma increases as one progresses down the sequence (17,23). ADH is associated with a twofold to fivefold increase in risk of developing breast cancer; although it is possible that some DCIS remains quiescent or may even involute, DCIS is regarded as a direct precursor lesion (17). In contrast, lobular carcinoma *in situ* (LCIS) is thought to be a risk factor rather than an anatomic precursor. LCIS is associated with an increase of 6.9 to 12 times an increase in relative risk, which is equal in both breasts (4).

''Agenda differences'' between patients and providers are common (24). Patient concerns commonly include personal risk, risk to children, and how to screen for and prevent malignancies (6). Patients have different reasons to choose to attend a familial cancer clinic, ranging from personal risk to family risk, and these groups differ significantly in psychological variables (25). Whereas counseling provides additional information, it may not alter the decision to undergo testing (26,27).

Women tend to overestimate personal risk, and even expert counseling has little impact on this (26,27).

It may be helpful to conceptualize women as being, on average, at moderately increased or high risk for breast cancer. Women at average risk (which in the United States is stated as 12% lifetime risk) need to follow generally accepted screening and health-promotion guidelines (28). Women at moderate risk may be in greatest need of reassurance and close surveillance; chemoprevention may be an option for some, as exemplified by the National Surgical Adjuvant Breast Project Study of Tamoxifen and Raloxifene trial (29).

It is the group of women at highest risk for whom the choice is less certain. There are three basic approaches: intensive surveillance, chemoprevention, and prophylactic mastectomy (30). No single correct answer can be correct all the time. All the data are category III (expert consensus) and have not been validated for women with identified genetic mutations such as *BRCA1* carriers (31). Prospective randomized trials would be ideal (32), but it appears unlikely that women would consent to a study that would randomize prophylactic mastectomy against other options (33). Thus, data most likely will emerge through registries and carefully designed comparative trials (22,30). A trial combining preoperative imaging modalities such as magnetic resonance imaging (MRI) with careful pathologic examination of resected tissue would be of great value (30).

What is meant by intensive surveillance? The general consensus is that monthly breast self-examination, twice-annual specialist breast examination, and breast imaging should begin early (19,34). But how early should mammography be undertaken (16,19,20,34)? The risks of increased radiation exposure (particularly to young women, when the breast appears most vulnerable) must be balanced against the odds of early detection (12,15,30). A sensible approach would appear to be a mammogram at age 40 or five years earlier than the youngest first degree relative with breast cancer, whichever comes first. The quality of this mammogram (density) should then be evaluated before deciding upon continued annual or twice-annual mammography (19). MRI provides an alternative that shows great promise in limited studies (35). UK guidelines specify early mammography if breast cancer has occurred in two relatives between the ages of 40 and 49, or one relative under age 40. While a strong family history, including a family history of ovarian cancer increases the readiness to begin early intensive surveillance, the role of specific genetic mutations (e.g., AT) that lead to radiation-sensitivity must be sought before this can be a general recommendation (10,13, 14,16,36, 37). Increased mammographic density in younger women not only renders this screening modality less effective but may correlate with an increased risk of breast cancer because it is due to a greater percentage of epithelial/stromal cells compared with fat (38).

Several approaches are being taken to chemoprevention, an approach preferred by many women (39, 40). Tamoxifen, raloxifene, and similar agents have shown benefit in women at increased risk, but this finding has not been validated in women with known mutations (20,26,27,39,40). Raloxifene was associated with the best compromise between quality of life and life extension in one mathematical model

(39,40). Several studies using retinols are under way (19). Leuprolide is being investigated as a way to decrease ovarian hormone production and may be combined with estrogen and progesterone. In one study, oophorectomy reduced the risk of breast cancer in high-risk women, even when estrogen and progesterone were given. Other innovation approaches include inducing an early "pseudopregnancy" or seeking an ideal combination oral contraceptive that might induce terminal differentiation and provide advantages analogous to early pregnancy (37).

What about prophylactic surgery? For any prophylactic surgery to be useful, the procedure must be effective, the population at risk should be identifiable, and there should be a favorable cost-to-benefit analysis (both financial and from the standpoint of quality of life) (41,42). Prophylactic mastectomies have been performed for decades for varying indications. In the 1960s and 1970s, bilateral prophylactic mastectomy was used for mastodynia and in women in whom physical examination was unreliable because of multiple previous biopsies or nodularity, particularly those with cancerophobia (42). Most of these women were actually not at significantly increased risk by today's standards.

Prophylactic removal of the contralateral breast (in women with breast cancer of one breast) has been selectively used for decades (43). In a representative large series of 500 women who underwent prophylactic contralateral mastectomy, 8.4% were found to have unsuspected DCIS, LCIS, or invasive carcinoma on the "unaffected" side (43). Prophylactic contralateral mastectomy was generally reserved for women with a strong family history, with multicentric disease in the affected breast, or who have "precancerous mastopathy" on biopsy of the contralateral breast. Finally, it was generally considered appropriate only for women whose known breast cancer, age, and overall health status did not exclude at least a 20-year life expectancy (43). From this early experience, a cohort of 296 women was identified and studied for issues that caused them to regret the decision for prophylactic surgery. Regret was expressed by 6% of these women; issues included a poor cosmetic result, diminished sexuality, and lack of education about alternatives. Regret appeared slightly more common in women who had undergone reconstructive surgery (44). This seemingly paradoxical result may reflect the limitations of reconstruction or unrealistic expectation.

Prophylactic contralateral mastectomy is no longer *generally* advocated. For most women, the risk of mortality from the known primary exceeds the potential risk from an unknown second primary. Only 4.1% of women with breast cancer will have developed a contralateral breast cancer at 4 years and 7% at 10 years, and alternative strategies of close observation and chemoprevention have been developed (45). It *is* appropriate to consider prophylactic contralateral mastectomy in special cases. For example, exceptions might be made for young women who have developed breast cancer following Hodgkin disease and mantle radiation or known *BRCA* mutation carriers with cancer of one breast (12). For instance, affected carriers of *BRCA1* face a 60% risk of developing cancer in the opposite breast as well as an increased risk of ovarian cancer and both prophylactic contralateral mastectomy and prophylactic oophorectomy (see later discussion) may be considered (12). It is appropriate to consider this in selected cases. The Society of Surgical Oncology guidelines support the use in women with diffuse microcalcifications and large breasts that are difficult to evaluate as well as in situations associated with increased risk (4).

The suggestion that prophylactic mastectomy might benefit carefully selected women at high risk because of strong family histories has long been present (12). Only recently, however, did a study confirm that prophylactic mastectomy does decrease the incidence of breast cancer in high-risk women (compared with Gail model predictions and actual experience in sisters) (46). A flurry of media interest and Internet sites for women interested in prophylactic mastectomy followed. A recent Internet search on the phrase *prophylactic mastectomy* yielded more than 1,200 hits. Many of these sites describe, in poignant detail, individual women's experiences with the highly personal decision to undergo prophylactic mastectomy, frequently in response to the death of a sister from breast cancer. Others give news items or information for the lay public about the procedure (47,48).

Balanced against this is the undeniable fact that modern techniques of breast conservation therapy are applicable to approximately 80% of women with breast cancer, rendering the prophylactic operation more radical than the curative procedure (45). Calculations of increased life expectancy must be interpreted particularly carefully. All are derived from complex mathematical models that often have unknown specific relevance. Not all mutation carriers develop breast cancer. Such a woman experiences substantial morbidity and no increase in life expectancy from prophylactic mastectomy; whereas the woman destined to develop breast cancer may benefit substantially more. The statistical *average* increase in life expectancy in one case far overstates and in the other vastly understates the potential individual benefit (49). Further studies appear to be needed before prophylactic mastectomy can be considered the "answer to the genetically endangered maiden's prayer" (50).

Finally, prophylactic mastectomy does not completely eliminate the risk of breast cancer. To understand that particular issue, it is important to clarify the distinction between two types of mastectomy (*subcutaneous* and *total*) that have been performed for prophylaxis. Currently, skin-sparing *total* mastectomy with autogenous reconstruction is the preferred prophylactic approach in the United States (42,45,51–55). Reviews of European centers have revealed no clear pattern of technical preference, with the option of skin and/or nipple–areola preservation available in every case (34,56). Despite the modern preference in the United States for total mastectomy, women are still encountered who have undergone subcutaneous mastectomy decades previously. The two operations are briefly described here.

Subcutaneous mastectomy is performed through an incision in the inframammary crease. Flaps are developed and the nipple–areolar complex is retained. As much breast tissue as possible is removed. The nipple–areola complex is rich in lymphatics and ductal tissue. Significant at-risk tissue remains. Generally, only 90% to 95% of breast tissue can be removed through this approach; breast tissue remains under the nipple–areolar complex, within the flaps, in the tail of Spence, and in the infraclavicular fossae (4). The retained nipple–areolar complex is insensate, the nipple is incapable of erection, and the cosmetic result is frequently inferior due to scarring and tethering to underlying tissue. The chest wall is insensate. Modern reconstructive surgical techniques yield a superior cosmetic result by creating a new nipple–areolar complex rather than attempting to retain it (4). Reconstruction is frequently performed by implant placement.

In contrast, *total mastectomy* is performed through a skin-sparing incision that excises the entire nipple–areolar complex. The technique of mastectomy is similar to that used for cancer, but the intercostobrachial nerve and axillary nodes are spared. Flaps are cut thin, the thickness depending on the thickness of subcutaneous fat. Frozen-section control may be needed to avoid leaving breast tissue behind, particularly on the inferior flap. The boundaries of the dissection are the clavicle superiorly, the rectus abdominis muscle inferiorly, the sternum medially, and the latissimus dorsi muscle laterally. Removal of pectoralis major fascia and even a thin layer of muscle fibers assists in complete removal of breast tissue. Even when a careful attempt is made to remove all breast tissue, some may remain and women should be counseled that continued followup is required (4). Immediate reconstruction is usually offered, and bilateral free transverse rectus abdominus myocutaneous flap reconstruction is emerging as the preferred option (15,57–59).

It has been difficult to quantitate the amount of risk reduction associated with a significant (but not complete) extirpation of breast tissue. Animal experiments using a carcinogen-induced model of breast cancer failed to show a decreased risk with 50% to 100% mastectomy, or, at best, an early reduction in risk that was not maintained (60–62). In contrast, studies of women who had undergone reduction mammoplasty have shown decreased risk of breast cancer, roughly proportional to the amount of breast tissue removed, but generally only in women who underwent the procedure after age 40 (63–65). This was thought to be consistent with reduction in number of potential foci (65). A study from Toronto showed a 0.61 standard incidence ratio independent of age at reduction (66). Breast cancer has been reported to develop after prophylactic (often subcutaneous) mastectomy, in one instance 42 years after surgery (46,56,67–70). Most often, such recurrences are subcutaneous, but the occasional patient presents with metastatic disease (56,68,69). All the recurrences in a recent series occurred after subcutaneous, rather than total, mastectomy (46), confirming that the residual risk appears to be related to the amount of breast tissue left behind (56). The efficacy of the procedure in women with genetically identified syndromes remains unknown. Women who undergo prophylactic mastectomy must be advised that careful follow-up is still necessary.

Does the benefit outweigh the negatives of the procedure? On the plus side, prophylactic mastectomy is associated with decreased morbidity and mortality rates from breast cancer and breast cancer treatment, decreased anxiety, and less morbidity from surveillance or chemoprevention. This must be balanced against the significant negatives of psychological distress, altered quality of life, continued risk of breast cancer (or other malignancies), and morbidity from the surgery itself (71). Satisfaction with prophylactic mastectomy may be high, whereas satisfaction with the results of reconstruction less favorable (57).

Prophylactic mastectomy is thought to offer the greatest potential benefit to young women with a strong family history (12). For a woman with an estimated lifetime risk of 40%, prophylactic mastectomy would add almost 3 years of life; with an estimated lifetime risk of 85%, prophylactic mastectomy would add more than 5 years (20). As previously noted, these "average" figures may mean little to a particular woman. Prophylactic mastectomy may be the best choice for a woman at significantly increased risk, from a family where women die from breast cancer (24). The benefits decrease with age and are minimal when prophylactic mastectomy is performed in 60-year-old women (49).

Women who seek out familial cancer clinics have been shown to be more highly educated and from higher socioeconomic status than those who do not (72), and they may be more likely to want prophylactic mastectomy (25,70). Even women who do not wish genetic testing may express interest in prophylactic surgery (57). Models of shared decision making and other studies stress the importance of patient education and delay in assuring that the patient has made a deliberate, informed choice (39,51,73). Decision making is heavily influenced by subjective perception of risk, history of biopsy, and anxiety concerning breast cancer (57). In one study of 333 women awaiting initial appointment for risk assessment and genetic counseling, 19% would consider prophylactic mastectomy. This percentage increased with hypothetical positive genetic testing results, and correlated with high levels of breast cancer anxiety and overestimation of personal risk (74). Wagner reported that 21% of Austrian mutation carriers would choose prophylactic mastectomy and that most expected it would decrease their quality of life (9). In another study, 17% of unaffected BRCA1 carriers planned to have prophylactic mastectomy (8).

Delay is good because it allows a thorough assessment of risk (43) and may give time for the emotional reaction that surrounds a diagnosis of breast cancer or death of a close friend or relative [events which may motivate a woman to seek prophylactic mastectomy to subside (45)]. As mentioned, the theme of reaction to a sister's breast cancer or death is particularly striking in Internet sites posted by individual women who have chosen prophylactic mastectomy. A sobering case report of Münchausen syndrome manifested by factitious family history led to the reminder that "this is one of few ablative procedures done on history alone" (75).

Schnabel and Estabrook reminded readers that there is no one correct answer to the two related questions: When should the physician offer prophylactic mastectomy? And when should the physician consider prophylactic mastectomy at the patient's request (19)? In a decision analysis model, both chemoprevention and prophylactic mastectomy and oophorectomy were cost-effective or cost-saving compared with surveillance alone (39,40). Specific mutations may be associated with lesser disease severity or may predispose to ovarian cancer (as opposed to breast cancer), making prophylactic mastectomy less relevant for affected persons (76). Even the effect of lifestyle modification and controllable risk factors, such as hormone administration, may not be the same in mutation carriers as the general population (10,19,76). The lack of a clear clinical preference for one of the three management options makes psychologic factors even more important.

Just as women vary in the degree to which they are willing to accept prophylactic mastectomy, physicians vary in their likelihood to offer the procedure. In a survey of Maryland surgeons, plastic surgeons were more likely than general surgeons to recommend the procedure, and both types of surgeons were more likely than gynecologists (55). Of note, the percentage of female physicians selecting prophylactic mastectomy in response to standard high-risk clinical vignette increased significantly if they were asked what they would choose if they were the patient (77). In at least one study, physicians were more likely to recommend than women were to choose prophylactic mastectomy (24). Finally, in one study, only 50% of insurance carriers provided coverage for prophylactic mastectomy (78).

Several studies of the excised breast tissue have shown a high incidence of abnormalities, which would seem to confirm the wisdom of the ablative procedure. In one study of patients with a positive family history but no personal history of breast cancer, there was a 33% incidence of high-risk findings (ADH or higher) on prophylactic mastectomy (79). In the most recent report, two invasive cancers were found in 639 prophylactic mastectomies, one of which was associated with clinically significant disease (46). Clonal abnormalities have been identified in a large percentage of prophylactic mastectomies performed on patients with known genetic abnormalities (80,81). The significance of this is not known, particularly in the era of better options for chemoprevention.

Even though several studies outline psychologic reactions to prophylactic mastectomy (44,59,82–84), data reflecting modern practices in both counseling and surgery are sparse (4). Of 25 consecutive patients who underwent bilateral subcutaneous mastectomy, a high percentage have postoperative anxiety or debilitating depression. Lack of social support, history of psychiatric treatment, or a tendency to deny cancer correlated with poor adjustment (82). In contrast, Stefanek found satisfaction with prophylactic mastectomy to be acceptable in women with strong support systems and who underwent formal risk counseling prior to surgery (70). The spectrum of reactions was highlighted by Goin, who noted that although ten women expressed a sense of loss, two women with large, pendulous breasts expressed a sense of relief (83). Even with immediate reconstruction, the new breast is not immediately incorporated into body image (83). Desire for protection against cancer and a good result from reconstruction were best predictors of happiness in one study (59). In the Memorial Sloan Kettering experience, regrets were expressed by only 21 of 370 women who underwent prophylactic mastectomy. These women cited severe emotional trauma and lack of psychologic support or rehabilitation, complications of surgery or reconstruction, and dissatisfaction with the cosmetic result as the leading regrets. Of note, all the women who regretted their decision indicated that a physician had initiated the discussion about prophylactic mastectomy (84).

Should breast cancer be managed differently in women who are known mutation carriers? Data conflict as to whether *BRCA1* tumors are higher or lower in grade (12,71) and are more or less prone to recurrence (71). Medullary forms are relatively more common in *BRCA1*, and DCIS and LCIS are less common; moreover, tumors are more likely to be estrogen and progesterone receptor negative (12,71). *BRCA2* tumors are predominately ductal without the increase in medullary forms noted with

BRCA1 (71). Because mutations of these genes decrease the ability to repair radiation-induced DNA damage, there may be implications for radiation therapy and 12 of 16 European centers were more apt to recommend modified radical mastectomy than breast conservation for known mutation carriers (12,34). The extremely rare AT homozygote is pathologically sensitive to radiation and may develop tissue necrosis; implications, if any, for the 1% of the population heterozygous for this trait are unknown (13,14). Molecular prognostic indicators such as *HER-neu* overexpression, *p53*, erbB oncogene, loss of heterozygosity, chromosomal aberrations, microsatellite instability, transforming growth factor (TGF)-α, and the presence of the multiple drug resistance gene show promise for fine-tuning prognosis and guiding therapy (17,18,85).

Because of the association between breast and ovarian cancer, it is important to ask the woman with a family history of breast cancer about this malignancy as well. In the Mayo Clinic series of high-risk women, two of 639 women developed ovarian cancer after prophylactic mastectomy (46). Neither sonography nor periodic CA-125 screening has altered the mortality from ovarian cancer, and even prophylactic oophorectomy does not diminish the risk to zero as peritoneal rests remain (19). Carriers of genes associated with increased risk of ovarian cancer face limited choices. Because screening is so ineffective, prophylactic oophorectomy may offer benefit for carriers especially if there is a strong family history of ovarian cancer (12). The procedure can be performed laparoscopically. Acceptance of the procedure has ranged from 33% to 50% of mutation carriers (8,9). It has been suggested that *BRCA2* carriers might benefit from prophylactic oophorectomy at menopause (45–50) and *BRCA1* carriers at age 35 to 40 (86). Surgery at a later age was not protective (87). Dorum et al. speculated that if prophylactic oophorectomy prevents ovarian cancer, prophylactic oophorectomy at age 45 would have prevented 75% of cancers in high-risk women (88). Chemoprevention is being investigated for this malignancy as well.

Data continue to emerge about other malignancies in these families. Male carriers of *BRCA1* have a threefold increase in the incidence of prostatic cancer but are not prone to breast cancer (15), in contrast to male carriers of *BRCA2*, who may be at increased risk of breast cancer. The incidence of colon cancer in *BRCA* mutation carriers is unknown (15). Li-Fraumeni syndrome is associated with brain, soft-tissue, adrenal, and hematologic malignancies. AT homozygotes are at increased risk of lymphoma and leukemia, ovarian, oral, stomach, pancreatic, and bladder cancer. Cowden syndrome is associated with gastrointestinal polyps and thyroid nodules (19).

One last question that the physician is likely to hear is, What about hormone replacement therapy? The effect on patients with hereditary breast cancer syndromes is largely unknown. A survey of European centers revealed that hormone replacement therapy was used after surgical, but not after natural, menopause in these women (34). In general, the absolute benefit of hormone replacement therapy falls as the risk of breast cancer increases. In one mathematical model, hormone replacement therapy did not increase life expectancy for a woman with a lifetime risk of breast cancer exceeding 30% and an average risk of cardiac events, and these researchers suggest that raloxifene may be a better option for women with substantially increased risk (20). Prophylactic oophorectomy decreased the incidence of breast cancer in patients with *BRCA1*, and this effect was not negated with hormone replacement therapy (87).

In summary, strategies for management of the woman at high risk for breast cancer are still evolving. Women tend to overestimate their personal risk. Risk assessment should be incorporated into health maintenance practices. Several tools are available for risk assessment. Women who are found to be at high risk face a decision between intensive surveillance, chemoprophylaxis, and prophylactic mastectomy. Further studies are needed to determine the relative cost-to-benefit ratios of each strategy. Management of breast cancer may be altered in some high-risk women. Finally, some of these women are at increased risk for other malignancies as well.

REFERENCES

1. Bishop DT. BRCA1 and BRCA2 and breast cancer incidence: a review. *Ann Oncol* 1999;10:113–119.
2. van Golen K, Milliron K, Davies S, et al. BRCA-associated cancer risk: molecular biology and clinic practice. *J Lab Clin Med* 1999;134:11–18.
3. Shattuck-Eidens D, Oliphant A, McClure M, et al. BRCA1 sequence analysis in women at high risk for susceptibility mutations. *JAMA* 1997;278:1242–1250.
4. Bilimoria MM, Morrow M. The woman at increased risk for breast cancer: evaluation and management strategies. *CA Cancer J Clin* 1995;45:263–278.
5. Eeles RA. Screening for hereditary cancer and genetic testing, epitomized by breast cancer. *Eur J Cancer* 1999;35:1954–1962.
6. Clark S, Iglehart JD. Genetic counseling for breast cancer. *Adv Surg* 1999;33:199–215.
7. Rosenthal TC, Puck SM. Screening for genetic risk of breast cancer. *Am Fam Physician* 1999;59: 99–104,106.
8. Lerman C, Narod S, Schulman K, et al. BRCA1 testing in families with hereditary breast-ovarian cancer: a prospective study of patient decision making and outcomes. *JAMA* 1996;275:1885–1892.
9. Wagner TM, Moslinger R, Langbauer G, et al. Attitude towards prophylactic surgery and effects of genetic counseling in familiar with BRCA mutations. *Br J Cancer* 2000;82:1249–1253.
10. Coughlin SS, Khoury MJ, Steinberg KK. BRCA1 and BRCA2 gene mutations and risk of breast cancer. Public heath perspectives. *Am J Prev Med* 1999;16:91–98.
11. Neuhausen SL. Ethnic differences in cancer risk resulting from genetic variation. *Cancer* 1999;86: 2575–2582.
12. Mann GB, Borgen PI. Breast cancer genes and the surgeon. *J Surg Oncol* 1998;67:267–274.
13. Jongmans W, Hall J. Cellular responses to radiation and risk of breast cancer. *Eur J Cancer* 1999; 35:540–548.
14. Sakorafas GH, Tsiotou AG. Genetic disposition to breast cancer: a surgical perspective. *Br J Surg* 2000;87:149–162.
15. Solomon JS, Brunicardi CF, Friedman JD. Evaluation and treatment of BRCA-positive patients. *Plast Reconstr Surg* 2000;105:714–719.
16. Eccles DM, Evans DG, Mackay J. Guidelines for a genetic risk based approach to advising women with a family history of breast cancer. *J Med Genet* 2000;37:203–209.
17. Hayes DF. Tumor markers for breast cancer: current utilities and future prospects. *Hematol Oncol Clin North Am* 1994;8:485–506.
18. Menard S, Tagliabue E, Campiglio M, Role of HER2 gene overexpression in breast carcinoma. *J Cell Physiol* 2000;182:150–162.
19. Schnabel FR, Estabrook A. Surgical treatment of patients at high risk of cancer, and with unusual neoplasms and clinic presentations. In: Roses DF, ed. *Breast Cancer.* Philadelphia: Churchill Livingstone, 1999:579–591.

20. Armstrong K, Eisen A, Weber B. Assessing the risk of breast cancer. *N Engl J Med* 2000;342: 564–571.
21. American Society of Clinical Oncology. Statement of the American Society of Clinical Oncology: genetic testing for cancer susceptibility. *J Clin Oncol* 1996;14:1730–1736.
22. Eisinger F, Alby N, Bremond A, et al. INSERM-FNCLCC collective expert's report. Recommendations for management of women having a genetic risk of developing breast and/or ovarian cancer. *Ann Endocrinol (Paris)* 1998;59:470–484.
23. Lakhani SR. The transition from hyperplasia to invasive carcinoma of the breast. *J Pathol* 1999; 187:272–278.
24. Geller G, Bernhardt BA, Doksum T, et al. Decision-making about breast cancer susceptibility testing: how similar are the attitudes of physicians, nurse practitioners, and at-risk women? *J Clin Oncol* 1998;16:2868–2876.
25. Brain K, Gray J, Norman P, et al. Why do women attend familial breast cancer clinics? *J Med Genet* 2000;37:197–202.
26. Elwood JM. Public health aspects of breast cancer gene testing in Canada. Part 1: risks and interventions. *Chronic Dis Can* 1999;20:3–13.
27. Elwood JM. Public health aspects of breast cancer gene testing in Canada. Part 2: selection for and effects of testing. *Chronic Dis Can* 1999;20:14–20.
28. Smith RA, Mettlin CJ, Davis KJ, Et al. American Cancer Society Guidelines for the Early Detection of Cancer. *CA Cancer J Clin* 2000;50:34–49.
29. Chlebowski RT. Reducing the risk of breast cancer. *New Engl J Med* 2000;343:191–198.
30. Weber BL, Giusti RM, Liu ET. Developing strategies for intervention and prevention in hereditary breast cancer. *J Natl Cancer Inst* 1995;17:99–102.
31. Burke W, Daly M, Garber J, et al. Recommendations for follow-up care of individuals with an inherited predisposition to cancer. II. BRCA1 and BRCA2. *JAMA* 1997;277:997–1003.
32. Palmieri C. Trial of prophylactic mastectomy is needed (letter). *BMJ* 1999;318:1556–1557.
33. Tambor ES, Bernhardt BA, Geller G, et al. Should women at increased risk for breast and ovarian cancer be randomized to prophylactic surgery? An ethical and empirical assessment. *J Womens Health* 2000;9:223–233.
34. Vasen HF, Haites NE, Evans DG, et al. Current policies for surveillance and management in women at risk of breast and ovarian cancer: a survey among 16 European family cancer clinics. *Eur J Cancer* 1998;34:1922–1926.
35. Kuhl CK, Schmutzler RK, Leutner CC, et al. Breast MR imagining screening in 192 women proved or suspected to be carriers of a breast cancer susceptibility gene: preliminary results. *Radiology* 2000; 215:267–279.
36. Bennett LM. Breast cancer: genetic predisposition and exposure to radiation. *Mol Carcinog* 1999; 26:143–149.
37. Love RR. Prevention of breast cancer in premenopausal women. *J Natl Cancer Inst* 1994;16:62–65.
38. Boyd NF, Lockwood GA, Martin LJ, et al. Mammographic densities and risk of breast cancer among subjects with a family history of this disease. *J Natl Cancer Inst* 1999;91:1404–1408.
39. Grann VR, Jacobson JS, Sundararajan V, et al. The quality of life associated with prophylactic treatments for women with BRCA1/2 mutations. *Cancer J Sci Am* 1999;5:283–292.
40. Grann VR, Jacobson JS, Whang W, et al. Prevention with tamoxifen or other hormones versus prophylactic surgery in BRCA1/2-postivie women: a decision analysis. *Cancer J Sci Am* 2000;6: 13–20.
41. Winchester DP. Putting prophylactic mastectomy in proper perspective (editorial). *CA Cancer J Clin* 1995;45:261–262.
42. Lopez MJ, Porter KA. The current role of prophylactic mastectomy. *Surg Clin North Am* 1996;76: 231–242.
43. Leis HP Jr. Managing the remaining breast. *Cancer* 1980;46:1026–1030.
44. Montgomery LL, Tran KN, Heelan MC, et al. Issues of regret in women with contralateral prophylactic mastectomies. *Ann Surg Oncol* 1999;6:546–552.
45. Morrow M. Insurance policies for prophylactic surgery: to cover or not to cover? [Editorial]. *Ann Surg Oncol* 2000;7:321–322.
46. Hartmann LC, Schaid DJ, Woods JE, et al. Efficacy of bilateral prophylactic mastectomy in women with a family history of breast cancer. *N Engl J Med* 1999;340:77–84.
47. http://mayohealth.org/mayo/9901/htm/breastop.htm.
48. http://www.cancer.org/media/story/011399.html.

49. Schrag D, Kuntz KM, Garber JE, et al. Decision analysis—effects of prophylactic mastectomy and oophorectomy on life expectancy among women with BRCA1 or BRCA2 mutations. *N Engl J Med* 1997;336:1465–1471.
50. Fentiman IS. Prophylactic mastectomy: deliverance or delusion? We don't know, so we need to start registering all cases now [Editorial]. *BMJ* 1998;317:1402–1403.
51. Stalmeier PF, Unic IJ, Verhoef LC, et al. Evaluation of a shared decision making program for women suspected to have a genetic predisposition to breast cancer: preliminary results. *Med Decis Making* 1999;19:230–241.
52. Snyderman RK. Prophylactic mastectomy: pros and cons. *Cancer* 1984;53:803–808.
53. Wapnir IL, Rabinowitz B, Greco RS. A reappraisal of prophylactic mastectomy. *Surg Gynecol Obstet* 1990;171:171–184.
54. Temple WJ, Lindsay RL, Magi E, Urbanski SJ. Technical considerations for prophylactic mastectomy in patients at high risk for breast cancer. *Am J Surg* 1991;161:413–415.
55. Houn F, Helzlsouer KJ, Friedman NB, Stefanek ME. The practice of prophylactic mastectomy: a survey of Maryland surgeons. *Am J Public Health* 1995;85:801–805.
56. Evans DG, Anderson E, Lalloo F, et al. Utilisation of prophylactic mastectomy in 10 European centres. *Dis Markers* 1999;15:148–151.
57. Stefanek ME, Helzlsouer KJ, Wilcox PM, et al. Predictors of and satisfaction with bilateral prophylactic mastectomy. *Prev Med* 1995;24:412–419..
58. Morris RJ, Koshy CE, Zambacos GJ. Prophylactic mastectomy, oophorectomy, hysterectomy, and immediate transverse rectus abdominis muscle flap breast reconstruction in a BRCA2-negative patient [Letter]. *Plast Reconstr Surg* 2000;105:473.
59. Kroll SS. Prophylactic mastectomy with few regrets [Editorial]. *Ann Surg Oncol* 1998;5:569–570.
60. Nelson H, Miller SH, Buck D, et al. Effectiveness of prophylactic mastectomy in the prevention of breast tumors in C3H mice. *Plast Reconstr Surg* 1989;83:662–669.
61. Wong JH, Jackson CF, Swanson JS, et al. Analysis of risk reduction of prophylactic partial mastectomy in Sprague-Dawley rats with 7,12-dimethylbenzantracene-induced breast cancer. *Surgery* 1986; 99:67–71.
62. Klamer TW, Donegan WL, Max MH. Breast tumor incidence in rats after partial mammary resection. *Arch Surg* 1983;118:933–935.
63. Boice JD Jr, Friis D, McLaughlin JK, et al. Cancer following breast reduction surgery in Denmark. *Cancer Causes Control* 1997;8:253–258.
64. Baasch M, Nielsen SF, Engholm G, et al. Breast cancer incidence subsequent to surgical reduction of the female breast. *Br J Cancer* 1996;73:961–963.
65. Lund K, Ewertz M, Schou G. Breast cancer incidence subsequent to surgical reduction of the female breast. *Scand J Plast Reconstr Surg Hand Surg* 1987;21:209–212.
66. Brown MH, Weinberg M, Chong N, et al. A cohort study of breast cancer risk in breast reduction patients. *Plast Reconstr Surg* 1999;103:1674–1681.
67. Willemsen HW, Kaas R, Peterse JH, et al. Breast carcinoma in residual breast tissue after prophylactic bilateral subcutaneous mastectomy. *Eur J Surg Oncol* 1998;24:331–332.
68. Goodnight JE Jr, Quagliana JM, Morton DL. Failure of subcutaneous mastectomy to prevent the development of breast cancer. *J Surg Oncol* 1984;26:198–201.
69. Jameson MB, Roberts E, Nixon J, et al. Metastatic breast cancer 42 years after bilateral subcutaneous mastectomies. *Clin Oncol R Coll Radiol* 1997;9:119–121.
70. Stefanek ME. Bilateral prophylactic mastectomy: issues and concerns. *J Natl Cancer Inst* 1995;17: 37–42.
71. Gauthier-Villars M, Gad S, Caux V, et al. Genetic testing for breast cancer predisposition. *Surg Clin North Am* 1999;79:1171–1187.
72. Steel M, Smyth E, Vasen H, et al. Ethical, social and economic issues in familiar breast cancer: a compilation of views from the E.C. Biomed II demonstration project. *Dis Markers* 1999;15:125–131.
73. Unic I, Stalmeier PF, Verhoef LC, et al. Assessment of the time-tradeoff values for prophylactic mastectomy of women with a suspected genetic predisposition to breast cancer. *Med Decis Making* 1998;18:268–277.
74. Meiser B, Butow R, Friedlander M, et al. Intention to undergo prophylactic bilateral mastectomy in women at increased risk of developing hereditary breast cancer. *J Clin Oncol* 2000;18:2250–2257.
75. Grenga TE, Dowden RV. Munchausen's syndrome and prophylactic mastectomy. *Plast Reconstr Surg* 1987;80:119–120.

76. Rebbeck TR. Inherited genetic predisposition in breast cancer: a population-based perspective. *Cancer* 1999;86:2493–2501.
77. Stefanek M, Enger C, Benkendorf J, et al. Bilateral prophylactic mastectomy decision making: a vignette study. *Prev Med* 1999;29:216–221.
78. Kuerer HM, Hwang S, Anthony JP, et al. Current national health coverage policies for breast and ovarian cancer prophylactic surgery. *Ann Surg Oncol* 2000;7:325–332.
79. Khurana KK, Loosmann A, Numann PJ, et al. Prophylactic mastectomy: pathologic findings in high-risk patients. *Arch Pathol Lab Med* 2000;124:378–381.
80. Petersson C, Pandis N, Mertens F, et al. Chromosome aberrations in prophylactic mastectomies from women belonging to breast cancer families. *Genes Chromosomes Cancer* 1996;16:185–188.
81. Teixeira MR, Pandis N, Gerdes AM, et al. Cytogenetic abnormalities in an *in situ* ductal carcinoma and five prophylactically removed breasts from members of a family with hereditary breast cancer. *Breast Cancer Res Treat* 1996;38:177–182.
82. Meyer L, RiØngberg A. A prospective study of psychiatric and psychosocial sequelae of bilateral subcutaneous mastectomy. *Scand J Plast Reconstr Surg Hand Surg* 1986;20:101–107.
83. Goin MK, Goin JM. Psychological reactions to prophylactic mastectomy synchronous with contralateral breast reconstruction. *Plast Reconstr Surg* 1982;70:355–359.
84. Payne DK, Biggs C, Tran KN, et al. Women's regrets after bilateral prophylactic mastectomy. *Ann Surg Oncol* 2000;7:150–154.
85. Dahiya R, Deng G. Molecular prognostic markers in breast cancer. *Breast Cancer Res Treat* 1998; 52:185–200.
86. Moller P, Evans G, Haites N, et al. Guidelines for follow-up of women at high risk for inherited breast cancer: consensus statement from the Biomed 2 Demonstration Programme on Inherited Breast Cancer. *Dis Markers* 1999;15:207–211.
87. Rebbeck TR, Levin AM, Eisen A, et al. Breast cancer risk after bilateral prophylactic oophorectomy in BRCA1 mutation carriers. *J Natl Cancer Inst* 1999;91:1475–1479.
88. Dorum A, Heimdal K, Lovslett K, et al. Prospectively detected cancer in familial breast/ovarian cancer screening. *Acta Obstet Gynecol Scand* 1999;78:906–911.

24

Medicolegal Pitfalls in Breast Cancer Diagnosis and Management

Janet Rose Osuch and Vence L. Bonham, Jr.

Breast cancer is the most common cancer in women (1), and failure to diagnose it in a timely manner is the second most common successful malpractice claim paid by malpractice carriers on behalf of the physicians they insure (2). An understanding of the common allegations made when a malpractice suit is filed for failure to diagnose breast cancer can provide insight into the risk management of a physician's practice and simultaneously improve patient care so that mistakes in diagnosis and management are minimized. Many physicians are unaware of the legal process involved in a malpractice suit until it affects them or a close colleague. At this point, objective perspective is often impossible. Nonetheless, it is inevitable that many, if not most, physicians will find themselves a defendant in a medical malpractice suit at some point in their career for a less-than-perfect patient outcome, whether medical negligence has occurred or not. This chapter outlines the common allegations of misdiagnosis or mismanagement of breast cancer, reviews the process of legal proceedings common to a malpractice suit, reviews the issues likely to arise in the defense of a case, and provides recommendations on the steps to take when facing malpractice litigation.

MAGNITUDE OF THE PROBLEM

In 1995, the Physician's Insurance Association of America (PIAA) published a report from their Data Sharing Project summarizing the 10-year history between January 1985 and December 1994 of indemnity claims of the 36 medical malpractice insurance companies that are members of the association (2). This report, along with a subsequent more detailed analysis of it (3), provides the best overview of the magnitude of the malpractice problem. Its data source was national rather than regional or local, and PIAA provided malpractice insurance to more than 90,000 physicians at the time the study was published. During this time, more than 117,000 claims for medical malpractice were filed and 35,700 closed. The report analyzed the closed claims and found that the most common condition resulting in a successful medical malpractice suit was related to breast cancer (8%), followed by brain-damaged infants (7%) and pregnancy-associated issues (5%). It is interesting to review the three most common diagnostic or treatment errors resulting in successful claims by specialty. The rank-order for general surgery is breast cancer, appendicitis, and spinal fracture. For radiology, it is breast cancer, lung cancer, and spinal fracture. For obstetrics and gynecology, it is breast cancer, ectopic pregnancy, and pregnancy. For family practice, it is myocardial infarct, breast cancer, and appendicitis, and for internal medicine, it is lung cancer, myocardial infarct, and breast cancer. This list provides insight into medical malpractice claims in general and reasons why breast cancer–related allegations are so common. The conditions listed are notorious for being difficult to diagnose under many circumstances, lack definitive or immediate diagnostic criteria, and result in a devastating impact on the life of the person affected by the condition.

It should not be surprising that radiologists, surgeons, and obstetricians/gynecologists have breast cancer diagnostic failures as number one in rank-order frequency for claims paid. The sheer numbers of women undergoing screening mammography for breast cancer, coupled with the prevalence of the disease, would predict for a high frequency of medical malpractice suits among radiologists. Because general surgeons are most responsible for the management of symptomatic breast problems, the number-one rank order for this discipline also can be explained intuitively on the basis of prevalence. Prevalence alone, however, does not account for the frequency of allegations for failure to diagnose breast cancer. Kern, in a nationwide study of 338 cases of missed diagnosis of cancer, demonstrated that the frequency of allegations for failure to diagnose breast cancer is twice as high as the proportion of breast cancer cases in the general population (4). Part of the explanation for this situation relates to the expectation of the public that if a diagnosis of breast cancer is made in a timely fashion, cure is guaranteed and if not, that the patient's survival has by definition been compromised. In addition, the PIAA study demonstrated that women most likely to sue are much younger than the average woman who is diagnosed with breast cancer and are more likely to have a negative or equivocal mammogram finding (2). This finding correlates with the fact that obstetricians/gynecologists, who see a large number of young women in their practices, have breast cancer diagnostic failures as number one in rank-order frequency for claims paid among the errors in diagnosis for their discipline.

COMMON ALLEGATIONS IN THE DIAGNOSIS OR MANAGEMENT OF BREAST CANCER

Although physicians are not immune from treatment-related allegations, the vast majority of malpractice claims related to breast cancer allege a failure in the diagnosis rather than a treatment-related problem. Successful suits have been filed, however, when physicians fail to provide "reasonable skill and care" in the administration of drugs, radiation therapy, or surgery for breast cancer treatment, just as with any medical condition. In addition, litigation for claims of unnecessary surgery are not uncommon, especially if nonsurgical treatment alternatives were not disclosed (5). Many states have laws that require physicians to provide patients with a standardized written summary of their treatment options if breast cancer is diagnosed, and some specify penalties for noncompliance with the legislation (5). It is possible, for instance, for a patient to sue her physician for lack of informed consent if she claims lack of full disclosure, did not receive the standardized materials required in her state, and had a mastectomy for treatment but later learned she might have been a candidate for breast-preservation therapy. In this scenario, and if the physician believed that the patient had received full disclosure, the standardized brochure could become a strong part of the physician's defense, if it had been provided. On the other hand, a patient who was eligible for breast-preservation therapy and who chose it would be far less likely to claim successfully a lack of informed consent, even if the standardized written materials were not provided to her, unless she could claim and prove harm related to her treatment (5). The legal principles behind these scenarios are discussed in a later section.

The best source detailing the common allegations related to failure to diagnose breast cancer come from the nationwide PIAA study cited earlier (2). It documented 487 paid claims from 33 member companies, many involving indemnity payment to the claimant from more than one physician. Only data related to these paid claims were reported. A narrative summary describing the plaintiffs' major allegations was examined by a Breast Cancer Committee at the company to assess the source of the diagnostic error(s). The most frequent reason for a delay in diagnosis was a failure of the physician to be impressed with the clinical findings (35% of cases). Poor physical examination by the physician was reported in an additional 10% of cases. The second most common reason for a diagnostic delay was the failure to follow up with the patient in a timely manner (31% of cases); when follow-up did occur, the physical examination failed to impress the clinician in an additional 11% of cases. Mammography also contributed to diagnostic errors. In 13% of cases, a mammogram was not ordered. Of the 407 patients who had mammograms, 52% were negative, and 28% were equivocal. Of the negative mammograms, 23% were misinterpreted films. In 14.7% of cases, the mammogram was correctly interpreted as suspicious or malignant, but the physician failed to react to the finding. These physician-related errors resulted in an average delay in diagnosis of 14 months, with a range between 1 month and 96 months (with a 120-month outlier); the average indemnity payment per case was $301,460.

The study also documented patient delays. Even in recent studies, the average patient delay from symptom to medical consultation is about 3 months (6,7). In the PIAA study, no patient delay was documented in 63% of cases. There were a variety of reasons suspected for patient delays that did occur, including fear, procrastination, socioeconomic reasons, or denial. Additionally, 11% of patients failed to keep follow-up appointments. Many physicians are surprised to learn that this patient behavior does not excuse their responsibility in an allegation of diagnostic delay. This issue relates to the topic of duty, the first of four components of a medical malpractice case.

ELEMENTS OF MEDICAL MALPRACTICE

Medical malpractice law has been viewed by some as convoluted in its rules and regulations (8). This view reflects the fact that the comprehension of the topic by those not trained in law is, at best, challenging. One legal scholar describes medical malpractice law as "a maze of judicial mistakes one century in the making" (8). Nonetheless, understanding the current elements of medical malpractice is necessary to those it may affect. Although some physicians may believe that they are immune from malpractice litigation because they practice exemplary medicine, this is an incorrect assumption. Any physician involved in the practice of medicine may find herself or himself a defendant in a medical malpractice lawsuit, and becoming knowledgeable of the litigation process before it occurs will serve a physician better than denying that malpractice litigation is a possibility.

The liability of physicians is governed by general negligence principles. *Malpractice* usually is defined as unskillful practice resulting in injury to the patient and failure to exercise the required degree of care, skill, and diligence under the circumstances (9). To have a claim of negligence, four elements must be present: duty plus a breach of the standard of care plus causation plus damages.

Duty

A *duty* in negligence cases may be defined as a legal obligation, statutory or common law, to conform to a particular standard of conduct or standard of care toward another (10). A physician–patient relationship establishes a duty for the physician to provide care in compliance with the standard of care for a reasonable physician of that specialty. The patient must prove that a duty of the physician existed (11). A duty does not exist to provide care if there is no physician–patient relationship. The existence of the relationship is a question of fact to be determined by a jury. A physician–patient relationship exists when a doctor renders professional services to a person who has contracted for such services (12), and this is both a professional and a legal obligation. The courts have recognized that the acceptance or undertaking of treatment of the patient by a physician creates the physician–patient relationship (13). The issue of duty is not an area of dispute in most medical malpractice cases.

Standard of Care

Once the physician–patient relationship is established, the physician has a duty to exercise the same degree of care and skill in managing the patient as would be exercised by a competent physician in a similar situation. To establish a breach of duty, the patient must prove that the physician failed to comply with the standard of care. Courts refer to the degree of care and skill that should be exercised as the *standard of care* (11).

Proximate Cause

An essential element of the patient's medical malpractice action is that there be causal connection between the act or omission of the doctor and the harm that the patient has suffered. This connection usually is handled by the courts in terms of what is called *proximate cause* or *legal cause* (10). The test for a direct causal connection or cause-in-fact between the patient's injury and the doctor's negligence usually is described by the courts in terms of the "but for" test. The patient must prove that "but for" the doctor's act(s) or omission(s), the patient's injuries would not have occurred. Under the "but for" test, a patient cannot establish proximate cause unless an improved outcome (>50%) was more likely than not, absent the physician's actions. This test of causation has been problematic in delay of diagnosis cases, and many states have established different causation tests (9,14). Alternatives include the substantial factor test and the loss of chance doctrine. These are discussed in more detail in an upcoming section of this chapter.

Damages

If a plaintiff can prove that a duty existed and that the duty was breached and was the cause of an injury or harm, then a defendant will be liable for compensatory damages. There are two types of compensatory damages: special and general. *Actual* or *special damages* represent reimbursement for actual economic payment for medical care and related expenses, incurred losses, and disability (15). General noneconomic damages are losses from pain, suffering, inconvenience, physical impairment, or physical disfigurement that cannot be measured exactly in monetary terms. As part of malpractice tort reform, some states have put a cap on noneconomic losses. Each state has developed its own statutory basis for limiting damages.

MALPRACTICE ISSUES RELATED TO BREAST CANCER

Standard of Care: Legal and Clinical Issues

Most malpractice cases related to breast cancer focus on whether there was violation of the standard of care. Physicians are held to an objective standard of care specific to the case in question. The courts have recognized that perfection is neither realistic nor expected in the practice of medicine. It also has been acknowledged, however, that it is not enough for physicians to do their best if their conduct does not rise to the level of care required of similar members of the profession practicing under circumstances similar to the case in question (16).

The standard of care to which a physician is held is a national standard in most state courts. The court has established that "The duty of care . . . takes two forms: (a) a duty to render a quality of care consonant with the level of medical and practical knowledge the physician may reasonably be expected to possess and the medical judgment he may be expected to exercise and (b) a duty based upon the adept use of such medical facilities, services, equipment and options as are reasonably available'' (17).

Rarely, a court will impose its own value judgment on physicians; an exception is the case of *Helling v Carey*. The trial court ruled that compliance with customary practice within the medical profession is not conclusive evidence that a physician was not negligent (18). It is unusual for a court to disagree expressly with the standard of care that prevails among physicians. *Helling v Carey* is important because it is not the rule but an aberration. Most courts reject the *Helling* court approach of establishing the standard of care as a matter of law. Typically, the standard of care is not set by the judge or the jury but by the medical profession (8) through expert witness testimony.

In recent years, one of the tools used by expert witnesses includes the citing of clinical practice guidelines published by professional organizations. Medical and legal commentators have been debating the role of clinical practice guidelines in the establishment of the standard of care since guidelines became widely used. Because clinical practice guidelines are not written to include the circumstances of individual clinical scenarios, expert witness testimony is necessary to establish the standard of care, as reflected in the following statement from a health law treatise:

> American physicians and specialty groups have expended substantial efforts on standard settings in recent years, specifying treatments for particular diseases. . . . Such guidelines provide a particularized source of standards against which to judge the conduct of the defendant physician and their production by national medical specialty societies and the government will be influential. A widely accepted clinical standard may be presumptive evidence of due care, but expert testimony will still be required to introduce the standard and establish its sources and its relevancy (9).

Some commentators believe the use of clinical guidelines as practice standards may benefit physicians by providing definition as to the standard of care and thus limit lawsuits for bad outcomes. Others believe that using clinical guidelines to establish the standard of care will restrict the practice of medicine. In cases of medical malpractice, it is likely that clinical guidelines will be taken into consideration as expert witnesses describe the standard of care. The standard of care changes with the individual circumstances of a case, advances in medicine over time, and changes in societal expectations, as reflected in the following statement:

> The standard of care does incorporate objective evaluations of medical science, and can be determinate to the extent that medical science is determinate, but it also incorporates normative societal values and goals. The standard is capable of evolving to accommodate advances in medicine and changing societal concerns (19).

Medical malpractice lawsuits alleging a delay in the diagnosis of breast cancer often become a battle of the experts regarding the definition of the standard of care. Expert witnesses are hired by opposing sides of a case and are often at odds with one another regarding the conduct of a physician and whether that conduct meets the standard of care for an individual case. As a consequence, an *expert witness* serves a far more important function than what one usually thinks of when one thinks of the word *witness*. Not simply an observer of events (as in a marriage), or one who substantiates the truth (as in a criminal trial), the expert witness establishes the standard of care for the court. Because the expert witness helps establish the standard of care for a given case, his or her testimony has a profound influence on its outcome. Expert witnesses have a professional responsibility to provide objective and unbiased opinions based on medical fact and judgment rendered as a result of meticulous preparation of a case. Although it should not matter whether an individual expert is hired by the plaintiff's or the defendant's attorney, because the testimony of that expert should be the same for the circumstances of a given case, it often does matter. One way a defendant physician may have input into his or her case of medical malpractice involves the careful consideration of which expert witnesses should be used to assist in defense of the case. Those capable of giving ethical, objective, and credible testimony will be of greatest advantage to the defendant physician. This topic is considered in more detail later.

Proximate Cause and Legal Issues

Establishing causation is a primary focus in a breast cancer medical malpractice suit. Historically, the "but for" definition has been applied to establish causation and already has been discussed. An alternative definition established by some state courts is called the *substantial factor test*, which allows recovery when the breach of the standard of care is a substantial factor in producing injury, even if the plaintiff's chances at a better outcome absent the negligent action was less than 50%. This definition was first applied by the New Jersey Supreme Court in a delay in the diagnosis of breast cancer case (20). This case has been recognized for expanding the causation rules for the delay in the diagnosis of breast cancer cases (21).

Another alternative definition of causation is referred to as the *loss of chance doctrine*. This represents a legal doctrine to establish causation when the plaintiff cannot prove that but for the doctor's actions or omissions, the patient's injury (decrease in chance of survival or death) would not have occurred. The doctrine was designed specifically to address problems arising in medical malpractice cases, and its use has been limited almost exclusively to such cases (22). When a physician is negligent in diagnosing a disease, and the resulting delay reduces the plaintiff's chances of survival (even though the chance of survival was below 50% before the missed diagnosis), many states have adopted a loss of a chance doctrine. The rationale for adaptation of this principle was discussed in a law review article as follows:

> As one court explained, loss of a chance doctrine . . . developed in part because of the difficulty in the medical malpractice area of proving precise degrees of causation, and in part because of the perceived unfairness in denying recovery when a doctor's negligence, although not shown to be the probable cause . . . significantly decreased the patient's chance of recovery (23).

In a typical "lost chance" case, a patient is initially at risk for some injury or perhaps death, through no fault of the defendant. Some negligent act by the defendant physician, however, causes the plaintiff to incur an increase in risk for that same injury, and the plaintiff in fact subsequently suffers the injury. The most difficult cases are those in which the plaintiff had a very high initial risk of injury ($>50\%$) and experts are unable to testify that the defendant's negligence (as opposed to the preexisting condition) probably caused the plaintiff's injury (24). This doctrine is particularly important in delay in diagnosis of breast cancer cases.

Regardless of the legal guidelines regarding causation, the expert witness hired to testify regarding proximate cause will be asked to predict the survival of the patient from the disease both at the time it *could have been* diagnosed and the time it *was* diagnosed. Predictions of survival then will be estimated based on circumstances of no diagnostic delay and compared with those of the case under consideration. The heterogeneous behavior of breast cancer makes these estimates of probability less definitive than the simplistic view of breast cancer biology that is often taken. In this regard, the public health message encouraging women to obtain yearly breast cancer screening correctly communicates that a diagnosis in an asymptomatic phase of the disease can result in improved survival. The inverse, however, does not necessarily follow: that mammography in asymptomatic women reduces mortality from breast cancer is often erroneously equated with the notion that a delayed diagnosis in the symptomatic disease phase will automatically result in increased mortality. Survival from breast cancer is a complicated issue, and definitive predictions regarding the disease course in an individual patient can be very difficult. It is even more difficult to convey these concepts to those that must weigh the evidence to determine the legal issue of proximate cause. Because of this, the defense of a case will be much easier if it can be proven that the standard of care was not violated. It is important to understand the issues that will be raised by the expert witnesses surrounding the issue of proximate cause.

Proximate Cause: Clinical Issues

Proximate cause, as discussed, refers to the burden of proof that the plaintiff possesses to establish that she was harmed in a direct way by the defendant's actions. In other words, it is not enough that the plaintiff's attorney proves that the defendant physician violated the standard of care, but it must also be proved that the violation resulted in harm to the patient. For example, assume that a 1-cm mammographic abnormality is followed up for a year, and biopsy is performed with free margins when it reaches 1.2 cm. Histologically, the lesion is composed entirely of ductal carcinoma *in situ*. It is possible that a patient who has experienced such a delay may contemplate a suit alleging, perhaps, that the biopsy should have been done in a more timely fashion. Even if the plaintiff established that allegation as true, it would be extremely difficult to prove that any harm had occurred directly linked to the diagnosis of a disease that has no ability to metastasize and for which she would have the full complement of treatment options available. Under these circumstances, the case would have likely been dismissed.

The topic of proximate cause depends on the biology of the disease in question and typically is linked to treatment and survival. For some diseases, this might be relatively straightforward, but such is not the case for breast cancer. This has to do with the complexity of treatment options available for breast cancer as well as the heterogeneous biology of the disease. In the past, treatment arguments often centered around the issue of whether or not a patient would have needed chemotherapy if her diagnosis would have been made in a more timely manner. This is much less often an issue since it has become common for most women with invasive disease of 1 cm or larger to receive some form of systemic therapy (25).

Proximate cause arguments may take local treatment forms if it has been necessary for a patient to have a mastectomy rather than breast preservation for treatment, and that necessity can be proved to be linked to a delayed diagnosis, as has already been discussed. Regardless of treatment issues related to proximate cause, however, survival predictions almost always are considered in cases alleging a delay in diagnosis. These predictions become critical in the calculation of damages if the prior components of the allegations are proved.

Prognosis and Survival

The question the court will be attempting to answer during proximate cause arguments centers on the prediction of an individual patient's prognosis and survival. There is no prognostic measure short of clinical evidence of metastatic disease that will predict for this with certainty. Instead, the expert witness will rely on a battery of prognostic indicators to predict the biological behavior of the tumor in a given case. The most common of these include time between symptom onset and diagnosis, tumor size at symptom onset and at diagnosis, axillary lymph node status and number of lymph nodes involved, tumor stage according to the TNM (tumor, node, metastasis) system of classification, tumor grade, nuclear grade, estrogen and progesterone receptor status, and, when available, flow cytometry data, including ploidy and S-phase analysis (26). Not all these markers are independent of one another, and not all carry the same level of evidence in terms of their predictive ability for survival from breast cancer. Many other markers are available with even less evidence of usefulness (27). Each of these factors, however, can help the expert estimate the biological behavior of the individual tumor and the likelihood of survival. Knowledge of these factors, as well as a thorough understanding of the complexity of the natural history of breast cancer and the biologic heterogeneity of its behavior, is critical to the credible testimony of a given expert.

Proximate Cause, Screening, and the "Early Diagnosis" of Breast Cancer

It is important for the expert witness to have a clear concept of the strengths and limitations of breast cancer screening as it relates to the concept of the early diagnosis of breast cancer. Prior to mammography, the diagnosis depended on physical signs, such as a lump in the breast or nipple discharge. This period is referred to as the *clinical phase* of the disease. All diseases also have a period during which the biological processes causing the eventual symptoms are present but not clinically apparent. This period is referred to as the *latent phase*. Some diseases have an extremely short latent phase, notably bacterial infectious diseases. In contrast, the latent period for most cancers, including breast cancer, evolves over years of time. Diseases with a long latent phase are possible candidates for screening tests, the goal of which is to diagnose the disease during the *asymptomatic*, or preclinical, phase. The *preclinical phase* is that portion of the latent phase during which the disease is detectable using the screening test.

One of the most important criteria in the decision to use a test to detect a disease in an asymptomatic population is its ability to intervene in the natural history of the disease and affect outcome by reducing mortality (28). The results of multiple randomized, controlled clinical trials evaluating screening mammography have demonstrated an average 30% mortality reduction in women aged 50 and older (29). Although this issue is more controversial, a meta-analysis of studies done in women aged 40 to 49 shows an 18% mortality reduction from mammography in that age group (30). These facts are often used in medical malpractice cases to establish that an earlier diagnosis would have resulted in a better prognosis. What the logic of this argument fails to recognize is that the inverse is also true. A 30% reduction in mortality in screened women by mammography also implies that in 70% of the screened population destined to die from breast cancer, mammography makes no difference in outcome. What accounts for this? To answer that question, the concepts of angiogenesis, metastasis, and ''biological predeterminism'' must be introduced.

Angiogenesis and Biological Predeterminism

Breast cancer mortality is directly linked to *metastasis*, or the spread of the cancer to distant organ sites. As with any cancer, not all breast cancer cases possess the biological ability to metastasize (31). In fact, a complex, ten-step process is involved. This process depends on (a) the proliferation of cancer cells following neoplastic transformation, which depends on the presence of growth factors; (b) the process of *angiogenesis*, that is, the formation of new blood vessels, to support the growth of a tumor mass beyond 1 to 2 mm; (c) invasion of tumor cells into the stroma of the organ of origin and subsequent vascular invasion; (d) embolization of tumor cells from the vasculature to larger vessels; (e) survival of tumor cells in the circulation; (f) adherence of tumor cells in the capillary beds of distant organs; (g) extravasation of tumor cells into the parenchyma of distant organs; (h) proliferation of tumor cells in the parenchyma of distant organs; (i) evasion of immune mechanisms of the host at the primary and distant sites; and (j) neovascularization of the tumor bed at the distant sites (31). This complicated process depends on the proper microenvironment at each step. If the cascade is interrupted at any one step, metastasis cannot be established.

Whether or not a tumor possesses the necessary biological components to establish the metastatic process is not obvious at the point of diagnosis of most cases of breast cancer, and metastasis can occur even 40 years after the initial treatment (32). This makes the establishment of proximate cause problematic. Conversely, biologically, metastasis has often occurred long before it is clinically detectable. Angiogenesis, for example, has been shown to be established and, in fact, necessary when the tumor burden reaches 1 to 2 mm (33), well before our current detection capabilities of either primary or metastatic disease. These principles relate directly to the concept of biological predeterminism, which were originally developed by MacDonald. In a study in 1951, MacDonald observed that 56% of breast tumors that were 1 cm or smaller had already spread to axillary lymph nodes, whereas 23% of tumors that were 5 cm or larger had not done so (34). This paradox caused him to question the generally held belief that tumor size and lymph node status were cause-and-effect phenomena. He postulated that many tumors already had developed the ability to metastasize before their primary diagnosis. This concept was expanded on by Heuser et al. and applied to the Breast Cancer Detection Demonstration Project data, a study conducted in the 1970s that focused on breast cancer screening (35). They concluded that some of the cancers diagnosed in the study grew extremely slowly and essentially never would have had the ability to metastasize, whereas others grew so fast that no matter what intervention was applied, death would have been the eventual outcome. In other words, metastasis would have been biologically impossible even in the clinical phase of the disease in the former case and biologically established even before the preclinical phase of the disease in the latter. In either case, screening mammography would have made no difference on the disease outcome. The 30% mortality reduction with the use of screening mammography is a laudable accomplishment in breast cancer control, but the large number of women who undergo the screening test and in whom the test makes no difference in outcome points to the need for more efficacious detection tools for breast cancer. Studies related to screening, however, have helped to define the biology of the disease and have underscored the concept that the biological behavior of breast cancer is complicated and difficult to predict with certainty (36).

Diagnostic Delay, Survival, and Symptomatic Breast Cancer

Although allegations of failure to screen occur, far more often, the allegation of failure to diagnose breast cancer in a timely manner occurs in the setting of a palpable mass (3). The concept that a diagnostic delay automatically predicts a decrease in an individual woman's life expectancy has been debated for years. Hundreds of studies have been done with conflicting results. An excellent discussion of the individual studies and their conclusions can be found in a textbook chapter by Kern (37). More recently, two studies of the topic, both from the United Kingdom but conducted in quite different ways, were published in the same journal. These two studies reached opposite conclusions. The first, by Sainsbury et al., examined more than 35,000 patients with breast cancer listed in the Yorkshire Cancer Registry between 1976 and 1995, approximately 4% to 5% of whom had diagnostic delays of greater than 90 days. The study found no adverse effect of diagnostic delay on survival. In fact, patients treated within 30 days had a decreased survival compared with the remaining patients (38). The other study was a systematic review of 87 observational studies of more than 100,000 patients with a diagnostic delay of breast cancer. In the 38 studies and more than 50,000 patients in whom a quantitative survival outcomes analysis could be done, they found that patients with delays of 3 months or longer had a 12% lower 5-year survival compared with the group with shorter delays and that those with delays between 3 and 6 months had a 7% lower survival rate compared with those with shorter delays (39). The study found that in this first group, which included studies from 1907 through 1996, those that included inoperable disease and those that included only operable disease had similar results. This finding contrasted with the second group of studies analyzed (21 studies and more than 25,000 patients), all of which were conducted after 1970. This group did not include actual 5-year survival data. Fourteen studies confirmed that delay in diagnosis of 3 months or more resulted in shorter survival than delays of less than 3 months (both inoperable and operable cases). Seven studies in this group showed no decreased survival, and four of these seven included only operable patients. The third group of studies analyzed in this review included 28 studies of more than 20,000 patients; 25 of these analyzed operable disease only. Ten of these 25 studies showed worse survival in those with diagnostic delays, whereas 15 of the 25 showed no impact of delay on survival. These researchers also tested a secondary hypothesis that longer delays were associated with more advanced stage. The 13 studies that were analyzed supported the hypothesis, but in three studies that analyzed survival within individual stages, none found a decrease in survival among patients with stage I disease, and one study found improved survival among patients with stage III disease. Correcting for lead-time bias, the overall conclusions of this group is that the survival rate decreases by about 5% for those with diagnostic delays of 3 to 6 months. They acknowledge that for many patients, a diagnostic delay of 3 to 6 months will have no impact on survival, but for a minority of patients, it will have an effect. This group is theorized to be the group in which the disease progresses to a more advanced stage during the diagnostic delay. This may or may not be the correct conclusion. Certainly, a group of patients exists in whom a diagnostic delay is of no consequence because the disease remains without metastatic potential, and another group exists in whom metastasis has occurred in the preclinical phase of the disease and therefore cannot be influenced by early detection efforts (it is possible that this is the reason for worse outcomes in the study of Sainsbury et al. in the patients treated promptly). There is a third group of patients with varying biologic behavior, some of whom may be harmed by diagnostic delay. The challenge in a given case is to predict which patients may fall into this category.

LITIGATION PROCESS

Doctors often misunderstand the litigation process. The process is cumbersome, drawn out, and too often not clearly explained to the parties of a lawsuit. For purposes of understanding the legal process, it can be divided into six phases.

1. The preinitiation of the lawsuit
2. Filing of the lawsuit
3. Discovery Phase
4. Motion Practice
5. Trial
6. Appeal

Litigation in the United States is a method of using a formal system to resolve disputes. For many individuals, when they think of "litigation," they think of a trial seeking "truth." Only 3.8% of the delay in the diagnosis of breast cancer cases reported to the PIAA were decided at a trial by a jury (3). Most lawsuits are resolved prior to trial, either by the claims being dismissed voluntarily or by settlement by the parties based on a judicial decision.

The *prediscovery phase* of litigation is a phase of informal discovery of the facts. In this phase of litigation, the plaintiff and his or her lawyer analyze whether they believe the matter is meritorious, determining whether they believe the elements for a medical malpractice claim has been met. This phase involves obtaining and reviewing the primary medical records in the case and consulting with a physician expert to determine whether the claim is meritorious. A reference book for lawyers on litigation and trial techniques states the following:

> Discovery may be a good way to learn what a witness will say and may be a good way to hold a witness or a party to a particular version of the facts, but it is a very inefficient way to get information. The suggestion is not to ignore discovery, but rather to stop ignoring informal methods of investigation. . . . Instead, this discussion is about learning facts in other ways—by doing . . . "trolling," or nosing about for essential information. Doing it well is one of the marks of a good trial lawyer (40).

This process of informal discovery is important to a plaintiff's lawyer to determine whether there is merit to filing a lawsuit. Tort reform laws in many states require a greater level of evidence of violation of the standard of care before a cause of action or lawsuit can be initiated (41).

The *filing* of the lawsuit is the second phase of the litigation process; it begins with serving of the summons and complaint on the defendant. A summons is an instrument used to commence a civil action. The summons may be personally served by a process server, or it can be mailed to the defendant, depending on the laws of an individual state. Many physicians have heard horror stories of sheriffs going to their offices disrupting the staff and patients to serve a summons. This is not a common occurrence. It is more likely that the summons and complaint will be mailed to the physician or an individual will, in a professional manner, personally serve the summons and complaint.

The *complaint* and *answer* are called *pleadings*, which are the formal allegations by the parties of their respective claims and defenses (42). A complaint is the initial pleading, which sets forth a claim for relief. A complaint shall set forth the allegations that are the basis of the lawsuit and is the plaintiff's general statement of the allegations. Most medical malpractice cases are decided by state courts. The defendant must respond to the allegations in a legal document that is called the *answer,* which is a concise response to each allegation made in the complaint. These two pleadings, the complaint and the answer, begin the formal litigation process.

The third phase of litigation is the *discovery phase.* In this phase, the parties discover the facts and the arguments of both parties: ''Parties may obtain discovery of any relevant, unprivileged information, unless the court limits discovery. This may include information, which is not itself admissible, as long as it may lead to admissible evidence. Thus the scope of discovery is very broad (43).'' This is the stage of the litigation process that often takes the longest time and involvement of both parties. Various tools are used for discovery, including interrogatories, depositions, request for documents, and request for admission. Interrogatories are a set or series of written questions drawn up for the purpose of being answered by a party, witness, or other person having information related to the lawsuit (42). They are an inexpensive method of discovery and are binding on the person giving the answers (43). A deposition is a discovery device by which one party asks oral questions of the other party or of a witness for the other party. A *deposition* is recorded testimony taken under oath. The person who is deposed is called the *deponent.* A court reporter or stenographer is present to record the testimony. A word-for-word transcript is made of the deposition. This is a common discovery technique. A *request for documents* is a discovery tool that is often used to obtain production of medical records, office policies, clinical guidelines, contractual arrangements and other documents related to the medical practice and the care provided the patient. *Request for admission* is a written statement of facts concerning the case submitted to the opposing party. That party then is required to admit or deny the statement. The statements are treated by the court as having been established and need not be proved at trial (42).

The fourth phase is described as *motion practice.* A *motion* is a written or oral application to the court for a ruling or order. Various types of motions can be made to the court, including motions to add parties, motion to amend the complaint, and motions for summary judgment. A motion for summary judgment is a motion that there is no dispute of fact and, based on the law, the moving party is entitled to prevail as a matter of law. Motions are argued orally before the court. Some motions include written legal arguments by the parties that are presented to the judge, who makes a ruling based on the law.

The fifth phase is the *trial,* during which a jury makes a determination about whether there was a violation of the standard of care that caused an injury to the patient. A medical malpractice trial is not substantially different from other civil trials. Between 7% and 10% of medical malpractice cases go to trial (44). The remainder of cases are resolved by the plaintiff voluntarily dismissing the lawsuit, the Court dismissing the case, or the parties reaching an out-of-court settlement.

The sixth phase is the *appeal process.* Most medical malpractice cases that go to trial will not be appealed because, after final judgment by the trial court, an appeal can be taken only on questions of law, not on questions of fact. Typically, questions of law relate to the trial judge's rulings and the admissibility of evidence (43).

WHAT ARE THE COMMON QUESTIONS LAWYERS ASK?

Understanding the common questions asked by plaintiff (45) or defense attorneys can provide insight into good risk management practices. The following are examples of common questions:

Did you document all complaints made by a patient?

Do you have a system to track mammograms and diagnostic reports?

Do you have a system for follow-up of your patients?

What was the date the problem was discovered, and what were all prior and subsequent examination dates?

If the problem was a mass, what were the size and location of the mass at each visit?

Who was present in the examining room during each visit?

What was said and done by the doctor and any nurses on each visit?

Were breast self-examination instructions given to the patient?

Did you document all patient interactions with the office, including telephone calls?

Did the time from the first complaint to diagnosis result in increase in the stage of the disease?

PHYSICIAN–PATIENT AND PHYSICIAN–PHYSICIAN COMMUNICATION

Effective communication between the patient and her physician is an important aspect of the physician–patient relationship. The patient is much more likely to feel satisfied with her care if she feels her complaints have been taken seriously, that she has reason to be concerned, and that the provider shares her concerns (11). Beckman et al. showed that perceived lack of caring and/or collaboration in the delivery of health care often is associated with a patient's decision to sue her doctor (46). This viewpoint has been underscored more recently by Levinson et al., who stated the following:

> Patient dissatisfaction is critical. The combination of a bad outcome and patient dissatisfaction is a recipe for litigation. When faced with a bad outcome, patients and families are more likely to sue a physician if they feel the physician was not caring and compassionate. Breakdowns in communication between physicians and patients lead to patient anger and dissatisfaction and possible litigation. Conversely, effective communication enhances patient satisfaction and health outcomes (47).

These same researchers showed that the length of routine primary care visits is predictive of malpractice risk and that physicians with shorter routine visits are more likely to have been sued (47). Recommendations should be communicated clearly, and reasons should be provided for the recommendations.

It is important to recognize communication problems and take affirmative action to improve the physician–patient relationship. When this becomes impossible, referral to a physician who may be able to establish a more positive relationship with

TABLE 24.1. *Common allegations for failure to diagnose breast cancer and recommended steps in risk management*

Allegation	Recommendations for risk management
Failure to screen	Perform clinical breast exam according to guidelines. Order mammography according to guidelines. Teach patients breast self-exam. Communicate recommendations. Document each step above.
Failure to have knowledge of abnormal mammogram results	Track result of tests. Communicate abnormal results and recommendations to patient. Document each step above.
Failure to follow up on complaint; failure to take patient complaint seriously	Perform focused history and clinical breast exam. Follow complaint to resolution or refer. Communicate findings/recommendations. Track patient follow-up appointments. Document each step above.
Failure to verify a patient complaint on physical exam	Perform careful history and clinical breast exam. Compare and confirm results of clinical breast exam with results of breast self-exam. Repeat exam at best phase of menstrual cycle if ovulating. Follow complaint to resolution or refer. Communicate findings/recommendations. Track patient follow-up appointments. Document each step above.
Failure to follow up on a physical exam with abnormal findings	Follow physical finding to resolution or refer. Communicate findings/recommendations. Track patient follow-up appointments. If referred, establish follow-up responsibility with referring provider and patient. Document each step above.
Failure to refer	Refer any persistent breast abnormality to a specialist, no matter what the mammogram result. Communicate area of concern to persistent and specialist. Establish follow-up responsibility. If surgical intervention deferred, establish clear follow-up plan. Document each step above.
Misinterpretation of abnormal findings of physical exam as benign or breast lump with normal mammogram as benign	Refer any persistent breast abnormality to a specialist.
Failure to perform a biopsy	Communicate area of concern to patient and specialist. Establish follow-up responsibility. Document each step above. Perform a biopsy for any persistent abnormality. If surgical intervention deferred, establish clear follow-up plan. Communicate plan to patient and provider. Establish follow-up responsibility. Document each preceding step.

Modified from Osuch JR, Bonham VL. The timely diagnosis of breast cancer. *Cancer* 1994;74:271–278, with permission.

the patient is advised. Poor communication, and the failure to establish an effective physician–patient relationship, too often is the root of a decision to sue a physician (11). Communication with the patient is necessary in understanding the patient's complaints. In this regard, many women who have breast complaints are not really sure that they feel a mass and are filled with fear and apprehension. Many seek reassurance rather than problem confirmation (11). This being said, it must be recognized that most women who file suit for failure to diagnose breast cancer discovered the mass instead of their physician (3). Assisting a patient in determining whether a mass is present or not, initiating appropriate workup and follow-up of findings, and communication of workup and follow-up plans are the keys to patient satisfaction of care in this setting.

In addition to patient-physician communication, communication between providers is essential to providing quality care and managing risk of liability (11). Failure for providers to communicate diagnostic results or treatment plans to one another can potentially result in a successful claim alleging a delay in the diagnosis of breast cancer.

In summary, numerous medical errors can occur in the diagnosis or treatment of breast cancer. All too commonly, the errors are ones of communication, follow-up, or tracking. Common allegations related to the failure to diagnose breast cancer, and recommended steps in managing risk and improving quality of care, are identified in Table 24.1 (11).

COPING WITH A LAWSUIT

Being sued can have a significant impact on the personal and professional life of a physician. Shapiro et al. showed that sued physicians find the practice of medicine more challenging, rewarding, and satisfying prior to being sued but after a claim against them, sued physicians find medicine more frustrating (48). They also demonstrated that the more personally involved the physician felt, the stronger the self-reported anger, inner tension, depression, and sense of defeat engendered in the physician by the claim (48).

It is important to recognize that the filing of a malpractice lawsuit is not evidence of a failure to provide quality care, nor does it denote physician incompetency. Errors occur in medicine, as in any profession, and litigation is a part of our society in the United States.

WHAT TO DO WHEN YOU ARE SUED

Receiving a summons and complaint or being contacted by a plaintiff's lawyer should trigger certain steps on the part of a defendant physician:

1. If you receive a letter or telephone call from an attorney advising you that he or she represents your patient and wants information, contact your insurer and advise your insurer of the letter or communication.

2. If you receive a notice of intent to sue or a summons and complaint, contact your insurer immediately. There are time limits that must be addressed in response to the complaint.

3. Do not alter any medical records under any circumstances. This includes removing words, progress note sections, reports, or any other records. Additions to the medical record, even if intended as clarifications, should also be avoided under all circumstances.

4. Discuss the selection of your attorney with your insurer. You have a right to participate in the selection of your attorney. Obtain recommendations on good defense malpractice attorneys from other physicians.

5. Do not discuss the patient and the case with your colleagues and friends because to do so might become an issue in the litigation. Any conversations with a colleague or friend may be discoverable.

6. Cooperate with your lawyer and your insurer.

7. Do not expect that you can bring a counterclaim against your patient.

8. Be an active participant in your case. Educate your lawyer about the clinical aspects of the case.

9. Have input when expert witnesses are selected to defend your case. Do not choose friends and close colleagues to defend your case but rather respected physicians in the field with whom you do not have a personal relationship. Chosen experts should be able to demonstrate respect for the legal process, be familiar with the current medical literature, testify for both plaintiffs and defendants, and be able to articulate their opinions well.

10. Keep everything in perspective. Being sued does not equate with being an incompetent physician.

SUMMARY

The diagnosis and management of breast cancer require an understanding of the common allegations of negligence in the care of patients with breast cancer. Taking steps to manage the risk of liability will reduce the risk of misdiagnosis of breast cancer and mismanagement of a patient and will improve the quality of care provided. Being sued for delay in diagnosis of breast cancer is one of the most common reasons primary care physicians and surgeons are sued. Understanding the litigation process and actively participating with your lawyer in your defense may increase the chances of a satisfactory outcome when faced with malpractice litigation.

REFERENCES

1. Greenlee RT, Murray T, Bolden S, et al. Cancer Statistics, 2000. *CA Cancer J Clin* 2000;50:7–33.
2. Physician's Insurance Association of America (PIAA). Breast Cancer Study. Data Sharing Reports, Executive Summary. Washington, DC: PIAA, 1995.
3. Physician's Insurance Association of America (PIAA). Data Sharing Reports, Executive Summary. Washington, DC:PIAA, 1995.

4. Kern KA. Medicolegal analysis of the delayed diagnosis of cancer in 338 cases in the United States. *Arch Surg* 1994;129:397–403.
5. Arnold R, Klingman R. Medical malpractice liability for errors in breast cancer diagnosis and treatment. In: Donegan W, Spratt J, eds. *Cancer of the breast.* Philadelphia: WB Saunders, 1995:795–808.
6. Anderson B, Cacioppo J. Delay in seeking a cancer diagnosis: delay stages and psychophysiological comparison processes. *Br J Social Psychol* 1995;34:33–52.
7. Lauver D. Care-seeking behavior with breast cancer symptoms in Caucasian and African-American women. *Res Nurs Health* 1994;17:421–431.
8. Kacmar DE. The impact of computerized medical literature databases on medical malpractice litigation: time for another *Helling v. Carey* wake up call? *Ohio St. L.J.* 1997;58:617.
9. Furrow BR, Greany TL, Johnson SH, et al. *Health law* St. Paul, MN: West Publishing Company, 1995.
10. Prosser WL. *Law of torts.* St. Paul, MN: West Publishing Company, 1978.
11. Osuch J, Bonham VL. The timely diagnosis of breast cancer. *Cancer* 1994;74:271–278.
12. *Oja v Kin,* 229 Mich. App. 184, 581 N.W. 2d 739 (1998).
13. Rigelhaupt JL. What constitutes physician-patient relationship for malpractice purposes. *ALR* 2000; 17:132.
14. *Glicklich v Spievack,* 16 Mass App 488 (1983).
15. Sandbar SS, Gibofsky A, Firestone MH, et al. *Legal medicine.* St. Louis: Mosby, 1995.
16. King, JH. Reconciling the exercise of judgment and the objective standard of care in medical malpractice. *Oklahoma Law Review* 1999;52:49–84.
17. *Hall v Hilbun,* 466 So.2d 856, 872-73 (Miss. 1992).
18. *Helling v Carey,* 519 P.2d 981 (Wash 1974).
19. Hirshfeld EB. Economic considerations in treatment decisions and the standard of care in medical malpractice litigation. *JAMA*1990;70:2004–2012.
20. Evers v. Dollinger, 95 N.J. 399 (1984).
21. Gabin JH. The Evers case:1984 decision has lasting impact. *New Jersey Med* 1993;90:536–537.
22. Aagarrd TS. Identifying and valuing the injury in lost chance cases. *Mich L. Review* 1998;96: 1335–1361.
23. Ellis LR. Loss of chance as technique: toeing the line at fifty percent. *Texas Law Review* 1993;72: 369–402.
24. Walker VR. Direct inference in the lost chance cases: factfinding constraints under minimal fairness to parties. *Hofstra Law Review* 1994;23:247–307 .
25. National Institutes of Health Consensus Conference: Treatment of early-stage breast cancer. *JAMA* 1991;265:391–395.
26. Hayes DF, Trock B, Harris AL. Assessing the clinical impact of prognostic factors: when is "statistically significant"; clinically useful? *Breast Cancer Res Treat* 1998;2:305–319.
27. ASCO Expert Panel. 1997 update of recommendations for the use of tumor markers in breast and colorectal cancer. *J Clin Oncol* 1998;16:793–795.
28. Cole P, Morrison AS. Basic issues in cancer screening. In: Miller AB, ed. *Screening in cancer,* vol 40. Geneva: UICC, 1978;7.
29. Shapiro S. Screening: assessment of current studies. *Cancer* 1994;74:231–238.
30. Hendrick RE, Smith RA, Rutledge JH III, et al. Benefit of screening mammography in women aged 40-49: a new meta-analysis of randomized controlled trials. *J Natl Cancer Inst Monogr* 1997;22: 87–92.
31. Fidler IJ. Critical factors in the biology of human cancer metastasis: twenty-eighth G.H.A. Clowes Memorial Award Lecture. *Cancer Res* 1990;50:6130–6138.
32. Rutqvist LE, Wallgren A. Long-term survival of 458 young breast cancer patients. *Cancer* 1985; 55:658–665.
33. Folkman J. Tumor angiogenesis. *Adv Cancer Res* 1985;43:175–203.
34. MacDonald I. Biological predeterminism in human cancer. *Surg Gynecol Obstet* 1951;92:443–452.
35. Heuser L, Spratt JS, Polk HC, Jr. Growth rates of primary breast cancers. *Cancer*1979;43:1888–1894.
36. Tabar L, Duffy SW, Vitak B, et al. The natural history of breast carcinoma: what have we learned from screening? *Cancer* 1999; 86:449–462.
37. Kern K. The delayed diagnosis of symptomatic breast cancer. In: Bland K, Copeland E, eds. *The breast: comprehensive management of benign and malignant disease*, vol 2. Philadelphia: WB Saunders, 1998:1588–1631.

38. Sainsbury R, Johnston C, Haward B. Effect on survival of delays in referral of patients with breast-cancer symptoms: a retrospective analysis. *Lancet* 1999;353:1132–1135.
39. Richards MA, Westcombe AM, Love SB, et al. Influence of delay on survival in patients with breast cancer: a systematic review. *Lancet* 1999; 353:1119–1126.
40. McElhaney JW. *McElhaney's trial notebook,* 2nd ed. American Bar Association, 1987.
41. Mich. Comp. Laws Sec.600.291 2d (2000).
42. Black HC. *Black's law dictionary.* St. Paul, MN: West Publishing Company, 1979.
43. Danner D, Varn LL, Mathias SJ. *Medical malpractice: checklist and discovery.* New York: CBC, 1994.
44. Vidmar N. *Medical malpractice and the American jury.* Ann Arbor, MI: The University of Michigan Press 1995.
45. Ellerin IM, Frieder MI, Hillerich GR. Handling a failure to diagnose breast cancer. *Trial* 1996:31–37.
46. Beckman HB, Markakis KM, Suchman AL, et al. The doctor-patient relationship and malpractice: Lessons from plaintiff definitions. *Arch Intern Med* 1994;154:1365–1370.
47. Levinson W, Roter DL, Mullooly JP, et al. Physician-patient communication: the relationship with malpractice claims among primary care physicians and surgeons. *JAMA* 1997;277:553–559.
48. Shapiro RS, Simpson DE, Lawrence SL, et al. A survey of sued and nonsued physicians and suing patients. *Arch Intern Med* 1989;149:2190–2196.

Index

Page numbers followed by an *f* indicate figures; page numbers followed by a *t* indicate tables.

A

Abscess(es), breast, during breast–feeding, 120
Absolute risk reduction, defined, 310
Age
  as factor in adjuvant polychemotherapy for breast
    cancer, 311–313, 312t, 313t
  as factor in breast cancer, 506
    in males, 420–421, 420t
  as factor in mammographic screening, 186–188
  as factor in nipple discharge, 358
  at menarche, as factor in breast cancer, 152–153
  at menopause, as factor in breast cancer, 153
Alcohol consumption, as factor in breast cancer,
    164–165, 164t, 166f
Amastia, 9, 40–41
American Cancer Society, 438
Androgen(s), for metastatic breast cancer, 368
Angiogenesis
  and biological predeterminism of breast cancer,
    528–529
  defined, 528
Angiolipoma(s), 424
Anthracycline(s), for breast cancer, 313–314
Antiestrogen(s)
  for breast cancer, 321
    metastatic, 366–367
  in chemoprevention of breast cancer, 492–493
Anxiety, in breast cancer patients, psychosocial
    support for, 449–450
Appeal process, in litigation process, 532
Areola(s), 2–4, 4f
Aromatase inhibitors
  for breast cancer, 321–323, 322t
    metastatic, 367–368
  in chemoprevention of breast cancer, 493
Ataxia–telangiectasia, and breast cancer, 506
Athelia, 40–41
Atypical hyperplasia
  of breast, histologic criteria for, 252–254, 253t
  defined, 136
Autotransplantation, for breast cancer in males,
    430–431
Axilla, management of, 298–302
Axillary lymph node(s), of breast, 7–8
Axillary lymph node dissection, 298
Axillary relapse, 300–301
Axillary tail, 1

B

Bias
  lead–time, 179, 180f
  length, 179
  selection, 179, 181
Biochemical markers, in breast evaluation, 67–69
Blood, occult, in breast evaluation, 66–67
Bone metabolism
  raloxifene effects on, 490–491
  tamoxifen effects on, 488

BRCAPro, in breast cancer predisposition, 465
Breast. *See also* Mammary glands.
  amastia, 40–41
  anatomy of, 28, 55
    gross, 1–13
    microscopic, 10–13, 11f–13f
  asymmetry of, 8–9
  athelia, 40–41
  atypical hyperplasia of, histologic criteria for,
    252–254, 253t
  axillary nodes of, 7–8
  burns of, 43, 44f
  core needle biopsy of, 223–225, 224f
  cyst. *See* Cyst(s), breast.
  cysts of. *See* Cyst(s), breast.
  development of, 14–15, 25–28, 26f. *See also*
    Thelarche.
  embryology of, 14–15
  enlargement of, during pregnancy, 27
  gigantomastia, 45–48, 45f, 47f. *See also*
    Gigantomastia.
  gynecomastia, 30–32, 31f, 417–418, 418t
  iatrogenic deformities of, 42–44, 43f, 44f
  idiopathic asymmetry of, 33–36, 34f–36f
  immunohistochemistry of, 13–14
  inverted nipples of, 42
  macrocysts of, 353
  male
    benign conditions of, 417–419, 418t
    described, 417
  MRI of, 225–226, 226f
  nipple–type, 32
  nodular deformities in, 44
  physiology of, 15–19, 17f, 18f, 20f–22f, 55
  Poland syndrome, 36–38
  polymastia, 38–40, 39f
  polythelia, 38–40, 39f
  premature thelarche, 28–30
  prenatal examination of, 99–100
  reconstructive surgery for, 296–298
  seatbelt injuries, 42, 43f
  skin of, innervation of, 5
  Snoopy–nose, 32
  sonographic anatomy of, 220–221, 220f
  symmastia, 41–42, 41f
  tuberous, 32–33, 33f
  tubular, 32–33, 33f
  vascular supply of, 5
Breast abscess, during breast–feeding, 120
Breast cancer. *See also* Mammography screening
    trials.
  age and, 506
  age at menarche and, 152–153
  age at menopause and, 153
  agenda differences in, 507–508
  alcohol consumption and, 164–165, 164t, 166f
  anxiety with, 449–450
  Canadian trials, 184–185

539